BASIC ANATOMY
OF THE
HEAD AND NECK

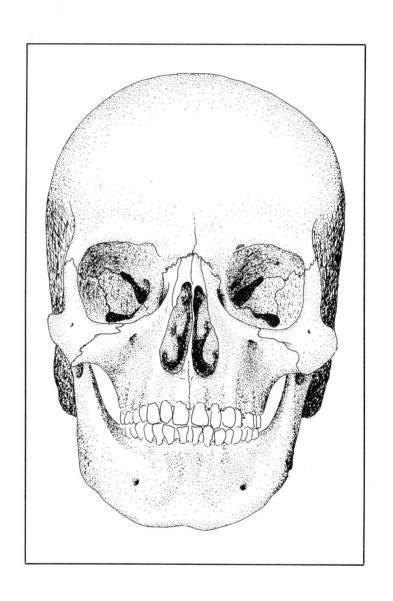

BASIC ANATOMY OF THE HEAD AND NECK

MARTHA GARDNER, Ph.D.

Assistant Professor of Anatomy
School of Dentistry
Oregon Health Sciences University

Philadelphia   LEA & FEBIGER   London
1992

Lea & Febiger
200 Chester Field Parkway
Malvern, Pennsylvania   19355-9725
U.S.A.
(215) 251-2230

Executive Editor: George H. Mundorff
Project Editor: David Amundson
Production Manager: Elizabeth S. Frazier

Library of Congress Cataloging-in-Publication Data

Gardner, Martha.
    Basic anatomy of the head and neck / Martha Gardner.
        p.   cm.
    Includes index.
    ISBN 0-8121-1448-5
    1. Head—Anatomy.   2. Neck—Anatomy.   I. Title.
    [DNLM: 1. Head—anatomy & histology.   2. Neck—anatomy &
histology.   WE 705 G227b]
    QM535.G36   1992
    611′.91—dc20
    DNLM/DLC   91-27304
    for Library of Congress   CIP

Reprints of chapters may be purchased from Lea & Febiger in quantities of 100 or more.

Print number: 5   4   3   2   1

To Harry H. Wilcox

CONTENTS

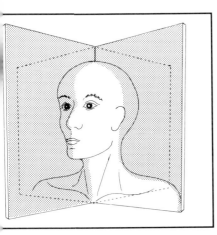

CHAPTER 1

INTRODUCTION

This book is written for students undertaking a study of the basic gross anatomy of the head and neck regions of the body and for those desiring to review these areas. Although an attempt has been made to present the essentials and reduce the details, there is no easy way to discuss these complex areas. Without any detail, they become incomprehensible.

Since the head and neck are not isolated parts functioning independently from the remainder of the body, they cannot be understood without some knowledge of the thorax. Of particular importance is knowledge of the vasculature through which blood flows from and back to the heart, the organization of the spinal cord, general principles of sensory and motor innervation of body structures, the pathway followed by sympathetic nerve fibers destined for head and neck innervation, and the vertebral column and its surrounding musculature. Many students undertaking this study will have had some background in these topics. For those who have not, I have tried to include enough background information to make head and neck anatomy understandable.

In studying gross anatomy, one of the major difficulties is the vast terminology that must be mastered. The place to begin is to learn that descriptions of structures are always based on a body oriented in the **anatomic position.** In Fig. 1–1A, the anatomic position for the head and neck can be seen. It is simply the normal posture while standing, with the head positioned so the eyes look straight ahead.

A student of anatomy must be able to describe the location of a body structure and its position relative to other structures. If descriptions are always based on a body in the anatomic position, the location will be clear even if the body being described is standing on its head or lying on its back or its stomach.

Certain terms are particularly useful, indeed essential, in anatomic descriptions.

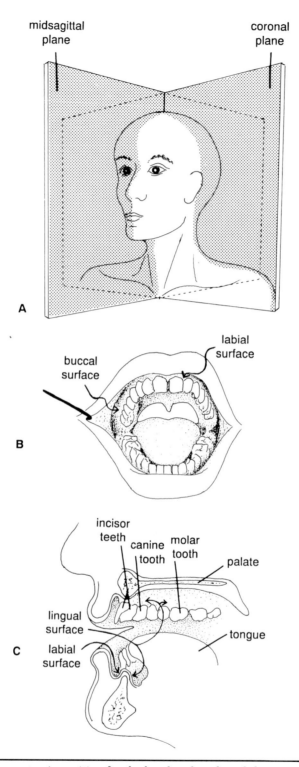

FIG. 1–1. A. The anatomic position for the head and neck and the two major planes of section. **B.** An anterior view into the oral cavity. The gingival surfaces are named according to what lies adjacent to them. **C.** A midsagittal section to show gingival surfaces and the relation of the palate to the tongue.

superficial, deep. The skin is superficial, relative to all other parts. It can also be said that everything is deep relative to the skin. Beneath the surface, however, some structures are closer to the surface than others and therefore are superficial relative to them.

lateral, medial, median. Structures located in the midline of the body are described as being median in position. Structures to the right or left are lateral to the midline, but some are more lateral than others. For instance, both the cheek and the third molar tooth are lateral to the midline, but the molars are medial to the cheek.

midsagittal plane, parasagittal plane. A plane passing through the midline dividing the body into right and left sides is a midsagittal plane. Planes parallel but lateral to the midsagittal are parasagittal.

anterior (ventral), posterior (dorsal). A structure on the front side of the body is anterior, or ventral, and one on the back side is posterior, or dorsal. These terms are also used to describe relative positions. For instance, the canine teeth are posterior to the incisors but anterior to the molars.

frontal (coronal) plane. A frontal or coronal plane is perpendicular to a sagittal plane and divides the body into an anterior part and a posterior part.

superior, inferior. A structure closer to the top of the head, or rostral end, is superior to a structure closer to the tail, or caudal end. For example, although the palate is inferior to the nasal cavity, it is superior to the tongue. One can also say the tongue is inferior to the palate.

transverse plane. A transverse plane is horizontally oriented and divides a body or a structure into superior and inferior parts.

It is also possible to distinguish a specific surface of a structure according to what lies adjacent to it. For instance, within the oral cavity, an area of obvious interest to those specializing in areas related to dentistry, the terms **buccal, labial,** and **lingual** are used to indicate the different surfaces of gingiva, which lie adjacent to the cheeks, lips, and tongue (Fig. 1–1B,C).

Numerous illustrations are provided so that the student can refer to them while reading. As much as possible, they are placed near the text most closely describing them. Because one area within the head and neck does not function in isolation from others, however, many illustrations are useful in several places. Therefore I have attempted to indicate particularly relevant figures from other chapters.

These abbreviations are used in labeling the illustrations.

m — muscle
a — artery
v — vein
n — nerve
V1 — ophthalmic division of the trigeminal nerve
V2 — maxillary division of the trigeminal nerve
V3 — mandibular division of the trigeminal nerve

The drawings are my own. I drew most of them from illustrations in *Gray's Anatomy,* 30th edition, with the kind permission of Lea & Febiger Publishers.

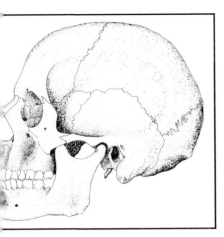

CHAPTER 2

THE SKELETON OF THE HEAD AND NECK

The skeletal support of the soft tissues of the head and neck is the skull and the cervical vertebrae. This chapter presents the major features of the bones comprising them. Other details necessary for understanding the anatomy of particular regions are discussed in the chapters on those regions.

SUPERIOR VIEW OF THE SKULL (Fig. 2–1)

The bones seen in a superior view of the skull underlie the scalp. They form a broad, flat arched surface that contributes to the cranial vault for housing and protecting the brain. They go by the name of skull cap, or **calvaria,** the part that can be removed in most of the skulls used for studying anatomy.

All the bones are covered on their surfaces with a layer of connective tissue called periosteum. Most of the joints between adjacent bones of the skull are sutures. This means they are immovable joints. The periosteum extends between the two bones forming the suture, creating a fibrous covering of the joint surfaces and helping to hold them together.

The **frontal bone** is the anterior bone of the calvaria. It articulates at the coronal suture with the two **parietal bones.** They articulate with each other at the sagittal suture and usually have a parietal foramen on one or both sides of the suture. Posteriorly they articulate with the **occipital bone** at the lambdoidal suture. Small, irregular bones within the latter suture are frequently present and are called sutural, or Wormian, bones.

5

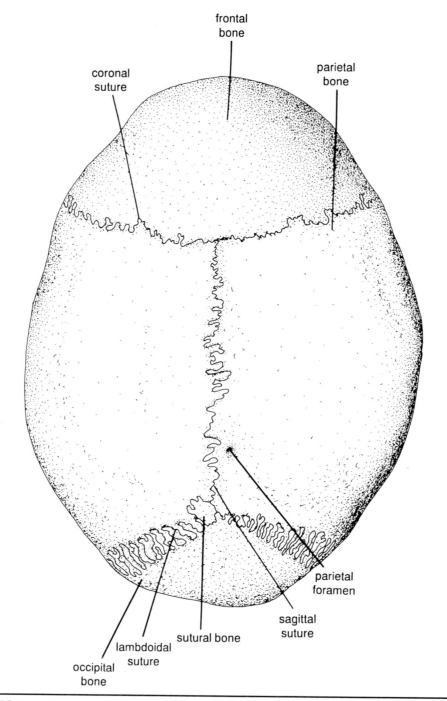

FIG. 2–1. A superior view of the calvaria.

ANTERIOR AND LATERAL VIEWS OF THE SKULL
(Figs. 2-2 and 2-3)

In an anterior view, the bones of the skull presenting a surface underlying the superficial face can be seen. Some are paired; others are single. They are complex in shape in order to provide bony rims for the orbits, the nasal cavity, and the mouth. The **frontal bone** underlies the forehead and forms the superior part of the orbital rim. Superciliary arches create elevations above the rim and are particularly apparent in males. Between them the smooth prominence is the glabella. In a mature skull the frontal bone is unpaired. During fetal development, however, it forms from two separate centers of ossification, and it is not unusual to see a small suture remaining anteriorly as the metopic suture.

The **zygomatic bones** form the lateral and much of the inferior orbital rims, and their malar prominence creates the high part of the cheek. Projecting from the main body of the bone is a frontal process directed toward the frontal bone, a temporal process into the zygomatic arch toward the temporal bone, and a maxillary process toward the maxilla.

The paired **maxillae** contribute to borders of all three of the major openings on the face. They form much of the lower and medial rims of the orbits; the borders of the piriform aperture, the opening into the nasal cavity, except for the superior narrow part, which is formed by the two **nasal bones;** and their alveolar process, containing the roots of the maxillary teeth, forms the entire bony upper border of the entryway into the oral cavity proper. Inferior to the piriform aperture in the midline, the anterior nasal spine is a sharp bony projection. Over the root of the canine tooth the bone is elevated to form the canine eminence. The depression medial to the eminence is the incisive fossa, and the one lateral to it is the canine fossa. Extending from the zygomatic bone to the first molar tooth is a thick ridge of bone called the zygomaticoalveolar crest.

In a lateral view of the temporal region of the skull, the thin squamous part of the **temporal bone** can be seen. Its zygomatic process forms a major part of the zygomatic arch; the thick rounded mastoid process points inferiorly, and the external auditory meatus lies just superior and anterior to it. The anterior wall of the meatus is formed by the tympanic plate. It is possible to look down into the meatus and see the small space of the middle ear cavity within the petrous part of the temporal bone. In a living person, three tiny bones, the ossicles, which are the malleus, incus, and stapes, are housed within this cavity (see Chapter 13 and Fig. 13-3).

The broad depression on the lateral side superior to the zygomatic arch is the temporal fossa. The greater wing of the unpaired **sphenoid bone** articulates in the temporal fossa with the frontal, parietal, and squamous part of the temporal bones. The fossa extends to the temporal lines.

The region inferior to the zygomatic arch and deep to the mandibular ramus is the infratemporal fossa. The lateral pterygoid plate of the sphenoid bone limits the fossa medially; the posterior surface of the maxilla limits it anteriorly.

The **occipital bone** can be seen posteriorly. In the posterior midline its external occipital protuberance is palpable through the soft tissues of the scalp. Promi-

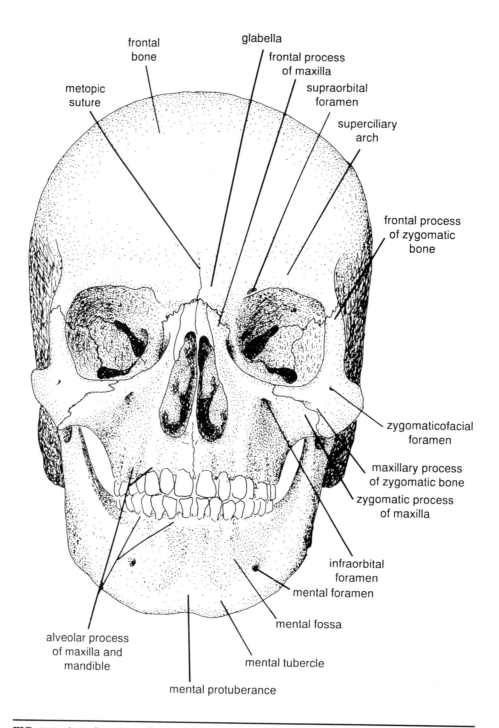

frontal bone

glabella

frontal process of maxilla

supraorbital foramen

superciliary arch

metopic suture

frontal process of zygomatic bone

zygomaticofacial foramen

maxillary process of zygomatic bone

zygomatic process of maxilla

infraorbital foramen

mental foramen

mental fossa

alveolar process of maxilla and mandible

mental tubercle

mental protuberance

FIG. 2–2. Anterior view of the skull.

8   THE SKELETON OF THE HEAD AND NECK

nent superior nuchal lines are bony ridges that extend laterally from the protuberance.

Inferiorly, the unpaired **mandible** contributes the lower border of the entryway into the oral cavity proper, and its alveolar process houses the roots of the mandibular teeth. The more horizontally elongated part of the mandible is the body, and the more vertical part is the ramus. At the junction of these two parts is the angle. On the ramus is a process projecting upward composed of the condyle, or head, sitting on the mandibular neck and bearing a surface that articulates with the temporal bone just superior to it. More anteriorly situated is the coronoid process. The gap between the two processes is the mandibular

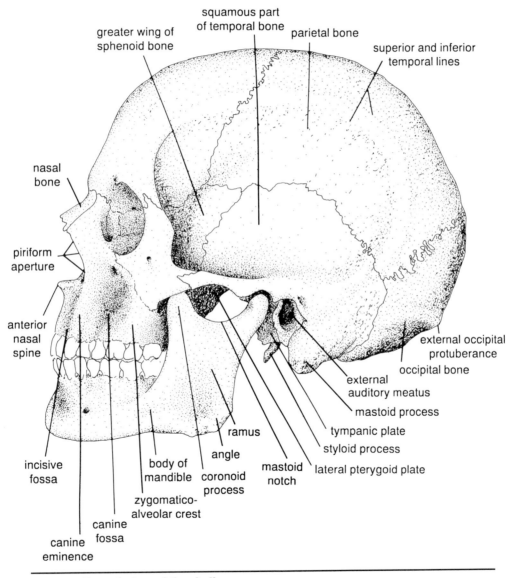

FIG. 2–3. Lateral view of the skull.

notch. In the anterior midline the mental protuberance projects forward, as do the mental tubercles on either side of it. Above them the mental fossa is a depressed area related to the roots of the mandibular incisors.

Cutaneous nerves and vessels emerge onto the face through several important foramina. Just above the superior rim of the orbit in the frontal bone is the **supraorbital foramen,** frequently a notch rather than a foramen. Inferior to the orbit in the maxilla is the **infraorbital foramen.** In almost the same vertical plane as these two foramina is the **mental foramen** in the mandible. Two foramina open on the zygomatic bone; the **zygomaticofacial** on the malar prominence and the **zygomaticotemporal** on the frontal process. The latter is not seen in these views because it opens on the deep surface of the process.

THE BASE OF THE SKULL (Fig. 2–4)

Anteriorly lies the **maxilla.** Its arched alveolar process contains the maxillary teeth. It forms most of the hard palate. In the suture between the two maxillae lies the incisive foramen. A smaller contribution to the hard palate is made by the **palatine bones,** which form the posterior part and contain the greater and lesser palatine foramina. On their free edge in the midline they form the sharply pointed posterior nasal spine.

Posterior to the last molars and maxillae can be seen the pterygoid processes of the **sphenoid bone,** each having a medial and a lateral pterygoid plate. The hamulus is the hook-like projection on the medial pterygoid plate. The body is the mid portion of the sphenoid. The small, unpaired, midline **vomer** articulates with it, forming part of the nasal septum. The part of the greater wing of the sphenoid bone seen in this view forms the roof of the infratemporal fossa. It shows two foramina, the foramen ovale and the foramen spinosum, which has the spine of the sphenoid just posterior to it.

Posterior to the greater wing of the sphenoid is the **temporal bone.** Its more lateral part bears the mandibular fossa and other joint surfaces that participate in the articulation with the mandible and the mastoid process with its deep digastric notch. The petrous part, an irregularly shaped piece of bone containing a prominent opening into the carotid canal, lies more medially. Posterior to the canal and between the petrous temporal and the occipital bones are the jugular fossa and foramen. Lateral to the foramen is the long, slim styloid process, which is separated from the mastoid process by the stylomastoid foramen.

The **occipital bone** presents a large surface inferiorly. It contains the foramen magnum with an occipital condyle on either side for articulation with the first cervical vertebra. Anterior to the foramen is the basilar part of the occipital bone. The small elevation on it is the pharyngeal tubercle. Anterior and posterior to each condyle are an anterior and posterior condylar canal; the posterior ones are not always present.

Between the occipital, the petrous temporal, and the sphenoid bones is an irregularly shaped opening called the **foramen lacerum;** in life it is sealed by cartilage and is not a foramen, although some small nerves do pass through the cartilage.

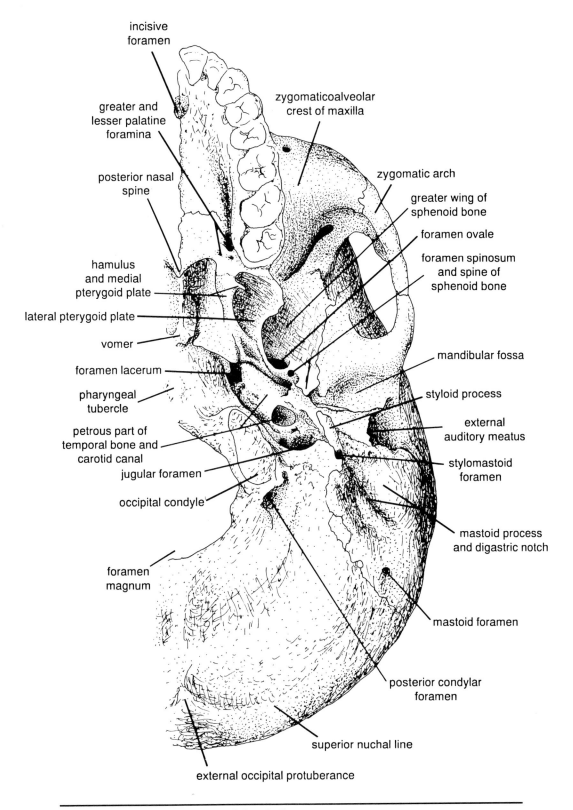

FIG. 2–4. Left side of the base of the skull.

incisive foramen

zygomaticoalveolar crest of maxilla

greater and lesser palatine foramina

posterior nasal spine

zygomatic arch

greater wing of sphenoid bone

foramen ovale

foramen spinosum and spine of sphenoid bone

hamulus and medial pterygoid plate

lateral pterygoid plate

vomer

mandibular fossa

foramen lacerum

pharyngeal tubercle

styloid process

external auditory meatus

petrous part of temporal bone and carotid canal

jugular foramen

stylomastoid foramen

occipital condyle

foramen magnum

mastoid process and digastric notch

mastoid foramen

posterior condylar foramen

superior nuchal line

external occipital protuberance

THE CRANIAL CAVITY (Fig. 2–5)

The cranial cavity provides protective housing for the brain. The bones of its roof were discussed above as the calvaria. Its floor has three easily distinguished regions, the anterior, middle, and posterior cranial fossae. They conform rather closely to the shape of the base of the brain. The bones of the floor provide openings through which cranial nerves pass to get from their origin on the brain to regions outside the cranial cavity and through which the blood supply for the cranial contents enters.

Except for the floor, the walls consist of broad, rather thin, flat bone contributed to by the frontal, parietal, temporal, sphenoid, and occipital bones. Both the outer and inner layers of these bones are compact bone. Between the layers is spongy bone referred to as diploë. It is characterized by irregular trabeculae of bone with intervening irregular marrow spaces.

In the anterior cranial fossa the major part of the floor is formed by the **frontal bone,** specifically its orbital plate, so named because it forms most of the roof of the underlying orbit. In the midline, the **ethmoid bone** contributes the cribriform plate and the projecting crista galli. Posteriorly lies the **sphenoid bone,** its lesser wings projecting laterally and its anterior clinoid processes pointing posteriorly. They form a sharp border between the anterior and middle cranial fossae.

In the middle cranial fossa the **sphenoid bone** contributes a large part to the floor. Its body forms the sella turcica, or hypophyseal fossa, where the pituitary gland sits and, more anteriorly, shows the chiasmatic groove leading into the optic foramen, which opens into the orbit. Lateral to each side of the body is the greater wing of the sphenoid, containing the foramina rotundum, ovale, and spinosum. A groove in the bone leading laterally from the foramen spinosum and showing a branching pattern is formed by the middle meningeal artery. Between the greater and lesser wings is the superior orbital fissure, leading into the orbit.

The **temporal bone** is the other major contributor to the middle cranial fossa. It is the only paired bone in the floor of the cranial cavity and the only one that does not contribute to the median part of the floor. More anteriorly is its thin squamous part, and more posteriorly is its petrous part. On the latter is a sharp ridge, or apex, forming the border with the posterior cranial fossa. Opening from the petrous part adjacent to the body of the sphenoid is the carotid canal. Looking down through the canal the irregular shape of the foramen lacerum can be seen between the temporal, sphenoid, and occipital bones. A small foramen on the petrous temporal, the hiatus of the facial canal, opens into a narrow groove directed toward the carotid canal.

In the posterior cranial fossa in the anterior midline, the dorsum sellae of the **sphenoid bone** can be seen, bearing two upwardly projecting posterior clinoid processes, which form part of the boundary with the middle cranial fossa. The dorsum sellae articulates with the basilar part of the **occipital bone.** Just lateral to the foramen magnum are the anterior condylar canals, also known as hypoglossal canals. More lateral are the petrous and mastoid parts of the **temporal bone.** The petrous part contains the internal auditory meatus. In the suture between it and the occipital bone the jugular foramen can be seen.

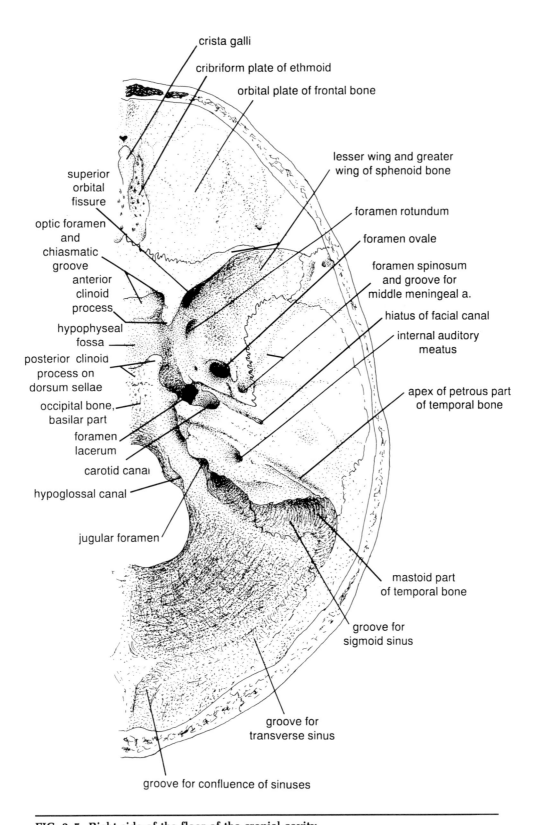

crista galli

cribriform plate of ethmoid

orbital plate of frontal bone

lesser wing and greater wing of sphenoid bone

foramen rotundum

foramen ovale

foramen spinosum and groove for middle meningeal a.

hiatus of facial canal

internal auditory meatus

apex of petrous part of temporal bone

superior orbital fissure

optic foramen and chiasmatic groove

anterior clinoid process

hypophyseal fossa

posterior clinoid process on dorsum sellae

occipital bone, basilar part

foramen lacerum

carotid canal

hypoglossal canal

jugular foramen

mastoid part of temporal bone

groove for sigmoid sinus

groove for transverse sinus

groove for confluence of sinuses

FIG. 2–5. Right side of the floor of the cranial cavity.

The usually prominent grooves in the posterior cranial fossa formed by the dural venous sinuses are discussed in Chapter 4.

OPENINGS IN THE SKULL AND THEIR CONTENTS

Table 2-1 names the openings in the skull that are cited in later chapters and lists the major structures they contain.

TABLE 2–1. OPENINGS IN THE SKULL AND THEIR CONTENTS	
OPENING	CONTENT OF OPENING
Anterior ethmoidal foramen	Anterior ethmoidal nerve
	Anterior ethmoidal artery and vein
Auditory (or eustachian) tube	Auditory tube
Carotid canal	Internal carotid nerve
	Internal carotid artery
Foramen cecum	Emissary vein
Foramen lacerum	Cartilage
	Greater petrosal nerve
	Deep petrosal nerve
Foramen magnum	Spinal cord and meninges
	Spinal accessory nerve
	Vertebral artery
	Anterior spinal artery
	Posterior spinal artery
Foramen ovale	Mandibular nerve
	Emissary vein
	Lesser petrosal nerve (variable)
Foramen rotundum	Maxillary nerve
Foramen spinosum	Middle meningeal artery
	Meningeal branch of mandibular nerve
Hiatus of the facial canal	Greater petrosal nerve
Hypoglossal canal	Hypoglossal nerve
	Emissary vein
Incisive canal	Sphenopalatine artery
	Nasopalatine nerve
Inferior orbital fissure	Infraorbital artery and vein
	Infraorbital nerve
	Zygomatic nerve
Infraorbital foramen	Infraorbital artery and vein
	Infraorbital nerve
Internal acoustic meatus	Labyrinthine artery
	Facial nerve
	Vestibulocochlear nerve
Jugular foramen	Jugular bulb
	Glossopharyngeal nerve
	Vagus nerve
	Spinal accessory nerve
Lesser palatine foramen	Lesser palatine artery and vein
	Lesser palatine nerve
Mandibular foramen	Inferior alveolar artery and vein
	Inferior alveolar nerve

TABLE 2–1. Continued

OPENING	CONTENT OF OPENING
Mandibular notch	Artery and vein to masseter muscle
	Nerve to masseter muscle
Mastoid foramen	Mastoid emissary vein
Mental foramen	Mental artery and vein
	Mental nerve
Optic foramen (or canal)	Ophthalmic artery
	Optic nerve
Palatine canal	Descending palatine artery
	Greater palatine nerve
	Lesser palatine nerve
Parietal foramen	Parietal emissary vein
Petrotympanic fissure	Anterior tympanic artery
	Chorda tympani nerve
Pharyngeal canal	Pharyngeal artery
	Pharyngeal nerve
Posterior condylar canal	Emissary vein
Posterior ethmoidal foramen	Posterior ethmoidal artery and vein
	Posterior ethmoidal nerve
Pterygoid canal	Artery of the pterygoid canal
	Nerve of the pterygoid canal
Pterygomaxillary fissure	Maxillary artery
	Posterior superior alveolar nerve
Sphenopalatine foramen	Sphenopalatine artery
	Nasopalatine nerve
Stylomastoid foramen	Facial nerve
Superior orbital fissure	Superior ophthalmic vein
	Oculomotor nerve
	Trochlear nerve
	Abducens nerve
	Ophthalmic nerve
Supraorbital foramen (or notch)	Supraorbital artery and vein
	Supraorbital nerve
Vestibular aqueduct	Endolymphatic duct
Zygomaticofacial foramen	Zygomaticofacial artery and vein
	Zygomaticofacial nerve
Zygomaticoorbital foramen	Zygomaticoorbital artery and vein
	Zygomaticofacial nerve

THE CERVICAL VERTEBRAE (Figs. 2-6, 2-7, and 2-8)

In the neck region there are seven vertebrae. The articulations between them allow flexion, extension, lateral bending, and rotation of the neck. Articulations between them and the occipital condyles on the skull allow head movements.

A **typical cervical vertebra** has a small vertebral body. From each side arise two projections. The more posterior are the pedicles, which, together with the laminae, form the neural arch. The transverse process extends laterally from the junction of lamina and pedicle. The more anterior is the costal process. It is a remnant of cervical ribs possessed by man's ancestral vertebrates. It is connected to the transverse process by the costotransverse bar, which leaves an opening called the transverse foramen. The vertebral artery and its surrounding venous plexus traverse this opening in the sixth cervical vertebra and ascend through consecutive vertebrae and then through the foramen magnum to the cranial cavity. The vertebral body and the neural arch border the vertebral foramen. The sequence of all the vertebral foramina of the vertebral column creates the vertebral canal, which houses the spinal cord. Intervertebral foramina, formed by notches in adjacent vertebrae, provide passageways for spinal nerves to emerge from the vertebral canal. A slender, short, bifid spinous process projects posteriorly. The first one to be easily palpable belongs to the seventh vertebra, which is often referred to as the vertebra prominens.

For articulation with adjacent vertebrae, each transverse process bears a superior articular process with an articular facet facing in a posterosuperior direction and an inferior articular process with an articular facet facing in an anteroinferior direction. The orientation of these facets allows for movements between vertebrae. They form freely moveable, or synovial, joints (see Chapter 9).

Articulation also occurs between adjacent vertebral bodies. In the type of joint seen here, movement is much more restricted and it is classified as a symphysis. The articular surfaces are covered with hyaline cartilage. The interval between them is filled with an intervertebral disk. This structure consists of an outer annulus fibrosus composed of fibrous and fibrocartilaginous tissue and a central, gelatinous nucleus pulposus. The disk cushions the shock between vertebrae and allows for some movement between the vertebral bodies.

The first vertebra, the **atlas,** and the second, the **axis,** are atypical. Although the atlas has transverse processes that project further laterally than those of any other cervical vertebra, its spinous process is represented by only a posterior tubercle on the posterior arch. The superior surface of the arch has a groove along which runs the vertebral artery on its way from the transverse foramen to the foramen magnum. The atlas also lacks a vertebral body. During development it fuses with the vertebral body of the axis, forming the dens and leaving the atlas with an anterior arch instead. The dens is held against the anterior arch by a strong transverse ligament and acts as a pivot around which rotatory movements can take place, which result in side-to-side rotation of the head. The facets on the inferior articular processes of the atlas and the superior articular processes of the axis are oriented so as to permit this rotation.

Superiorly, the atlantooccipital articulation is constructed for flexion, or forward bending, and extension, or backward bending, of the head. The superior articular processes have elongated and somewhat saddle-shaped concave facets that conform to the elongated, convex facets on the occipital condyles.

THE HYOID BONE (Fig. 2–9)

The hyoid is a small but important bone in the anterior neck. It is somewhat U-shaped, although the limbs of the U are widely spread. The anterior central part is the body. Projecting dorsally from each of its lateral borders is a greater horn, which is 20 mm or more in length. At the junction of body and greater horn is the lesser horn.

The hyoid bone is unusual in that it does not articulate with any other bone and maintains its position by the attachment of ligaments, fibrous membranes, and the supra- and infrahyoid muscles of the neck (see Chapter 8).

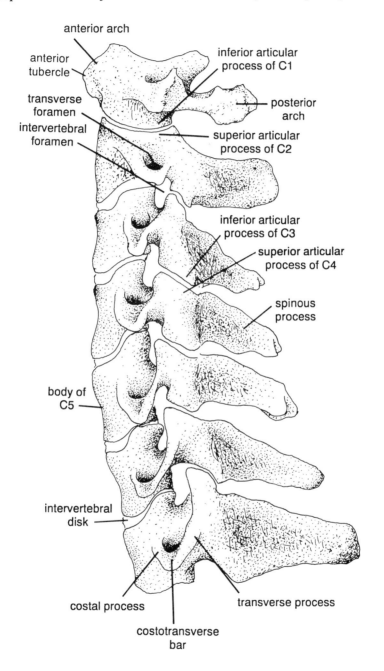

FIG. 2–6. Lateral view of the cervical vertebrae.

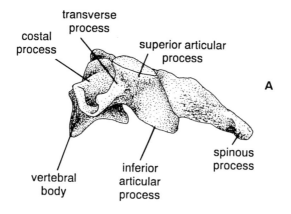

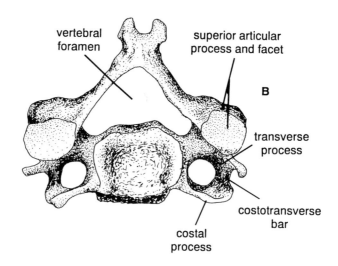

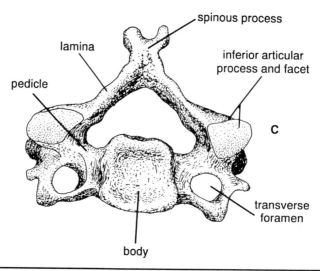

FIG. 2–7. A typical cervical vertebra.
A. Lateral view. B. Superior view. C. Inferior view.

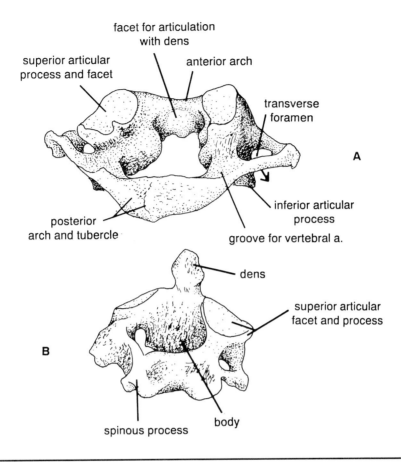

FIG. 2–8. The first two cervical vertebrae.
A. The atlas. B. The axis.

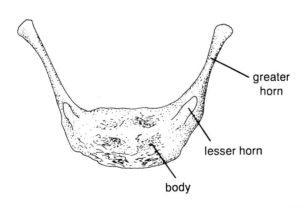

FIG. 2–9. Anterosuperior view of the hyoid bone.

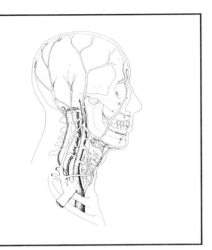

CHAPTER **3**

BLOOD SUPPLY OF THE HEAD AND NECK

Oxygenated blood destined for the head and neck regions—and for all other regions of the body—leaves the left ventricle of the heart and enters the aorta. Within the thorax, the aorta ascends and then curves from an anterior position to a posterior position as the aortic arch. The remainder of the aorta descends through the thorax and abdomen. It is from the aortic arch that the branches to the head and neck arise.

Venous blood from the head and neck, and other parts of the body as well, is collected within the thorax by the superior vena cava and returned to the right atrium of the heart.

A broad description of the distribution of arteries from the aortic arch into the head and neck and the veins that return blood to the superior vena cava is given in the paragraphs below. A more detailed description follows in the chapters on the various regions of the head and neck.

ARTERIAL SUPPLY FOR THE HEAD AND NECK
(Figs. 3-1 and 3-2)

The first branch to arise from the aortic arch is the **brachiocephalic trunk,** which divides as it leaves the thorax into right common carotid and right subclavian arteries. The second branch to arise from the aortic arch is the **left common carotid.** The third, and last, branch of the arch is the **left subclavian.** The common carotids are the major suppliers of oxygenated blood to the head and neck. The subclavians, although mostly carrying blood to the upper limb, give rise to some branches important in the head and neck.

On both sides of the neck the common carotid arteries ascend to the level of the upper border of the thyroid cartilage, where they terminate as internal and external branches. The **internal carotid artery** continues upward to traverse the base of the skull through the carotid canal in the petrous part of the temporal bone. It emerges from the canal within the cranial cavity and, after a short course, makes a sharp bend, at which point the **ophthalmic artery** branches from it and travels into the orbit. The remainder of the internal carotid supplies major arterial branches to the brain. The ophthalmic artery supplies the orbital contents and sends some branches out into the face.

The **external carotid artery** has far reaching branches arising in the neck and retromandibular areas. Their names are, for the most part, descriptive of their destinations. There are two posteriorly directed branches, the **occipital** and **posterior auricular,** heading toward the posterior neck and scalp; the **ascending pharyngeal** branch, arising on the medial, or deep, surface of the external carotid; and the four anteriorly directed branches, the **superior thyroid** for the thyroid gland, the **lingual** for the tongue, the **facial** for the superficial face, and

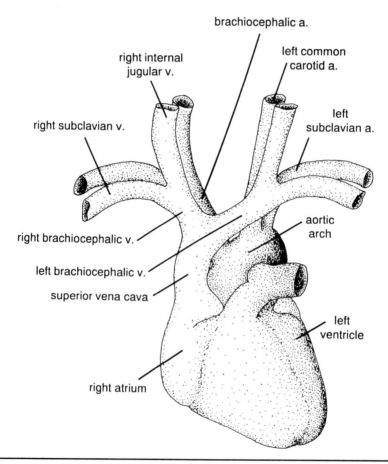

FIG. 3–1. Anterior view of the heart and the major vessels carrying blood to and from the head and neck.

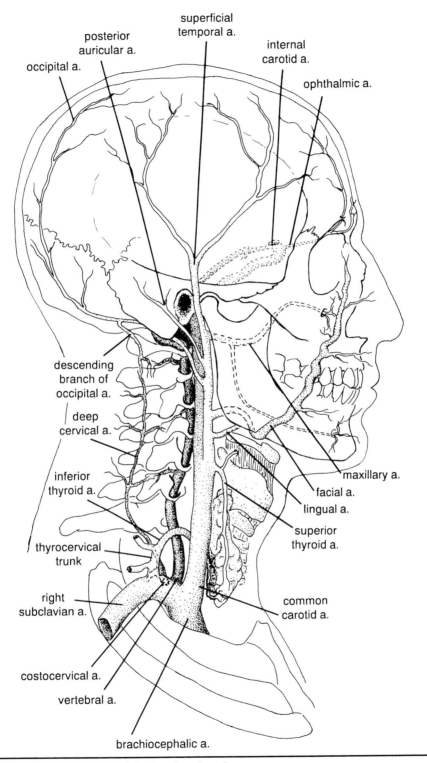

occipital a.

posterior
auricular a.

superficial
temporal a.

internal
carotid a.

ophthalmic a.

descending
branch of
occipital a.

deep
cervical a.

inferior
thyroid a.

thyrocervical
trunk

right
subclavian a.

costocervical a.

vertebral a.

brachiocephalic a.

maxillary a.

facial a.

lingual a.

superior
thyroid a.

common
carotid a.

FIG. 3–2. Arterial supply of the head and neck.

a terminal branch, the **maxillary,** for the deep face. Another terminal branch is the superiorly directed **superficial temporal,** heading toward the lateral side of the head and scalp.

The first branch to arise from the **subclavian artery** is the **vertebral** artery. It ascends in the neck by passing through the transverse foramina in the first six cervical vertebrae and then enters the cranial cavity through the foramen magnum. It is a major supplier of blood to the brain. The **costocervical** branch, from the posterior side of the subclavian, gives off its **deep cervical** branch, which ascends between muscle layers in the deep neck, anastomosing with branches of the occipital and vertebral arteries. And finally, the **thyrocervical trunk** arises from the subclavian, with its important **inferior thyroid** branch, which has anastomoses within the gland with the superior thyroid artery.

Wherever the ends of the branches from one source come close to those from another source, anastomoses can occur, such as those between the thyroid arteries within the thyroid gland or within the scalp between the branches of the superficial temporal and occipital arteries. Arteries from the right and left sides anastomose across the midline, as occurs with the branches of the right and left facial arteries or with those of the right and left superficial temporal arteries. These are only a few examples of the many anastomoses that occur in the head and neck. Should blood flow be decreased or lost in one artery, its anastomosis with another provides a route whereby the tissues it nourished can still be supplied with blood.

VENOUS DRAINAGE OF THE HEAD AND NECK (Fig. 3–3)

The **superior vena cava** is formed in the thorax by the **left and right brachiocephalic veins,** which carry blood returning from the two sides of the head and neck. Each brachiocephalic vein forms at the point where the subclavian vein joins with the internal jugular vein, which occurs at the junction of the inferior part of the neck and the thorax.

The **internal jugular vein** begins at the base of the skull in the jugular foramen. Inside the cranial cavity, venous blood from the brain is collected in venous sinuses within the dura mater. Most of this blood drains into the jugular bulb, a slight dilation of the internal jugular vein at the foramen. As the internal jugular vein descends in the neck it receives other tributaries such as those from the pharynx and the thyroid gland.

The **subclavian vein** is the major collecting vessel for blood from the upper limb, but it also has the external jugular and vertebral veins as tributaries from the head and neck.

The **external jugular vein** forms at the junction of the **posterior auricular vein,** from the scalp behind the ear, with a posterior division of the retromandibular vein, descending just posterior to the mandible. The **retromandibular vein** drains the superficial side of the head via its superficial temporal tributary and the deep face via its maxillary tributary. It has an anterior division, which meets with the facial vein, descending from the tissues of the superficial face; together they make up the common facial vein, which empties into the internal jugular. The external jugular receives tributaries from upper limb structures and the **anterior jugular** from the anterior superficial neck.

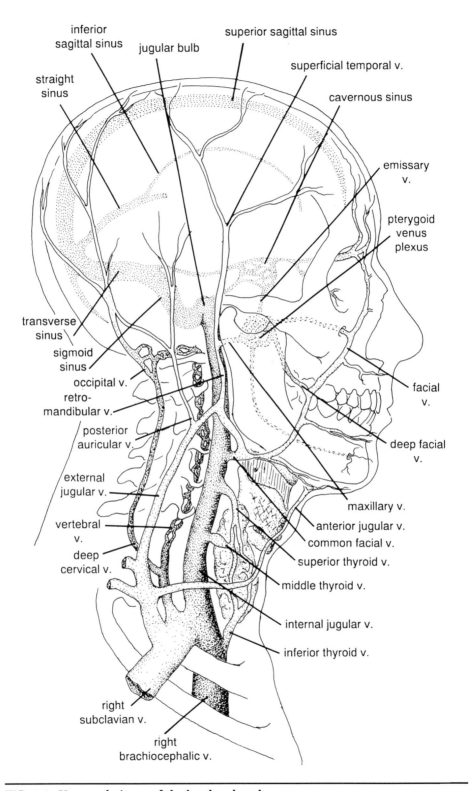

FIG. 3–3. Venous drainage of the head and neck.

Close to its termination, the subclavian vein is joined by the **vertebral vein.** The latter forms a plexus around the vertebral artery and has anastomoses with the occipital and deep cervical veins in its most superior part. The **deep cervical vein** drains the deep neck musculature and terminates in the lower part of the vertebral vein.

Within the infratemporal fossa lies the **pterygoid venous plexus.** Although it empties into the **maxillary vein,** it has connections with the superficial face via the **deep facial vein** and with the cavernous venous sinus via an **emissary vein** that penetrates the skull. By means of this venous network, bacteria from an infection in one area, for example the superficial face, can spread to deeper areas and even into the cranial cavity. This can have serious or even fatal consequences. Other connections also exist, such as the anastomosis between the veins on the face and the ophthalmic veins of the orbit, by which infection can be transferred to deeper structures.

Students reading this text during a course including dissection of the head and neck will become aware of variations that occur from one human to another. Variations are particularly frequent in the vascular system and are especially apparent in the veins of the neck. Not only does one individual differ from another, but one side commonly differs from the other in the same individual.

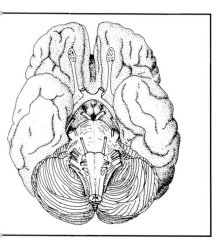

CHAPTER 4

INTRODUCTION TO THE NERVOUS SYSTEM

A basic knowledge of what the nervous system does is essential for understanding human anatomy. In order to acquire this knowledge, it is necessary to begin by studying how the nervous system is organized.

The nervous system has two major divisions. One, the **central nervous system,** includes the brain and the spinal cord. The other, lying outside the brain and spinal cord, is the **peripheral nervous system.**

The functional unit of these two divisions is the nerve cell, usually called a **neuron** (Fig. 4–1). It is composed of two major parts, the **cell body** and its **processes,** which are axons and dendrites. Within the cell body are the nucleus and the components essential for protein synthesis and maintenance of the life of the cell. Its processes receive information from one location and transmit it to another. In general, dendrites are thought of as the processes that receive the information and axons, the ones that deliver it to another location. Neurons vary in shape and size, depending on where they are and what their purpose is. Their dendrites vary in number, length, and degree of branching. Axons vary in these respects too, except there is only one for each cell.

Neuron cell bodies are not scattered at random throughout the nervous system but occur clustered together in groups. Such a group within the central nervous system is known as a **nucleus.** One nucleus of neurons sends information to others by way of many neuron processes. Processes that travel together form a **tract** in order to reach a common destination. Within the peripheral nervous system, a group of cell bodies is known as a **ganglion,** and processes traveling together form a **nerve.** The central and peripheral divisions of the nervous system do not function independently of one another. As will subsequently be seen, many neurons found to have their cell body located in one extend their axon into the other.

An understanding of the nervous system depends on knowing where groups of cell bodies are located, where their dendrites or peripheral processes pick up the information they transmit, where they deliver it, and what kinds of information a particular group of processes is carrying. An understanding of a body region or structure depends on a knowledge of two different kinds of nuclei or ganglia: (1) those whose processes pick up information about what is currently going on *from* the region and carry it back to the central nervous system, and (2) those whose processes deliver information *to* the region so it can react in an appropriate way.

The kinds of information being carried by the numerous processes that comprise a nerve fall into two broad categories, **sensory (afferent)** and **motor (efferent)**. It is important to realize that one nerve can carry both, in which case it is a **mixed nerve.**

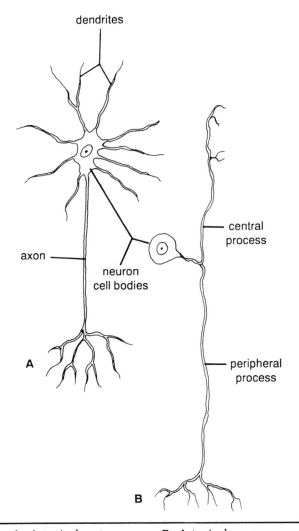

FIG. 4–1. **Neurons. A.** A typical motor neuron. **B.** A typical sensory neuron.

The central nervous system is informed about what is going on in the body by general sensory stimuli such as heat, cold, touch, pressure, and proprioception, which is the sense of position and movement. The sensory information is carried over some of the processes within peripheral nerves to the central nervous system.

Motor information is transmitted from the central nervous system back to the body. Examples of the result of impulses carried along a motor axon include contraction of a skeletal muscle in a limb, the body wall, the head, or the neck; contraction of a smooth muscle in the wall of a blood vessel or visceral organ; and secretion by a gland.

This book discusses the peripheral nervous system in greater detail than the central nervous system. Only those features of the latter essential for understanding peripheral nerve functions are mentioned. For more information about the central nervous system one should consult a neuroanatomy text.

THE SPINAL CORD AND SPINAL NERVES (Figs. 4-2, 4-3, and 4-4)

The spinal cord is contained in the **vertebral canal** within the vertebral column. It is separated from the walls of the canal by layers of membranes and spaces. The outermost of these, the **epidural space,** contains a venous plexus

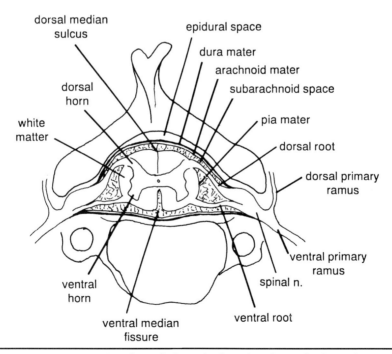

FIG. 4-2. Transverse section through the spinal cord and vertebral canal.

The spinal cord is contained in the **vertebral canal** within the vertebral column. It is separated from the walls of the canal by layers of membranes and spaces. The outermost of these, the **epidural space,** contains a venous plexus embedded in fat and connective tissue, which serve as protective padding and support for the cord. The epidural space is limited on its deep surface by the outermost membrane layer, the **dura mater,** a tough tubular sheet of connective tissue whose superior and inferior attachments to periosteum help to anchor the spinal cord in its proper position. Pressed against the dura on its deep surface and thus conforming to its tubular shape is the **arachnoid mater,** a thin, filmy meningeal layer. The **subarachnoid space,** which lies deep to the arachnoid membrane, is filled with **cerebrospinal fluid.** Pressure of this fluid holds the two layers in apposition. Trabeculae of connective tissue extend across the space and connect the arachnoid membrane to the deepest meningeal layer, the **pia mater,** which covers the surface of the spinal cord.

On the dorsal surface of the spinal cord, a shallow midline groove extends its entire length; the grove is called the **dorsal median sulcus.** A similar but much deeper groove, the **ventral median fissure,** extends along the ventral midline. Along the dorsolateral surface of each side of the cord, a series of 31 **dorsal roots** arises. Along the ventrolateral surface of each side, a series of 31 **ventral roots** arises. At each intervertebral foramen a dorsal and a ventral root join to form a **spinal (segmental) nerve,** which leaves the vertebral canal by passing through the foramen. Of the 31 pairs of spinal nerves thus formed, the

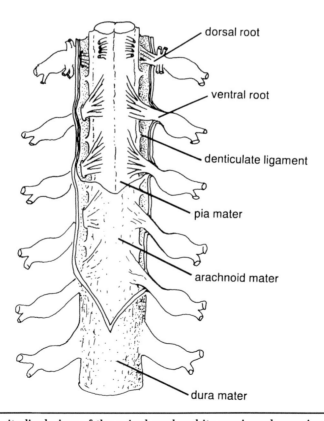

dorsal root

ventral root

denticulate ligament

pia mater

arachnoid mater

dura mater

FIG. 4–3. Longitudinal view of the spinal cord and its meningeal coverings.

first 8 are **cervical spinal nerves,** the next 12 are **thoracic,** followed by 5 **sacral** pairs and 1 **coccygeal** pair.

If a section through the spinal cord is examined, **white matter** can be seen around the periphery and **gray matter** deeper, arranged in a butterfly-shaped pattern. White matter contains tracts, ascending to carry information to a higher level in the central nervous system or descending to carry information to more inferior levels of the cord. Gray matter contains all the neuron cell bodies in the cord. They give rise to many of the processes that ascend or descend in the tracts. The **ventral horns** of the gray matter contain neurons with a motor function. They send their axons out to the spinal nerves by way of the **ventral roots.** They carry the motor information destined for skeletal muscles, which stimulates their contraction. In the thoracic and upper lumbar segments of the cord, there is also a **lateral horn;** it too contains motor neurons whose axons utilize the ventral roots to leave the cord. Their function is autonomic and causes contraction of smooth muscles or secretion of glands (Chapter 5).

The **dorsal horns** of the gray matter are involved with processing sensory information coming into the cord through the **dorsal roots,** which are composed of processes coming from sensory neuron cell bodies located on each dorsal root within a **dorsal root ganglion.** All these neurons are called **primary afferent (sensory) neurons** because they are the first neuron in the sensory pathway.

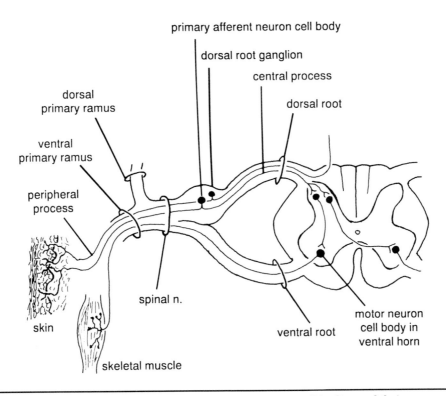

FIG. 4–4. **The location of sensory and some motor neuron cell bodies and their processes in and around the spinal cord.**

They are unusual in that they lack dendrites. Their one process divides into two branches. One of them, the **peripheral process,** enters the spinal nerve and travels, for example, to the periphery, where its endings are stimulated by sensations such as a painful pin prick, by the touch or pressure of something against the skin, or by movement of joints or contraction or stretch of skeletal muscles. The stimulus is passed along the peripheral process back to the other branch, the **central process,** which carries the impulse through the dorsal root into the spinal cord. Its ending contacts the dendrites of a second neuron within the central nervous system and transfers information across this contact, which is called a synapse. If the sensory information is transmitted within the cord to a motor neuron, a reflex contraction of muscles results. This is what happens when a person touches a hot object with the fingers and rapidly withdraws the hand. Other central processes bringing in sensory information ascend in the cord before synapsing in order to deliver the information to a higher level.

Spinal nerves, through which all this incoming sensory and outgoing motor information must pass, are themselves very short and on emerging from the intervertebral foramina divide immediately into two branches called the **dorsal and ventral primary rami.** The spinal nerves of only the cervical and upper thoracic regions and their roots and primary rami carry innervation for structures of the head and neck; they are therefore the ones having a distribution that is described further in this and in following chapters of this book.

DISTRIBUTION OF THE CERVICAL SPINAL NERVES IN THE HEAD AND NECK   (Figs. 4–5, 4–6, and 4–7)

Cervical spinal nerves provide the innervation for the skin over the back of the head, some of the side of the head, and all of the neck. They also supply much of the neck musculature. It is important to compare the distribution of their dorsal rami with that of their ventral rami.

Dorsal rami of cervical spinal nerves travel posteriorly from the intervertebral foramina and immediately enter and innervate the postural musculature of the deep back and neck. No branches to skin (cutaneous branches) are given off by the dorsal ramus of the first cervical spinal nerve (C1). Most of the others do have cutaneous branches. They emerge into the superficial fascia, the connective tissue layer just deep to the skin, close to the posterior midline. The **greater occipital nerve,** the C2 dorsal ramus, has the greatest area of skin to innervate, ascending all the way to the vertex of the scalp. The **third occipital,** the C3 dorsal ramus, supplies neck and scalp up to the external occipital protuberance. Other cervical dorsal rami are limited in distribution to a small area of the posterior neck and upper back. The lower two usually lack a cutaneous branch.

Ventral rami of C1 through C4 contribute to the cervical plexus. Each ventral ramus sends off fibers that communicate with the adjacent ventral rami; thus short connecting loops are formed between them that can give rise to branches containing fibers from more than one ventral ramus. These ventral rami, their connecting loops, and their branches comprise the cervical plexus.

Four cutaneous branches arise from the plexus: the **great auricular** distributes to skin over the lower part of the auricle and adjacent skin of face and lateral head; the **lesser occipital** to scalp posterior to the ear; the **transverse cervical** to skin over the anterior neck; and the **supraclavicular** nerves to skin over the base of the neck as well as over the shoulder and anterior thorax.

The infrahyoid group of muscles in the neck receives its motor innervation from the cervical plexus. A nerve loop, the **ansa cervicalis,** is formed by a superior limb from the C1 ventral ramus and an inferior limb from the C2 and C3 ventral rami. The level at which they join in the neck is highly variable. The uppermost part of the superior limb runs for a way through the neck with the XIIth cranial nerve, the hypoglossal, before it descends to make the loop. Part of the C1 fibers continue further with the hypoglossal, some leaving it in the vicinity of the thyrohyoid muscle and the others at the geniohyoid muscle.

The C3 and C4 ventral rami also serve as the major contributors to the **phrenic** nerve. This is the motor nerve of the diaphragm. Because this muscular structure divides the thoracic cavity from the abdominal cavity, the nerve has a long way to go to reach its destination.

THE BRAIN (Figs. 4–8 and 4–9)

The brain is housed inside the skull in the cranial cavity. Most of the space is occupied by the **cerebral hemispheres,** the largest, most obvious parts of the brain. They are separated from each other by the longitudinal fissure. On their surfaces are prominent rounded folds, the gyri, separated by grooves called fissures or sulci. A hemisphere is divided into frontal, temporal, occipital, and parietal lobes, each named according to the bone of the skull with which it is

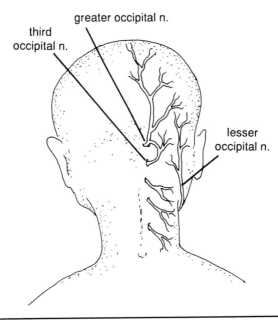

FIG. 4–5. The cutaneous distribution of dorsal primary rami of cervical spinal nerves.

most closely related. Functions of the cerebral hemispheres are varied and numerous. Much of the control of voluntary muscle function, understanding of the significance of sensory information, memory, the ability to make plans and carry them out, and the thoughts that go into setting moral standards are located within the cerebral hemispheres.

The **diencephalon** is a center where sensory information, brought into the central nervous system by the spinal and cranial nerves, converges and then is passed on to the cerebral hemispheres. It also plays an important role in regulation of visceral functions such as hunger, thirst, respiration, cardiovascular responses, and body temperature. It is closely related physically and functionally to a major endocrine organ, the pituitary gland. Part of the latter develops in the embryo as an outgrowth of the diencephalon; hormone production by the other part of the gland is under the control of chemical substances produced by the diencephalon.

The part of the brain consisting of **midbrain, pons,** and **medulla** is called the brain stem. These parts give rise to 10 of the 12 pairs of cranial nerves. Some tracts within the brain stem convey sensory information, brought in by cranial

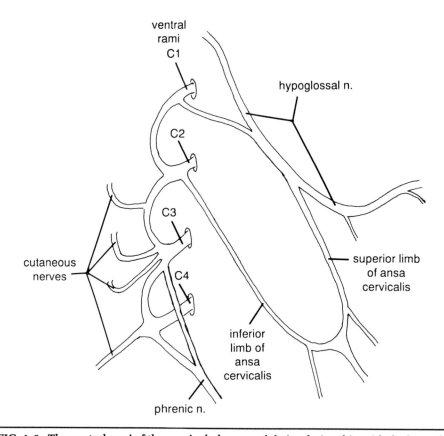

FIG. 4–6. The ventral rami of the cervical plexus and their relationship with the hypoglossal nerve.

and spinal nerves, to the diencephalon. Some carry information to motor neurons in the brain stem or spinal cord.

The **cerebellum** is the part of the brain concerned with coordination of the body's muscular activity. It has two hemispheres, which show many folds, called folia, but they are very narrow and sheet-like, not broad, as are the gyri of the cerebral hemispheres.

MENINGEAL COVERINGS OF THE BRAIN

The meningeal coverings and spaces around the brain are continuous with and similar to those found around the spinal cord. There are the same three layers of connective tissue: dura mater, arachnoid mater, and pia mater, with a subarachnoid space between the latter two.

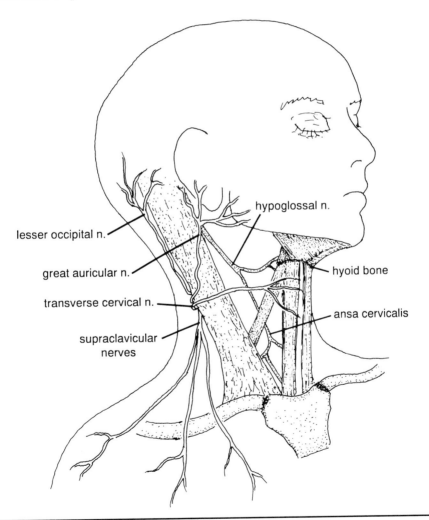

FIG. 4-7. The distribution of the branches of the cervical plexus.

THE DURA MATER AND ITS VENOUS SINUSES (Figs. 4–10, 4–11, and 4–12)

The major differences between the meninges around the brain and those around the spinal cord have to do with the **dura mater.** The dura of the spinal cord has only one layer; over the brain it consists of two. The outermost is the **periosteal layer.** It is a layer of connective tissue adhering to the inner surface of the bones that form the cranial cavity, conforming to all their surface irregularities. Therefore the fat-filled epidural space found external to dura around the spinal cord is lacking.

The innermost layer, called the **meningeal layer,** or the true dura, is fused to the outer layer. Over most of their extent the layers cannot easily be separated and there is no intervening space. In areas where the periosteal and meningeal layers are separated, the spaces between are filled with blood. These are the **dural venous sinuses.** Tributaries to them come from several sources: cerebral veins from the brain, diploic veins from the trabecular spaces within the bones surrounding the cranial cavity, and emissary veins that traverse foramina in the skull, connecting veins in the scalp with the venous sinuses.

The most superior of the venous sinuses, the **superior sagittal sinus,** extends from the crista galli anteriorly to the internal occipital protuberance posteriorly. It is formed as the true dura separates from the periosteal layer along the midsagittal plane to form a large sheetlike infolding called the **falx cerebri.** It extends into the longitudinal fissure between the medial surfaces of the right

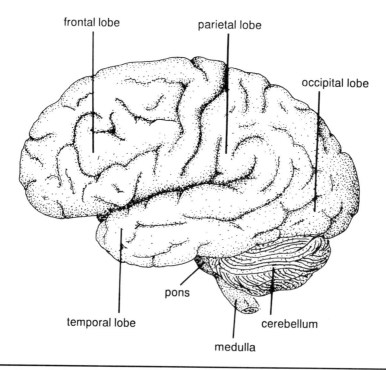

FIG. 4–8. Lateral view of the brain.

and left cerebral hemispheres. Within its inferior free edge is an elongated but very-small-diameter **inferior sagittal sinus.** Posteriorly it meets with the **tentorium cerebelli** in the midsagittal plane, and the so-called **straight sinus** is created along their line of junction. The tentorium is an extensive infolding of meningeal dura, more or less horizontally oriented, that separates the occipital lobes of the cerebral hemispheres from the cerebellar hemispheres inferior to them. Within the junction of the tentorium and the periosteal dura lining the occipital bone is the **transverse sinus.** In the occipital midline inferior to the tentorium is the **falx cerebelli.** This infolding of meningeal dura forms a partial septum between the two cerebellar hemispheres. The small space between its two layers is called the **occipital sinus.** A large dilated space lies in the region of the internal occipital protuberance. It is the **confluence of sinuses.** The straight, superior sagittal, and occipital sinuses drain into the confluence. Blood from it is collected by the transverse sinuses, which pass laterally from the midline. As they reach the temporal bone, each one turns inferiorly to become a **sigmoid sinus,** which terminates at the jugular foramen by emptying its venous blood into the jugular bulb, forming the beginning of the internal jugular vein.

Along each side of the body of the sphenoid bone in the cranial cavity, separation of the two dural layers forms a **cavernous sinus.** This sinus is of particular interest because the internal carotid artery, while traveling through it on its way to supply blood to the brain, is closely associated with several cranial nerves: the third, fourth, and sixth, all of which control movements of

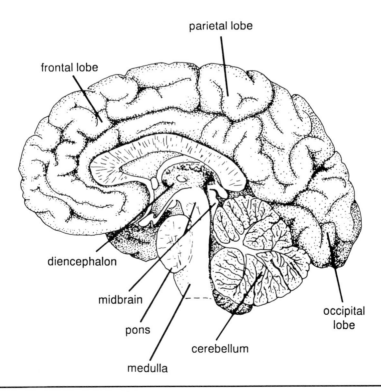

FIG. 4–9. Medial view of the brain.

the eyeball, lie within it or in its lateral wall, formed by the meningeal layer of dura; and the ophthalmic and maxillary divisions of the trigeminal nerve lie in its lateral wall. The proximity of the pituitary gland to these nerves is of great significance in patients with pituitary tumors because enlargement of the gland can put pressure on the nerves and prevent their normal functioning. The sinus is also of significance because it has connections with areas lying outside the cranial cavity (Fig. 9-15). Ophthalmic veins from the orbit empty their blood into the cavernous sinus. Because they have anastomoses with veins on the face, they create a path for spread of infections from the face to the meninges and brain.

The right and left cavernous sinuses are connected with each other by **inter-cavernous sinuses,** passing from side to side within the diaphragma sella around the pituitary gland.

Draining into the cavernous sinus anteriorly is the **sphenoparietal** sinus, which lies along the sharp border of the lesser wing of the sphenoid bone. Blood draining from the cavernous sinus can flow posteriorly by two different routes: by way of the **inferior petrosal sinus,** which follows the temporo-occipital suture to reach the jugular foramen, and by way of the **superior petrosal sinus,** which

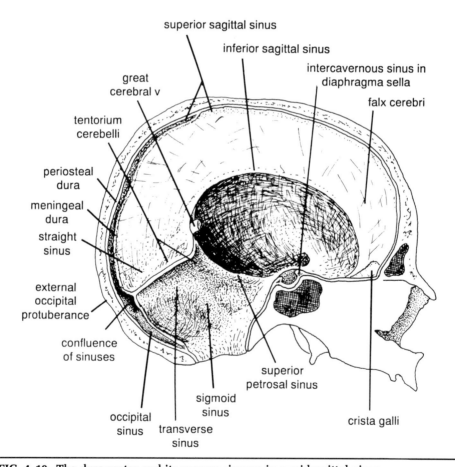

FIG. 4–10. The dura mater and its venous sinuses in a midsagittal view.

extends along the superior edge of the petrous part of the temporal bone to reach the point where the transverse sinus turns into the sigmoid.

Within the dura covering the basilar part of the occipital bone is the **basilar sinus,** which has connections with the internal jugular vein and the venous plexus in the epidural space around the spinal cord.

THE ARACHNOID MATER AND THE PIA MATER

Lying against the inner surface of the dura with only a potential space between it and the dura is the arachnoid mater. It is a thin, filmy layer, pressed against the dura by the pressure of cerebrospinal fluid, which fills the underlying subarachnoid space. The fluid helps to cushion the brain against shocks and to support and hold it in its proper position. In some areas the arachnoid forms small fingerlike extensions of **arachnoid villi,** which project into a venous sinus. They are particularly easily seen along the superior sagittal sinus. The innermost membrane, the pia mater, is closely adherent to the surface of the brain, following across its gyri and down into the depths of its sulci and fissures.

THE VENTRICLES OF THE BRAIN AND CEREBROSPINAL FLUID
(Figs. 4–13 and 4–14)

In addition to the fluid-filled subarachnoid space surrounding the brain, there is a series of fluid-filled interconnected spaces called ventricles within the brain. The largest are the **lateral ventricles,** within the cerebral hemispheres. Each communicates by way of the **foramen of Monro** with the unpaired **third ventricle** in the diencephalon. A very-small-diameter channel, the **cerebral aqueduct,** passes through the midbrain to connect the third ventricle with the **fourth ventricle.** The latter lies along the dorsal surface of the pons and medulla, both of which contribute to its floor. Its roof is formed mostly by the cerebellum.

Cerebrospinal fluid is produced within the lateral, third, and fourth ventricles by **choroid plexuses.** These are thin infoldings of a layer of pia and a layer of epithelium, which lines the ventricles, separated by a third layer consisting of connective tissue containing capillaries. Its composition of water, proteins, glucose, and electrolytes provides a stable chemical environment over the brain's surfaces. Openings from the fourth ventricle allow for flow of the cerebrospinal fluid out of the ventricles and into the subarachnoid space, where it can circulate around both the brain and the spinal cord. Constant production of cerebrospinal fluid within the ventricles requires its constant elimination. It is transferred to the venous system through the thin **arachnoid villi,** also called arachnoid granulations, which are composed of a layer of greatly attenuated dura.

BLOOD SUPPLY OF THE BRAIN (Fig. 4–15)

The arteries that supply the brain approach its ventral surface. They come from two pairs of arteries: the **vertebrals** and the **internal carotids.**

The vertebral arteries enter the cranial cavity through the foramen magnum and join to form the **basilar artery** at the junction of pons and medulla. Before

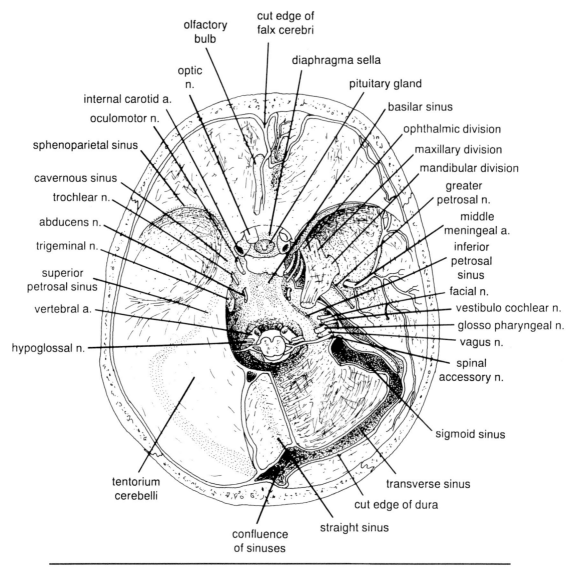

olfactory
bulb

cut edge of
falx cerebri

optic
n.

diaphragma sella

pituitary gland

internal carotid a.

basilar sinus

oculomotor n.

ophthalmic division

sphenoparietal sinus

maxillary division

mandibular division

cavernous sinus

greater
petrosal n.

trochlear n.

middle
meningeal a.

abducens n.

inferior
petrosal
sinus

trigeminal n.

superior
petrosal sinus

facial n.

vertebral a.

vestibulo cochlear n.

glosso pharyngeal n.

hypoglossal n.

vagus n.

spinal
accessory n.

sigmoid sinus

tentorium
cerebelli

transverse sinus

cut edge of dura

straight sinus

confluence
of sinuses

FIG. 4–11. The cranial cavity. The dura covering the bones of the right middle cranial fossa has been removed; the right tentorium cerebelli has been removed so the posterior cranial fossa can be seen. The venous sinuses on the right side have been opened.

joining, they give rise to **posterior and anterior spinal branches** as well as the **posterior inferior cerebellar arteries.** Among the branches of the basilar artery are the **anterior inferior cerebellar arteries;** the **labyrinthine arteries,** to the inner ear of each side; several right and left **pontine arteries;** the **superior cerebellar arteries;** and the two terminal branches, the **posterior cerebral arteries.**

The internal carotid arteries approach the brain from the cavernous sinuses. Their **middle cerebral** branch enters the lateral fissure and gives off branches to the lateral side of the cerebral hemisphere. Their **anterior cerebral** branch passes anteriorly between the frontal lobes and is joined to the same artery on the other side by the very short **anterior communicating** artery. Their **posterior**

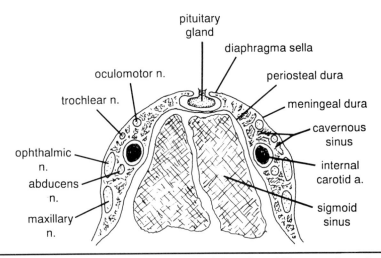

FIG. 4–12. Coronal section through the body of the sphenoid bone to show the relations of the cavernous sinus on each side.

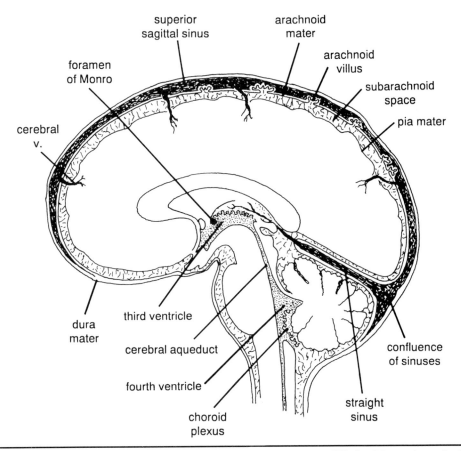

FIG. 4–13. Midsagittal view of the brain showing the spaces filled with cerebrospinal fluid.

communicating branch passes posteriorly to connect with the posterior cerebral. Thus an arterial circle, the **circle of Willis,** is formed. From it, smaller vessels for the brain arise.

Cerebral veins empty into the dural venous sinuses, especially the superior sagittal, and by way of the **great cerebral vein,** the straight sinus.

BLOOD SUPPLY AND INNERVATION OF THE DURA

Most of the dura receives its blood from the **middle meningeal artery,** which enters the skull through the foramen spinosum. It lies on the outer surface of the dura against the bone, and pressure from the blood within the vessel causes obvious grooves in the hard tissue. It also serves as a major source of nutrient branches to the bone.

Meningeal nerves for the dura arise mainly from the three branches of the trigeminal nerve. In the posterior cranial fossa small branches from the cervical spinal nerves supply the innervation. They enter the cranial cavity with the tenth and twelfth cranial nerves.

Meningeal veins drain mostly into the dural venous sinuses. The **middle meningeal vein,** accompanying the artery, drains into the pterygoid venous plexus (see Chapter 9).

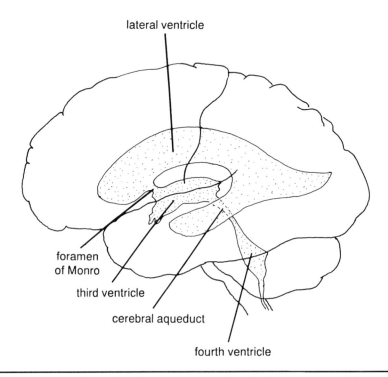

lateral ventricle

foramen
of Monro

third ventricle

cerebral aqueduct

fourth ventricle

FIG. 4–14. Lateral surface of the brain showing the relative positions of the ventricles.

THE CRANIAL NERVES (Fig. 4–16)

Arising from the brain are 12 pairs of cranial nerves. They are conventionally designated either by name or by Roman numerals I through XII.

Many of the kinds of functions they perform are the same as those of spinal nerves: they carry the same general sensations of pain, body temperature, touch, pressure, and the sense of muscle and joint position; they send out motor impulses that cause contraction of skeletal muscle and general visceral motor impulses that cause contraction of smooth muscles and glandular secretion. In addition they perform some special sensory functions that spinal nerves cannot do: they receive visual and auditory stimuli, they carry information about equilibrium, and they are stimulated by smell and taste. No one cranial nerve performs all these general and special functions. Some can perform only one of them, others as many as five.

A cranial nerve with a sensory function is similar to a spinal nerve in that it must have a ganglion outside the central nervous system to house its primary afferent neuron cell bodies; the cell bodies give rise to a single process that

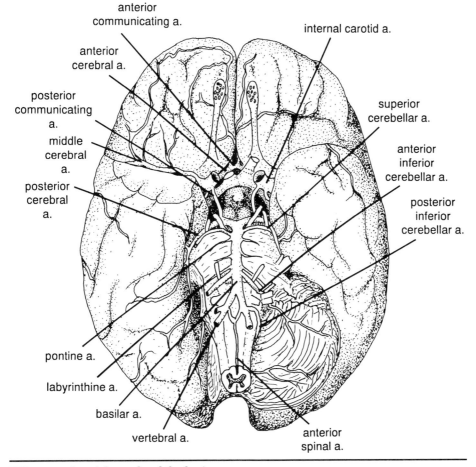

FIG. 4–15. Arterial supply of the brain.

divides into a peripheral and a central process. A cranial nerve with a motor function must have a nucleus within the gray matter of the brain to house the motor neuron cell bodies. Their dendritic processes are short and their axon is long, just as in the spinal nerves.

A brief introduction to some of the distinguishing features of each cranial nerve pair follows. Included are mention of where it emerges from the brain, its motor distribution to skeletal muscle, and its sensory function. More details are provided in the chapters on the various regions of the head and neck. For the motor distribution to smooth muscles and glands see the section on the autonomic nervous system.

CRANIAL NERVE I, THE OLFACTORY NERVE (Fig. 4–17)

The olfactory nerve carries the special sense of smell. Primary sensory neuron cell bodies and their extremely short dendrites lie in a specialized **olfactory epithelium** in the superior part of the nasal cavity. The olfactory epithelium

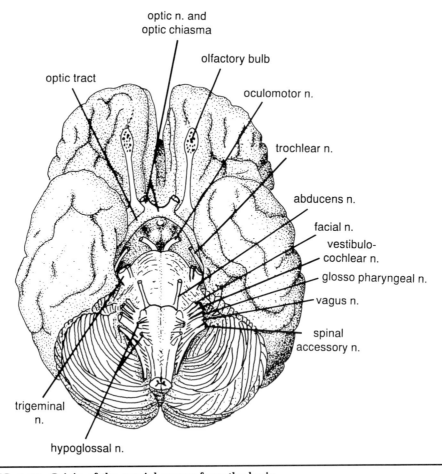

FIG. 4–16. Origin of the cranial nerves from the brain.

serves as the "ganglion" for this nerve. The short dendrites receive the stimulus. The longer axon carries the information from the epithelium to the olfactory bulb, which lies over the cribriform plate of the ethmoid bone, and synapses. The term "olfactory nerve" is somewhat misleading because it is not a single nerve; it is numerous, separate **olfactory filaments,** each containing some central processes. From the bulb the information is conveyed through the olfactory tract to the brain. Because the olfactory bulbs develop in the embryo as outgrowths of the cerebral hemispheres, the pathway for the sense of smell from periphery to cerebral cortex does not pass through and include a synapse in the diencephalon, as it does for all other sensations.

CRANIAL NERVE II, THE OPTIC NERVE (Fig. 4–18)

The optic nerve conveys the special sense of vision. Its primary sensory neuron cell bodies are the ganglion cells in the retina within the eyeball. Their peripheral processes are very short. Their central processes make up the optic nerve. As the two nerves approach the brain, some of the fibers from each one cross in the optic chiasma to the other side. The remainder of the pathway to the diencephalon is the optic tract.

CRANIAL NERVE III, THE OCULOMOTOR NERVE (Fig. 4–19)

The oculomotor nerve emerges from the ventral side of the midbrain. Its destination is the orbit. It must perform two kinds of motor activities. (1) Skeletal muscle function. There are six skeletal muscles within the orbit. Of these, four that move the eyeball are innervated by the third nerve: the superior, medial, and inferior rectus muscles and the inferior oblique. The one that elevates the upper eyelid, the levator palpebrae superioris, also is innervated by the third nerve. (2) Parasympathetic autonomic function (see Chapter 5).

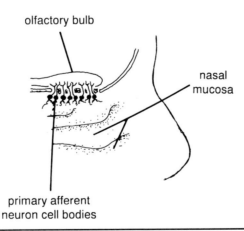

olfactory bulb

nasal mucosa

primary afferent neuron cell bodies

FIG. 4–17. The olfactory nerve.

CRANIAL NERVES IV AND VI, THE TROCHLEAR AND ABDUCENS NERVES (Fig. 4–20)

The trochlear nerve emerges from the midbrain. It has the distinction of being the only cranial nerve arising from the dorsal surface of the brain. The abducens nerve emerges from the pons at its junction with the medulla just lateral to the midline. The function of both these nerves is motor, each supplying one of the skeletal muscles that moves the eyeball: the fourth supplies the superior oblique muscle; the sixth, the lateral rectus muscle.

CRANIAL NERVE V, THE TRIGEMINAL NERVE (Figs. 4–21 through 4–23)

The trigeminal nerve emerges from the ventral side of the pons. It has a large sensory root and a small motor root. The sensory root contains central processes originating from primary sensory neuron cell bodies in the trigeminal ganglion (also called the semilunar or gasserian ganglion). From the ganglion peripheral processes enter the three divisions of the nerve: the ophthalmic, or V1; the maxillary, or V2; and the mandibular, or V3. The latter is joined by the entire motor root, whose axons originate from cell bodies in the pons. Therefore V3 is the only division with a motor function. Branches of the three divisions are so widespread that the trigeminal has a broader distribution in the head than any other cranial nerve.

Although the trigeminal is not one of the cranial nerves with an autonomic function, some of the branches of each of its divisions do pick up autonomic fibers belonging to other nerves and carry them for a distance. This function is discussed in Chapter 5.

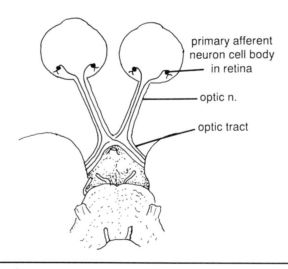

primary afferent
neuron cell body
in retina

optic n.

optic tract

FIG. 4–18. The optic nerve.

The ophthalmic division gives rise to its meningeal branch and then enters the orbit. Its branches supply general sensory innervation to the eyeball, skin on the upper face and anterior scalp, and some mucosa in the nasal cavity.

The maxillary division gives rise to its meningeal branch and then enters the pterygopalatine fossa. It distributes general sensory innervation to some skin on the side of the face, cheek, and upper lip, most of the mucosal lining of the nasal cavity and hard and soft palates, and all the maxillary teeth and gingiva.

The mandibular division enters the infratemporal fossa. From within the fossa it gives rise to a meningeal branch and branches that supply general sensory innervation to skin of the lower face, the lateral side of the head and scalp, mucosa of much of the oral cavity, and all the mandibular teeth and gingiva. Its motor innervation supplies the four muscles of mastication, the anterior belly of the digastric and the mylohyoid muscles in the neck, the tensor tympani muscle in the middle ear cavity, and the tensor veli palatini muscle of the soft palate.

CRANIAL NERVE VII, THE FACIAL NERVE (Fig. 4–24)

The facial nerve emerges from the pons close to its junction with the medulla. In function it is a mixed nerve, having both sensory and motor components. Primary sensory neuron cell bodies, mainly for the special sensation of taste, are

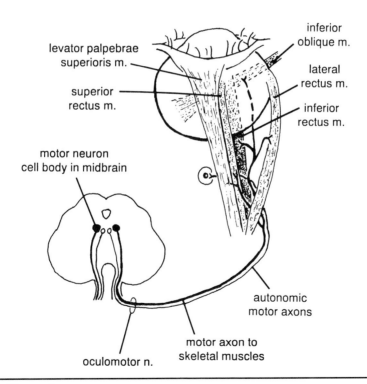

FIG. 4–19. The oculomotor nerve.

grouped together to form the geniculate ganglion. They extend their peripheral processes from the ganglion to the anterior two-thirds of the tongue. Motor neuron cell bodies in the pons send axons to several locations. Some pass to the face to innervate the group of skeletal muscles known as the muscles of facial expression, some extend to the middle ear cavity to the stapedius muscle, and others extend to the neck to supply the posterior belly of the digastric and stylohyoid muscles. The other motor function of the facial nerve is parasympathetic autonomic and is discussed in Chapter 5.

CRANIAL NERVE VIII, THE VESTIBULOCOCHLEAR NERVE
(Fig. 4–25)

The vestibulocochlear nerve conveys the special senses of hearing and equilibrium from tiny receptor organs located in the inner ear. Two ganglia contain the primary sensory neuron cell bodies, the cochlear, or spiral, for hearing and the vestibular for equilibrium. The ganglia lie adjacent to the inner ear organs their peripheral processes supply. Central processes of the cell bodies enter the ventral side of the pons near its junction with the medulla immediately lateral to the facial nerve.

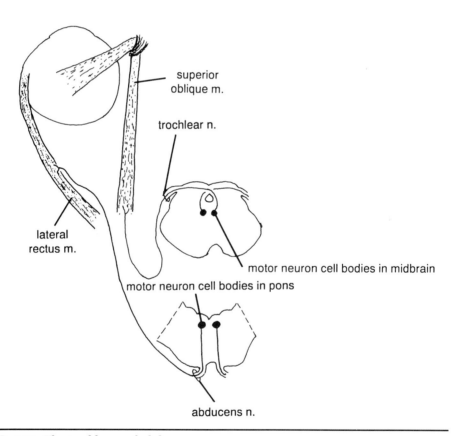

superior oblique m.

trochlear n.

lateral rectus m.

motor neuron cell bodies in midbrain

motor neuron cell bodies in pons

abducens n.

FIG. 4–20. The trochlear and abducens nerves.

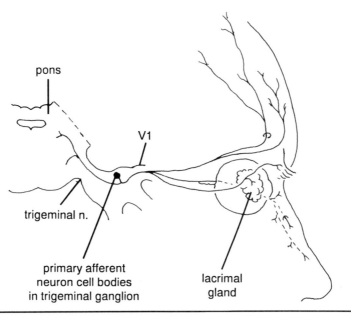

pons

V1

trigeminal n.

primary afferent
neuron cell bodies
in trigeminal ganglion

lacrimal
gland

FIG. 4–21. The ophthalmic division (V1) of the trigeminal nerve.

CRANIAL NERVE IX, THE GLOSSOPHARYNGEAL NERVE
(Fig. 4–26)

The glossopharyngeal nerve emerges from the ventrolateral surface of the medulla close to its junction with the pons. It is a mixed nerve, carrying both sensory and motor information. Primary sensory neuron cell bodies lie in its superior and inferior ganglia. They send peripheral processes to the posterior part of the tongue for general sensations and the special sense of taste; to mucosa of the middle ear cavity; to most of the mucosa of the pharynx; and to the carotid sinus and body for reception of information about blood pressure and oxygen–carbon dioxide content of blood. From motor neuron cell bodies in the brain axons distribute to the stylopharyngeus, the only skeletal muscle innervated by IX. The other motor function of the glossopharyngeal nerve is parasympathetic and is discussed in Chapter 5.

CRANIAL NERVE X, THE VAGUS NERVE (Fig. 4–27)

The vagus nerve emerges from the ventrolateral surface of the medulla caudal to the glossopharyngeal nerve. It carries both sensory and motor innervation. Primary sensory neuron cell bodies lie in the vagal superior and inferior ganglia. Their peripheral processes receive sensory input from visceral organs of the thoracic cavity, mucosa of the larynx and lower part of the pharynx, and much of the gastrointestinal tract. Cell bodies in one motor nucleus within the medulla distribute to skeletal muscles in the pharynx, esophagus, soft palate, and larynx

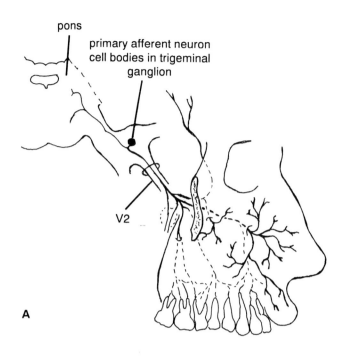

A

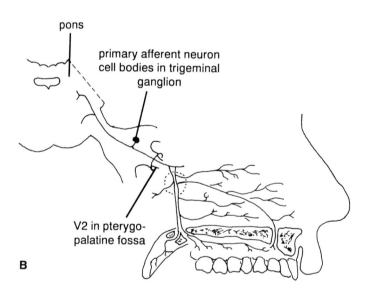

B

FIG. 4–22. The maxillary division (V2) of the trigeminal nerve.
A. The more lateral distribution. B. The more medial distribution.

(but see a further discussion of the laryngeal motor distribution under cranial nerve IX below). The vagus also has a parasympathetic autonomic motor function, which is discussed in Chapter 5. This book describes only those vagus nerve fibers distributing to the head and neck areas.

CRANIAL NERVE XI, THE SPINAL ACCESSORY NERVE (Fig. 4–28)

The spinal accessory nerve supplies motor innervation to skeletal muscles. It is unusual because many of its axons have their origin from neuron cell bodies located in the upper cervical part of the spinal cord. After exiting the cord they ascend along its lateral side as the spinal root of the eleventh nerve. On reaching

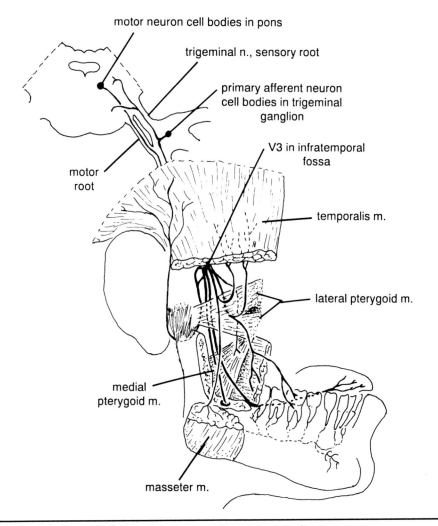

FIG. 4–23. The mandibular (V3) division of the trigeminal nerve.

the level of the medulla, they are joined by motor fibers arising from the same nucleus in the medulla that supplies motor fibers to the vagus nerve. After a short distance, these motor fibers leave the spinal accessory nerve and join the vagus. They are destined for the muscles of the larynx. The spinal root fibers supply motor innervation to the sternocleidomastoid and trapezius muscles.

CRANIAL NERVE XII, THE HYPOGLOSSAL NERVE (Fig. 4–29)

The hypoglossal nerve supplies motor innervation to the skeletal musculature responsible for tongue movement. From neuron cell bodies in nuclei in the medulla, axons leave and form the hypoglossal nerve. It emerges from the ventral surface of the medulla in a more medial position than cranial nerves IX,

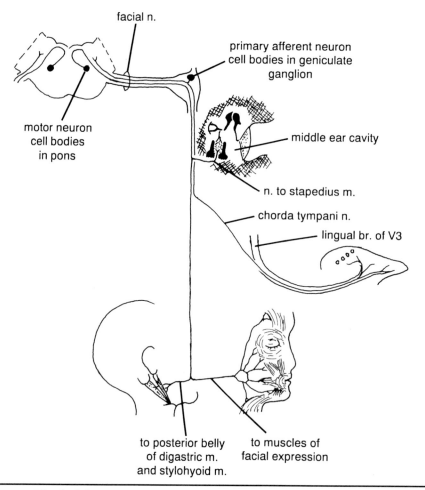

FIG. 4–24. The facial nerve.

X, and XI and descends into the neck before curving anteriorly to reach the tongue.

LOCATION OF OPENINGS IN THE SKULL UTILIZED BY CRANIAL NERVES (Figs. 4–11 and 2-5)

Each cranial nerve, as it travels from the brain to its peripheral destination, must pass through one or more openings in the skull. They are situated in the skull as close as possible to the area outside the cranial cavity where each nerve will undergo its most profuse branching.

In the floor of the anterior cranial fossa, just over the nasal cavity, lies the **cribriform plate** of the ethmoid bone with its numerous perforations for the small filaments of the olfactory nerve.

The middle cranial fossa contains openings for six of the cranial nerves. All are within the sphenoid bone. The **optic foramen** carries the optic nerve, accompanied by the ophthalmic artery, into the orbit. Also entering the orbit, but via the **superior orbital fissure,** are the oculomotor, trochlear, and abducens nerves. All three divisions of the trigeminal nerve arise from the semilunar ganglion in the middle cranial fossa. The superior orbital fissure directs the ophthalmic nerve into the orbit; the **foramen rotundum** directs the maxillary division into the pterygopalatine fossa; and the **foramen ovale** directs the mandibular division into the infratemporal fossa.

The last six cranial nerves exit from the posterior cranial fossa. Both the facial and the vestibulocochlear nerves enter the **internal auditory meatus.** The facial nerve continues on in the facial canal, where its geniculate ganglion is located; the canal tunnels through the petrous part of the temporal bone, terminating at the **stylomastoid foramen,** where the facial nerve exits the skull. In the canal the facial nerve gives rise to its greater petrosal, nerve to the

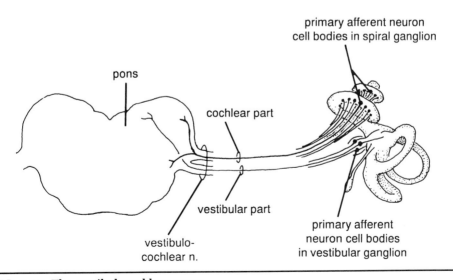

FIG. 4–25. The vestibulocochlear nerve.

stapedius, and chorda tympani branches. The vestibulocochlear nerve ends at its vestibular and cochlear ganglia just inside the meatus.

The **jugular foramen** is the opening for the glossopharyngeal, vagus, and spinal accessory nerves. Both glossopharyngeal and vagus nerves have their superior and inferior ganglia just external to the foramen. The spinal accessory nerve passes from the spinal cord into the cranial cavity through the **foramen magnum** and leaves again through the jugular foramen.

The **hypoglossal foramen,** or canal, carries the hypoglossal nerve.

FUNCTIONAL COMPONENTS OF NERVES

Any one cranial or spinal nerve has within it many processes coming from many different neuron cell bodies. Because the cell bodies can lie in different locations and if they do they vary in function, a nerve can have more than one

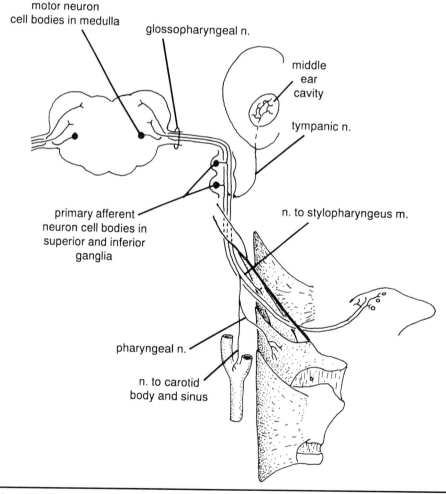

FIG. 4–26. The glossopharyngeal nerve.

function. The functional components a nerve might carry are cited below. Some nerves carry only one of them. A few nerves carry as many as five.

General Somatic Efferent. The general somatic efferent (GSE) component designates motor fibers that go to most of the skeletal muscles of the body. These are the voluntary muscles over which we have control of movement. Nerve impulses traveling over GSE fibers cause contraction of these muscles. The neuron cell bodies that give rise to them are located in the brain or the spinal cord. GSE fibers are carried by all spinal nerves and by cranial nerves III, IV, VI, the spinal part of XI, and XII.

Special Visceral Efferent. Special visceral efferent (SVE) motor fibers to skeletal muscles are derived embryologically from pharyngeal (branchial) arches. Histologically and functionally, these are the same as the skeletal muscles mentioned above. The only difference is the embryologic derivation. That is what makes them special. All neuron cell bodies that give rise to SVE fibers

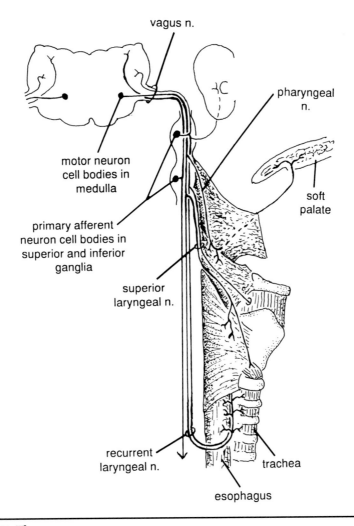

FIG. 4-27. The vagus nerve.

are located in the brain and they supply all muscles innervated by the Vth, VIIth, IXth, and Xth cranial nerves.

General Visceral Efferent. General visceral efferent (GVE) motor fibers cause contraction of smooth muscles and secretion of glands. These are functions over which we have no control and are spoken of as involuntary or autonomic. Parasympathetic autonomic GVE fibers are carried by cranial nerves III, VII, IX, and X and the second, third, and fourth sacral spinal nerves. Sympathetic autonomic GVE fibers leave the spinal cord with all thoracic spinal nerves and the first two or three lumbar spinal nerves.

General Somatic Afferent. General somatic efferent (GSA) fibers carry general sensory information about pain, temperature, touch, and pressure from ectodermally derived epithelium. This includes the epithelium of all skin and the mucosa lining the oral cavity. GSA fibers also carry proprioceptive information from such places as skeletal muscles and joints about the position of body parts such as the limbs, fingers, trunk, head, and mandible. Cranial nerves V, VII, IX, and X and all spinal nerves carry this component.

General Visceral Afferent. The general visceral afferent component is carried by fibers conveying general sensory information from endodermally derived epithelium, visceral organs, glands and blood vessels. It includes information about blood pressure and oxygen and carbon dioxide content of blood. Cranial nerves IX and X and all spinal nerves carry these fibers.

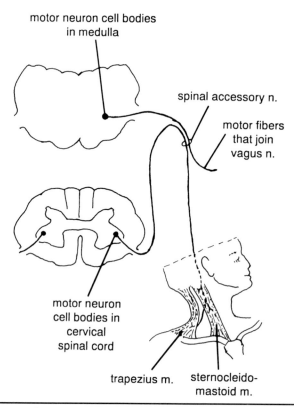

FIG. 4–28. The spinal accessory nerve.

Special Somatic Afferent. Special somatic afferent fibers are special sensory fibers carried by the optic nerve for vision and the vestibulocochlear nerve for hearing and equilibrium.

Special Visceral Afferent. The special visceral afferent component includes special sensory information carried by the olfactory nerve for smell and by the facial and glossopharyngeal nerves for taste.

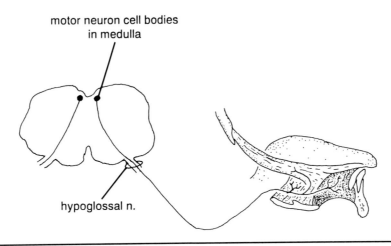

FIG. 4–29. The hypoglossal nerve.

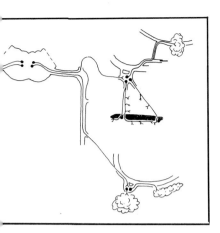

CHAPTER **5**

THE AUTONOMIC NERVOUS SYSTEM

The autonomic nervous system carries motor impulses resulting in contraction of smooth and cardiac muscle and in secretion of glands. These motor functions occur, for the most part, without our being conscious of them and are not under voluntary control. Smooth muscles are widespread in the body. They occur in the wall of most internal visceral organs and in the wall of blood vessels, where their contraction alters the diameter of the lumen; in the skin, where they cause erection of hair; and in the iris of the eye, where they constrict and dilate the pupil. Glands are found in skin for sweat secretion; within the mucosal lining of the nasal cavity and respiratory and gastrointestinal tracts for secretion of mucous and other substances; near the mouth and within its mucosal lining for production of saliva; and in the orbit for tear secretion. Only the details of the autonomic nervous system relevant to innervation of the smooth muscles and glands of the head and neck are described in this book.

In contrast to the motor innervation of skeletal muscle, which utilizes only one axon from the central nervous system to the muscle, autonomic motor innervation reaches the smooth muscle or gland by passing along a sequence of two neurons. The first neuron cell body in the sequence belongs to the **preganglionic neuron,** and it always lies within the central nervous system. Its axon leaves the central nervous system and goes to an autonomic ganglion, where it synapses on the second neuron, called the **postganglionic neuron.** It sends its postganglionic process to the muscle or gland to be innervated.

The autonomic nervous system has two subdivisions: the **sympathetic** and the **parasympathetic.** Their effects are frequently opposite. For instance, the sympathetic causes dilation of the pupil and inhibition of secretion of digestive glands, but the parasympathetic constricts the pupil and increases digestive gland secretion. Both stimulate salivary glands to secrete, however. The quality of the secretion is thick and ropy as a result of sympathetic stimulation and thin and watery as a result of parasympathetic stimulation.

GENERAL PLAN OF SYMPATHETIC INNERVATION OF THE HEAD AND NECK (Fig. 5–1)

Sympathetic autonomic innervation to the head and neck regions arises from preganglionic neuron cell bodies located in the **lateral horn** gray matter in the upper thoracic region of the spinal cord. Preganglionic fibers exit the cord in the **ventral root**, then pass through the **spinal nerve** to its **ventral ramus,** which they leave by passing through the white communicating ramus to enter the thoracic part of the **sympathetic chain.** Within the chain the fibers ascend to its cervical part, where they synapse on postganglionic neuron cell bodies located in the superior, middle, or inferior cervical ganglion. Most fibers carrying innervation for the head synapse on postganglionic neurons located in the **superior cervical ganglion.**

From the superior cervical ganglion many postganglionic axons enter the **carotid nerves,** which form a plexus on the walls of the internal and external carotid arteries, ascending in the immediate vicinity. As these arteries give off their branches, sympathetic postganglionic fibers accompany them wherever they go. Other postganglionic axons from all three cervical ganglia travel by way of **gray communicating rami** to ventral and dorsal rami of all the cervical spinal nerves. As the latter distribute branches to skin and skeletal muscles for general sensation and muscle contraction, they distribute the postganglionic fibers to smooth muscles in the walls of vessels and sweat glands and smooth muscles for hair erection in the same areas.

GENERAL PLAN FOR PARASYMPATHETIC INNERVATION OF THE HEAD AND NECK

Parasympathetic autonomic innervation to the head and neck arises from preganglionic neuron cell bodies located in nuclei within the brainstem. **Only four pairs of cranial nerves leave the brain carrying preganglionic axons: the third, the seventh, the ninth, and the tenth.** Except for those in the tenth nerve, the vagus, these processes synapse on postganglionic neuron cell bodies within one of the four parasympathetic ganglia of the head: the ciliary, the pterygopalatine, the submandibular, or the otic. From the ganglia, postganglionic fibers pass to the organ to be innervated. The vagus nerves distribute their major mass of parasympathetic fibers to regions outside the head and neck.

PARASYMPATHETIC DISTRIBUTION OF THE OCULOMOTOR NERVE (Fig. 5–2)

The parasympathetic preganglionic neuron cell bodies of the oculomotor nerve lie within a nucleus in the midbrain. Their postganglionic processes leave the central nervous system as part of the oculomotor nerve. After the nerve enters the orbit, the preganglionic fibers branch off to enter the **ciliary ganglion,**

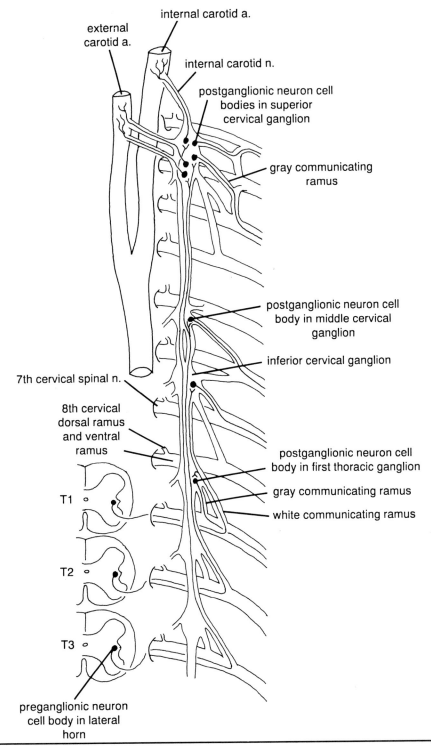

FIG. 5–1. The source of sympathetic autonomic innervation to the head and neck. The first three thoracic spinal cord segments contain the preganglionic neuron cell bodies.

PARASYMPATHETIC DISTRIBUTION OF THE OCULOMOTOR NERVE   **61**

where they synapse on postganglionic neuron cell bodies. The latter send their postganglionic fibers into the eyeball to innervate the sphincter pupillae muscle of the iris and the ciliary muscle of accommodation. Contraction of the sphincter causes the pupil to become smaller, which occurs when light shines into the eye. Contraction of the ciliary muscle reduces tension on the periphery of the lens and allows it to become rounder. Both these parasympathetic effects take place when the eyes are being used for near-vision activities, such as reading a book.

PARASYMPATHETIC DISTRIBUTION OF THE FACIAL NERVE (Fig. 5–3)

Of the four cranial nerves with parasympathetic fibers, the facial nerve has the most complicated distribution. Preganglionic cell bodies in the pons give rise to preganglionic fibers that belong to the facial nerve. The nerve enters the facial canal within the petrous part of the temporal bone, where it gives rise to two branches carrying preganglionic parasympathetic fibers.

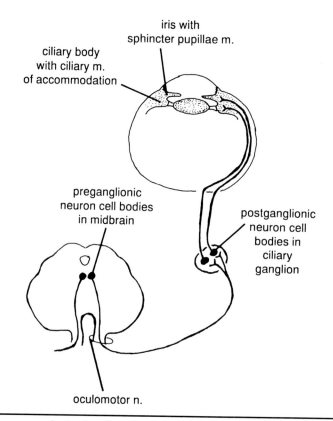

FIG. 5–2. Parasympathetic distribution of the oculomotor nerve.

The first branch is the **greater superficial petrosal nerve,** which exits the canal at the hiatus of the facial canal and enters the cranial cavity. From there it travels to the pterygopalatine fossa, where its preganglionic fibers synapse on postganglionic neuron cell bodies located in the **pterygopalatine ganglion.** The postganglionic fibers coming from them have a widespread distribution. Some leave the ganglion and travel first with the zygomatic branch of the maxillary (V2) division of the trigeminal nerve and then with the lacrimal branch of the ophthalmic (V1) division of the trigeminal nerve in order to reach the **lacrimal gland** in the orbit. Their function is to cause secretion of tears. Other postganglionic fibers join the branches of the maxillary division, traveling to mucosa of the nasal and oral cavities in order to stimulate secretion of mucous glands in these locations.

The second branch is the **chorda tympani nerve.** It leaves the canal, travels through the middle ear cavity across the surface of the tympanic membrane, and exits to enter the infratemporal fossa through the petrotympanic fissure. There it joins the lingual branch of the mandibular division of V. As the lingual nerve approaches the floor of the oral cavity, the parasympathetic preganglionic

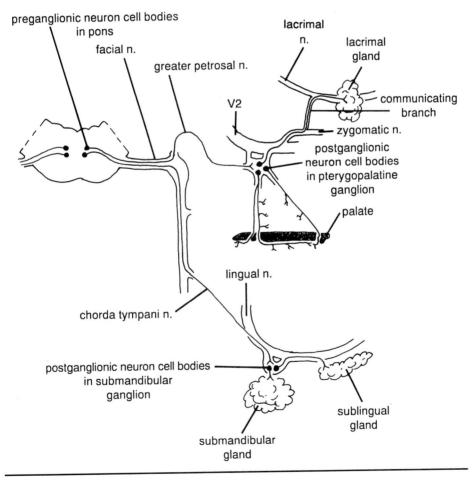

FIG. 5–3. Parasympathetic distribution of the facial nerve.

fibers leave it to synapse on postganglionic neuron cell bodies in the **submandibular ganglion.** Some of their postganglionic fibers pass directly to the adjacent submandibular gland. Others rejoin the lingual nerve, travel with it to the floor of the oral cavity, and again leave it to innervate the sublingual gland. Thus the facial nerve is responsible for glandular secretion in two of the three large salivary glands.

PARASYMPATHETIC DISTRIBUTION OF THE GLOSSOPHARYNGEAL NERVE (Fig. 5–4)

The glossopharyngeal nerve carries the parasympathetic innervation for the parotid salivary gland. Its preganglionic neuron cell bodies lie in the medulla. Their preganglionic fibers travel into the infratemporal fossa as the **lesser petrosal nerve** to synapse on postganglionic neuron cell bodies located in the **otic ganglion.** Postganglionic fibers from the ganglion join the auriculotemporal branch of the mandibular (V3) division of the trigeminal nerve; they leave it as it curves from a deep position to a superficial one and begins to ascend anterior to the ear to reach skin of the lateral side of the head. The parasympathetic fibers of IX enter the parotid gland.

PARASYMPATHETIC DISTRIBUTION OF THE VAGUS NERVE (Fig. 5–5)

The vagus nerve carries parasympathetic innervation for the visceral organs of the thorax, many of those in the abdomen, and a few in the pelvic region. Its preganglionic neuron cell bodies lie in the medulla. Their preganglionic axons

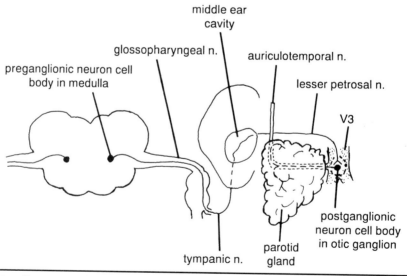

FIG. 5–4. Parasympathetic distribution of the glossopharyngeal nerve.

are a large part of the vagus nerve and are some of its longest fibers. They travel to synapse on postganglionic neurons located very near or more commonly, within the wall of the organ to be innervated. Because these organs lie outside the head and neck, details of their innervation are not presented in this text.

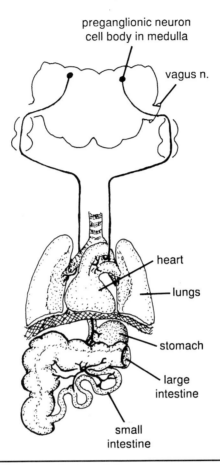

FIG. 5–5. Parasympathetic distribution of the vagus nerve.

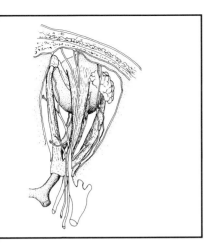

CHAPTER **6**

THE ORBIT

The eyeball, the organ responsible for the special sense of vision, is housed within the space in the skull known as the orbit. Many of the contents of the orbit are present because they are essential for proper functioning of the eyeball: skeletal muscles for production of eyeball movements; vessels for blood supply; and nerves for contraction of the muscles, for reception of touch from the cornea, and for vision. Another nerve stimulates the lacrimal gland to secrete tears. Other structures within the orbit are simply passing through to reach some of the skin over the face and scalp. All these structures are held firmly in place by loose connective tissue containing a large amount of fat and filling all the intervening space.

THE BONY BOUNDARIES OF THE ORBIT (Fig. 6–1)

The seven bones of the orbit form a prominent orbital rim and bound a conically shaped space closely related on three sides to other important cranial spaces. The cranial cavity is superior to the orbit, the maxillary sinus is inferior to it, and the nasal cavity is medial to it.

The **frontal bone** contributes the most to the orbital boundaries, forming the superior parts of the rim and walls from the medial to the lateral side. Its orbital plate, in the roof of the orbit, separates the orbital contents from the overlying cranial cavity and frontal lobe of the brain.

The **zygomatic bone** forms the remainder of the lateral side of the orbital rim and continues on around its inferior margin. It is also a major contributor to the lateral wall and floor of the orbit.

The **maxilla** completes the inferior and medial rim and the remainder of the floor of the orbit. The latter part is also the roof of the maxillary sinus. The infraorbital groove and canal pass across the floor. On the medial wall the maxilla articulates with the **lacrimal bone.** Together they form the **lacrimal fossa,** which contains the opening into the nasolacrimal canal, leading from the orbit to the nasal cavity.

Completing the medial wall of the orbit is the **ethmoid bone,** and posterior to that, a very small contribution by the **palatine bone.** In the frontoethmoid suture the **anterior and posterior ethmoidal foramina** can be seen.

The posterior part of the roof and lateral wall of the orbit are completed by the **sphenoid bone.** It contains, or contributes to, the three major openings in the orbit through which vessels and nerves enter. The **superior orbital fissure** lies between the lesser and greater wings of the sphenoid bone. The **inferior orbital fissure** is between the greater wing of the sphenoid and the maxilla, and the **optic foramen** is at the junction of the lesser wing and body of the sphenoid.

The periosteum lining these bones forms a tough connective tissue sheath for the orbital contents called the **periorbita.** At the orbital rim it is continuous with the periosteum over the bones of the face.

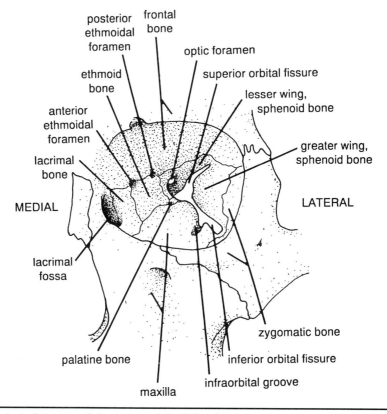

FIG. 6–1. Anterior view of the bones of the left orbit.

THE LACRIMAL APPARATUS (Fig. 6–2)

The lacrimal apparatus includes the **lacrimal gland,** which secretes tears, and the structures that convey excess tears into the nasal cavity. The lacrimal gland lies in the superolateral part of the orbit just posterior to the orbital rim. Its secretions flow downward across the anterior surface of the eye to keep it moistened. Excess fluid escapes in the medial corner of the eye through two small **lacrimal puncta,** or openings. Each leads into a **lacrimal canaliculus** that empties into the **lacrimal sac** situated in the lacrimal fossa. From here the **nasolacrimal duct** continues to the nasal cavity.

THE EYEBALL (Fig. 6–3)

The eyeball is a sphere with a diameter of about 2.5 cm. Most of its wall is three-layered, and it contains within its posterior four-fifths a clear, semigelatinous substance called the vitreous body.

The outermost white layer is the **sclera.** In order to give some protection to the inner contents, it is tough and fibrous. The **cornea** is the anterior part of this layer. It is more strongly curved and is transparent in order to allow passage of light to the interior. Over its anterior surface, the **conjunctiva** contributes a thin layer of epithelium, which continues around to line the posterior surface of the eyelids and makes a transition to become the skin over their anterior surface.

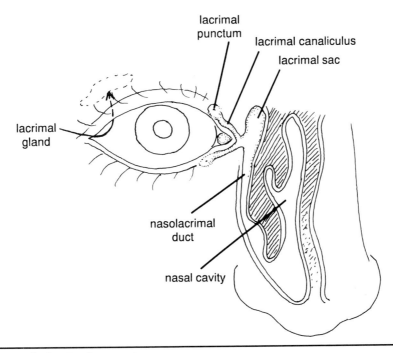

FIG. 6–2. The lacrimal apparatus.

Posteriorly the sclera is perforated by fibers of the optic nerve and other closely associated nerves and vessels destined for the interior of the eyeball.

The middle layer is the **choroid.** It is a darkly pigmented coat containing the nerves and blood supply to the internal structures of the eye. Adjacent to the junction of sclera and cornea, the choroid layer thickens to become the **ciliary body.** Suspensory ligaments pass from ciliary processes on the ciliary body to the periphery of the lens. When stretched, they pull on the periphery, tending to flatten the lens. Contraction of smooth muscles within the ciliary body causes relaxation of these ligaments and the lens rounds up. This is essential for near vision. Anterior to the ciliary body the choroid layer forms the **iris,** a thin membrane having the **pupil** as a central opening in it. The diameter of the pupil is altered by contractions of the sphincter pupillae and dilator pupillae muscles, which are smooth muscles within the iris. The space between the lens and the cornea is divided by the iris into an **anterior chamber** and a **posterior chamber.** The minute, finger-like projections of the ciliary processes on the ciliary body are covered with epithelium and elaborate a watery fluid, the **aqueous humor,**

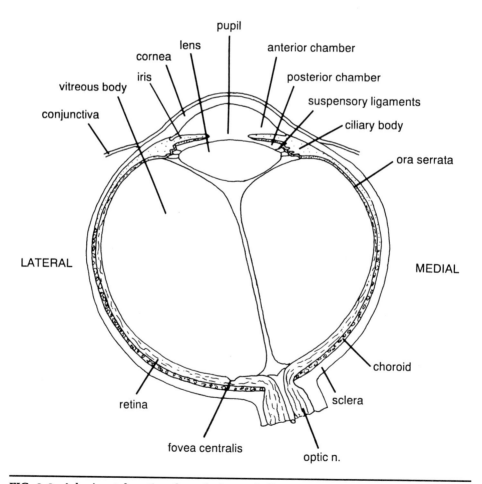

FIG. 6–3. A horizontal section through the eyeball.

that fills the chambers. Drainage is accomplished by a network of veins lying at the junction of iris and cornea. If these veins become blocked, the fluid accumulates and causes pressure on the retina. Blindness can result. This is what produces glaucoma, one of the leading causes of blindness.

The innermost of the three layers is the **retina.** It has two parts, which differ from each other in function. The neural part coats the choroid layer over the posterior half of the eye and forward to the **ora serrata.** It is responsible for receiving light and visual images. Light entering the eye passes through the cornea, aqueous humor, pupil, lens, vitreous humor, and all the cell layers of the retina to reach light receptors within it called rods and cones. Visual impulses are then transmitted from the rods and cones back through the layers of retinal cells to enter the axons that form the optic nerve and carry the visual information to the brain. Light passing straight through the pupil and striking the posterior pole falls on a spot of the retina called the **macula lutea.** At its midpoint there is a small depression, the **fovea centralis,** where only cones are found. They are the receptors responsible for the greatest visual acuity.

The nonneural part of the retina lies anterior to the ora serrata and lines the ciliary body and posterior part of the iris. It contains pigmented cells, which, along with pigment in the choroid contribution to the iris, give the iris its color.

THE ORBITAL MUSCULATURE (Figs. 6–4 and 6–5)

Contained within the eyeball are the small smooth muscles mentioned in the preceding section, the **sphincter pupillae** and the **dilator pupillae** within the iris and the **ciliary muscle of accommodation** within the ciliary body.

Conspicuous within the orbit, however, are seven skeletal muscles. One of them, the levator palpebrae superioris, is responsible for elevation of the upper eyelid. The other six, commonly referred to as the extrinsic muscles of the eye, have the function of turning the eyeball so that one can look upward, downward, medially, and laterally, in addition to looking straight ahead.

The **medial rectus, lateral rectus, superior rectus,** and **inferior rectus** muscles are named for their relative positions within the orbit and attachment sites on the eyeball. Their origin is from a common ring tendon located in the posterior part of the orbit. They pass straight from their origin to insert a few millimeters posterior to the cornea into the scleral coat of the eyeball. The other two muscles, the **superior oblique** and the **inferior oblique,** approach the eyeball from the medial side. Although the superior oblique arises posteriorly in the orbit just superior to the ring tendon and passes straight forward in a superior and medial position, it turns through a fibrous pulley, the trochlea, attached to the frontal bone, and heads diagonally on the superior side of the eyeball to the posterolateral quadrant, where it inserts on the sclera. The inferior oblique muscle arises from the maxilla in the anteromedial floor of the orbit and passes diagonally inferior to the inferior rectus muscle to insert posterior to the equator of the eyeball more laterally than the superior oblique.

From its posterior origin just above the ring tendon the **levator palpebrae superioris** muscle passes straight forward superior to the superior rectus muscle. It enters the upper eyelid, where some of its fibers insert into the **tarsal plate.**

This is a tough fibrous structure that gives shape to the eyelid. Other fibers insert into the superficial fascia beneath the skin of the lid, where they interdigitate with fibers of the orbicularis oculi muscle, which is responsible for closing the eye. The upward pull of the levator on the structures to which it is attached serves to hold the upper eyelid in the elevated, or open, position.

As the result of contraction of the extrinsic muscles, the eyeball can be rotated about three different axes. (1) Rotation about its vertical axis results in medial or lateral gaze. (2) Rotation about its horizontal axis results in upward or downward gaze. (3) Rotation about its anterior-posterior axis moves the superior point on the equator of the eyeball in a nasal or temporal direction. Figure 6–6 summarizes these movements for each muscle.

THE NERVES IN THE ORBIT (Figs. 6–7 and 6–8; also Figs. 4-18 to 4-21)

The **optic nerve,** for the special sense of vision, is the largest nerve in the orbit. Emerging from the posterior part of the eyeball, it passes to the optic foramen, where it exits the orbit and continues on, conveying visual information

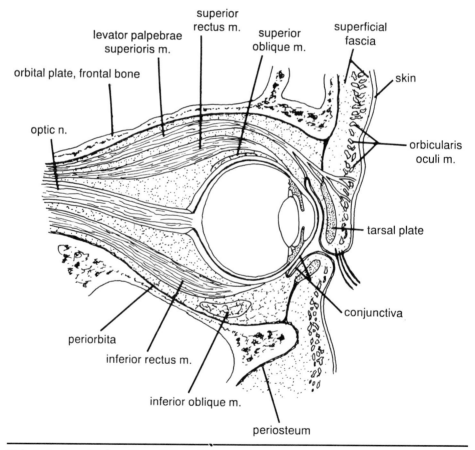

FIG. 6–4. A sagittal section of the orbit.

to the brain. It contains processes that arise from ganglion cells located in the neural part of the retina and terminate in the diencephalon. As they converge in the posterior retina on the slight swelling of the **optic disk,** they cause a **blind spot** where there are no rods and cones. Because the retina develops in the embryo as an outgrowth of the brain, the optic nerve is enclosed by meninges all the way to the eyeball.

Three cranial nerves enter the orbit through the superior orbital fissure for the purpose of motor innervation of the skeletal musculature. The **trochlear nerve** supplies the superior oblique muscle, the **abducens nerve** supplies the lateral rectus muscle, and the **oculomotor nerve** supplies the other five. It has a superior branch to the levator palpebrae superioris and superior rectus muscles and an inferior branch to the inferior oblique, inferior rectus, and medial rectus muscles.

In addition to the above, the **oculomotor** nerve carries parasympathetic innervation destined for the sphincter pupillae muscle and the ciliary muscle of accommodation. Preganglionic parasympathetic axons arise from neurons located in the midbrain. On reaching the posterior part of the orbit, they leave the inferior branch of the oculomotor nerve to enter the **ciliary ganglion,** located between the lateral rectus muscle and the optic nerve. They synapse in the ganglion on postganglionic neurons. The latter send postganglionic axons via the **short ciliary nerves** into the posterior part of the eyeball. They run forward within the choroid layer to reach the muscles. (See also Chapter 5 and Fig. 5–2.)

Innervation for the general sensations of pain, touch, and pressure is supplied by the **ophthalmic division of the trigeminal nerve.** Its branches are the frontal,

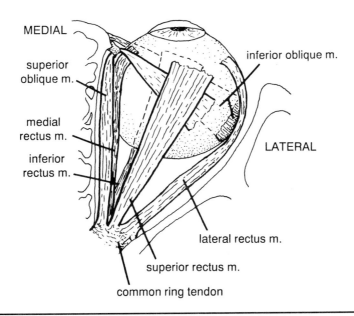

FIG. 6–5. **Superior view of the right orbit showing the extrinsic muscles.**

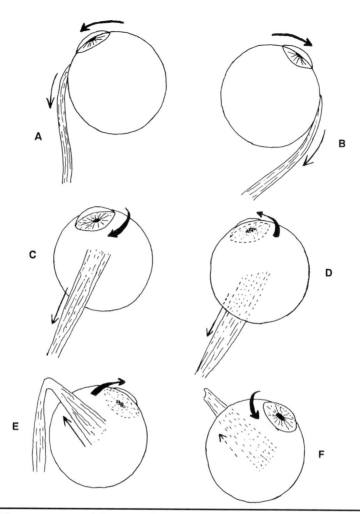

FIG. 6–6. The movements of the eyeball. Each shows a superior view of the right eyeball.
A. The medial rectus muscle produces adduction of the cornea. **B.** The lateral rectus muscle produces abduction of the cornea. **C.** The superior rectus muscle produces upward gaze and adduction of the cornea and medial rotation of the eyeball. **D.** The inferior rectus muscle produces downward gaze and adduction of the cornea and lateral rotation of the eyeball. **E.** The superior oblique muscle produces downward gaze and abduction of the cornea and medial rotation of the eyeball. **F.** The inferior oblique muscle produces upward gaze and abduction of the cornea and lateral rotation of the eyeball.

lacrimal, and nasociliary nerves, which enter the orbit through the superior orbital fissure.

The **frontal nerve** merely passes through the orbit in a position superior to the levator palpebrae superioris muscle on its way to a cutaneous destination in the forehead and scalp. Anteriorly it divides into its **supraorbital** and **supratrochlear** branches. They pass around the superior orbital rim as they leave the orbit, the supratrochlear nerve lying just above the trochlea, the supraorbital nerve traversing the supraorbital foramen or notch.

The **nasociliary nerve** crosses from a lateral position in the posterior part of the orbit to a medial position and continues anteriorly, giving rise to branches along its pathway. General sensory information from the eyeball, such as touch on the cornea, is conveyed through several **long ciliary branches** and also by fibers that traverse the **sensory root** to the ciliary ganglion and the short ciliary nerves. The fibers of both the short and the long ciliary nerves penetrate the posterior part of the eyeball and traverse the choroid layer to reach their destinations. The general sensation of touch from the cornea is particularly important because it is essential in maintaining the blink reflex, which protects the cornea from damage. Along the medial wall of the orbit the nasociliary nerve gives rise to a **posterior ethmoidal branch** to supply ethmoid air cells and the sphenoid sinus. A short distance onward, the **anterior ethmoidal nerve** arises to supply some of the ethmoid air cells and then continue on into the nasal cavity for further distribution. The terminal branch of the nasociliary nerve is the **infratrochlear nerve** for cutaneous distribution.

In addition to its sensory function, the nasociliary nerve carries **sympathetic postganglionic nerve fibers**. These fibers come from the sympathetic plexus on

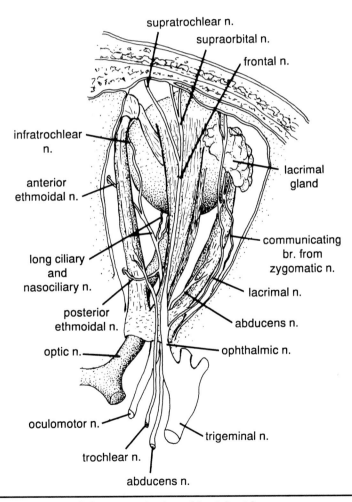

FIG. 6–7. Superior view of the nerves in the orbit, right side.

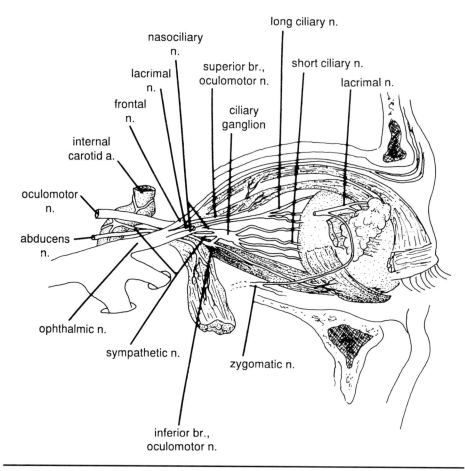

long ciliary n.

nasociliary n.

superior br., oculomotor n.

short ciliary n.

lacrimal n.

lacrimal n.

frontal n.

ciliary ganglion

internal carotid a.

oculomotor n.

abducens n.

ophthalmic n.

sympathetic n.

zygomatic n.

inferior br., oculomotor n.

FIG. 6–8. Lateral view of the right orbit showing the nerves.

the internal carotid artery and gain access to the nasociliary nerve in the cavernous sinus. As it gives rise to its long ciliary branches and its sensory root to the ciliary ganglion, the sympathetic fibers are able to use these branches as pathways to the eyeball. Passing forward within the choroid layer, they reach the dilator pupillae muscle of the iris.

The **lacrimal branch** of the ophthalmic nerve passes through the superolateral part of the orbit to the lacrimal gland. Terminally, it gives rise to a cutaneous palpebral branch that continues into the upper eyelid.

In the floor and lateral wall of the orbit two branches of the maxillary division of the trigeminal nerve run their course to a destination that is in large part cutaneous. Both enter the orbit through the inferior orbital fissure. The **zygomatic nerve,** after a short course along the lateral wall of the orbit, gives off its communicating branch to the lacrimal nerve, mentioned above, before entering the zygomatic bone, where it divides into its zygomaticotemporal and zygomaticofacial branches for cutaneous distribution (Fig. 7–4). The **communicating branch** contains the parasympathetic fibers for lacrimal gland secretion. They belong to the seventh cranial nerve, but, posterior to the orbit, they join the zygomatic nerve in order to gain access to the orbit (Fig. 5–3). The other branch of the maxillary nerve, the **infraorbital nerve**, lies in the infraorbital groove. After only a short distance, the groove becomes the infraorbital canal, which transports the nerve to the face (Fig. 7–4).

VESSELS IN THE ORBIT (Figs. 6–9 and 6–10)

In the middle cranial fossa the **ophthalmic branch** of the internal carotid artery arises. It enters the orbit through the optic foramen along with the optic nerve and supplies all the orbital contents, as well as some more peripheral areas. Many of its branches accompany the nerves within the orbit and are similarly named, such as the **lacrimal, anterior and posterior ethmoidal, supraorbital, supratrochlear,** and **palpebral** branches.

Other branches vary in name or distribution pattern from that found for the nerves. The **central artery of the retina** penetrates the optic nerve and runs within it to enter the eyeball at the optic disk. **Posterior ciliary arteries** enter the eyeball posteriorly along with the ciliary nerves. **Muscular arteries** supply the

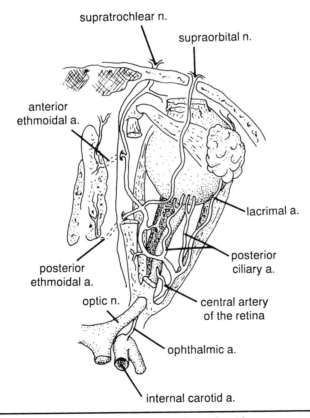

FIG. 6–9. Superior view of the arteries of the orbit right side.

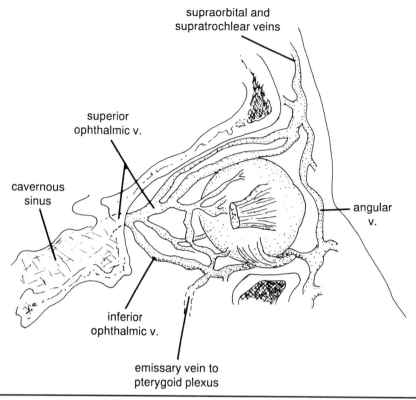

supraorbital and
supratrochlear veins

superior
ophthalmic v.

cavernous
sinus

angular
v.

inferior
ophthalmic v.

emissary vein to
pterygoid plexus

FIG. 6–10. Lateral view of the veins of the right orbit.

extrinsic musculature, running forward within the muscles' connective tissue sheaths and giving rise to anterior ciliary arteries, which penetrate the sclera just posterior to its junction with the cornea.

The **superior and inferior ophthalmic veins** collect blood from the orbit. They receive the various tributaries that accompany the arteries as well as the vorticose veins of the eyeball. Veins in the choroid coat are tributaries to four or five large **vorticose veins,** which penetrate the sclera of the posterior half of the eyeball. Anteriorly, the ophthalmic veins have anastomoses with veins on the face. The inferior ophthalmic vein, through the inferior orbital fissure, has an anastomosis with the pterygoid plexus of veins in the infratemporal fossa (see also Fig. 9–15). Usually, the inferior ophthalmic vein empties into the superior ophthalmic vein, which, in turn, drains into the cavernous sinus, although both can be separate tributaries to the sinus.

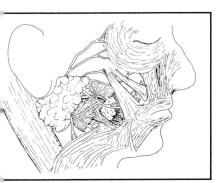

CHAPTER 7

THE SUPERFICIAL PART OF THE FACE AND THE SCALP

A study of the head, or of any other area of the body, most logically begins with the superficial part, the part closest to the surface. This includes the skin and the **superficial fascia** underlying it. Superficial fascia is a layer of loose connective tissue containing fat that varies in amount from person to person and from one spot to another in the same individual. There are structures of great importance in superficial fascia. In the head they include the muscles of facial expression, the nerve supply to the muscles, and the cutaneous nerves and vessels that must travel through the superficial fascia to reach the skin.

THE SUPERFICIAL PART OF THE FACE

The soft tissues comprising the superficial part of the face form a thin covering external to the facial bones of the skull. The nerves and vessels that supply the skin and those that supply the superficial musculature are branches of deeper lying parent vessels and nerves. Many of those for skin enter the superficial fascia on exiting foramina in the skull. Other branches come from within the orbit or the infratemporal fossa, also known as the deep face, located on the lateral side of the face deep to the ramus of the mandible.

MUSCLES VISIBLE ON THE FACE (Fig. 7–1)

Almost all the musculature visible on the face belongs to the group known as the **muscles of facial expression.** Their location within the superficial fascia is a unique feature. They form a thin, interrupted sheetlike layer. They take origin either on bones or from superficial fascia and insert into skin and superficial fascia. When they contract, the orientation and insertion of most of them are

79

such as to cause movement around the eyes, nose, or mouth. This creates the expressions seen on the face and accounts for their group name. Actions of these muscles are best understood if the ones oriented around each of the large openings on the face are studied as a unit.

Encircling the orbits and the palpebral fissures are the muscles that close the eyes or cause squinting. They are the **orbicularis oculi** muscles. Their bony origins are from the frontal bone and maxilla, along the medial margin of the orbit. The broadest part of the muscle is the orbital part; the palpebral part is within the eyelids. Located deep to their superior medial part are the **corrugator supercilii muscles,** which take origin from the bone between the eyebrows and pass laterally to insert into the skin. Their contraction causes the vertically oriented corrugations between the eyebrows that are indicative of worry or concern.

Situated over the bridge of the nose, the **procerus** muscle arises from fascia over the nasal bone and inserts into skin between the eyebrows. It causes horizontal wrinkles in the skin over the bridge. The more transversely oriented **nasalis** muscle takes origin from bone superior to the incisive fossa. The fibers

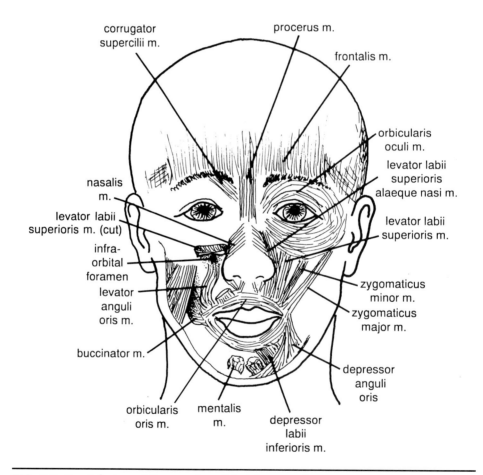

FIG. 7–1. Frontal view of the muscles of facial expression.

from each side are joined by an aponeurosis that spans the bridge of the nose. When contracted, it compresses the sides of the nose and the nostrils. Other fibers of the nasalis pass upward to the alae and septum of the nose, and they depress them when they contract.

More facial muscles are oriented around the mouth than around the other major openings. Completely encircling it is the **orbicularis oris.** It is a widely spread muscle, which causes closing of the lips or pursing of the lips, as in whistling. Many of its fibers come from merging fibers of the surrounding musculature. Others arise from skin or bone around the incisors, and they insert into deeper tissues of the lip or blend with other entering muscle fibers. Elevation of the upper lip is carried out by a series of three muscles arising from superiorly lying bony origins: the **levator labii superioris alaeque nasi,** the **levator labii superioris,** and the **zygomaticus minor.** Their origins lie in a series, the most medial being from the frontal process of the maxilla, then laterally across the maxilla superior to the infraorbital foramen to the zygomatic bone. Upward pull on the angle of the mouth, as in smiling, is carried out by two muscles: the **levator anguli oris** muscle takes the deeper origin, from the maxilla just inferior to the infraorbital foramen, and passes inferiorly to reach the angle in a position deep to the levator labii superioris. The **zygomaticus major** muscle approaches the angle obliquely from an origin on the zygomatic bone. Widening of the mouth, or pulling on the angle laterally, can be contributed to by the small horizontally oriented **risorius** muscle, although it is absent in a large number of people. It takes its origin from the superficial fascia and inserts into the skin over the angle. In addition the **platysma** muscle, which originates in the superficial fascia over the anterior thorax or chest region, passes upward to insert along the inferior border of the mandible and blend into the musculature of the angle of the mouth and the lower lip. Downward pull on the angle is carried out by the **depressor anguli oris** muscle, which approaches from the oblique line of the mandible (Fig. 9–6B). Medial to this arises the **depressor labii inferioris** muscle, which ascends to merge with the musculature of the lower lip and pull downward on the lip when it contracts. Arising from the mental fossa just inferior to the mandibular incisor teeth is the **mentalis** muscle. It inserts into the skin of the chin. When contracted it causes the puckering of the chin and protrusion of the lower lip seen so often in young children on the verge of crying.

The muscle of facial expression having the deepest origin is the **buccinator.** Its fibers arise from the pterygomandibular raphe (see Chapter 11 and Fig. 12–5) and the lateral sides of the maxilla and mandible in the region of the molar teeth. They pass anteriorly in the cheek to a more superficial position, their fibers blending with those of the orbicularis oris and other musculature around the mouth. The major function of the buccinator muscle is to give firmness to the cheek while exerting enough pressure against the teeth to keep food on their occlusal surfaces while chewing.

The group of muscles known as the **muscles of mastication** has two representatives visible on the face, the masseter and the temporalis. They lie deep to the superficial fascia, separated from it by a sheetlike covering of connective tissue known as **deep fascia.** Their function is to move the mandible. The **temporalis** is the major muscle superior to the zygomatic arch on the lateral side of the head. Its external surface is covered by a tough layer of temporal fascia and auricular muscles that move the ear but are rudimentary in most humans. The latter belong to the facial expression group. The **masseter** muscle is inferior to the zygomatic arch and external to the mandible. Much of it is hidden from view by the parotid gland. The muscles of mastication are discussed in detail in Chapter 9.

The **buccal fat pad** extends from the superficial face into the infratemporal fossa, passing through a narrow gap between the buccinator and masseter muscles. Enclosing the fat pad is a capsule formed from the same deep fascia as mentioned above.

Nerves and most of the blood vessels for the masticatory muscles enter on their deep surface and are not visible in the superficial face.

THE FACIAL NERVE AND THE PAROTID GLAND (Figs. 7–2 and 7–3)

The largest part of the parotid salivary gland is situated on the lateral side of the face inferior to the zygomatic arch, overlying the posterior part of the masseter muscle and ramus of the mandible. Its posterior extension is limited

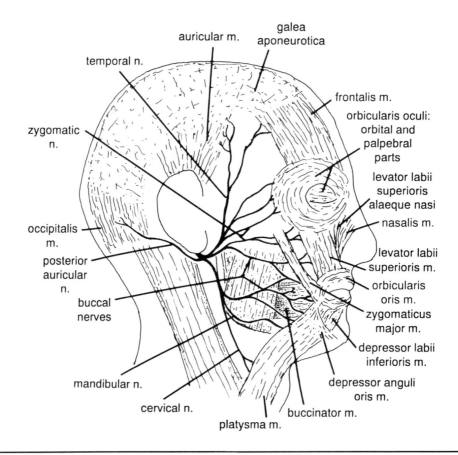

FIG. 7–2. The branches of the facial nerve and the muscles of facial expression.

by the sternocleidomastoid muscle of the neck and the external auditory meatus. Passing from it anteriorly is the parotid duct, also called Stenson's duct, which penetrates the buccinator muscle just anterior to the masseter muscle in order to empty its saliva into the oral cavity. A deeper part of the gland, not visible on the face, extends medially as far as the styloid process (see Chapter 9). Around the gland the deep fascia of the muscles of mastication forms a capsule, which sends connective tissue fibers into the gland, dividing it into lobules.

The **facial nerve** innervates the muscles of facial expression. Shortly after it emerges from the skull through the stylomastoid foramen it gives off the posterior auricular nerve and enters the parotid gland, where it divides into branches. They emerge from the anterior border of the gland and pass through the superficial fascia to reach the facial muscles they supply. The branches are named for the general region they travel toward: temporal, zygomatic, buccal, mandibular, and cervical.

Musculature around the nose and mouth receives innervation from the **buccal branches;** musculature of the lower lip is also contributed to by the **mandibular** branch; **zygomatic** and **temporal** branches share innervation of the musculature oriented around the orbit and eyelids. The **cervical** branch distributes to the platysma.

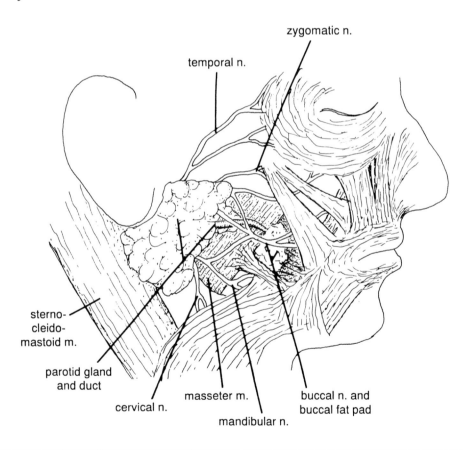

FIG. 7–3. The parotid gland and the facial nerve branches.

INNERVATION AND BLOOD SUPPLY OF THE SKIN (Figs. 7–4 and 7–5)

Most of the skin over the face is innervated by cutaneous branches arising from one of the three divisions of the trigeminal nerve. Most of these branches reach the face by passing through a foramen.

Five branches destined for the skin arise from the **ophthalmic division of the trigeminal nerve** in the orbit.

1. The **supraorbital** branch passes from the orbit through the supraorbital foramen or notch and ascends the forehead to reach the vertex of the head.
2. Just medial to the supraorbital nerve, and also emerging from the orbit and ascending, is the **supratrochlear** nerve.
3. The **infratrochlear** nerve exits the medial side of the orbit to reach nearby skin of the lower eyelid and side of the nose.

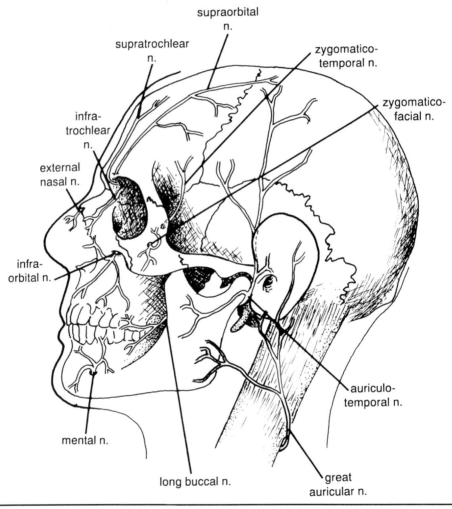

FIG. 7–4. Cutaneous innervation of the face.

4. The **palpebral** branch leaves the lateral side of the orbit and gives branches to the lateral extent of the upper eyelids.
5. The **external nasal** branch takes an indirect path from the orbit and arrives at the skin over the lower part of the nose by emerging from beneath the nasal bone.

There are three cutaneous branches from the **maxillary division of the fifth nerve.**

1. The largest of these is the **infraorbital** nerve. After passing across the floor of the orbit, first in the infraorbital groove and then in the infraorbital canal, it reaches the face by passing through the infraorbital foramen. Immediately

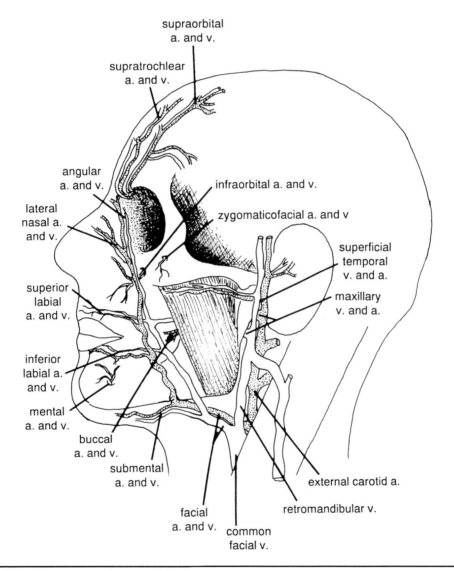

FIG. 7–5. Arteries and veins of the face.

it gives rise to branches that radiate upward to the lower eyelid, medially to the nose, and inferiorly to the upper lip.

2. The **zygomaticofacial** nerve passes through the foramen of the same name on the malar surface of the zygomatic bone and supplies skin in the overlying area.

3. The **zygomaticotemporal** branch emerges from the zygomatic bone, but the zygomaticotemporal foramen, lying on the deep surface of the frontal process, is hidden from sight in frontal and lateral views of the skull. This nerve supplies skin over the anterior part of the temporal region.

The **mandibular division of the trigeminal nerve** gives rise to three nerves with a cutaneous distribution.

1. The only one to enter the superficial fascia via a foramen is the **mental** branch, which arises in the mandibular canal from the inferior alveolar nerve. It supplies the skin over the chin and the lower lip.

2. The **buccal branch of V3**, also known as the **long buccal nerve**, passes from deep within the infratemporal fossa toward an area of skin on the cheek. Some of its branches penetrate the buccinator muscle to supply sensation within the oral cavity.

3. The **auriculotemporal** branch leaves the infratemporal fossa by passing posterior to the neck of the mandible and then ascends anterior to the ear. It distributes its branches widely to some of the skin of the ear and lateral side of the face and head. Branches to the parotid gland for parasympathetic innervation are given off as it turns upward. The nerve fibers in these branches, however, belong to the ninth cranial nerve. In the infratemporal fossa they leave the ninth nerve and join the auriculotemporal (see Fig. 9–12 and Fig. 5–4).

The branches of the ophthalmic division of the trigeminal nerve, except for the infratrochlear nerve, are accompanied by arteries and veins of the same name. The arteries derive from the **ophthalmic artery** within the orbit (Fig. 6–9). The veins are tributaries of the **ophthalmic veins,** also within the orbit, which drain into the cavernous sinus (Fig. 6–10). The vessels that accompany the three branches of the maxillary nerve are named similarly. The arteries are branches of the **maxillary artery.** The veins empty into the **pterygoid venous plexus.**

Two of the branches of the mandibular division of the trigeminal nerve, the long buccal and mental nerves, are accompanied by arteries that are branches of the **maxillary artery.** The veins drain into the **pterygoid venous plexus** or into the more superficial **facial vein** or its tributaries. The auriculotemporal nerve is accompanied by the **superficial temporal branch** of the external carotid artery and the **superficial temporal vein,** which is tributary to the retromandibular vein.

In addition to the above-mentioned vessels, the **facial branch of the external carotid artery** is a major contributor to the blood supply of the superficial face. As it passes from the neck onto the face over the lower border of the mandible anterior to the masseter muscle, its pulse is easily detected by a finger placed lightly against the skin. Particularly in the lower part of the face, it leads a tortuous course. As it ascends toward the medial corner of the eye, branches are given off for the skin, superficial fascia, and musculature along its path.

The medially directed branches anastomose across the midline with the same branches from the other side. The terminal part, the angular artery, forms anastomoses with the branches of the ophthalmic artery around the medial corner of the eye and the angular artery of the opposite side.

Accompanying the facial artery but in a slightly more posterior position is the **facial vein.** It receives tributaries having the same names as their accompanying arterial branches. Although the facial vein drains inferiorly into the internal jugular vein, it is connected with the pterygoid venous plexus by way of the **deep facial vein.** Because there are no valves, blood can flow in either direction. Thus there is an easy route for an infection in the superficial face to spread to deeper areas (see Fig. 3-3, Chapter 9, and Fig. 9–15).

THE SCALP (Figs. 7–6 through 7–9)

The layers of soft tissues comprising the scalp area of the head exhibit some features different from those of the superficial face. The superficial fascia is dense. Its fibers of connective tissue run in all directions and tightly attach to the overlying skin and an underlying tough sheetlike layer of connective tissue called the **galea aponeurotica.** Cutaneous nerves, abundant vessels, and the hair follicles from which the scalp hair grows lie in the superficial fascia. Some of the connective tissue fibers that join the outer three layers also attach to the arteries of the scalp and prevent their retraction if the scalp is lacerated. This accounts for the often surprising amount of bleeding that occurs in such cases. The layer formed by the galea aponeurotica includes the epicranius muscle, which belongs to the facial expression group of muscles. The epicranius muscle

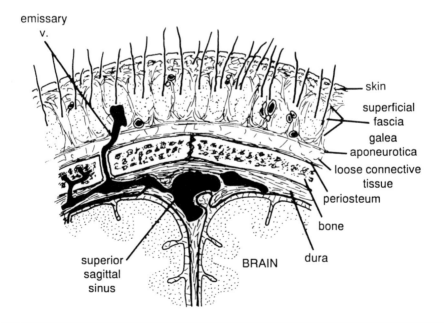

FIG. 7–6. A coronal section through the layers of the scalp.

has two parts, the **occipitalis** and the **frontalis.** The former originates from the superior nuchal line posteriorly and passes upward to insert into the galea aponeurotica. Originating from the galea aponeurotica on its anterior end is the frontalis muscle, which passes beneath the skin of the forehead to merge with the musculature around the orbit. Its contraction elevates the eyebrows and causes wrinkles to form horizontally across the forehead. Innervation of the occipitofrontalis muscle, because it belongs to the muscles of facial expression group, is by branches of the facial nerve. The temporal branch supplies the frontalis muscle, and the posterior auricular supplies the occipitalis muscle.

The muscle–galea aponeurotica layer is bound to the underlying periosteum of the skull by loose strands of connective tissue, which allow the superficial three layers of the scalp considerable freedom of movement over the bone. Should an infection reach this layer of loose connective tissue, there is little to impede its spread.

The deepest layer of the scalp is formed by the dense connective tissue of the **periosteum,** which adheres tightly to the skull.

Innervation and blood supply of the skin of the scalp is by cutaneous branches that ascend from below. More than half the scalp anteriorly is supplied by trigeminal branches and their accompanying arteries and veins. The supraor-

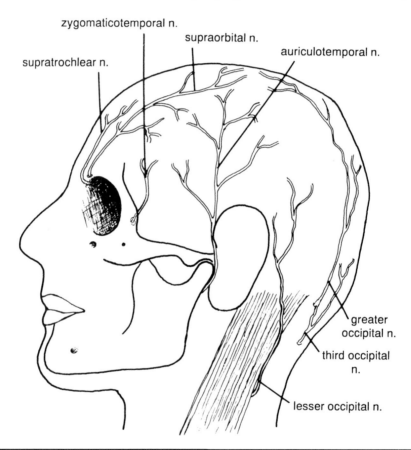

FIG. 7–7. Cutaneous nerves of the scalp.

bital group ascends to the highest point, the vertex. Along its way, it has anastomoses laterally with the zygomaticotemporal and auriculotemporal branches; medially, anastomoses occur with the supratrochlear branches as well as the supraorbital branches from the opposite side.

Posteriorly, the scalp is innervated by branches from cervical spinal nerves. The **greater occipital nerve** from the dorsal primary ramus of the second cervical spinal nerve supplies the greatest area. It ascends to the vertex in the company of the occipital artery and vein. In its lower part, it has an anastomosis with the dorsal ramus of the third cervical spinal nerve.

Passing through the skull are **emissary veins.** Externally they are connected with veins of the scalp, internally with dural venous sinuses in close proximity to the brain. Because there are no valves, blood can flow in either direction. They provide an easy route for an infection in the scalp to spread into the cranial cavity.

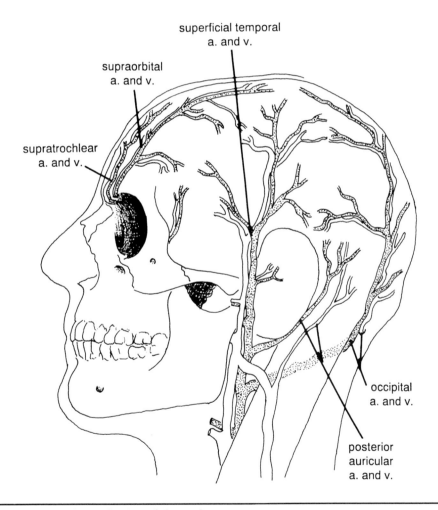

FIG. 7–8. Arteries and veins of the scalp.

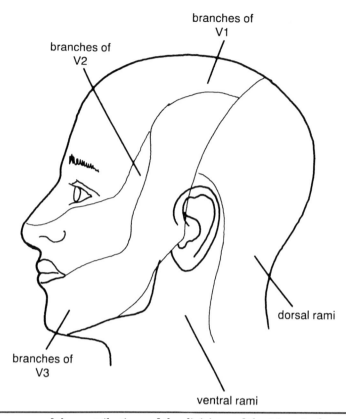

FIG. 7–9. Summary of the contributions of the divisions of the trigeminal nerve and the primary rami of the cervical spinal nerves to cutaneous innervation of the head.

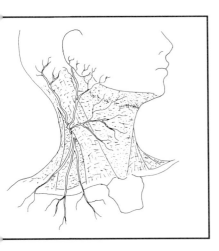

CHAPTER **8**

THE NECK

The neck has a general shape rather like that of a cylinder. It includes the part of the body between the lower border of the mandible, mastoid process, superior nuchal lines, and external occipital protuberance superiorly and the sternum, clavicle, superior margin of the scapula, and spinous process of the seventh cervical vertebra inferiorly.

Many structures packed into this narrow region serve as passageways between the head and the thorax. The larynx, pharynx, and esophagus carry air and food. Lateral to them arteries ascend to bring nutritive blood to the head and neck; veins descend, collecting blood from their tributaries and returning it to the heart; some cranial nerves enter and branch, including the vagus nerve, which continues on into the thorax. The cervical sympathetic chains carry ascending nerve fibers participating in innervation of the glands and smooth muscles of vessels in the head and neck. Posteriorly, the vertebral column and its surrounding musculature form a longitudinal axis for support of the head and neck.

THE SUPERFICIAL NECK (Figs. 8–1 through 8–3)

As elsewhere in the body, the most superficial layers of the neck are **skin** and its underlying **superficial fascia,** a loose connective tissue allowing the skin considerable flexibility. The **platysma muscle,** passing through the neck from an anterior thoracic origin to reach mandibular and facial insertions, lies in the superficial fascia over much of the anterior and lateral sides of the neck.

Important cutaneous veins and nerves travel toward their destinations through the superficial fascia deep to the platysma muscle. The major veins are tributaries to the external jugular vein or the deeper lying internal jugular.

The **external jugular vein** drains the superficial lateral sides of the head and the deep part of the face by way of its posterior auricular and retromandibular tributaries. The joining of these two veins posterior to the angle of the mandible forms the beginning of the external jugular vein. It descends superficial to the sternocleidomastoid muscle passing deep in the lower part of the neck to empty into the subclavian vein.

The **anterior jugular vein** begins in the superficial fascia under the chin and descends close to the anterior midline. As it approaches the clavicle it turns laterally, passes deep to the sternocleidomastoid muscle, and empties into the external jugular vein.

The **facial vein,** after descending from the superficial part of the face, crosses the lower border of the mandible and continues into the superficial neck. It receives the **submental vein** and then is joined by a communication from the retromandibular vein to form the **common facial vein.** The latter passes deep to empty into the internal jugular and frequently has a long communicating vein connecting it with the anterior jugular.

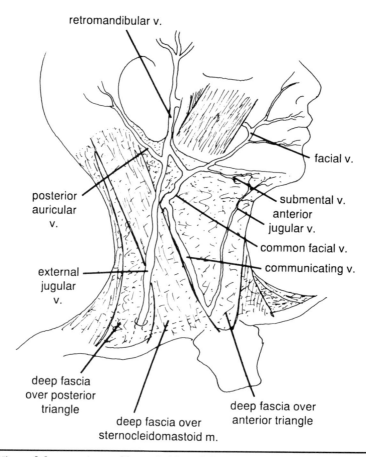

FIG. 8–1. View of the anterior and lateral sides of the neck showing the superficial layer of deep fascia and the superficial veins.

Anastomoses among veins across the midline and with other veins on the same side are to be expected, but the pattern of anastomoses and connections between veins is highly variable.

Innervation of the skin on the lateral and anterior sides of the neck is supplied by branches of the cervical plexus, which lies deeper in the neck. The branches penetrate the deep fascia (see following section) and emerge into the superficial fascia along the posterior border of the sternocleidomastoid muscle. Their names indicate their destination. The **transverse cervical nerve** passes anteriorly to supply skin over the anterior neck. The **great auricular nerve** ascends toward the ear to supply branches that extend over the posterior and inferior parts of the ear and the lower posterior part of the face. Indeed, it is the only source of innervation to skin of the face not provided by the trigeminal nerve. The **lesser occipital nerve** follows the posterior border of the sternocleidomastoid muscle, ascending into the lower lateral part of the scalp. The **supraclavicular nerves** descend over the clavicle and shoulder and into the anterior thoracic region.

In the posterior neck, **branches of dorsal rami** of the second through the sixth cervical spinal nerves emerge along either side of the midline to supply the skin.

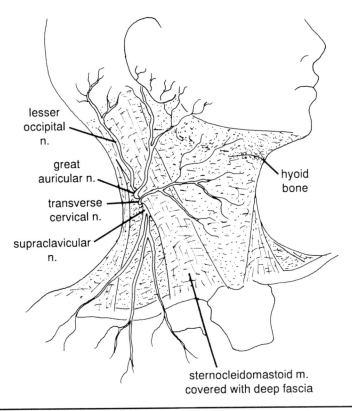

FIG. 8–2. View of the anterior and lateral sides of the neck showing the superficial layer of deep fascia and the cutaneous branches of the cervical plexus.

The second dorsal ramus, known as the **greater occipital nerve,** is the largest and ascends all the way to the vertex of the scalp.

FASCIAL COMPARTMENTS OF THE NECK (Figs. 8–1 and 8–4)

Deep to the skin and superficial fascia the various structural elements of the neck are compartmentalized by wrappings of a sheetlike layer of connective tissue called **deep fascia.** Wherever the deep fascia comes into contact with bone, it blends with the periosteum on the bone. In this way it serves to hold structures in their proper position. Thus the deep fascia, as well as the skeleton, is an important supporting element of the body. Its anterior bony attachments are to the mandible, hyoid bone, sternum, and clavicle, and its posterior attachments are to the spinous processes on the vertebrae and the superior nuchal lines on the skull.

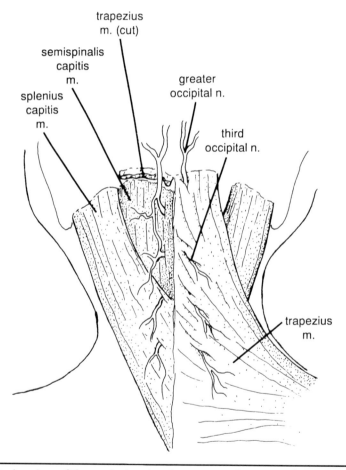

FIG. 8–3. Posterior view of the neck showing the segmental pattern of emerging cutaneous nerves. On the left side, the trapezius muscle has been removed.

The most superficial layer of deep cervical fascia is called the **enveloping,** or **investing, fascia.** It encircles the neck, splitting into two layers at the sternocleidomastoid and trapezius muscles so as to completely wrap them on both their superficial and deep sides.

Deep to the investing fascia in the anterior neck, **infrahyoid fascia** encloses the infrahyoid muscles and fuses laterally with the investing fascia.

Posterior to the infrahyoid fascia lies the cervical visceral compartment. It is enclosed by **cervical visceral fascia** and contains the pharynx, larynx, thyroid gland, trachea, and esophagus (see Chapter 12).

A tubular investment of fascia closely related laterally to the cervical visceral compartment is the **carotid sheath.** It contains the common carotid artery, or the internal carotid more superiorly, the internal jugular vein, and the vagus nerve. It surrounds and encloses these three structures all the way up to the jugular foramen and carotid canal on the base of the skull.

Posterior to the cervical visceral compartment is another cylindrical compartment surrounded by deep fascia called the **prevertebral fascia.** It encloses the vertebral column and its surrounding complex groups of musculature (Fig. 8–5).

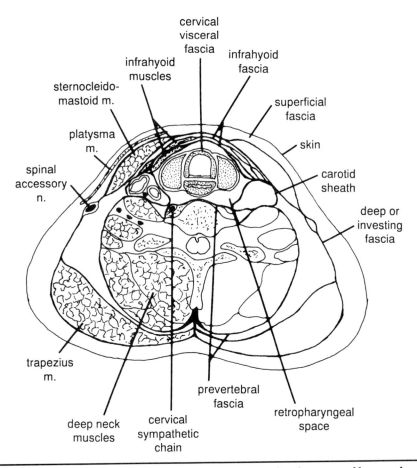

FIG. 8–4. Transverse section through the neck inferior to the pharynx and larynx showing the deep fascial compartments.

Some groups are responsible for the movements of flexion, extension, and rotation at the intervertebral joints. Their muscle fibers are of varying lengths, the shortest spanning only one joint and the longest spanning as many as six. Other groups of fibers attach to the skull and therefore cause these same kinds of movements at the joints between the vertebrae and the skull. On the anterior side of the vertebral column the longus colli, inserting on the vertebrae, and the longus capitis, inserting on the skull, are major examples of these muscles. On the posterior side are the deep neck muscles of the suboccipital region, which are discussed later in this chapter.

Intervening spaces between adjacent fascial compartments contain loose connective tissue. Should an infection reach one of these interfascial spaces, pressure building up as the infection progresses can cause it to spread along the paths of least resistance through the tissue. Perhaps the most important

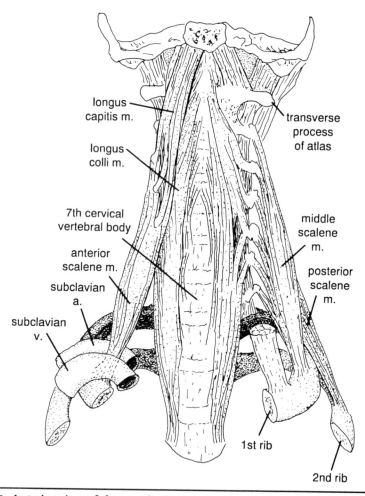

FIG. 8–5. Anterior view of the vertebral column and its prevertebral musculature. Note the relationships of the subclavian vein and artery to the insertion of the anterior scalene muscle.

interfascial space in this area from this standpoint is the **retropharyngeal space,** which lies between the cervical visceral compartment and the vertebral column and its prevertebral fascia. It extends from the base of the skull into the thorax. It is continuous, lateral to the pharynx in the head, with the lateral pharyngeal space. An infection in areas such as oral tissues or the tonsils, for instance, can work its way through the pharyngeal wall and gain access to this space and have far-reaching consequences.

THE TRIANGLES OF THE NECK (Figs. 8–6 through 8–8)

In undertaking a study of any region of the body, it is necessary first to understand its skeletal features and second to observe how its musculature is arranged. Then other structures can be fitted in on this framework. In the neck several of the bony parts and the muscles attached to them are oriented in such a fashion as to outline triangle-shaped areas called the anterior and the posterior triangles of the neck, and, in the suboccipital region, the very small suboccipital triangle. Within the borders of each triangle, important structures are located. A knowledge of these borders and the structures within the areas they delineate can aid the student in organizing and remembering the anatomy of the neck.

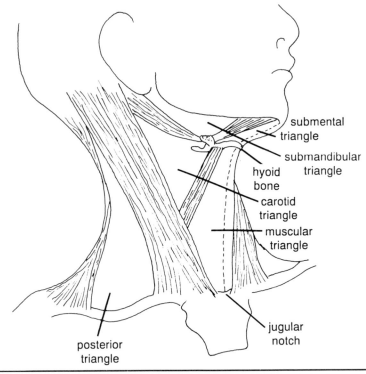

FIG. 8–6. A view of the neck showing the posterior triangle and the four small triangles that comprise the anterior triangle.

THE ANTERIOR TRIANGLES

The anterior triangle on each side of the neck is bounded by the lower border of the body of the mandible, the anterior border of the sternocleidomastoid muscle, and the anterior midline from mandible to jugular notch on the sternum. Each anterior triangle can be divided into four smaller ones: the submental, submandibular, muscular, and carotid triangles. The first two are superior in position to the hyoid bone, and the latter two are inferior.

1. The **submental triangle** is named for its position beneath the chin. Its borders are the hyoid bone, the anterior belly of the digastric muscle, and the anterior midline from the mandible to the hyoid bone.
2. The **submandibular triangle** is delineated by the lower border of the mandible, the anterior belly of the digastric muscle, and the posterior belly of the digastric muscle. Therefore it is often called the **digastric triangle.** The most obvious structure within it is the submandibular salivary gland.

The musculature of the two suprahyoid triangles is part of, or is closely related to, the floor of the oral cavity. The **mylohyoid muscle** is seen as the major structure of the submental triangle and also extends well into the submandibular triangle. It takes its origin from the mylohyoid line on the mandible and inserts into the connective tissue comprising the mylohyoid raphe and the hyoid bone. The **anterior belly of the digastric muscle** lies on the superficial side of the mylohyoid muscle and attaches to the digastric fossa on the mandible. It meets the **posterior belly of the digastric muscle,** which is coming from the mastoid

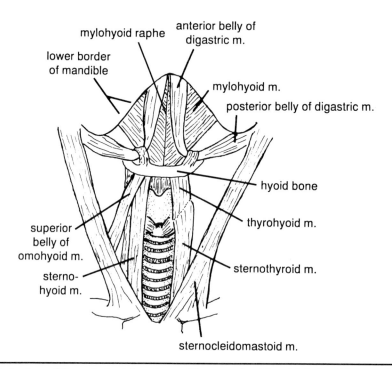

FIG. 8–7. A view of the anterior triangles and the suprahyoid and infrahyoid musculature.

98 THE NECK

process, in a central tendon anchored to the hyoid bone by fascia. When both bellies contract together and with the mylohyoid, they exert an upward pull on the hyoid bone. If the hyoid bone is stabilized by muscles pulling on it from below, they exert a downward pull on the mandible and thus assist in opening the mouth. The **stylohyoid** muscle passes anteriorly and inferiorly from the styloid process to the hyoid bone and splits around the central tendon of the digastric to help hold it to the bone and to participate in exerting the upward pull on the hyoid. Posterior to the mylohyoid, a small part of the **hyoglossus** muscle is visible arising from the hyoid bone. As it passes superior to the mylohyoid muscle it forms part of the musculature of the lateral side of the tongue.

3. The **muscular triangle** is the more medial of the two infrahyoid triangles. It is bordered by the superior belly of the omohyoid muscle, the sternocleido-mastoid muscle, and the anterior midline from the hyoid bone to the sternum. It is named after the important group of infrahyoid, or strap, muscles that it contains.

The **infrahyoid muscles** serve for anchoring or pulling down on the hyoid bone, which moves up and down during speech and swallowing. They occur in

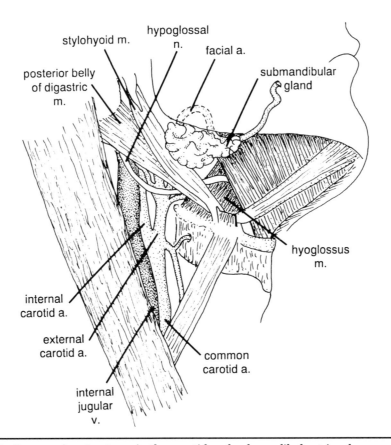

FIG. 8–8. Some major structures in the carotid and submandibular triangles.

two layers, the more superficial containing the **sternohyoid** and **superior belly of the omohyoid,** the deeper containing the **sternothyroid** and **thyrohyoid.** The first part of their names indicates the origin, the second part the insertion. "Omo" comes from omos, which is Greek for shoulder and refers to the shoulder bone, or scapular, origin of the omohyoid muscle. In the muscular triangles between the right and left omohyoid muscles the thyroid and parathyroid glands and the larynx and trachea can be approached.

4. The **carotid triangle** is bordered by the posterior belly of the digastric muscle, the superior belly of the omohyoid muscle, and the sternocleidomastoid muscle. The common carotid artery ascends in the neck wrapped in the carotid sheath along with the vagus nerve and the internal jugular vein. The lower one-third of the sheath lies deep to the sternocleidomastoid muscle. As the common carotid artery enters the carotid triangle, it divides into internal and external carotid branches (Fig. 8–9). These two arteries supply most of the blood for the head and neck. At the point of bifurcation, the carotid sinus lies within the dilation of the wall of the internal carotid. It has sensory

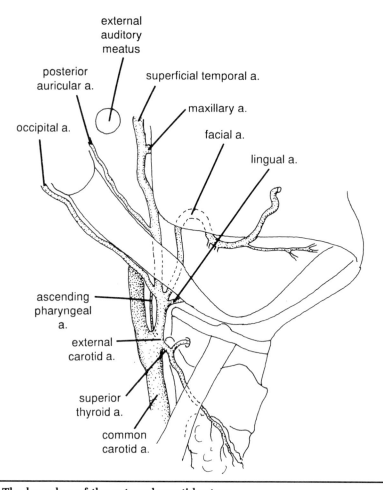

FIG. 8–9. The branches of the external carotid artery.

receptors that increasingly stimulate the glossopharyngeal nerve as blood pressure rises, which results in a fall in pressure. Adjacent to the bifurcation is the carotid body, a chemoreceptor for detecting a decline in the partial pressure of oxygen in the blood and resulting in increased respiration. It is supplied by the vagus and glossopharyngeal nerves.

The internal carotid artery has no branches in the neck. The external carotid gives rise to eight named branches, five of which arise in the carotid triangle. Just at its origin, two of the branches arise: the **superior thyroid artery** heads anteriorly and downward toward the superior pole of the thyroid gland, and the **ascending pharyngeal artery** ascends medial to the external carotid artery along the pharynx. The **lingual artery,** destined for the more anteriorly lying tongue, has only a short course in the neck and then passes from view deep to the hyoglossus muscle. The **facial artery** also passes anteriorly, takes a course deep to the submandibular gland, then curves over the lower border of the mandible and onto the face. In the neck it gives off a submental branch and several glandular branches to the submandibular gland. High in the carotid triangle the **occipital artery** arises and passes posteriorly along with the posterior belly of the digastric muscle to reach the occipital region. Leaving the carotid triangle, the external carotid ascends deep to the posterior belly of the digastric and gives off a second posteriorly directed branch, the **posterior auricular** artery. Its name indicates the region it supplies. The two terminal branches of the external carotid artery arise immediately posterior to the neck of the mandible. They are the **maxillary** and the **superficial temporal** arteries.

The internal jugular vein is the major venous drainage for the brain and the cranial cavity, and as it descends in the neck it receives tributaries from the face, the pharynx, the thyroid gland, and the larynx. Where it is hidden from view at its terminal end by the clavicle and sternocleidomastoid muscle, it joins with the subclavian vein to form the brachiocephalic.

Innervation of the Infrahyoid Muscles (Fig. 8–10). Innervation of the infrahyoid muscles is from the **cervical plexus** rather than from cranial nerves (see Chapter 4 and Fig. 4-6). From the first cervical ventral ramus (C1) of the plexus, nerve fibers join the hypoglossal nerve and travel with it to reach the carotid triangle. Some of these fibers leave the hypoglossal nerve as the **nerve to the thyrohyoid muscle.** Others leave as the **superior limb of the ansa cervicalis.** From C2 and C3 ventral rami of the plexus, the **inferior limb of the ansa cervicalis** is formed. It joins with the superior limb, and together they form a loop, the **ansa cervicalis.** It hangs down along the carotid sheath, caught within its fascia. Branches arise from the loop for innervation of the sternohyoid, omohyoid, and sternothyroid muscles.

Innervation of the Suprahyoid Muscles (Fig. 8–10). Several cranial nerves innervate the suprahyoid muscles. The **nerve to the mylohyoid and anterior digastric** muscles travels across the superficial surface of the mylohyoid muscle, giving off branches to it and then terminating in the anterior belly of the digastric muscle. It is from the inferior alveolar branch of the mandibular division of the trigeminal nerve.

Facial nerve branches innervate the stylohyoid and posterior belly of the digastric muscle close to their attachment to the styloid and the mastoid processes, respectively (Fig. 4-24).

The hyoglossus muscle is supplied by the **hypoglossal nerve,** the motor nerve of the tongue (Fig. 4-29). It emerges from the skull through the hypoglossal canal and descends to the carotid triangle, where it turns anteriorly to enter the submandibular triangle and disappear from view between the mylohyoid and hyoglossus muscles.

THE POSTERIOR TRIANGLES (Figs. 8–11 and 8–12)

The posterior triangles, one on either side, lie laterally in the neck, but their position is immediately posterior to the anterior triangle, and this relationship is the source of the name. In viewing someone's neck, the division between the

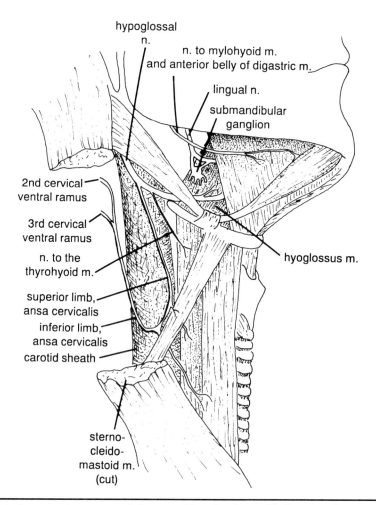

FIG. 8–10. Some major nerves of the carotid and submandibular triangles.

triangles is apparent because of the prominence of the sternocleidomastoid muscle, especially when the head is turned toward the side. The full extent of the muscle is visible from its sternal and clavicular origins to its insertion on the mastoid process. The borders of the posterior triangle are the entire posterior edge of the sternocleidomastoid muscle, the anterior border of the trapezius muscle, and the middle third of the clavicle. The investing layer of deep fascia spans the gap between the trapezius and the sternocleidomastoid muscles, forming a roof over the triangle and enclosing both muscles. Embedded within the fascial roof, the **spinal accessory nerve** passes across from the sternocleidomastoid muscle to the trapezius, innervating both. The **cutaneous branches arising from the cervical plexus** gain access to the superficial fascia by penetrating this fascial roof.

In the floor of the triangle, covered by prevertebral fascia, lies a series of muscles. Most superiorly, the **splenius capitis** muscle can be seen as it passes upward from the vertebral column to the skull (see further discussion in follow-

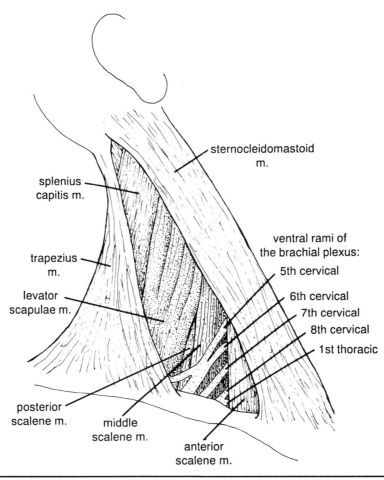

FIG. 8–11. A view of the posterior triangle showing its muscles and their relations to the cervical part of the brachial plexus.

ing section). Just inferior to it is the **levator scapulae** muscle, which extends inferiorly from its vertebral origin to its scapular insertion and has the function of elevating the scapula. The latter is a bone of the upper limb, and the levator is an upper limb muscle. Last in the series are the **posterior scalene,** the **middle scalene,** and most inferiorly, the **anterior scalene** muscles. They pass from the cervical vertebral column downward to insert on the first rib, for the anterior and middle scalenes and the second rib for the posterior. When contracted they pull upward on the ribs during respiration or, if the ribs are stabilized, they contribute to movements of the vertebral column.

Most of the anterior scalene muscle is hidden from view by the sternocleido-mastoid muscle and is therefore not actually within the posterior triangle. The **subclavian vein** passes across the first rib just anterior to the anterior scalene muscle. The **subclavian artery** passes across the rib, lying in a gap between the insertions of the anterior and middle scalene muscles. Emerging from this same gap are the **ventral rami of the fifth through the eighth cervical and the first**

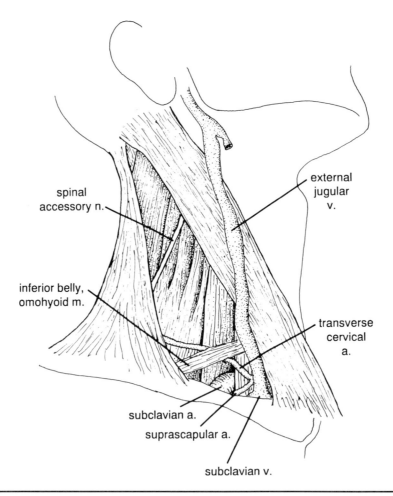

FIG. 8–12. The musculature of the posterior triangle and its relation to some of its major contents.

thoracic spinal nerves whose chief function is to form the brachial plexus for innervation of the upper limb. Two arteries from the thyrocervical branch of the subclavian artery, the transverse cervical and suprascapular, pass across to reach musculature around the scapula belonging to the upper limb. Study of the posterior triangle thus reveals that the neck is a passageway, not only for structures traveling between thorax and head and neck, but also between thorax and upper limb.

THE SUBOCCIPITAL REGION OF THE NECK (Fig. 8–13)

The most posterior part of the neck is the suboccipital region, named for its relationship to the occipital bone. If the trapezius muscle is cut from its attachment to the skull and vertebrae, the **deep neck musculature** underlying it is revealed. The **splenius muscle** passes from its origins on the seventh cervical and first six thoracic vertebral spinous processes obliquely upward, its capitis portion inserting on the mastoid process and superior nuchal line and its cervicis portion on the upper cervical transverse processes. Just on either side of the

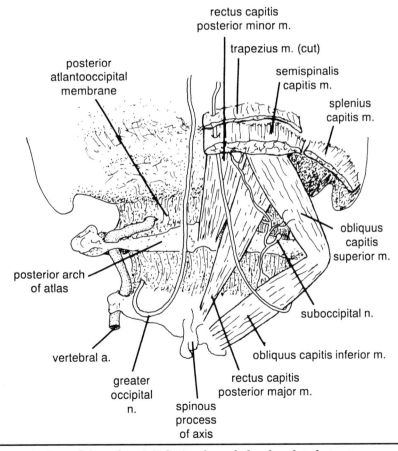

FIG. 8–13. A view of the suboccipital triangle and closely related structures.

midline and deep to the splenius muscle near its origin is the largest muscle mass of the neck, the vertically oriented **semispinalis capitis.** It arises from transverse processes of the seventh cervical through the sixth or seventh thoracic vertebrae and ascends to insert on the skull between the superior and inferior nuchal lines.

Reflection of the semispinalis reveals a group of four small muscles between the first two cervical vertebrae and the skull. The most medial one is the **rectus capitis posterior minor,** taking its origin from the posterior tubercle of the atlas and inserting on the skull. Just lateral to it the other three form the **suboccipital triangle.** Two of them arise from the spinous process of the axis: the **rectus capitis posterior major** inserts on the skull, and the **obliquus capitis inferior** inserts on the transverse process of the atlas. The latter bony process gives rise to the **obliquus capitis superior,** which inserts on the skull.

The functions of the muscles in this region, except the trapezius, whose action is on the upper limb, have to do with rotating the head and the vertebral column and maintaining an upright posture in the cervical region (see discussion of vertebrae in Chapter 2). These muscles are the cervical continuation of the deep muscles of the back, which have these same functions in the remainder of the vertebral column. They are discussed more thoroughly in gross anatomy texts dealing with the whole body.

An important structure within the suboccipital triangle is the **vertebral artery.** It arises as the first branch of the subclavian artery in the lowest part, or root, of the neck. It ascends by traversing the transverse foramina of the sixth cervical vertebra up through the first. Within the depths of the triangle it passes across the arch of the atlas and turns upward to enter the cranial cavity through the foramen magnum, where it serves as a major source of blood to the brain (Fig. 4-15). It is partially hidden from view by the **posterior atlanto-occipital membrane,** which spans the gap between the posterior arch of the atlas and the skull around the foramen magnum.

The dorsal ramus of the first cervical spinal nerve, often called the **suboccipital nerve,** emerges within the triangle superior to the arch of the atlas and innervates the four small muscles as well as supplying a branch to the overlying semispinalis muscle. The splenius and semispinalis muscles receive segmental innervation from other cervical dorsal rami. Inferior to the arch of the atlas emerges the dorsal ramus of the second cervical spinal nerve, called the **greater occipital nerve.** It curves around the lower margin of the obliquus capitis inferior muscle and ascends to perform its function as the major cutaneous innervation to the posterior part of the scalp all the way to the vertex of the skull.

Arterial supply to the suboccipital muscles comes from two major sources. Ascending from below is the **deep cervical branch of the costocervical** trunk from the subclavian artery. It anastomoses with a branch descending from the **occipital artery** as the latter passes toward the scalp (Fig. 3-2). Small branches arising segmentally from the vertebral artery also contribute to the blood supply. There is a rather extensive venous plexus in the area. It drains into the vertebral and deep cervical veins and sometimes the occipital vein.

THE CERVICAL SYMPATHETIC CHAINS (Figs. 8–14 and 5-1)

Embedded in the prevertebral fascia posterior to the carotid sheath on each side of the neck is the cervical sympathetic chain with its three ganglia. The **superior cervical ganglion** is large and elongated and lies high in the neck at the

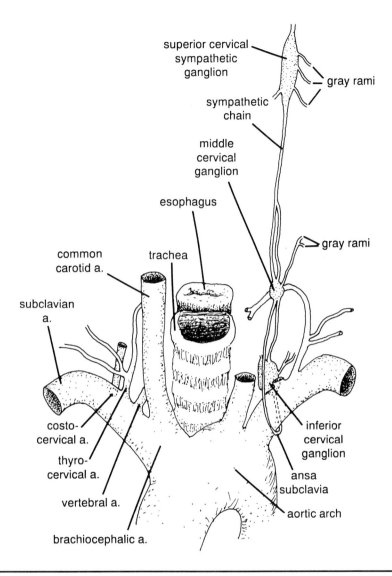

FIG. 8–14. Major structures in the root of the neck. The aortic arch and proximal parts of its three branches lie within the thorax.

level of the second cervical vertebra. The **middle ganglion** is smaller, often too small to be distinguished. Its location is variable, but in most persons it lies at the level of the highest part of the inferior thyroid artery and some distance from the superior ganglion. The part of the chain linking it with the inferior ganglion is shorter and usually in several strands, one looping around the subclavian artery to form the ansa subclavia. Frequently the **inferior ganglion** is fused with the first thoracic ganglion, in which case they form the stellate ganglion. An extension of the inferior ganglion is often present adjacent to the vertebral artery. Many postganglionic fibers, taking their origin in the three ganglia, form plexuses on the walls of adjacent vessels and run along with them to their destinations. Sympathetic plexuses accompanying the vertebral, internal, and external carotid arteries supply this type of innervation to the head and much of the neck. Other postganglionic fibers form gray communicating rami and distribute with the branches of the cervical spinal nerves, traveling with them to reach sweat glands and smooth muscles in the skin and smooth muscles in the walls of vessels supplying skeletal muscles and skin. Still others leave the chain and descend into the thorax. These are discussed in anatomy texts dealing with the innervation of the heart.

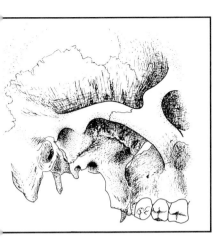

CHAPTER **9**

THE TEMPOROMANDIBULAR JOINT AND THE INFRATEMPORAL FOSSA

The deep part of the face, located medial to the ramus of the mandible, is the infratemporal fossa. It is an important area for several reasons. Three of the four major muscles responsible for movement of the jaws during chewing are there. It contains the mandibular nerve, which innervates the mandibular teeth and much of the oral cavity and skin of the face, and the maxillary artery, whose branches distribute with branches of the mandibular nerve.

STRUCTURE AND FUNCTION OF THE TEMPOROMANDIBULAR JOINT (Figs. 9–1 and 9–2)

When movement of the jaw occurs during chewing and opening and closing of the mouth, the articulating bones are the two condyles of the single mandible and both temporal bones. Movement on one side cannot take place without movement on the other. On the temporal bone superior to the condyle is the rather deeply concave **glenoid,** or mandibular, fossa. The bone there is exceedingly thin. No force is exerted against it when the joint is active. Anterior to the fossa is a thick ridge, the **articular eminence,** which extends in a medial direction from the **articular tubercle** on the zygomatic arch to the **entoglenoid process;** anteriorly, the eminence flattens out as the **preglenoid plane.** Because the condyle moves forward on opening and there is some side-to-side grinding movement during chewing, the articular eminence, the preglenoid plane, and the entoglenoid process on the temporal bone and the anteriosuperior and medial surfaces on the mandibular condyle bear the force exerted at the joint during activity.

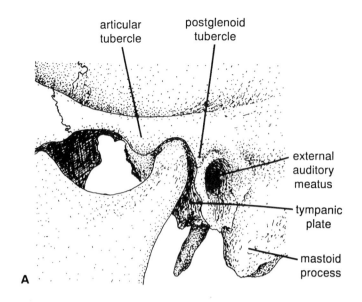

articular tubercle

postglenoid tubercle

external auditory meatus

tympanic plate

mastoid process

A

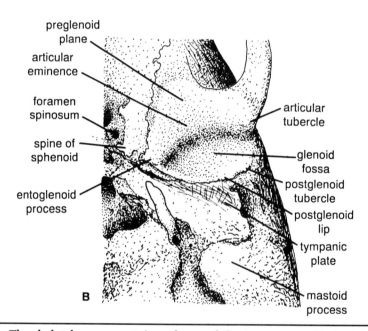

preglenoid plane

articular eminence

foramen spinosum

spine of sphenoid

entoglenoid process

articular tubercle

glenoid fossa

postglenoid tubercle

postglenoid lip

tympanic plate

mastoid process

B

FIG. 9–1. The skeletal components in and around the temporomandibular joint. **A.** Lateral view. **B.** Inferior view.

Closely related to the joint posteriorly, but not a part of it, is the tympanic plate of the temporal bone, which forms the anterior wall of the external auditory meatus. Its proximity is one of the main reasons the mandible must move forward in order for the mouth to open to the extent necessary.

Because this is a synovial joint, it has the structural features common to a joint of this type, but with some modifications from the usual.

1. The **fibrous capsule** common to all synovial joints encloses the joint components. On the mandible its posterior attachment is a distance down on the mandibular neck but anteriorly it is just below the articular surface of the

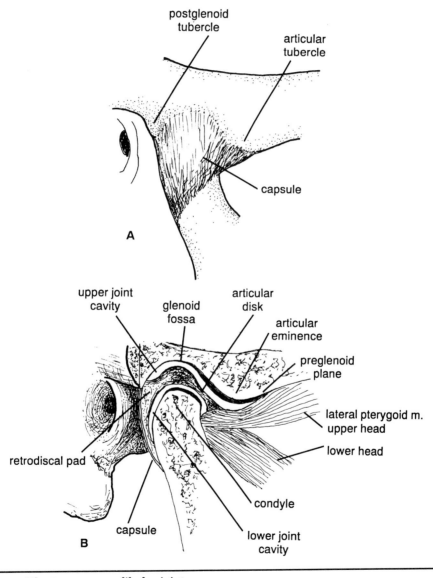

FIG. 9–2. The temporomandibular joint.
A. Lateral view of the joint capsule. B. Sagittal section through the joint.

condyle. On the temporal bone it attaches around the periphery of the joint. This includes lateral attachments along the zygomatic arch from the articular tubercle to the **postglenoid tubercle** and posterior attachments from the spine along the **postglenoid lip** to the entoglenoid process. Anteriorly, the capsule attaches around the border of the preglenoid plane.

2. As is usual in synovial joints, the capsule is strengthened by a ligament. In this case it is the **lateral temporomandibular ligament,** which extends from the articular tubercle to the lateral pole and posterior neck of the mandible. It prevents displacement of the mandible in posterior and inferior directions.

3. The inner surface of the capsule and the nonforce-bearing surfaces within the joint are lined by a **synovial membrane,** which produces the synovial fluid found in all synovial joints for lubricating the articular surfaces in order to eliminate friction between the moving parts.

4. A dense fibrous connective tissue with some fibrocartilage in its deepest layers covers the bony articulating surfaces in the temporomandibular joint. In most synovial joints the articulating surfaces are smoothed over by a thin covering of hyaline cartilage.

5. A **fibrous disk** separates the temporal surface from the condyle, thereby dividing the joint cavity into an upper and a lower joint space. Although this is not an unusual feature of synovial joints, many of them lack a disk. In the temporomandibular joint the disk is attached around its periphery to the capsule. Laterally and medially it is attached to the condyle itself so that whenever the condyle glides forward to protrude the mandible and then backward to restore its resting position or place the teeth in occlusion it must move the disk with it. The posterior attachment of the disk to the capsule is not a direct attachment but occurs by means of the **retrodiscal pad.** Within the pad are a superior and an inferior lamina of connective tissue fibers, which limit the extent of disk movement. Between the laminae is a layer of loose connective tissue containing most of the vessels and nerves that supply the joint.

LOCATION OF THE INFRATEMPORAL FOSSA ON THE SKULL (Fig. 9–3)

From the lateral side of the skull, the clearest view of the infratemporal fossa is obtained if the ramus of the mandible is removed. The fossa has bony boundaries in several directions: laterally, the mandibular ramus; anteriorly, the posterior part of the maxilla as far forward as the zygomaticoalveolar crest; medially, the deeply situated lateral pterygoid plate; and superiorly, a partial bony roof formed by the greater wing of the sphenoid bone and a small part of the squamous temporal bone. Along the lateral edge of the latter two bones is a ridge called the infratemporal crest. A horizontal plane extending from the crest to the zygomatic arch, an interval where there is no bone, also marks the roof of the infratemporal fossa. Above this plane lies the temporal fossa.

Several openings can be seen in the bones through which important vessels and nerves pass in order to enter or leave the fossa. The part of the roof formed by the sphenoid bone bears two of them, the foramen ovale and the foramen spinosum. More anteriorly the inferior orbital fissure connects the space of the fossa with that of the orbit; and the pterygomaxillary fissure connects it with the pterygopalatine fossa. One or more small posterior superior alveolar foramina perforate the maxilla.

ORIENTATION AND FUNCTIONS OF THE MUSCLES OF THE INFRATEMPORAL FOSSA (Figs. 9–4 through 9–7)

The four major pairs of muscles that move the jaw during chewing belong to the group known as the **muscles of mastication.** They are oriented around and

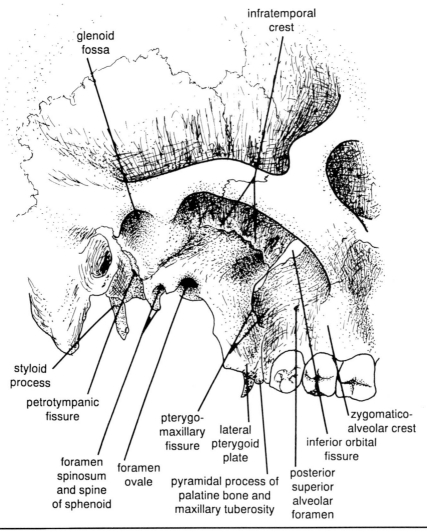

FIG. 9–3. A lateral view of the skeletal framework of the infratemporal fossa after the mandible is removed.

inserted on the mandible in a manner that will enable them to participate in moving the mandible through the positions it must assume during closing and opening. The condyles must engage in **rotation** against the disk in a hinge movement as the mandible is depressed and elevated. In addition, they, along with the disk, must slide forward over the articular eminences causing **protrusion** of the mandible and then backward (**retrusion**) to bring the teeth into full occlusion and to return the mandible to its resting position. These gliding movements are referred to as **translation.** Rotation and translation occur concurrently as the mandible opens and closes. The grinding movement occurring during mastication requires a lateral excursion of the mandible.

The **masseter** is the only one of the muscles of mastication lying completely outside the infratemporal fossa. It is described here because it is functionally a member of this muscle group. Its origin is the zygomatic arch. Most of its fibers pass obliquely in a posteroinferior direction and insert over the lateral side of the mandibular ramus and angle. They form a powerful muscle, active in rotating the mandible as it closes. The masseter has a deep head composed of a group of fibers that are vertically oriented in the closed position. They help to retrude the protruded mandible.

The **medial pterygoid** muscle works with the masseter. It takes its origin from the medial side of the lateral pterygoid plate, the pyramidal process of the

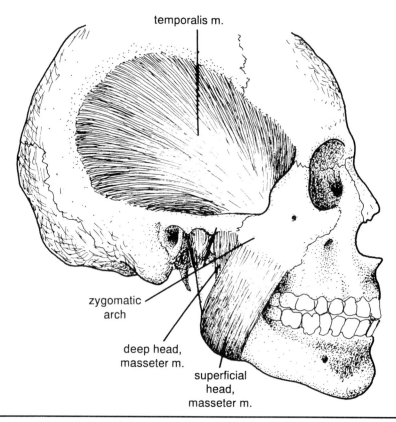

FIG. 9–4. A lateral view of the two most superficial muscles of mastication.

palatine bone, and the tuberosity of the maxilla in the infratemporal fossa. From these deep origins, its fibers pass obliquely downward and lateralward to reach the inner surface of the ramus and angle of the mandible. Lying against its lateral surface is the sphenomandibular ligament extending from the spine of the sphenoid to the lingula on the mandible. The medial pterygoid and masseter muscles, with their similarly oriented fibers, form a muscular sling that supports the mandible and elevates it.

The **temporalis** muscle works with the masseter and medial pterygoid muscles in rotation during closure, but it is also important in retrusion. It takes its broad origin in the temporal fossa. Its widespread fibers are arranged in an almost vertical orientation in its most anterior part and gradually shift to a horizontal orientation in its most posterior part. They converge to a narrower, thick muscle that passes into the infratemporal fossa to insert on the coronoid process. A superficial tendon continues down the anterior border of the ramus, and a deep tendon extends down the temporal crest. Both tendons can be palpated from within the oral cavity. The narrow gap between them is the retromolar fossa of the mandible. When the mandible is in the protruded position, contraction of the more horizontally directed fibers pulls it back into its retruded position. The more vertical fibers participate in rotation.

The **lateral pterygoid** muscle makes possible protrusion and lateral excursion of the mandible. It has two heads. The superior head takes its origin from the roof of the infratemporal fossa and passes horizontally and slightly laterally

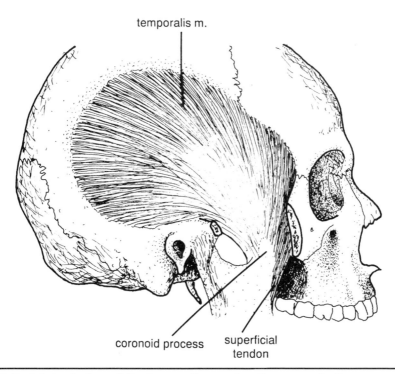

temporalis m.

coronoid process

superficial tendon

FIG. 9–5. A lateral view of the temporalis muscle after removal of a segment of the zygomatic arch.

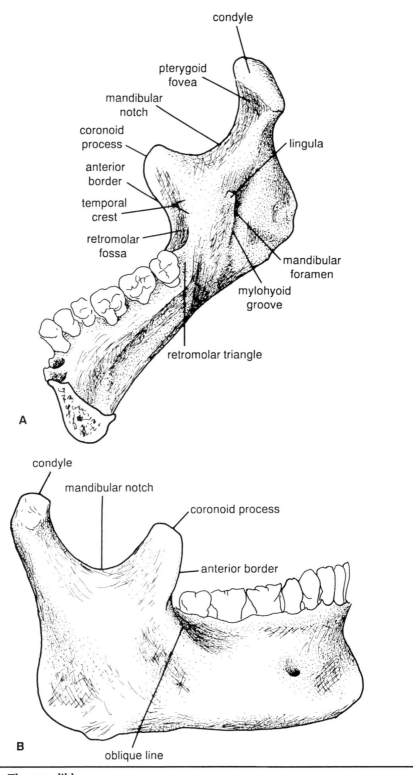

FIG. 9–6. The mandible.
A. The medial surface of the right side of the mandible. **B.** The lateral surface of the right side of the mandible.

toward a posterior insertion into the capsule and disk of the temporomandibular joint and the pterygoid fovea on the neck of the mandible. Because of these insertions, it plays an important part in maintaining the proper relationship of disk to condyle when the mouth is open. The inferior head is larger. It takes its origin from the lateral side of the lateral pterygoid plate, and its fibers travel posteriorly, superiorly, and quite a bit laterally to insert into the pterygoid fovea. If this muscle contracts simultaneously on both sides, the mandible is pulled forward into the protruded position. If only one side contracts, for instance the right lateral pterygoid, the deeper origin and more lateral insertion cause the right side of the mandible to be pulled medially and the entire mandible is shifted toward the left. Other muscle groups assist the four pairs of muscles of mastication in some of their actions, especially in opening. These are discussed with the suprahyoid region of the neck in Chapter 8.

One of the muscles of facial expression, the **buccinator,** lies partially within the infratemporal fossa. It has the function during eating of making the cheek firm and holding it pressed against the teeth so the food will be kept on the occlusal surfaces. From an origin on the pterygomandibular raphe (see Chapter 11 and Fig. 12–5) deep to the medial pterygoid muscle, the buccinator passes anteriorly across the infratemporal surface of the maxilla toward an insertion around the lips. Additional fibers arise from the bone adjacent to the maxillary and mandibular molar teeth.

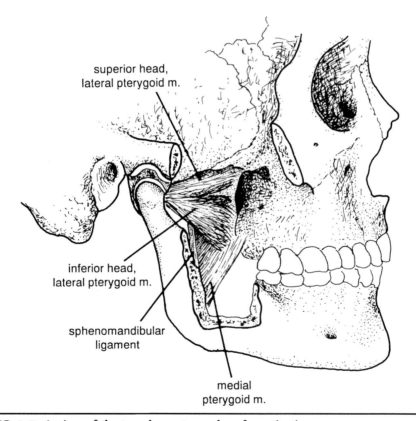

FIG. 9–7. A view of the two deepest muscles of mastication.

DEEP FASCIA AND THE MASTICATOR SPACE (Figs. 9–8 and 9–9)

Within the infratemporal fossa is a compartment called the **masticator space.** It is bounded by deep fascia covering the superficial surface of the masseter and the deep surface of the medial pterygoid. This deep fascia is a continuation of the superficial layer of deep fascia in the neck, the investing fascia, which attaches along the lower border of the mandible. Then it splits and continues upward to enclose a compartment containing the medial pterygoid and masseter muscles and all structures situated between them. Superior to the masseter, the deep fascia attaches to the zygomatic arch and continues upward over the temporalis muscle to the superior temporal line. Over the deep surface of the medial pterygoid muscle, the deep fascia ends superiorly by attaching to the pterygoid part of the sphenoid bone. As is true for all muscular deep fascia, its bony attachments help anchor the muscles and hold them in their proper position.

The buccal fat pad extends into the masticator space from the superficial fascia of the cheek. It pads the area and fills the spaces between muscles,

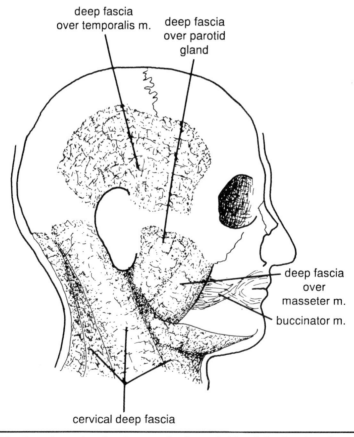

FIG. 9–8. The deep investing fascia over the lateral side of the head and neck.

nerves, and vessels. Infections in the superficial fascia of the face can utilize this route to spread into the infratemporal fossa. Abscesses around the molar teeth can erode through the bone and spread into this space. Further spread can continue along the anterior border of the medial pterygoid muscle into the lateral pharyngeal space, which is deep and medial to the muscle.

DEEP FASCIA AND THE PAROTID GLAND (Figs. 9–9, 9–10, and 7-3)

The parotid gland is completely enveloped by the same layer of deep fascia as is found over the masseter muscle. Its triangle-shaped **superficial part** overlies much of the masseter muscle. Its **deep part** extends medially, like a wedge between the mandible and the sternocleidomastoid muscle, as far as the styloid process and the deep surface of the medial pterygoid muscle. A thickening

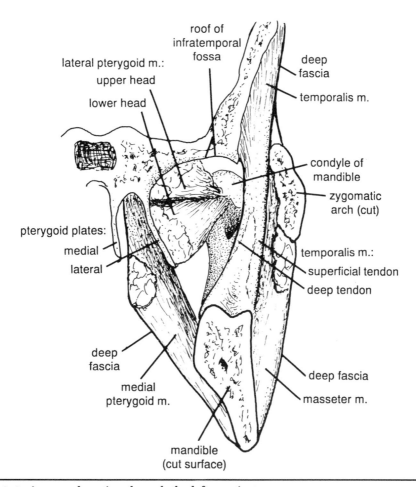

FIG. 9–9. A coronal section through the left masticator space.

of its deep fascia forms the **stylomandibular ligament,** which passes between attachments on the styloid process and the angle and ramus of the mandible. This ligament separates the parotid gland from the more inferiorly situated submandibular gland.

The deep part of the parotid has close relations with several important structures. As the external carotid artery ascends posterior to the mandible, it becomes surrounded by the gland. At the level of the neck of the mandible, it divides within the parotid tissue into its two terminal branches, the superficial temporal and the maxillary arteries. The maxillary artery turns into the infratemporal fossa, accompanied by the maxillary vein carrying blood out of the fossa. It joins with the superficial temporal vein in the parotid tissue to form the retromandibular vein. The latter descends into the neck in company with the external carotid artery. The facial nerve passes through the gland on its way to the face.

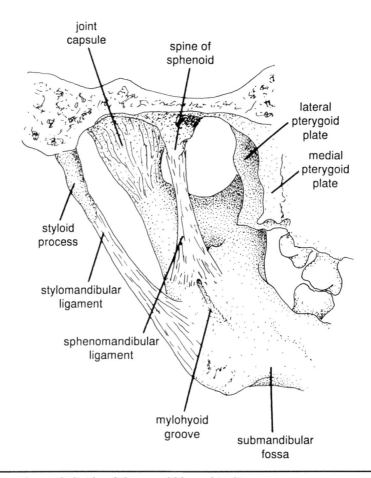

FIG. 9–10. The medial side of the mandible and its ligaments.

NERVES OF THE INFRATEMPORAL FOSSA (Figs. 9–11 through 9–13 and Figs. 4-22A and 4-23)

The great majority of nerves in the infratemporal fossa are branches of the mandibular division of the trigeminal nerve. The maxillary division of the trigeminal nerve is represented by its posterior superior alveolar branch. The glossopharyngeal nerve is represented by its otic ganglion and the facial nerve by its chorda tympani branch.

From the middle cranial fossa, the mandibular division (V3) enters the infratemporal fossa by passing through the foramen ovale. Lying next to its medial side is the otic ganglion. It immediately gives rise to a **meningeal** branch that re-enters the middle cranial fossa through the foramen spinosum and a **branch to the medial pterygoid muscle,** which also supplies the tensor tympani muscle of the middle ear cavity (see Chapter 13), and the tensor veli palatini muscle of the soft palate (see Chapter 12). Then V3 divides into an anterior part, which is variable in its branching pattern, and a posterior part.

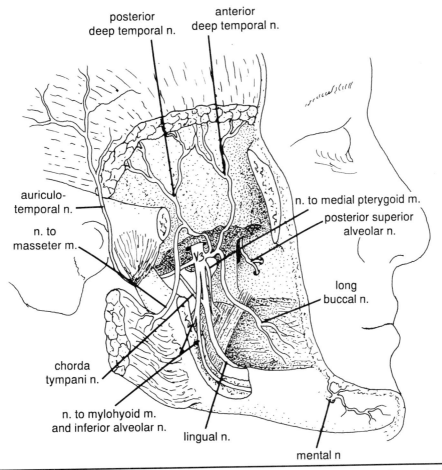

FIG. 9–11. Nerves of the infratemporal fossa seen if the lateral pterygoid muscle is removed.

The three branches of the posterior part of V3 are the auriculotemporal, the inferior alveolar, and the lingual nerves. They are mainly general sensory in function. Structures they innervate lie outside the fossa. The most posteriorly directed of these three branches is the **auriculotemporal** nerve, which travels between the sphenomandibular ligament and the mandibular neck to leave the fossa. It ascends anterior to the ear and posterior to the temporomandibular joint, for which it serves as the major source of sensory innervation. It supplies skin over the anterior ear and terminates in cutaneous branches that spread out over the broad temporal region of the head.

Fibers from the **otic ganglion** join the auriculotemporal nerve. The ganglion receives parasympathetic preganglionic axons from the lesser petrosal branch of the glossopharyngeal nerve. This branch arises from the tympanic plexus in the middle ear cavity (Figs. 5-4 and 13-5). From the plexus, it exits the petrous temporal bone and runs across the floor of the middle cranial fossa to the foramen ovale or spinosum, through which it passes to gain access to the otic ganglion. The axons synapse in the ganglion on parasympathetic postganglionic neuron cell bodies, whose postganglionic axons join the auriculotemporal nerve and leave it as it passes the parotid gland. Stimulation of these fibers results in salivary secretion into the parotid duct, which empties into the oral cavity.

The **inferior alveolar** nerve passes in a lateral and inferior direction, lying against the lateral surface of the medial pterygoid muscle until it reaches the mandibular foramen, where it exits the infratemporal fossa. As it traverses the mandibular canal, it gives off branches to mandibular teeth and most of their

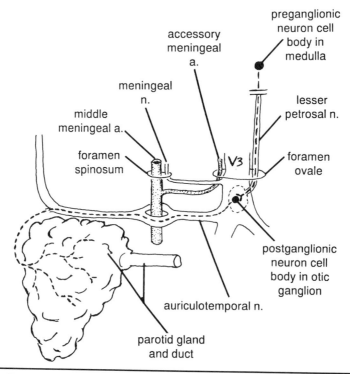

FIG. 9–12. Innervation of the parotid gland.

buccolabial gingiva. Two terminal branches arise within the canal in the vicinity of the second premolar tooth: the **mental branch,** which exits via the mental foramen to supply skin of the chin and lower lip, and the **incisive branch,** which continues in the canal to innervate the mandibular incisor teeth.

Arising from the inferior alveolar before it leaves the fossa is the **nerve to the mylohyoid and anterior belly of the digastric muscles.** This nerve follows the mylohyoid groove to innervate the two muscles for which it is named.

The **lingual nerve** descends on the medial pterygoid muscle anterior to the inferior alveolar nerve. It curves anteriorly as it approaches the mandible and leaves the infratemporal fossa to enter the tissue in the floor of the mouth immediately superior to the posterior border of the mylohyoid muscle. In the oral region the lingual fibers supply general sensation to the anterior two-thirds of the tongue and the mandibular lingual gingiva.

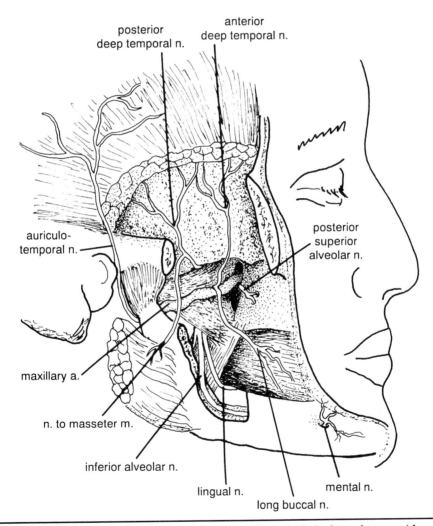

FIG. 9–13. The nerves visible in the infratemporal fossa with the lateral pterygoid muscle in place.

High in the infratemporal fossa the lingual nerve is joined by the **chorda tympani branch of VII.** Some of the chorda tympani fibers travel with the lingual nerve all the way to the tongue. They supply the special sense of taste to its anterior two-thirds (Fig. 4-24). The other fibers are for parasympathetic secretion of the submandibular and sublingual salivary glands (Fig. 5–3).

These branches of the mandibular nerve arise from its anterior part. Most are for innervation of muscles of mastication.

There is a short **branch to the lateral pterygoid** muscle.

The **posterior deep temporal** nerve ascends along the deep surface of the temporalis muscle.

The **nerve to the masseter muscle** usually arises from the posterior deep temporal nerve. It leaves the infratemporal fossa through the mandibular notch.

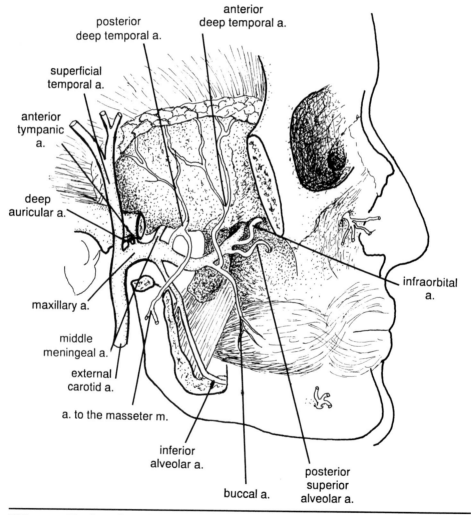

FIG. 9–14. The branches of the maxillary artery seen within the infratemporal fossa.

The **anterior deep temporal** nerve, like the posterior, ascends along the deep surface of the temporalis muscle but in a more anterior position.

The **long buccal nerve** usually arises from the anterior deep temporal nerve. It leaves the infratemporal fossa lateral to the buccinator muscle, passing across the retromolar fossa and penetrating the superficial tendon of the temporalis muscle on its way out. Some of its branches are sensory to skin of the cheek. Others penetrate the buccinator muscle without innervating it and supply general sensation to mucosa of the cheek and some buccal gingiva, generally around the mandibular second premolar and first molar teeth, although the exact gingival distribution is variable.

The **posterior superior alveolar** branch of the maxillary division of the trigeminal nerve (V2) can be seen on the posterior surface of the maxilla above the buccinator muscle. Arising from V2 in the nearby pterygopalatine fossa, it enters the infratemporal fossa through the pterygomaxillary fissure and, after a short course, leaves through the small foramen bearing the same name as the nerve. Frequently it branches while still in the fossa, in which case there will be more than one foramen. It supplies the maxillary molar teeth and their buccal gingiva with general sensation.

Because of the number of nerves in the infratemporal fossa destined for teeth and gingiva, it is an important area for those in the dental profession to understand. A needle inserted from the oral cavity must penetrate the buccinator muscle to enter the fossa. If the anesthetic is deposited just above the mandibular foramen between the bone and the sphenomandibular ligament, there will be anesthesia in the area supplied by the inferior alveolar nerve and the nearby lingual nerve. If the needle is directed to the posterior maxilla, the anesthesia will block nerve conduction in the posterior superior alveolar nerve; and if directed into the retromolar fossa between the temporalis tendons, the long buccal nerve. Thus, all the mandibular teeth and surrounding gingiva as well as the maxillary molars and their buccal gingiva can be anesthetized from within the infratemporal fossa.

VESSELS OF THE INFRATEMPORAL FOSSA (Figs. 9–13 through 9–15)

The artery of the infratemporal fossa is the **maxillary.** It is a large branch of the external carotid artery arising immediately posterior to the mandibular neck. It passes between the neck and the sphenomandibular ligament to enter the fossa, where it travels in an anterior direction, giving rise to branches that accompany most of the mandibular nerve branches. It does not end in the infratemporal fossa but continues on through the pterygomaxillary fissure into the pterygopalatine fossa. See Chapter 10 for these branches.

The first branches of the maxillary artery arise medial to the mandibular neck and are:

The **deep auricular** artery to the external auditory meatus.
The **anterior tympanic** artery to the tympanic membrane.

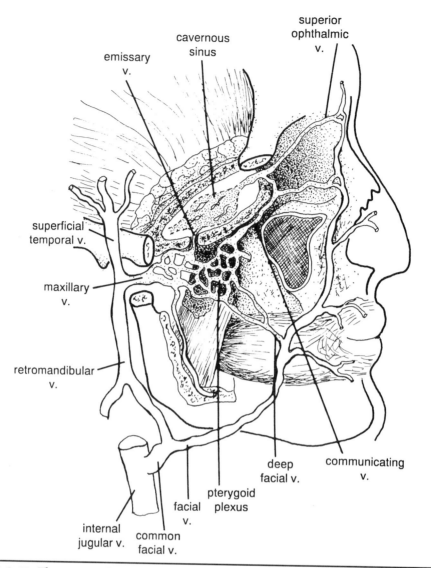

FIG. 9–15. The pterygoid venous plexus within the infratemporal fossa and its connections with adjacent areas.

The **middle meningeal** artery, which passes through the foramen spinosum to supply most of the dura mater.

The **accessory meningeal** artery, which passes through the foramen ovale to supply some dura. It frequently is a branch of the middle meningeal artery.

The **inferior alveolar** artery, which accompanies the inferior alveolar nerve and gives rise to the **artery to the mylohyoid and anterior digastric muscles.**

The other branches that arise within the infratemporal fossa are:

The **posterior deep temporal** artery, which accompanies the nerve of the same name and gives rise to the **masseteric** branch.

The **anterior deep temporal artery,** which also accompanies the nerve with the same name and gives rise to a **buccal branch** to accompany the long buccal nerve.

Short **branches to the medial and lateral pterygoid muscles.**

The **posterior superior alveolar** branch, which arises here or from the pterygopalatine part of the artery. It descends on the posterior surface of the maxilla in the company of the posterior superior alveolar nerve and has a similar distribution.

Within the fossa, closely associated with the maxillary artery and its branches, is a venous network called the **pterygoid venous plexus.** Veins accompanying the branches of the maxillary artery empty into this plexus, which can drain in several directions. Posteriorly it is a tributary of the maxillary vein. Anteriorly, the deep facial vein connects it with the facial vein on the superficial face. A communicating vein, through the inferior orbital fissure, connects it with ophthalmic veins in the orbit. Medially there are anastomoses with veins of the pharynx. And superiorly, an emissary vein connects it with the cavernous sinus within the middle cranial fossa. Because no valves exist in these veins, the blood can flow in either direction. Thus they can serve as routes for bacterial infection to spread from one area to another, eventually reaching the cranial cavity.

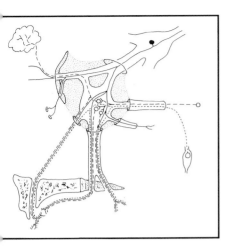

CHAPTER **10**

PTERYGOPALATINE FOSSA, NASAL CAVITY, AND PARANASAL SINUSES

The pterygopalatine fossa is a narrow and small, but important, space. Its importance is mainly due to the presence of the maxillary division of the trigeminal nerve, which gives rise to all but one of its branches there. The areas they supply with general sensory innervation include the maxillary teeth, mucosa, and gingiva; most of the nasal cavity; and a large region of skin on the face.

LOCATION OF THE PTERYGOPALATINE FOSSA ON THE SKULL (Fig. 10–1)

On each side of the skull the pterygopalatine fossa is located in the narrow gap between the pterygoid process of the sphenoid bone posteriorly and the palatine bone anteriorly. Students typically have difficulty locating the fossa, probably because they are looking for a much larger space. It is visible in several views of the skull but is easiest to locate if one examines the skull in lateral view, looks into the anterior depths of the infratemporal fossa, and locates the lateral pterygoid plate and the posterior part of the maxilla. Through the narrow gap between them, one can see the pterygopalatine fossa.

The walls of the fossa are perforated by numerous openings, all of which serve as passageways for nerves and vessels to enter or leave. In the lateral wall, the **pterygomaxillary fissure** is the gap just referred to above between pterygopalatine and infratemporal fossae. In the posterior wall, more laterally situated, is the **foramen rotundum**, through which the maxillary nerve enters from the cranial cavity; more medial is the opening for the **pharyngeal canal**, which leads to the nasopharynx; between them is the **pterygoid canal**. In the

129

medial wall the **sphenopalatine foramen** opens into the nasal cavity. In the anterior wall the **inferior orbital fissure** leads into the orbit. The opening in the floor is the entrance to the **palatine canal,** which passes inferiorly to divide and open on the hard palate as greater and lesser palatine foramina.

THE BONY STRUCTURE OF THE NASAL CAVITY (Figs. 10–2 through 10–4)

In a frontal view of the skull the large pear-shaped opening into the nasal cavity is the **piriform aperture.** It is bordered by the **nasal bones,** forming the bridge of the nose, and the **maxillae.**

Dividing the cavity into right and left (usually asymmetrical) sides is the **nasal septum,** comprised mainly of the **vomer** posteroinferiorly and the **perpendicular plate of the ethmoid bone** anterosuperiorly. The most anterior part of the septum is completed in a living person by septal cartilage. Some deviation of the septum to one side is almost always present. Too great a deviation of the septum can cause difficulty in breathing on the constricted side and can be surgically corrected.

In contrast to the smooth septum, the two **lateral walls** are irregular. They are formed in large part by the unpaired **ethmoid bone.** It contributes a superior and a middle concha (also called turbinate) to each side. They project into the

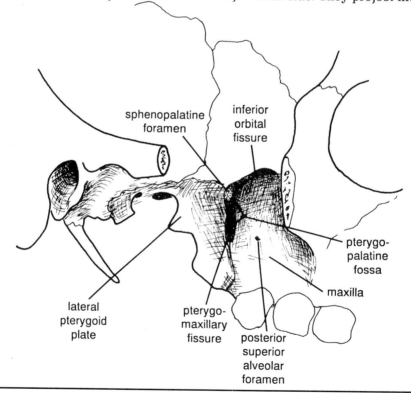

FIG. 10–1. The location on the skull of the pterygopalatine fossa.

nasal cavity, each creating a space beneath it called a meatus. The **superior turbinate** and its underlying superior meatus are very small. The **middle turbinate** and middle meatus are much larger. Projecting into the latter is a bulging, thin-walled bleb of the ethmoid bone called the **bulla ethmoidalis.**

The other major contributors to each lateral wall are the **maxilla** and the **inferior turbinate bone,** which has the inferior meatus below it. Ascending vertically along the posterior border of the lateral wall is the **vertical process of the palatine bone.** The **lacrimal bone** makes a small contribution anteriorly.

The roof of the nasal cavity is narrow. The **cribriform plate of the ethmoid bone** forms most of it. There is a small contribution from the **frontal bone** in the most anterior part and a small contribution from the **body of the sphenoid bone** posteriorly. The latter continues into the incomplete posterior wall.

The floor of the hard palate is made up, for the most part, of the **palatine process of the maxilla,** but there is an important contribution posteriorly from the **horizontal process of the palatine bone.**

Mucosa lines all the bony surfaces of the nasal cavity. Anterior and inferior to the bulla ethmoidalis in the middle meatus, a gap in the underlying bone causes the mucosa to have a deep groove, whose shape is reflected in its name, **hiatus semilunaris.** In the connective tissue beneath its epithelium course an

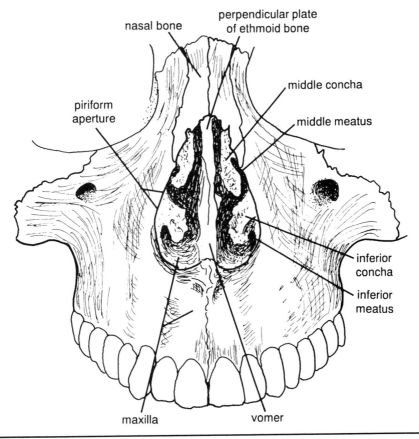

FIG. 10–2. An anterior view into the nasal cavity.

abundant blood supply and the nerves for general sensory innervation of the mucosa, autonomic innervation for secretion of small mucous glands within it, and contraction of smooth muscle within the walls of the vessels. The irregularities of the lateral nasal wall increase the mucosa-covered surface area, which is beneficial in warming inhaled air taken in through the nostrils, or anterior nares. The openings through which air passes at the posterior end of the nasal cavity are the **choanae,** or posterior nares. They open into the upper part of the nasopharynx (see Chapter 12).

THE PARANASAL SINUSES AND THEIR DRAINAGE SITES ON THE LATERAL NASAL WALLS (Fig. 10–5)

The sphenoid, ethmoid, and frontal bones and the maxillae contain hollow air-filled spaces called sinuses. The nasal mucosa continues into these spaces to provide a lining for their bony walls. Secretions from the mucosa normally drain from the sinuses through openings into the nasal cavity.

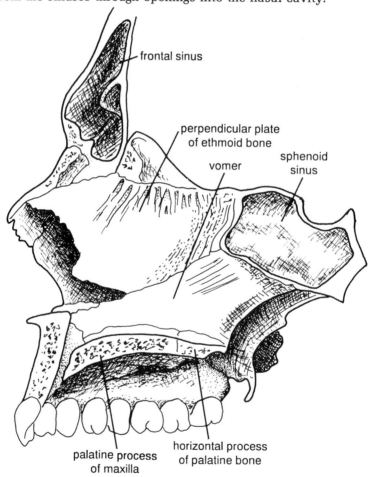

FIG. 10–3. The bony nasal septum.

Sinus trouble is not uncommon in individuals suffering from problems such as a cold or an allergy. Should the drainage sites be blocked by swelling of the mucosa that lines them, the result can be discomfort or pain as pressure builds within the closed space and the general sensory nerves passing through the mucosa become compressed.

The size and shape of the sinuses vary considerably from one person to another. Their function is questionable, but it is usually postulated that they serve as a means of decreasing the weight of the bones of the skull and as resonating chambers for the voice.

If midsagittally sectioned frontal bones are examined, the **frontal sinuses** can be seen to extend within the bone from a level between the eyebrows superiorly and laterally to variable degrees. The drainage site is seen within the most anterior part of the hiatus semilunaris, which is a slitlike curved opening in the mucosa of the middle meatus just inferior to the bulla ethmoidalis.

Within the body of the sphenoid bone is the **sphenoid sinus**. It is divided by an irregular partition of bone into asymmetrical right and left sides. Each side drains high in the posterior part of the nasal cavity into the sphenoethmoidal recess, located between the sphenoid body and the superior turbinate.

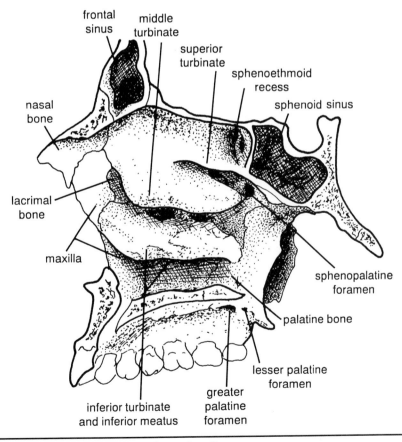

FIG. 10–4. The bones of the lateral nasal wall.

The **ethmoid sinuses** are not a single space but consist of small groups of air cells separated from one another by paper-thin septa. The air cells are organized into an anterior group, a middle group, and a posterior group, each having its own drainage site into the nasal cavity. In the middle meatus, anterior cells open into the hiatus semilunaris and middle cells open on the bulla ethmoidalis. Posterior ethmoid air cells open into the superior meatus.

The **maxillary sinuses,** situated lateral to the nasal cavity, are the largest. Their opening is in the hiatus semilunaris. Above their roof lies the orbit. Beneath their floor, which is well below the level of the nasal cavity floor, are the apices of the roots of the maxillary molar and premolar teeth. The nerve supply to the maxillary teeth enters the apical foramen in the tips of the roots. If the maxillary sinus in an individual is large, the nerves might be covered by only a very thin layer of bone or perhaps just the lining mucosa of the sinus. If drainage of the sinus is inadequate and increase of fluid content causes pressure on the nerves, the resulting discomfort can be interpreted mistakenly as tooth pain. Problems also can occur if a tooth is pulled and the overlying bone is too thin to remain intact or is nonexistent; the maxillary sinus can then drain through the resulting opening into the oral cavity. Surgical intervention might be necessary.

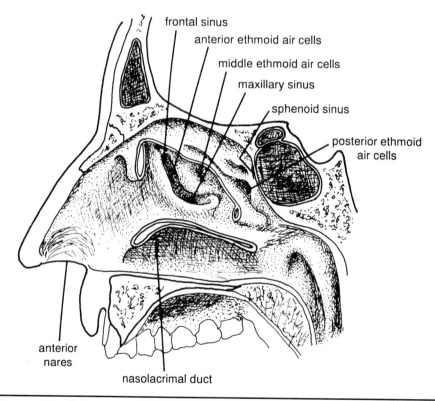

frontal sinus
anterior ethmoid air cells
middle ethmoid air cells
maxillary sinus
sphenoid sinus
posterior ethmoid air cells
anterior nares
nasolacrimal duct

FIG. 10–5. The drainage sites for the paranasal sinuses and tears. The middle and inferior turbinates have been partially removed.

The only opening in the nasal cavity serving as the drainage site for something other than mucus from a paranasal sinus is for tears. A surplus of tears that collects in the medial corner of the eye and does not run down the cheeks is carried through the **nasolacrimal duct,** which opens in the anterior part of the inferior meatus. This accounts for the runny nose while crying.

DISTRIBUTION OF NERVES AND VESSELS FROM THE PTERYGOPALATINE FOSSA

Three major structures enter the pterygopalatine fossa:

The **maxillary branch of the trigeminal nerve enters through the foramen rotundum** carrying general sensory innervation (Figs. 10–6 and 10–7, and 4-22A and B) and the nerve of the pterygoid canal (see next page).
The **maxillary branch of the external carotid artery enters through the pterygomaxillary fissure** (Figs. 10–8 and 10–9).

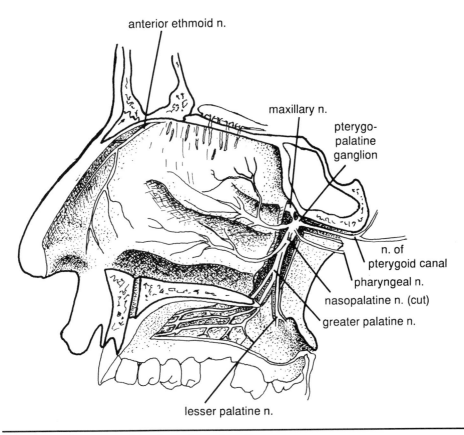

FIG. 10–6. The nerves of the lateral nasal wall.

The **nerve of the pterygoid canal enters through the pterygoid canal** carrying autonomic innervation. It is formed when two nerves join just before entering the canal. They are the greater petrosal nerve and the deep petrosal nerve (Figs. 10–10 and 10–11 and Fig. 5–3).

The following branches of the maxillary nerve and artery supply most of the nasal mucosa and some of the maxillary gingiva and mucosa in the oral cavity:

The **nasopalatine nerve,** accompanied by the **sphenopalatine artery,** leaves the fossa through the sphenopalatine foramen; they pass across the narrow roof of the nasal cavity and travel downward along the septum, giving off branches to the mucosa along their route. They pass through the incisive canal in order to reach the anterior part of the hard palate in the oral cavity.

Descending from the fossa through the palatine canal to the posterior part of the hard palate are the **greater and lesser palatine nerves** and accompanying **descending palatine artery.** While in the canal, small posterolateral nasal artery and nerve branches arise and exit to course anteriorly through the mucosa of the lateral nasal wall, and the descending palatine artery divides into greater and lesser palatine branches. The greater palatine nerve and artery exit through the greater palatine foramen and continue forward on the oral surface of the hard palate. The lesser palatine nerve and artery emerge through the lesser palatine foramen and travel posteriorly to supply mucosa of the soft palate.

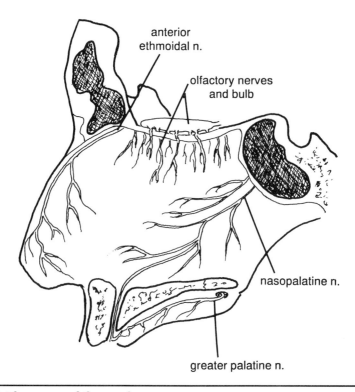

FIG. 10–7. The nerves of the nasal septum.

The **pharyngeal branch** of the maxillary nerve and the **pharyngeal artery** enter the pharyngeal canal to travel posteriorly to reach mucosa of the upper part of the nasopharynx.

The **zygomatic branch** passes anteriorly through the inferior orbital fissure to run along the lower lateral wall of the orbit. It enters the zygomatic bone through the zygomatic foramen and divides into the zygomaticofacial and zygomaticotemporal branches, which emerge through foramina of the same name to supply cutaneous innervation to some of the face and scalp.

The **posterior superior alveolar nerve and artery** exit laterally through the pterygomaxillary fissure onto the posterior part of the maxilla in the infratemporal fossa. A small foramen (or if they have already begun to branch, several small foramina) allows them to enter the maxillary sinus, where they course along its lateral wall, either through small canals in the bone or covered only by mucosa. Their destination is the maxillary molar teeth.

The remainder of the maxillary nerve continues anteriorly through the inferior orbital fissure as the **infraorbital nerve.** It traverses the floor of the orbit with the **infraorbital artery,** first in the infraorbital groove and then in the infraorbital canal, which opens at the infraorbital foramen. As they pass along the floor of the orbit, they give rise to two branches important for supplying maxillary teeth, the middle superior alveolar and the anterior superior alveolar. These too course in the wall of the maxillary sinus in order to reach the teeth.

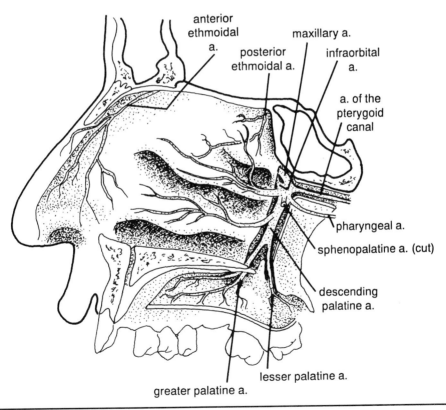

FIG. 10–8. The arteries of the lateral nasal wall.

The anterior parts of the nasal septum and lateral nasal wall are supplied not by the maxillary division of the trigeminal but by the **ophthalmic division** (Fig. 4-21). The **anterior ethmoidal nerve and artery** arise within the orbit, pass through the ethmoidal air cells that they supply, and have branches that descend in the anterior parts of the nasal mucosa. A **posterior ethmoidal artery** contributes to the supply of the posterior mucosa. The accompanying arteries are branches of the **ophthalmic artery.**

The **greater petrosal nerve** carries parasympathetic preganglionic fibers belonging to the facial nerve and coming from neuron cell bodies in the brain; they terminate by synapsing in the pterygopalatine ganglion, which lies in close association with the maxillary nerve in the pterygopalatine fossa. Two small pterygopalatine nerves link the ganglion and the maxillary nerve; they enable the maxillary nerve branches to pick up autonomic fibers and carry them along for whatever distance is required. The superior petrosal nerve branches from the facial nerve within the facial canal in the region of its geniculate ganglion. It emerges through the **hiatus of the facial canal** into the middle cranial fossa. After passing across its floor, they exit through the foramen lacerum and then enter the pterygoid canal on the base of the skull. From the ganglion, postganglionic parasympathetic fibers are able to join all the maxillary nerve branches that supply sensory innervation to mucosa in the nasal and oral cavities. They stimulate secretion of minor salivary glands within the oral mucosa. In addition, some of them go with the zygomatic nerve into the orbit and leave it by a communicating branch to the lacrimal nerve. Their destination is the lacrimal gland, which they stimulate for tear secretion.

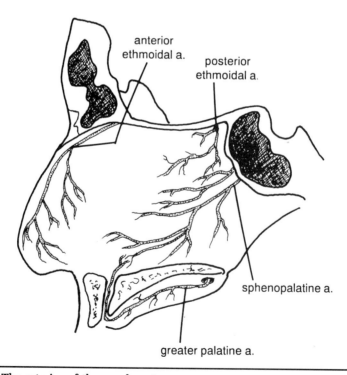

FIG. 10–9. The arteries of the nasal septum.

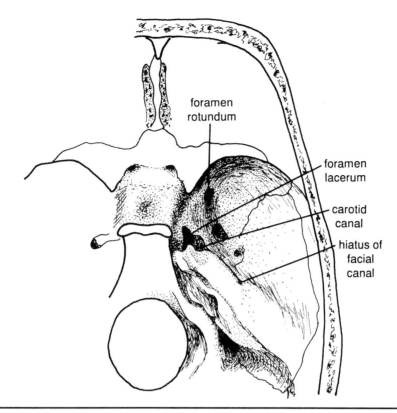

FIG. 10–10. The openings in the cranial cavity floor used by V2 and the greater petrosal nerve.

The **deep petrosal nerve** carries sympathetic postganglionic fibers, which come from neuron cell bodies in the superior cervical sympathetic ganglion. They enter the cranial cavity as part of the plexus on the internal carotid artery, and they exit through the foramen lacerum in order to enter the pterygoid canal. In the pterygopalatine fossa they simply pass through the pterygopalatine ganglion to reach the maxillary nerve branches, with which they travel to smooth muscle in the wall of blood vessels.

LOCATION OF OLFACTORY MUCOSA AND THE OLFACTORY NERVE (Fig. 4-17)

In addition to the general sensory innervation to the nasal mucosa described above, there is the **special sensory innervation** for olfactory sensation, or the sense of smell. The nerve endings, which serve as receptors for smell, are located in the mucosa of the roof and upper parts of the septum and lateral wall of the nasal cavity. The numerous nerve fibers that convey olfactory information to the central nervous system pass through the openings in the cribriform plate and enter the overlying olfactory bulb. These fibers comprise the **olfactory nerve.**

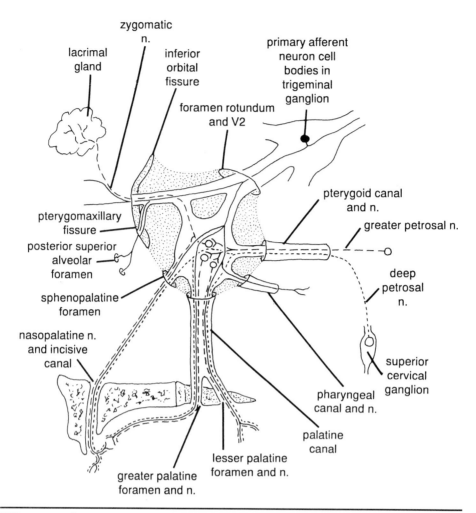

FIG. 10–11. The openings into the pterygopalatine fossa and their contents.

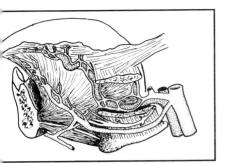

CHAPTER **11**

THE ORAL CAVITY

The mouth, or oral cavity, serves as the entryway into the digestive system. It is well adapted for taking in food and positioning it for mastication and swallowing. It is divided into the **vestibule,** limited anteriorly and laterally by the lips and cheeks, and the **oral cavity proper,** separated from the vestibule by maxillary and mandibular alveolar processes and teeth. The hard and soft palates form its roof. Within its floor are supporting muscles. Posteriorly, the gap bordered by the free edge of the soft palate, the right and left **anterior tonsillar pillars,** and the **sulcus terminalis** on the tongue, discussed below, indicate the extent of the oral cavity. The gap is called the **isthmus of the fauces.** Following mastication, food is pushed through the isthmus into the pharynx to be swallowed.

GENERAL FEATURES AND CONTENTS (Figs. 11–1 through 11–4)

The oral cavity is lined with mucosa. In the anterior midline of the vestibule, both superiorly and inferiorly, the mucosa is thrown into a vertically oriented fold called the **labial frenulum,** or **frenum,** extending from the alveolar process to the lips. The **lingual frenulum** passes between the ventral side of the tongue and the mandibular alveolar process.

The soft tissue over the hard palate is firmly attached to the underlying bone, especially along the midline raphe. Anteriorly, small horizontal folds called **rugae** extend laterally from the raphe and a slight papilla overlying the site of the incisive canal. The soft palate is distinguished by the **uvula,** suspended from its midline, and the folds of mucosa that arise from its lateral sides to form the tonsillar pillars. It is not fixed in position, as is the hard palate, but highly mobile, changing position constantly during eating, swallowing, and speaking.

On the dorsal side of the tongue, the mucosa of the anterior two-thirds has a velvety appearance due to slender **filiform papillae,** which are whitish. Scattered, more rounded **fungiform papillae** are red and have a few taste buds along their sides. Taste buds are too small to be seen with the unaided eye. **Foliate papillae,** which are not well developed in humans, are narrow folds on the lateral sides of the tongue, with many taste buds. At the junction of the anterior two-thirds and posterior one-third of the tongue, there is a V-shaped row of 8 to 12 **circumvallate papillae.** Lying immediately posterior to the V-shaped **sulcus terminalis,** each is encircled by a trough and has along its sides many taste buds. At the point of the V is the **foramen cecum,** indicating the site where the thyroid gland began its development in the embryo and from which it migrated to its final position. The posterior one-third of the tongue lacks papillae. Its mucosa has a lumpy appearance caused by underlying **lingual tonsils,** whose crypts open on the tongue surface. This part of the tongue does not lie within the oral cavity, but within the oral portion of the pharynx.

The mucosa of the ventral side of the tongue lacks the specialized features of the dorsal side. Through its thin epithelium large veins are visible.

Openings occur in the oral mucosa for the ducts of the three pairs of major salivary glands. The **parotid duct** opens in the cheek opposite the upper second molar tooth; a small protrusion of mucosa can usually be felt at that location. Under the anterior end of the tongue is the **sublingual caruncle,** where the **submandibular duct** opens. The sublingual salivary gland, in the floor of the mouth under the lateral side of the tongue, creates the **sublingual fold,** an elevation of the thin mucosa overlying it. Small bumps along the apex of the fold indicate the locations of openings of several short, small ducts from the sublingual gland rather than the single one possessed by the other two. Numerous small minor salivary glands lie within the mucosa and submucosa of the hard and soft palates, lips, cheeks, and tongue, and their tiny ducts open in those areas. They are responsible for keeping a constant moist environment for the mucosal surfaces of the mouth.

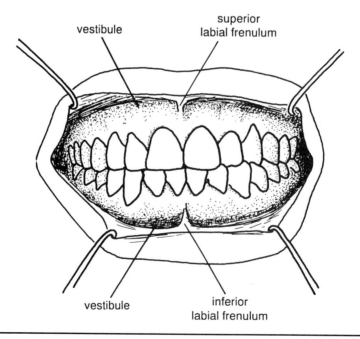

FIG. 11–1. The vestibule.

MUSCLES OF THE WALLS OF THE ORAL CAVITY (Figs. 11–5 and 11–6)

Within the tissues that form the walls and boundaries of the oral cavity are the muscles of the lips and cheeks. They belong to the **muscles of facial expression.** The **orbicularis oris** muscle within the lips causes their pursing and allows them to be pressed tightly together or held firmly against the teeth. Contraction of the **buccinator muscle** within the cheeks holds them firmly against the lateral sides of the teeth, thus keeping the food on the occlusal surfaces and preventing it from falling into the vestibule. The parotid duct must pierce the buccinator muscle in order to empty its secretions into the oral cavity. Because the posterior part of the buccinator muscle separates the oral cavity from the infratemporal fossa, routine injections in the dentist's office for anesthesia of nerves that innervate mandibular and some maxillary teeth involve piercing it with a needle in order to reach the appropriate site in the fossa (Fig. 9–11). The posterior extent of the buccinator muscle can be determined; its most posterior fibers arise from the **pterygomandibular raphe,** which is detectable in the oral cavity by a mucosal fold formed over it when it is stretched by opening the mouth. The connective tissue comprising the raphe extends from the pterygoid hamulus, which is palpable slightly medial and posterior to the maxillary alveolar pro-

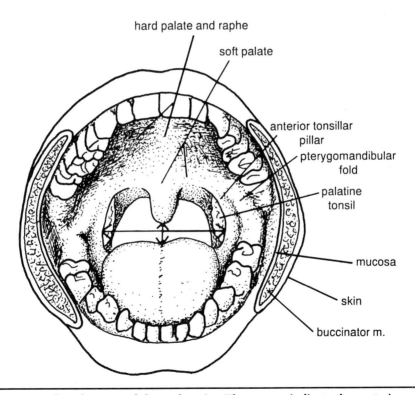

hard palate and raphe
soft palate
anterior tonsillar pillar
pterygomandibular fold
palatine tonsil
mucosa
skin
buccinator m.

FIG. 11–2. Surface features of the oral cavity. The arrows indicate the posterior extent of the oral cavity.

cess, to the retromolar triangle (Fig. 9–6A) just posterior to the last mandibular molar tooth. A needle mistakenly inserted posterior to the raphe will first pierce the superior pharyngeal constrictor muscle (see Chapter 12) and then the medial pterygoid muscle in the infratemporal fossa.

In the floor of the mouth the **mylohyoid muscle** forms a broad muscular support. It arises from the mylohyoid line on the mandible and inserts along the connective tissue which forms the mylohyoid raphe in the midline and on the hyoid bone. On its superior surface on either side of the midline are the **geniohyoid muscles** extending from the genial tubercle on the mandible to the hyoid bone. Contraction of these muscles pulls the hyoid bone upward and forward or tightens the floor of the mouth, thus giving firm support for the largest muscle mass in the oral cavity, the tongue. Resting on the mylohyoid muscle lateral to the tongue is loose connective tissue, which contains the sublingual gland; the deep part of the submandibular gland; the submandibular duct, passing from its posterior origin to the sublingual caruncle; and vessels and nerves of the area. If an infection from an abscessed tooth or some other source occurs in the loose connective tissue, it can have far-reaching consequences. It can spread downward over the posterior free edge of the muscle and enter the anterior neck. Or it can pass in a posterior direction lateral to the pharynx and into the retropharyngeal space (Fig. 8–4).

THE MUSCLES OF THE TONGUE (Figs. 11–6 and 11–7)

The tongue contains both extrinsic and intrinsic muscle masses. **Intrinsic muscles** lie completely within the tongue. They are organized into vertical, horizontal, and longitudinal groups. They are the muscles responsible for curling

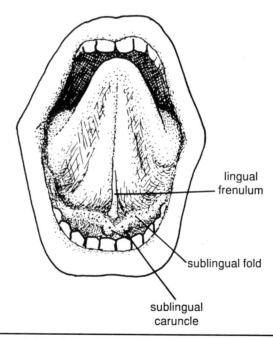

lingual
frenulum

sublingual fold

sublingual
caruncle

FIG. 11–3. The ventral side of the tongue.

or rolling, and flattening or thickening the tongue. **Extrinsic muscles** enter the tongue from origins outside the tongue. When they contract, they influence the position of the entire tongue. The **styloglossus muscle** arises from the styloid process and passes anteriorly to enter the lateral side of the tongue. Its contraction pulls the tongue in a posterior direction and retrudes a protruded tongue. The hyoid bone gives rise to the **hyoglossus muscle,** which passes upward to enter the lateral side of the tongue. Its contraction pulls downward and backward on the tongue and contributes to retrusion. The **genioglossus muscle** takes origin from the genial spine superior to the origin of the geniohyoid muscle. The two genioglossus muscles, one on either side of the midline of the tongue, make up its largest muscle mass. Their fibers fan out to span from anterior to posterior. Contraction of their more posteriorly directed fibers results in tongue protrusion; the anterior ones pull downward on the tip of the tongue. If the genioglossus muscle on just one side contracts, it causes the tongue to protrude to the opposite side. A fourth extrinsic muscle, the **palatoglossus muscle,** arises within the soft palate, courses downward within the anterior tonsillar pillar, and enters the posterior part of the tongue. Because the pillar is a elevation of mucosa caused by the underlying muscle, it is frequently called the **palatoglossal fold.** Contraction of both palatoglossus muscles draws the posterior part of the tongue and the soft palate together.

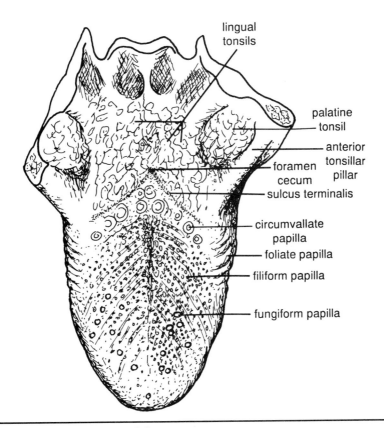

FIG. 11–4. The dorsal surface of the tongue.

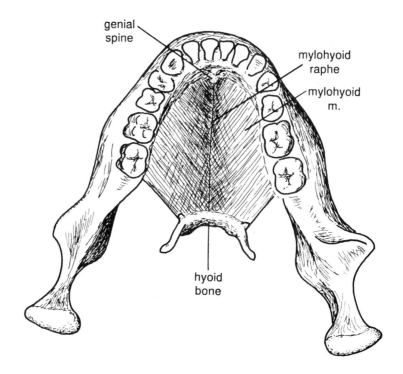

FIG. 11-5. The floor of the mouth in a superior view.

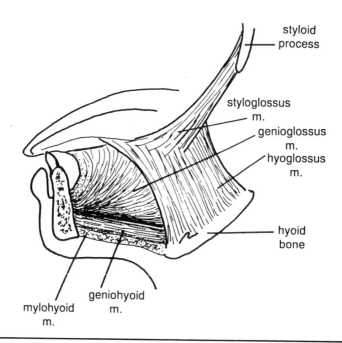

FIG. 11-6. The extrinsic muscles of the tongue seen from the left side and the floor of the mouth. The left side of the mandible has been removed.

INNERVATION OF THE ORAL CAVITY (Figs. 11–8 through 11–11)

The structures of the oral cavity that must be innervated include the muscles found within the lips, cheeks, tongue, and floor; mucosa, which forms the surface lining; teeth; taste buds; and major and minor salivary glands. Numerous nerve branches are involved in the innervation. They make their approach through the various tissues and bones in the walls and boundaries of the oral cavity. They approach from the superficial fascia of the face, from the submandibular region of the neck, from the infratemporal fossa, through the greater and lesser palatine and nasopalatine foramina, through the walls of the maxillary sinus, and from the area of the oropharynx.

Because the muscles of the cheeks and lips belong to the facial expression muscle group, they are innervated by **facial nerve branches**, which course through the superficial fascia of the face to reach them. They are discussed in Chapter 7.

All muscles of the tongue, except the palatoglossus, receive motor innervation from the hypoglossal nerve (Figs. 4-6, 4-29, and 8-10). It enters the tongue from the submandibular triangle of the neck along the lateral side of the hyoglossus muscle. As it approaches the geniohyoid muscle, the **nerve to the geniohyoid** is

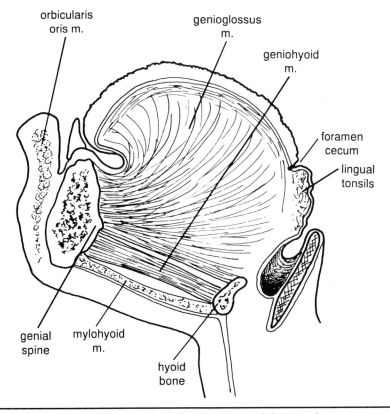

FIG. 11–7. Midsagittal section of the tongue and floor of the mouth.

given off. The fibers that make up this small branch arise from the ventral ramus of the first cervical spinal nerve; they join the hypoglossal nerve in the neck, and it carries them toward their ultimate destination. Innervation of the palatoglossus muscle is by the vagus nerve and is discussed with the muscles of the soft palate in Chapter 12.

Approaching the oral region from the infratemporal fossa is the **lingual branch of the mandibular nerve,** or V3. It enters the loose connective tissue in the floor of the mouth over the mylohyoid muscle immediately medial to the third mandibular molar tooth. Suspended from it at this point is the **submandibular ganglion.** As it continues anteriorly from the ganglion it is crossed by the **submandibular duct.** They are located along the lateral side of the hyoglossus muscle in a position superior to the hypoglossal nerve. Branches of the lingual nerve supply general sensory innervation to the anterior two-thirds of the tongue mucosa, the mucosa of the floor of the mouth, and the lingual gingiva of the mandibular molar teeth.

The lingual nerve is important for bringing other innervation into the oral region as well. While in the infratemporal fossa, it is joined by the **chorda tympani branch of the facial nerve,** which has two important functions: it supplies the fibers for the special sense of taste to the anterior two-thirds of the tongue, and it brings in preganglionic parasympathetic fibers to the submandibular ganglion, where they synapse (Fig. 5–3). The postganglionic fibers leave the ganglion, some going to the submandibular gland. The others rejoin the lingual nerve and leave via its sublingual branch to innervate the sublingual gland. Stimulation of the glandular branches causes secretion of saliva.

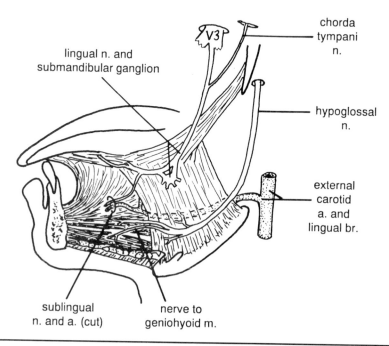

FIG. 11–8. Nerves in the floor of the oral cavity on the left side.

The **long buccal nerve** has been discussed (Chapter 7) as one of the cutaneous branches of V3 to the superficial face. Some of its fibers, however, penetrate the buccinator muscle to reach the mucosa lining the cheek and the buccal gingiva around the mandibular second premolar and first molar teeth. The gingival distribution is highly variable and can be either more or less extensive than this.

The **inferior alveolar branch** of V3 passes through the infratemporal fossa to the mandibular foramen (Figs. 4-23 and 9-11). Shortly before entering the foramen, it gives off the **nerve to the mylohyoid and anterior belly of the digastric muscles,** which descends in the mylohyoid groove to reach the superficial, or inferior, surface of the mylohyoid muscle in the suprahyoid region of the neck. The mandibular teeth and buccolabial gingiva, except the gingiva supplied by the long buccal nerve, receive innervation from the inferior alveolar nerve within the mandibular canal. The terminal branches of the inferior alveolar nerve are the **mental nerve,** which exits the mental foramen to supply skin and mucosa of the lower lip and skin of the chin, and the **incisive nerve,** which continues in the mandibular canal to supply the incisor teeth and their labial gingiva.

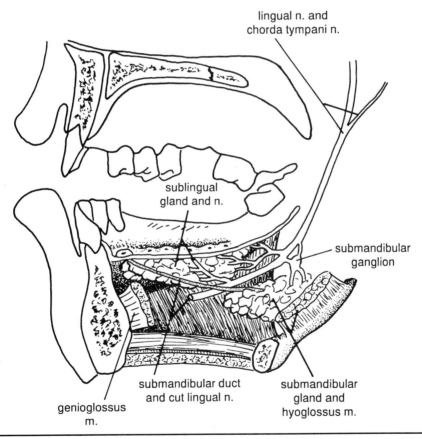

FIG. 11–9. The glands and their related structures on the right side in the floor of the oral cavity.

INNERVATION OF THE ORAL CAVITY   **149**

The maxillary division of the trigeminal nerve is the source of innervation for oral regions most closely related to the maxilla (Fig. 4-22). From within the bony floor and anterior wall of the maxillary sinus the **anterior superior alveolar, middle superior alveolar,** and **posterior superior alveolar** nerves supply branches to the maxillary teeth and their buccolabial gingiva. In general, the posterior superior alveolar nerve supplies the molar teeth, the anterior the incisors and canines, and the middle superior alveolar nerve the premolars and a small part of the first molar. Many people lack the middle superior alveolar nerve, in which case the anterior and posterior superior alveolar nerves share to varying degrees the innervation of this area.

From the posterior part of the hard palate the **greater palatine nerve** emerges from the greater palatine foramen (Fig. 10–6) and travels anteriorly to supply palatine mucosa and maxillary lingual gingiva as far forward as the canine. The **nasopalatine nerve** (Fig. 10–7), emerging through the nasopalatine foramen in the anterior part of the hard palate, supplies anterior palatine mucosa and lingual gingiva of the maxillary incisors, overlapping with the greater palatine nerve at the canine teeth. One or more small lesser palatine foramina transmit **lesser palatine nerves,** which head posteriorly to supply the oral mucosa on the soft palate.

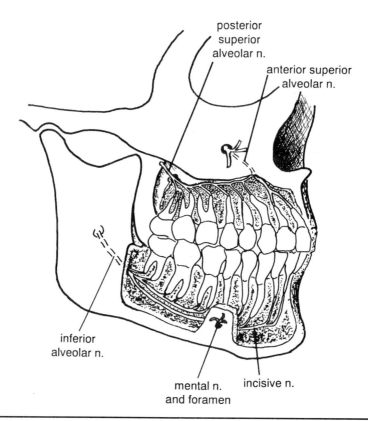

FIG. 11–10. Innervation of the teeth seen from the right side. The outer layer of bone of the mandible and maxilla has been removed.

Mucosa of the posterior one-third of the tongue is not within the oral cavity but the oropharynx. Both its general and special sensory innervations are provided by the glossopharyngeal nerve (Fig. 4-26), which can be located coursing toward the posterior tongue in the connective tissues of the palatine tonsillar bed.

BLOOD SUPPLY OF THE ORAL CAVITY (Figs. 11–11 and 11–12)

The maxillary artery or its branches supply the following arteries, which accompany and distribute with the nerves having the same names: **anterior, middle,** and **posterior superior alveolar** arteries; the **inferior alveolar artery** and its branches; the **buccal artery** with the long buccal nerve; and the **descending palatine artery,** which branches into the **greater** and **lesser palatine arteries.**

The nasopalatine nerve is accompanied by the **sphenopalatine** branch of the maxillary artery (Figs. 10-7 and 10-9). It sometimes traverses the incisive foramen to anastomose with the greater palatine artery on the hard palate; or branches of the greater palatine traverse the incisive foramen, in which case the anastomosis takes place on the nasal septum.

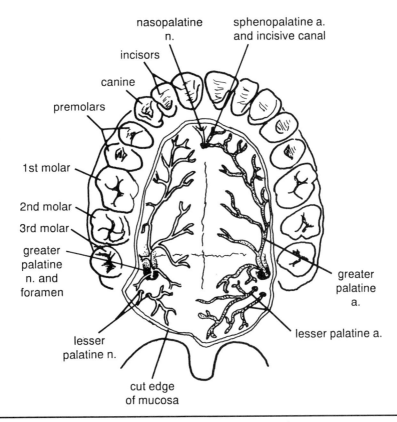

FIG. 11–11. **The nerves and arteries in the roof of the mouth.**

Arterial supply to the tongue is from the **lingual** branch of the external carotid (Fig. 8–9). The lingual artery arises in the carotid triangle of the neck and ascends to the submandibular triangle, where it takes a course deep to the hyoglossus muscle. A **dorsal lingual** and a **deep lingual** branch supply the tongue, and a **sublingual** branch passes across to reach the sublingual gland and surrounding mucosa.

Many of the veins from the oral region accompany the branches of the maxillary artery. They return the blood to the infratemporal fossa, where it enters the pterygoid venous plexus. The veins have the same names as the arteries they accompany. Blood from the **lingual vein** and from the **accompanying vein of the hypoglossal nerve** empties into the internal jugular vein.

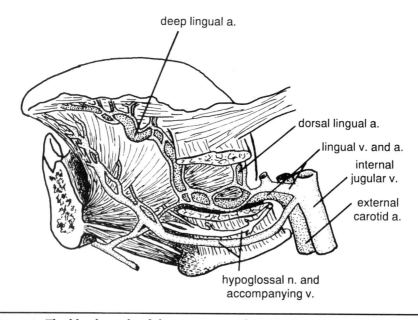

FIG. 11–12. The blood supply of the tongue seen from the left side.

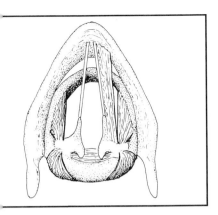

CHAPTER 12

THE VISCERAL COMPARTMENT OF THE NECK

Within the visceral compartment of the neck are the pharynx and upper part of the esophagus, the larynx and trachea, which are parts of the digestive and respiratory tracts, and the thyroid and parathyroid glands, which are endocrine organs. Enclosing these structures is the cylindrical sheath of deep fascia known as the **cervical visceral fascia.** The part of the fascia covering the posterior side of the pharynx and esophagus is called **buccopharyngeal fascia** (Figs. 8-4 and 12–1). The remainder, which encloses the trachea and the glands, is the **pretracheal fascia.** Loose connective tissue fills the narrow retro- and lateral pharyngeal spaces, which surround the muscular walls of the pharynx, allowing freedom for the movement occurring during swallowing. Through the retropharyngeal space the pharynx has a close relationship to the vertebral column and its prevertebral fascia; laterally its close relationship is with the deep fascia of the medial pterygoid muscle and infratemporal fossa.

THE PHARYNX (Fig. 12–2)

The relationships between the respiratory and digestive pathways can best be seen in a midsagittal section of the head and neck. Air breathed into the nasal cavity enters the most superior part of the pharynx, the **nasopharynx,** by passing through the posterior nares, or choanae. Food taken into the mouth enters the midportion of the pharynx, the **oropharynx,** through the oropharyngeal isthmus, or fauces.

The third, most inferior part of the pharynx is the **laryngopharynx,** related anteriorly to the larynx. In its upper half, the anterior aperture in its wall leads into the vestibule of the larynx and serves for passage of air on its way to and from the lungs. Food moves through the entire length of the laryngopharynx to reach the **esophagus.** The latter is a long muscular tube, which continues through the remainder of the neck and the thorax and terminates in the stomach almost immediately after entering the abdomen.

DISTINGUISHING FEATURES OF THE INTERIOR OF THE PHARYNX (Fig. 12–3)

The interior of the pharynx is lined with mucosa. The most superior part of the nasopharynx abuts against the sphenoid and occipital bones and is where the **pharyngeal tonsils,** the ones often referred to as adenoids, are located within the mucosa. Tonsils are lymphoid organs whose function is to provide a line of defense against infective organisms presented in abundance to the moist mucosal surface. Other tonsils, to be mentioned below, are situated nearby. In the lateral wall of the nasopharynx, the medial end of the cartilaginous part of the **auditory tube** protrudes beneath the mucosa, creating a prominent bulge called the **torus tubarius.** The lateral end of the auditory tube is through bone and opens into the middle ear cavity. Its purpose is to serve as the means by which air pressure in the middle ear cavity can be brought to equal external air pressure and prevent damage to the delicate structures within the ear. A fold of pharyngeal mucosa extends inferiorly from the posterior side of the torus tubarius. It is the **salpingopharyngeal fold,** caused by the underlying **salpingopharyngeus muscle.** A deep extension of the pharyngeal lumen posterior to the fold forms the **pharyngeal recess.**

Inferiorly in the nasopharynx, the **soft palate,** including the **uvula,** is suspended from the posterior midline, forming an obliquely oriented partition be-

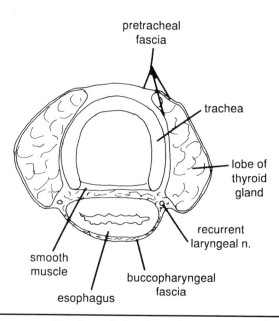

FIG. 12–1. A transverse section through the visceral compartment of the neck below the level of the pharynx and larynx.

tween it and the oral cavity. Passing from the lateral sides of the soft palate are two slightly diverging folds of mucosa created by underlying muscles. One, the **palatoglossal fold** over the **palatoglossus muscle,** marks the junction of oropharynx and oral cavity and lies more anteriorly. More posteriorly, the **palatopharyngeal fold** forms over the **palatopharyngeus muscle.** Between them is the bed for the **palatine tonsil.** The folds are often referred to as the anterior and posterior **tonsillar pillars.**

The posterior part of the tongue lies within the oropharynx. Its surface appears lumpy and irregular because of the presence of **lingual tonsils** in the mucosa. Posterior to the tongue the epiglottic cartilage of the larynx projects upward. In the midline a fold of mucosa called the **glossoepiglottic fold** stretches between epiglottis and tongue. The deep depression created on either side of the fold is the **vallecula epiglottica.**

The free edge of the epiglottis and the **aryepiglottic folds,** which pass posteriorly from its sides, rim the entryway into the larynx. Below, in the anterior wall of the laryngopharynx, the broad posterior surface of the **cricoid cartilage** of the larynx protrudes into the pharyngeal space, causing a deep crevice called the

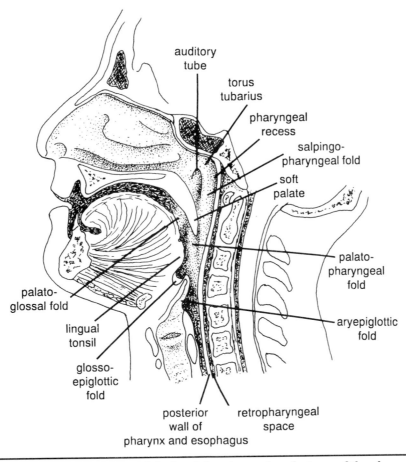

FIG. 12–2. Midsagittal section of the head showing surface features of the pharynx and its relations anteriorly to nasal, oral, and laryngeal cavities.

piriform recess to be created on each side. At the inferior level of the cricoid cartilage, the pharynx ends by becoming the esophagus.

MUSCULATURE OF THE PHARYNGEAL WALL (Figs. 12–4 and 12–5)

The major part of the muscular wall of the pharynx is composed of the **superior, middle,** and **inferior pharyngeal constrictor muscles.** They arise from anterolateral positions. Removal of the buccopharyngeal fascia covering their outer surfaces reveals that the muscles from both sides pass to the posterior midline to have a common insertion along a strip of connective tissue that extends from the pharyngeal tubercle on the occipital bone to the esophagus. It is called the **pharyngeal raphe.**

Their origins, more complicated and varied than their rather simple insertion, are as follows.

1. The **superior pharyngeal constrictor** muscle takes its origin laterally from several locations: the posterior edge of the medial pterygoid plate and its

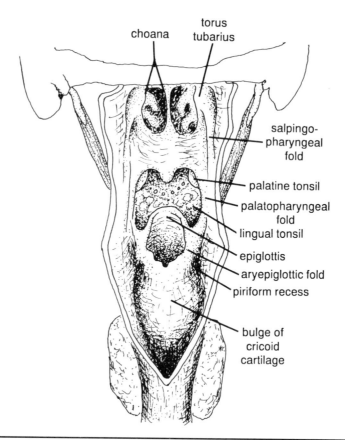

FIG. 12–3. A view into the pharynx from the posterior side. The wall of the pharynx has been opened with a longitudinal cut so that surface features can be seen.

hamulus, the pterygomandibular raphe, and the mylohyoid line. In a posterior view, through the gap between the muscle and the skull, a fascial layer that attaches to the skull can be seen. This layer continues between the mucosa and the muscular layers but is particularly strong where it spans this gap. It is called the **pharyngobasilar fascia.**

2. The **middle pharyngeal constrictor** muscle takes its origin from the stylohyoid ligament and the hyoid bone.

3. The **inferior pharyngeal constrictor** muscle takes its origin from the oblique line of the thyroid cartilage and the cricoid cartilage.

As the fibers of each constrictor muscle pass posteriorly, they spread as they approach their insertion along the pharyngeal raphe so that the upper fibers turn in a superior direction, the lower ones in an inferior direction. This results in some overlap between adjacent constrictors in such a way that the lower fibers of the more superior constrictor lie closer to the mucosal lining of the pharynx than the upper fibers of the one below it. During swallowing, the muscles contract in a sequential fashion, squeezing a bolus of food to successively lower levels.

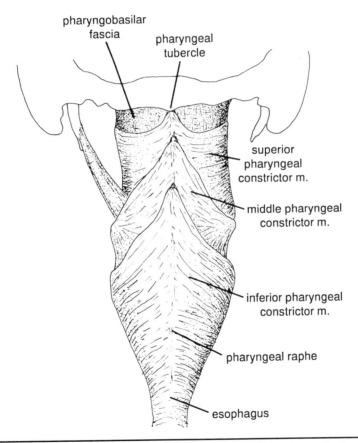

FIG. 12–4. A view of the posterior side of the pharyngeal muscular wall after the buccopharyngeal fascia has been removed.

Three other pharyngeal muscles, rather than having the more circular orientation of the constrictors, are oriented longitudinally. They are the stylopharyngeus, the palatopharyngeus, and the salpingopharyngeus. The **stylopharyngeus** arises from the styloid process, which is external to the pharynx. In order to contribute to the pharyngeal wall, it passes downward from its origin and through the gap between the superior and middle constrictor muscles. Its fibers spread out beneath the pharyngeal mucosa. They are joined by muscles arising internal to the pharynx, the **palatopharyngeus** from the soft palate and the **salpingopharyngeus** from the cartilage of the auditory tube. All the longitudinally oriented muscles have some of their fibers inserting on the superior and posterior borders of the thyroid cartilage of the larynx and others that simply

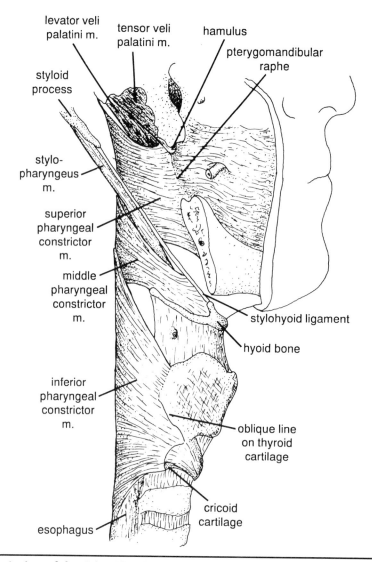

FIG. 12–5. A view of the right side of the pharynx.

spread out within the muscular wall of the pharynx. Contraction of the longitudinally oriented muscles pulls upward on the thyroid cartilage and the pharynx, thus shortening the pharynx.

MUSCULATURE OF THE SOFT PALATE (Fig. 12–6)

The soft palate contributes a significant part to the wall of the nasopharynx as well as the posterior roof of the oral cavity. It is a muscular structure. During quiet periods and when no food is being swallowed, it is in a relatively relaxed state. During swallowing or talking it must be made taut and drawn upward to close off access to the upper part of the pharynx. These two functions are performed by muscles that arise external to the pharynx. The **levator veli palat-**

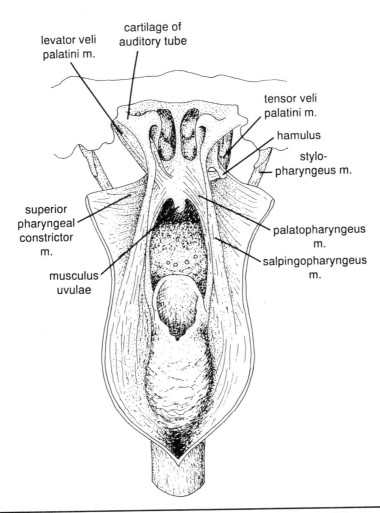

FIG. 12–6. A view into the pharynx from the posterior side. Some of the mucosa has been stripped away to reveal pharyngeal and soft palate musculature.

ini muscle arises from the cartilage of the auditory tube and adjacent petrous part of the temporal bone and enters the pharynx by passing over the upper border of the superior constrictor muscle. It descends only a short distance to enter the soft palate laterally on its superior surface. Thus, contraction of the right and left levator muscles pulls the soft palate upward and brings it into contact with the pharyngeal wall. The **tensor veli palatini** muscle, arising from the scaphoid fossa and the cartilage of the auditory tube, descends between the two pterygoid plates and makes a right-angle turn around the hamulus to enter the soft palate on its lateral side. The simultaneous contraction of the right and left tensor muscles serves to tighten the palate. The **musculus uvulae,** arising from the hard palate and connective tissue within the soft palate, seems to play little or no part in swallowing but might play a part in properly producing some sounds during phonation. The two remaining muscles, the **palatoglossus** and the **palatopharyngeus,** arise within the soft palate. The latter was mentioned above as one of the longitudinal muscles of the pharynx. The palatoglossus passes from the palate to the tongue, entering on the posterolateral side. It contributes to retraction of the tongue or depression of the soft palate (see Chapter 11).

INNERVATION OF THE PHARYNX AND SOFT PALATE (Fig. 12–7 and Figs. 4-26 and 4-27)

The **vagus** and **glossopharyngeal** nerves and the **cervical sympathetic chains** are the major sources of innervation to the pharynx and the soft palate. The **trigeminal** nerve has a relatively small contribution.

The vagus and glossopharyngeal nerves enter the neck through the jugular foramen in the skull. The glossopharyngeal nerve accompanies the stylopharyngeus muscle, which it innervates. Both these nerves and the sympathetic chain send pharyngeal branches downward toward the posterior part of the pharynx to form a **pharyngeal plexus** of nerves on the posterior surface of the middle pharyngeal constrictor muscle. From the plexus the following nerves arise: a **palatine branch of the vagus nerve,** motor in function to all muscles of the soft palate except the tensor veli palatini; **pharyngeal branches of the vagus nerve,** which supply motor innervation to the pharyngeal constrictors and salpingopharyngeus muscles and general sensory innervation to the mucosal lining of the laryngopharynx; **pharyngeal branches of the glossopharyngeal nerve** for general sensory innervation to the mucosal lining of the oropharynx and most of the nasopharynx; and **pharyngeal branches of the cervical sympathetic trunk** to the glands in the mucosal lining of the pharynx and smooth muscles in the walls of vessels.

The **trigeminal nerve** supplies the general sensory innervation to mucosa in the uppermost part of the nasopharynx with the **pharyngeal branch** from its maxillary division in the pterygopalatine fossa. The tensor veli palatini muscle is supplied by a small short branch from its mandibular division in the infratemporal fossa.

160   THE VISCERAL COMPARTMENT OF THE NECK

The larynx is a longitudinally oriented tubular structure that serves to conduct air from the laryngeal pharynx to the trachea. Its wall is, in large part, cartilaginous in order to maintain at all times an open respiratory passageway. The cartilages also serve as the skeletal structures for attachment of muscles of the larynx used in vocalization. Learning how the laryngeal cartilages are oriented with respect to one another is essential for understanding this region.

There are three **unpaired laryngeal cartilages:** the thyroid, the epiglottic, and the cricoid. The **thyroid** cartilage consists of two plates of cartilage that meet at an angle in the anterior midline, where they create the laryngeal prominence. The angle is more acute and noticeable in males and in layman's terms goes by

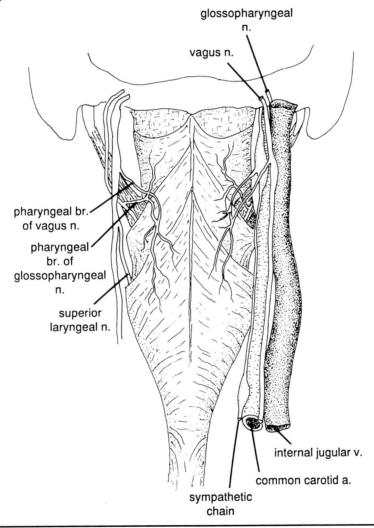

FIG. 12–7. A view of the posterior side of the pharynx to show the three contributions to the pharyngeal nerve plexus: the glossopharyngeal nerve, the vagus nerve, and the cervical sympathetic chain.

The angle is more acute and noticeable in males and in layman's terms goes by the name of "Adam's apple." The anterolateral surface of each thyroid lamina has a slight ridge, the **oblique line,** which serves for muscle attachments. Posteriorly the laminae diverge from each other, leaving a wide gap between their posterior borders, which are distinguished by prominent **superior** and **inferior horns** projecting from them. In the anterior midline the superior border has a deep **superior thyroid notch.** A tough fibrous **thyrohyoid membrane** spans the gap between the thyroid cartilage and the hyoid bone. Just below the superior thyroid notch on the posterior surface of the thyroid cartilage, a small thyroepiglottic ligament attaches to the **epiglottis,** a rather flattened spoon-shaped cartilage, which protrudes upward and slightly posteriorly from the attachment. The gap between the inferior border of the thyroid cartilage and the cricoid cartilage below is spanned by the tough cricothyroid membrane.

The **cricoid** cartilage is the only laryngeal cartilage that forms a complete ring. Anteriorly it is narrow. Posteriorly it flares out to become a broad lamina. On each side it articulates with the inferior horn of the thyroid cartilage by means of a small synovial joint strengthened by cricothyroid ligaments. Inferior to the cricoid cartilage, the trachea continues the respiratory tract through the lower part of the neck and into the thorax. It contains 16 to 20 C-shaped cartilages within its wall. The ends of each cartilage point posteriorly and have a

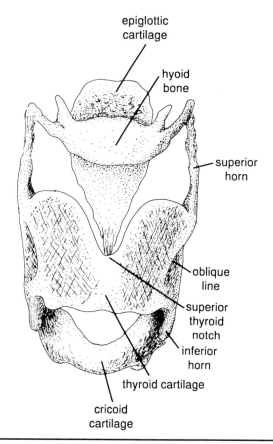

FIG. 12–8. Anterior view of the cartilages of the larynx.

band of smooth muscle spanning the gap between them. As it relaxes and contracts, it alters the diameter of the lumen of the trachea.

There are three **paired laryngeal cartilages:** the arytenoid, the corniculate, and the cuneiform. The two **arytenoids,** the largest and most important of the three, are somewhat pyramidal in shape. Each has a muscular process pointing laterally, a vocal process pointing anteriorly, and a superior process, or apex. They sit on the upper border of the broad lamina of the cricoid cartilage and articulate with it by means of a small synovial joint. The corniculate cartilages are joined by small ligaments to the apices of the arytenoid cartilages. The aryepiglottic folds of mucosa stretch between them and the sides of the epiglottis. Within the folds lie the **cuneiform** cartilages. In the posterior midline between the two arytenoid cartilages there is a small notch in the mucosa called the **interarytenoid notch.**

THE VOCAL FOLDS OF THE LARYNX (Fig. 12–11)

In addition to serving as part of the respiratory passageway, the larynx contains the vocal cords. Within the part of its lumen between the laminae of the thyroid cartilage, the mucosa is elevated over two pairs of vocal folds. The more superior ones are the **false vocal folds,** or the **vestibular folds;** the more inferior are the **true vocal folds,** or the vocal cords as they are commonly called. Between

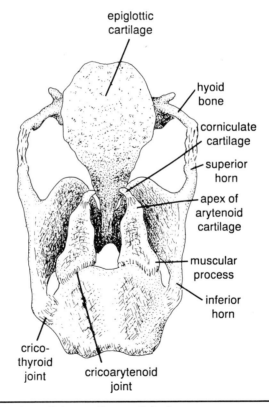

FIG. 12–9. Posterior view of the cartilages of the larynx.

the true and false folds on each side, the laryngeal lumen evaginates to create a small outpocketing called the **ventricle**. Within the true vocal folds is muscle. Within the false folds and ventricle are mucous glands. Their secretion flows downward, lubricating the vocal folds and preventing friction and irritation of the mucosa as a result of their constant movement occurring during speech and respiration.

The space in the lumen of the larynx between the right and left true vocal fold is called the **rima glottidis.** Its width changes whenever there is movement of the vocal folds. Between the entryway into the larynx, bordered by the aryepiglottic folds, and the rima glottidis, the lumen is called the **vestibule.** Inferior to the rima it is the **infraglottic space.**

MUSCLES OF THE LARYNX (Figs. 12–12 through 12–15)

The muscles of the larynx serve to thicken, stretch, tighten, spread apart, or bring closer together the true vocal folds in order to create changes in the voice or to allow greater or lesser amounts of air through to the lungs, the amount needed depending on the degree of physical exertion and the depth of respiration.

At their anterior ends, the vocal folds are attached to the inner surface of the thyroid cartilage on either side of its midline. Their posterior ends attach to the

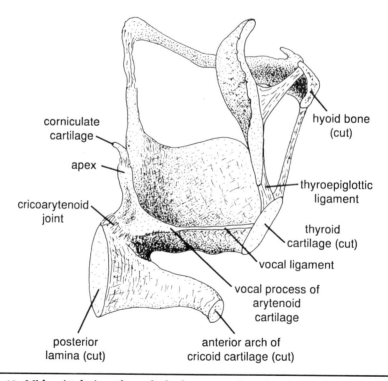

corniculate cartilage

apex

cricoarytenoid joint

hyoid bone (cut)

thyroepiglottic ligament

thyroid cartilage (cut)

vocal ligament

vocal process of arytenoid cartilage

posterior lamina (cut)

anterior arch of cricoid cartilage (cut)

FIG. 12–10. Midsagittal view through the larynx to show its supporting structures.

vocal processes of the arytenoid cartilages. Therefore, whenever the arytenoid cartilages move, there is movement of the vocal folds. When the arytenoid cartilages are pulled closer together or rotated so their muscular processes point inward, the vocal folds are brought closer together; the movement is called **adduction.** When the arytenoid cartilages are pulled apart or rotated so their vocal processes point more laterally, the vocal folds are spread apart; the movement is called **abduction.** Most of the laryngeal muscles are inserted on the arytenoid cartilages and thus are directly involved in producing movement of the vocal folds.

If the mucosa is stripped from the true vocal fold, the **vocal ligament** and the **thyroarytenoideus** muscle are seen passing from the internal surface of the thyroid cartilage to the vocal process of the arytenoid cartilage. Contraction of the muscle tilts the arytenoid cartilages forward and thickens the vocal cords, which in effect brings them closer together. The part of the thyroarytenoideus adjacent to the ligament is often called the **vocalis** muscle. Its contraction is thought to produce changes in vibration of small areas along the vocal cord.

The **transverse arytenoideus** muscle is attached to the posterior sides of both arytenoid cartilages. Its contraction pulls them toward each other, reducing the gap between the vocal folds. Working with them are the **oblique arytenoideus** muscles, which cross in the posterior midline. They have an attachment to the

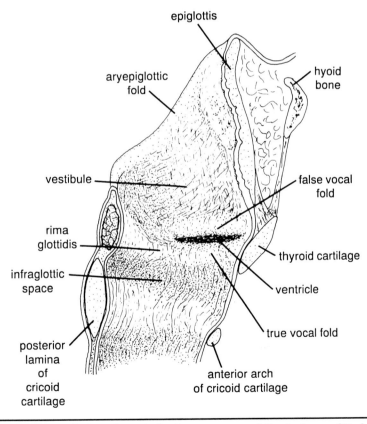

FIG. 12–11. Midsagittal view through the larynx to reveal the features of its lumen.

muscular processes but their fibers continue into the aryepiglottic folds as the aryepiglottic muscles. They contribute to pulling the epiglottis back over the entrance into the larynx during swallowing.

Posterior cricoarytenoideus muscles take a broad origin from the posterior lamina of the cricoid cartilage and pass obliquely to a narrow insertion on the muscular process of the arytenoid cartilage. Their contraction causes a rotation of the arytenoid cartilages so that the vocal process points more laterally. Thus they widen the gap between the two vocal folds and are abductors. The **lateral cricoarytenoideus** muscles originate laterally on the cricoid cartilage and pass posteriorly to insert on the muscular processes. When they contract, they rotate

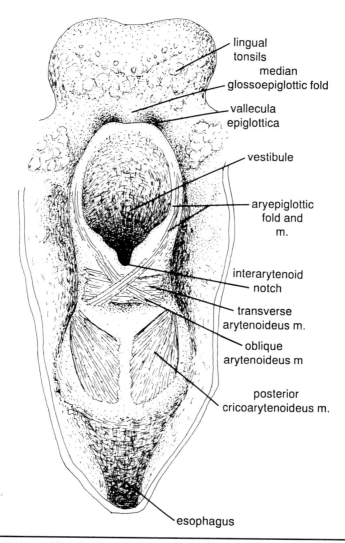

FIG. 12-12. A view of the pharyngeal surface of the larynx. The mucosa has been stripped away to reveal the laryngeal muscles.

the arytenoid cartilages so that the vocal processes point more medially. Therefore they are adductors.

On the anterior external surface of the larynx, the small **cricothyroid** muscles
originate on the arch of the cricoid cartilage and fan out superiorly to insert on
the thyroid cartilage. Their contraction pulls on the thyroid cartilage, tilting it
downward and away from the arytenoid cartilages, thus stretching and putting
tension on the vocal cords.

INNERVATION OF THE LARYNX (Figs. 12–15 and 4-27)

High in the cervical region the vagus nerve gives rise to its **superior laryngeal**
branch, which divides into external and internal laryngeal nerves. The **external
laryngeal** nerve innervates the cricothyroid muscle and contributes to innervation of the inferior pharyngeal constrictor muscle. The **internal laryngeal** nerve
pierces the thyrohyoid membrane and distributes within the larynx to supply
most of the laryngeal mucosa with general sensory innervation, extending
branches down as far as the true vocal fold.

In the most inferior part of the neck on the right side the vagus nerve crosses
the subclavian artery and gives off its **recurrent laryngeal** branch. On the left
side the recurrent laryngeal nerve arises from the thoracic part of the vagus and
travels upward to re-enter the cervical region. Both recurrent laryngeal nerves
ascend through the lower part of the neck, giving off branches to the esophagus
and the trachea. On reaching the cricothyroid joint they enter the larynx. In

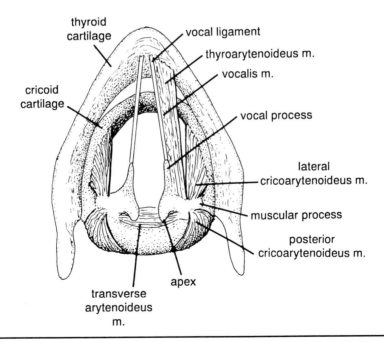

FIG. 12–13. A superior view of the larynx to show attachments and orientation of major
muscles used in vocalization.

addition to supplying motor innervation to all the laryngeal musculature except the cricothyroid muscle, they provide sensory branches to the inferior laryngeal mucosa up as far as the true vocal fold.

THE THYROID GLAND (Fig. 12–16)

The thyroid gland is one of the major endocrine glands of the body. It controls the rate of metabolism in the body tissues and thus influences a wide range of activities, including absorption in the intestines, body growth, and carbohydrate metabolism. The gland lies in the anterior part of the neck enclosed by pretracheal fascia. It has a **right lobe** and a **left lobe,** which extend superiorly to the

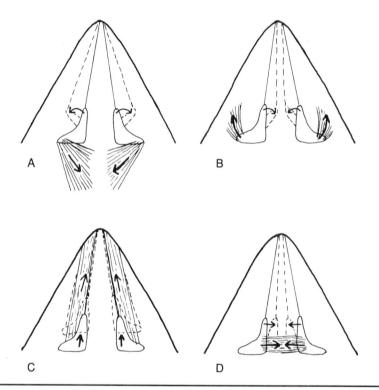

FIG. 12–14. Diagramatic illustrations of the thyroid and arytenoid cartilages and the muscles that attach to and move the latter, thus producing changes in spacing and tension of the true vocal folds.
A. The posterior cricoarytenoideus. When it contracts, the muscular process is pulled in the direction of the arrow and the vocal process rotates laterally, thus increasing the distance between the vocal folds. B. The lateral cricoarytenoideus. When it contracts, it pulls the muscular process anteriorly. The vocal process must rotate medially, thus bringing the folds closer together. C. The thyroarytenoideus. When it contracts, it pulls the arytenoid cartilage anteriorly, closer to the thyroid cartilage, thus thickening the folds and reducing tension on them. D. The transverse arytenoideus. When it contracts, it pulls both arytenoid cartilages closer to the midline, thus reducing the gap between the vocal folds.

oblique line on the thyroid cartilage. Their lower parts overlie the upper third of the trachea. The two sides are connected across the anterior midline by the glandular **isthmus,** which lies at the level of the second, third, and fourth tracheal rings. In some people a pyramidal lobe extends superiorly from the isthmus. Its length is variable.

Embedded within the posterior side of each lobe are two or more **parathyroid glands,** small, oval endocrine organs. They are important for maintaining normal calcium levels within the blood. Their absence is incompatible with life, and they must be carefully left in place in patients undergoing thyroid gland removal.

THE BLOOD SUPPLY OF THE PHARYNX, LARYNX, AND THYROID GLAND (Fig. 12–16)

Blood supply to the pharynx, larynx, and thyroid gland comes from three branches of the external carotid artery. The **ascending pharyngeal** artery, as its name implies, ascends along the lateral sides of the pharynx from its point of

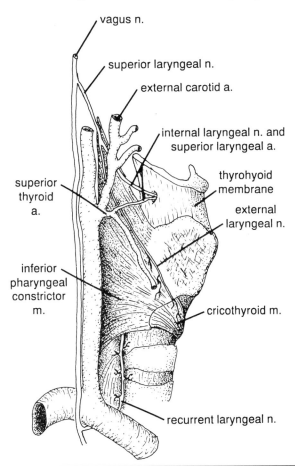

FIG. 12–15. Lateral view of the right side of the larynx and pharynx showing the nerves and some of the blood supply of the larynx.

origin; it is accompanied by the ascending palatine and tonsillar branches of the **facial** artery. The **superior thyroid** artery descends toward the superior pole of the thyroid gland, giving rise to its **superior laryngeal** branch, which enters the larynx through the thyrohyoid membrane, and terminal **thyroid** branches to the gland. In addition, the thyrocervical trunk from the subclavian artery gives rise to the **inferior thyroid** artery (Fig. 3-2), which passes to the inferior pole of the thyroid gland; its glandular branches anastomose with those of the superior thyroid artery, and it sends an **inferior laryngeal** branch into the larynx in company with the recurrent laryngeal nerve.

Venous return from these areas occurs along several routes. One route carries blood from the pharynx into the pterygoid plexus of veins in the infratemporal

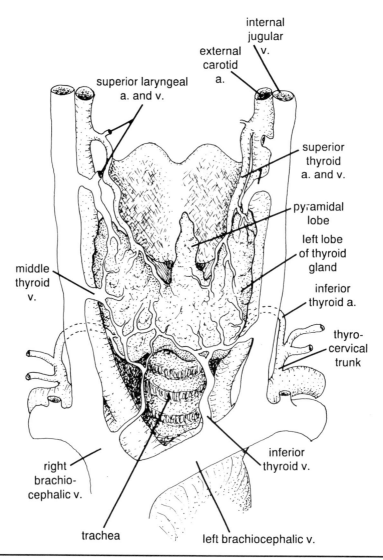

FIG. 12–16. Anterior view of the cervical visceral compartment and root of the neck. The common sources of blood supply to the thyroid gland and the larynx can be seen.

fossa, which lies just lateral to the upper part of the pharynx. Following another route, blood from pharyngeal veins passes into the internal jugular vein, which descends in the neck just lateral to the pharynx. The **superior** and **middle thyroid** veins also empty into the internal jugular (Fig. 3-3). The **inferior thyroid vein** or veins (they can be single or paired) enter the thorax to drain into the brachiocephalic veins. Both the superior and inferior thyroid veins receive a tributary from the larynx, the **superior** and **inferior laryngeal** veins, respectively.

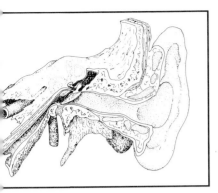

CHAPTER **13**

THE EAR

The ear is a complicated area organized for hearing. Two of its three parts, the external ear and the middle ear, are arranged so as to transmit vibrations created by sounds to the inner ear, where the cochlear nerve is stimulated. In addition, part of the inner ear is devoted to reception of the sensory information used for maintenance of equilibrium and stimulation of the vestibular nerve. Together, the cochlear and vestibular nerves make up the vestibulocochlear nerve, which transmits these two types of special sensory information from the inner ear to the brain. Except for a rather large part of the external ear, all the remainder is within the petrous part of the temporal bone.

THE EXTERNAL EAR (Fig. 13–1)

The external ear consists of the **auricle**, or pinna, and the **external auditory meatus**. The shape of the auricle is maintained with cartilage except in the **lobule** itself. It has a posterior projection overlying the external auditory meatus called the **tragus**. The deep depression posterior to the meatus is the **concha**. The concha is bordered posteriorly by a curved ridge, the **anthelix**, posterior to which is the **helix**, forming the rim around the upper and posterior margins. Superior to the lobule is the **antitragus**, separated from the tragus by the **intertragic notch**.

The external auditory meatus is a canal slightly more than an inch long leading to the cavity of the middle ear, from which it is separated by the tympanic membrane. The walls of the canal are cartilaginous in their outer one-third, and the glands of the skin lining it produce cerumen, commonly known as ear wax, which keeps the skin from drying. The remaining two-thirds of the canal lies within the temporal bone. Its anterior wall is formed by the tympanic plate of the temporal bone, situated just posterior to the mandibular neck and condyle.

General sensory innervation of the auricle is shared between the **auriculotemporal branch** of the mandibular division of the trigeminal nerve and the **great**

173

auricular branch of the cervical plexus. The external auditory meatus, including the external surface of the tympanic membrane, receives innervation from the auriculotemporal nerve. In addition, a small area of skin on the posterior auricle and meatus floor is supplied by the vagus, glossopharyngeal, and facial nerves.

THE MIDDLE EAR (Figs. 13–2 through 13–5)

The middle ear cavity is a small space whose bony walls are covered with a mucous membrane. It is most easily understood if thought of as having four walls, a roof, and a floor, although all these boundaries are irregular. The walls are medial, lateral, anterior, and posterior in position. The space is narrowest between the medial and lateral walls.

Most of the lateral wall is formed by the **tympanic membrane.** Its outer surface is covered with thin skin, the inner with mucosa, and in between is a layer of fibrous tissue that gives strength and support to the structure. Three tiny bones, or **ossicles,** articulate with each other across the space in a lateral to medial direction. The sites of articulation are synovial joints. The most lateral is the **malleus,** attached by a bony process called the **manubrium** to the tympanic membrane. It has a head process that articulates with the **incus.** A long process on the incus, in turn, articulates with the head of the **stapes.** The foot plate of the latter fits against an **oval window** on the medial wall of the middle ear cavity, closing the window. Vibrations are transmitted from the tympanic membrane via the three ossicles to the oval window. On the other side of the window, in the inner ear, lies the vestibule filled with perilymph fluid, which is set in motion by vibrations caused by movement of the footplate of the stapes. The

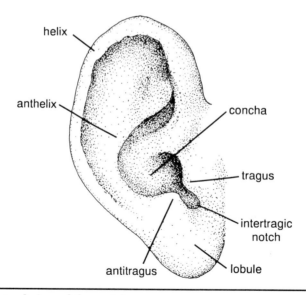

FIG. 13–1. A lateral view of the auricle.

pressure is released at the more inferiorly lying round window, which is closed by a membrane.

In the anterior wall of the middle ear cavity are two openings, one above the other. The more superior leads into a canal containing the **tensor tympani muscle.** It takes its origins from the wall of the canal, and its tendon inserts on the manubrium of the malleus. When the muscle contracts, it dampens the degree to which the tympanic membrane is deformed by the vibrations that strike it. The more inferior opening is for the **auditory tube,** also called the **eustachian tube.** It serves to connect the middle ear cavity with the pharynx so that pressure within the cavity can be kept equal to external pressure. However, it also creates a route by which infections in the pharynx can travel to the middle ear cavity. More inferiorly, the course of the **internal carotid artery** is related to the anterior wall. Because of its proximity to the auditory structures, its pulsations can sometimes be heard.

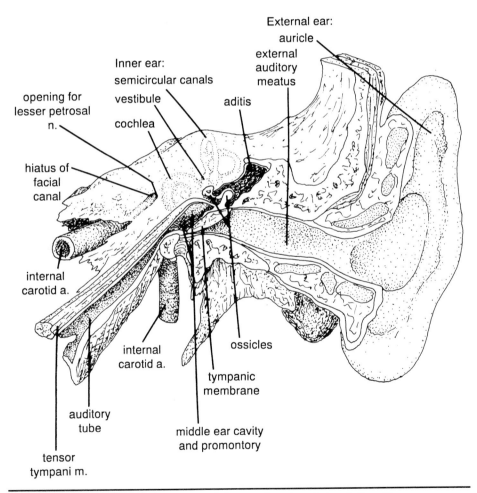

FIG. 13–2. A view of the three parts of the ear showing their relationships.

The medial wall is the bony partition between the middle ear and the inner ear. Thus, its **oval window** and **round window** mentioned above are concerned with conveying sound waves to the inner ear and relieving the pressure they cause. The protrusion of the **promontory** between the two windows into the middle ear cavity is caused by the position of the cochlea within the inner ear. The **tympanic plexus** of nerves lies against the promontory and is formed by the tympanic branch of the glossopharyngeal nerve for innervation of the mucosal lining of the middle ear. From this plexus the lesser petrosal nerve arises, which carries parasympathetic preganglionic fibers to the otic ganglion, where they synapse (Chapter 9 and Fig. 5–4). Above the oval window lies the **facial prominence,** caused by the facial canal, which curves downward when it reaches the posterior wall in order to carry the facial nerve through the temporal bone to its point of emergence from the skull at the stylomastoid foramen.

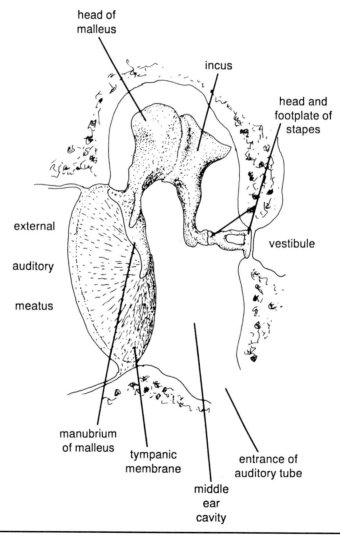

FIG. 13–3. The ossicles and the middle ear cavity.

The upper part of the posterior wall is incomplete; its opening, the **aditus ad antrum,** leads posteriorly into the **antrum,** which is the entryway into air cells within the mastoid part of the temporal bone. The mucosal lining of the middle ear cavity is continuous with the lining of the mastoid air cells. On the posterior wall is a small hollow elevation called the **pyramidal eminence,** within which arises the **stapedius muscle.** Its tiny tendon inserts into the neck of the stapes, and its contractions control the degree of movement of the footplate of the stapes against the perilymph fluid on the other side of the oval window. The facial nerve descends within the posterior wall, although the **facial canal** forms no prominence there. It gives rise to the **nerve to the stapedius** muscle and, still more inferiorly, to the **chorda tympani nerve** (Fig. 5–3), which enters the middle ear cavity, passes across the tympanic membrane, and exits anteriorly. This nerve carries taste sensations from the tongue and parasympathetic innervation for secretion of the sublingual and submandibular salivary glands.

The bony roof, called the **tegmen tympani,** is thin and separates the middle ear cavity from the middle cranial fossa. Infections within the middle ear can

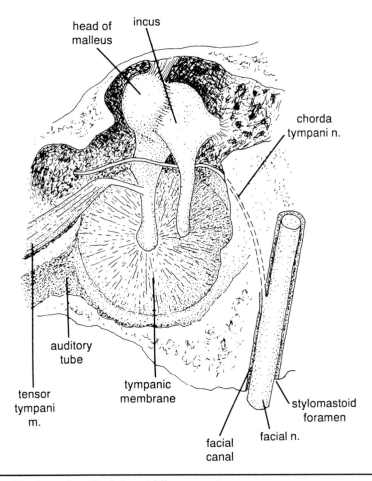

FIG. 13–4. The lateral wall of the middle ear cavity.

erode through the roof and endanger the meninges and brain within the cranial cavity.

The floor of the middle ear cavity is narrow. Just beneath it lies the **jugular fossa** containing the jugular bulb. This is where the internal jugular vein begins by receiving most of the venous drainage from the dural venous sinuses within the cranial cavity.

In addition to the **nerve to the stapedius muscle** from the facial nerve, there are branches from two other cranial nerves innervating structures within the middle ear. The **nerve to the tensor tympani** muscle is a branch from the trigeminal's mandibular division in the infratemporal fossa, which lies just lateral to the muscle's origin. The **tympanic branch**, mentioned above, arises from the glossopharyngeal nerve in the jugular foramen and penetrates the bone between the jugular fossa and carotid canal to enter the middle ear.

THE INNER EAR (Fig. 13–6)

The inner ear consists of a system of canals within the bone called the **bony labyrinth** in which is suspended a system of thin-walled ducts called the **membranous labyrinth. Perilymph,** the fluid within the canals, helps suspend

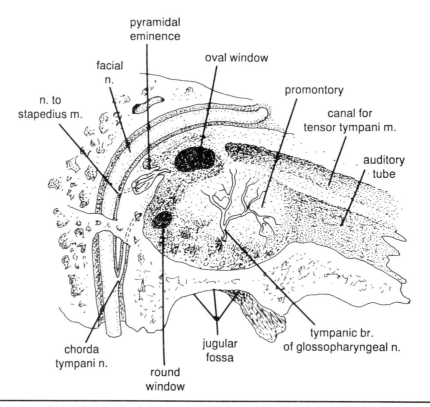

FIG. 13–5. The medial wall of the middle ear cavity.

the ducts and transmits the waves generated by the footplate of the stapes at the oval window. **Endolymph** fills the ducts.

The **cochlea** is the part of the bony labyrinth devoted to the special sense of hearing. It is spiralled like the shell of a snail for two and one-half turns. The membranous **cochlear duct** within it, likewise spiralled, contains sensory receptors bathed with endolymph. When the footplate of the stapes generates pressure in the perilymph at the oval window, flow of the perilymph causes movement of part of the cochlear duct and endolymph, resulting in stimulation of the receptors. The pressure is relieved at the round window, where the closing membrane bulges outward toward the middle ear cavity. The receptors transfer the stimulus to the short dendritic processes of the cochlear neurons, whose cell bodies lie within the spiral of the central bony core of the cochlea. For this reason, they make up what is known as either the **spiral ganglion** or the cochlear ganglion (see Fig. 4-25).

The remainder of the labyrinth system is devoted to the special sense of equilibrium. It consists of the membranous **semicircular ducts** suspended within the **semicircular canals** and the membranous **saccule** and **utricle** within the **vestibule.** There are three semicircular canals, an anterior, a posterior, and a lateral. Each has an enlarged end known as the **ampulla.** The canals open into the vestibule. The shape of the ducts and their ampullae conforms to that of the canals. Movement of the endolymph caused by turning the head, changing the position of the head, and rapid linear acceleration and deceleration stimulates special receptor cells located at specific spots within the ampullae, utricle, or saccule. These receptors stimulate the short dendrites of the vestibular neurons, whose cell bodies lie nearby in the **vestibular ganglion** inside the internal auditory meatus (see Fig. 4-25).

The vestibule is positioned between the cochlea anteriorly and semicircular canals posteriorly. The oval window, also called the **vestibular window,** is on its lateral wall. It is the perilymph at this location that receives the pressure from the footplate of the stapes. Within the vestibule the **utricle** receives endolymph from the semicircular ducts, the **saccule** has a small connection with the cochlear duct, and the **utriculosaccular duct** connects utricle and saccule. Thus the membranous labyrinths of the auditory and vestibular systems are connected. Excess endolymph is eliminated from the duct system via the **endolymphatic sac,** which extends from the utriculosaccular duct through the bony **vestibular aqueduct** in the petrous part of the temporal bone and comes to lie beneath the dura in the posterior cranial fossa. There is a separate drainage site for perilymph near the jugular foramen.

THE BLOOD SUPPLY OF THE EAR

The auricle and external auditory meatus receive their blood supply from the **superficial temporal** and **posterior auricular** branches of the external carotid artery (Fig. 8–9) and venous drainage from their accompanying veins (Fig. 8–1), which drain into the retromandibular and external jugular veins. The **deep auricular** branch of the maxillary artery also supplies the meatus in its most proximal part, and its accompanying vein drains into the pterygoid venous plexus in the infratemporal fossa.

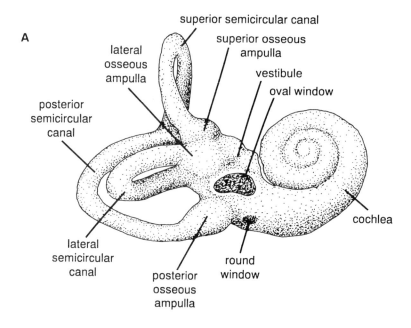

A

superior semicircular canal

superior osseous ampulla

lateral osseous ampulla

vestibule

oval window

posterior semicircular canal

cochlea

lateral semicircular canal

posterior osseous ampulla

round window

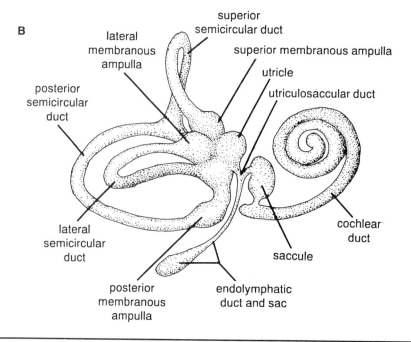

B

superior semicircular duct

lateral membranous ampulla

superior membranous ampulla

utricle

utriculosaccular duct

posterior semicircular duct

cochlear duct

lateral semicircular duct

saccule

posterior membranous ampulla

endolymphatic duct and sac

FIG. 13-6.
A. The right osseous labyrinth from the anterolateral side. **B.** The right membranous labyrinth from the anterolateral side.

Although numerous very small arteries supply the middle ear, its major arteries are the **anterior tympanic** branch of the maxillary artery (Fig. 9–14) and the **stylomastoid** branch of the posterior auricular. Veins accompany the arteries. The major drainage site is the pterygoid venous plexus.

The blood supply to the inner ear is from the **labyrinthine** branch of the basilar artery (Fig. 4-15); it enters the internal auditory meatus with the facial and vestibulocochlear nerves.

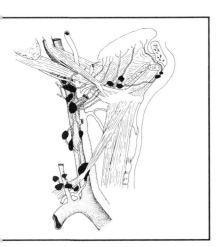

CHAPTER 14

OVERVIEW OF THE LYMPHATIC DRAINAGE OF THE HEAD AND NECK

Fluid is found within the tissues of the body filling in the space between the cells and the various fibrous components of connective tissue. It contains cell nutrients, which have come from the blood capillaries, and waste products from the cells. It is constantly being replenished and therefore must be eliminated into either the venous or the lymphatic capillaries. Once the fluid enters the latter, it is called lymph. It is watery and contains proteins and lymphocytes, or white blood cells. In addition, infectious material in the tissues, including bacteria and cancer cells, can be transported through the lymph vessels. The lymph capillaries drain into larger lymph vessels, which ultimately drain into the venous system. However, their paths are interrupted along the way by several groups of lymph nodes, where the lymph is filtered and many lymphocytes are added to the fluid. Bacteria sequestered within the lymph nodes can cause them to become sites of infection. Proliferation of the cancer cells that become trapped within them can block the entering lymph vessels and cause swelling in the tissues drained by those vessels.

The first nodes through which lymph drains from a particular area are called the primary nodes for that site. One group of nodes can be the primary nodes for lymph from one site but secondary or tertiary nodes for lymph from other sites. Pathologic nodes can become enlarged enough to be palpable through the skin. A knowledge of the areas drained by such nodes can lead to detection of the source of the problem. However, it is important to understand that areas adjacent to the midline of the body often have some lymph-collecting vessels that drain to the opposite side.

Ultimately the lymph on each side of the head and neck enters the venous system at the junction of the internal jugular vein with the subclavian, where the brachiocephalic vein forms. Lymph entering at this point on the left side enters via the **thoracic duct,** which is the largest lymphatic vessel in the body. It collects lymph from both lower limbs, the abdomen, and the left side of the thorax, the left upper limb, and the left side of the head and neck. On the right side, the **right lymphatic duct** empties into the venous system, collecting lymph from the right side of the thorax and head and neck and the right upper limb. Thus the veins play a major part in metastasis, or dispersal of cancer cells throughout the body.

Deep to the sternocleidomastoid muscle, the largest group of lymph nodes in the neck lies along the internal jugular vein. They form the **deep cervical chain of nodes** (Fig. 14–1). Those that lie superior to the omohyoid muscle comprise the **superior deep cervical nodes;** those lying inferior to it form the much smaller group of **inferior deep cervical nodes.** Lymph flows downward through the nodes

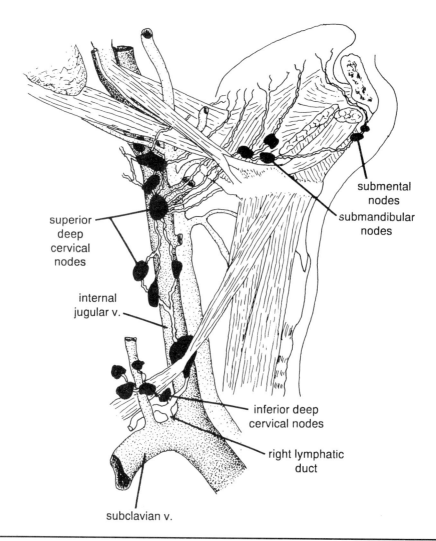

FIG. 14–1. Deep cervical lymph nodes.

and the lymphatic vessels that connect them toward the point where it enters the venous system. Tributaries to the vessels along their descending course bring in lymph from other parts of the head and neck.

In their most superior part, the superior deep cervical nodes receive lymph from the **superficial cervical nodes** (Fig. 14–2) situated along the external jugular vein just inferior to the ear and superficial to the sternocleidomastoid muscle. The groups of nodes that drain into this superficial group are located in the more superficial parts of the head. They are the occipital nodes draining the lymph vessels from the posterior scalp and the posterior auricular and preauricular (or parotid) nodes draining some of the scalp and the external ear.

Other groups of nodes draining into the superior deep cervical nodes are the **parotid nodes,** which lie within and around the parotid gland, draining the superficial face superior and anterior to the gland and, more deeply, some of the pharynx; **retropharyngeal nodes,** draining walls of the nasal cavity and nasopharynx; **deep facial nodes,** which lie in the infratemporal fossa along the maxillary artery and drain the fossa as well as some of the nasopharynx; and **submandibular nodes,** which lie closely associated with the submandibular gland. The superior deep cervical nodes also receive lymph from the palate and the upper parts of the larynx and are the primary nodes for the posterior part of the tongue.

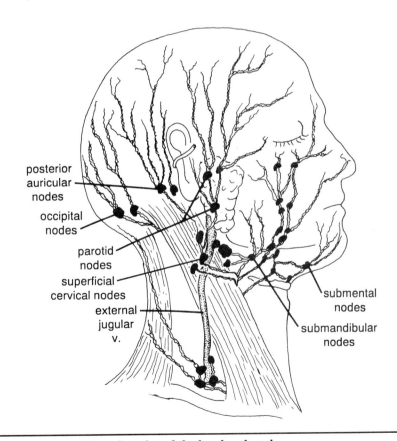

FIG. 14–2. Superficial lymph nodes of the head and neck.

The **submandibular nodes** are an important group. They drain the facial nodes of the superficial face, which receive lymph from the infraorbital region. They drain the **submental nodes,** which are primary nodes for lymph from the tip of the tongue, the mandibular incisors, and the anterior part of the floor of the mouth and lower lip. They are the primary nodes for the lateral part of the body of the tongue and most of the teeth. They receive lymph from the anterior nose, cheek, hard palate, upper lip, the lateral parts of the lower lip, and the floor of the mouth.

The **inferior deep cervical nodes** receive lymph vessels descending from the superior deep cervical nodes as well as the inferior parts of the larynx, the trachea, and some of the occipital region of the scalp. They are the last group through which lymph passes before entering the right lymphatic duct or the thoracic duct.

INDEX

Numbers in **BOLD** type refer to illustrations.

innervation of, 101
suprahyoid triangles and, 98

N

Nasal
  bones, 130
    anterior view and, 7
  cavity,
    bony structure of, 130-132
    head midsagittal section and, **155**
  nerve, external, skin innervation and, 84
  septum, 130
    arteries of, **138**
    nerves of, **136**
  wall,
    lateral,
      arteries of, **137**
      bones of, **133**
      nerves of, **135**
      sinus drainage sites on, 132-135, **134**
Nasalis muscle, facial expression and, 80
Nasociliary nerve
  branches, 75
  nerve fibers, sympathetic postganglionic and, 75-76
  orbit and, 74-75
Nasolacrimal duct, 69
Nasopalatine
  foramen, nasopalatine nerve and, 150
  nerve,
    oral cavity blood supply and, 151
    oral cavity innervation and, 150
    pterygopalatine fossa and, 136
Nasopharynx
  air breathed and, 153
  distinguishing features, 154-155
  innervation of, 160
  trigeminal nerve and, 160
Neck
  arterial supply for, 21-22, 24
    views of, **22**
  described, 91
  fascial compartments of, 94-97
    fascia of, deep, **95**, 95
  infrahyoid muscles of, innervation of, 101, **102**
  lymphatic drainage of, 183-186
  nervous system,
    parasympathetic and, 60
    sympathetic and, 60, **61**
  root of, structures of, **107**
  spinal nerves, cervical, 32-33
  suboccipital region of, **105**, 105-106
  superficial, 91-94

  cervical plexus cutaneous branches of, **93**
  cutaneous nerves and, **93**
  superficial veins of, **92**
  suprahyoid muscles of, innervation of, 101, **102**
  sympathetic chains of, cervical, **61**, 106, **107**, 108
  triangles of, 97
    anterior, **97**, **98**, 98-102
    carotid, 100-101, **102**
    digastric, 98
    posterior, **97**, 102-105
    submandibular, 98, **102**
    submental, 98
    suboccipital, 106
  venous drainage of, 24, 26
  visceral compartment of,
    blood supply to, 169-171
    larynx, 161-169
    pharynx, 153-159, 160
    soft palate, 159-160
    transverse section of, **154**
Nerve
  ganglion and, 27
  mixed, 28
  see also specific names of nerves
Nervous system
  autonomic. *See* Autonomic nervous system
  divisions of, 27
  see also Central nervous system; Peripheral nervous system
Neurons
  described, 27
  illustrated, **28**
Nose, facial muscles of, 80-81
Nucleus, neuron cell bodies and, 27

O

Oblique
  arytenoideus muscles, 165
  superior and inferior muscles, 71
    oculomotor nerve and, 73
    trochlear nerve and, 73
Obliquus capitis
  inferior, suboccipital triangle and, 106
  superior, suboccipital triangle and, 106
Occipital
  artery, carotid triangle and, 101
  auricular artery, 22
  bone,
    basilar sinus and, 39
    dorsum sellae and, 12
    lateral view and, 7, 9
    nasopharynx and, 154
    skull base and, 10

Z

Zygomatic
  arch, 109
    infratemporal fossa and, 112
  bone,
    anterior view and, 7
    orbit and, 67
    zygomaticofacial foramen and, 10
    zygomaticotemporal foramen and,
      10
  nerve,
    orbit and, 76
    parotid gland and, 83

pterygopalatine fossa and, 137
Zygomaticoalveolar crest, infratemporal
    fossa and, 112
  lateral view of skull and, **9**
Zygomaticofacial
  foramen,
    contents of, 15t
    zygomatic bone and, 10
  nerve, skin innervation and, 86
Zygomaticotemporal
  nerve, skin innervation and, 86
  zygomatic bone and, 10
Zygomaticus major and minor muscles
    facial expression and, 81

Volume II   1877 to the Present

American Experiences

Readings in American History

Second Edition

Volume II   1877 to the Present

American Experiences

Readings in American History

Second Edition

■

Randy Roberts
Purdue University

■

James S. Olson
Sam Houston State University

SCOTT, FORESMAN/LITTLE, BROWN HIGHER EDUCATION
A Division of Scott, Foresman and Company
Glenview, Illinois   London, England

3 Library of Congress, Brady Collection **8** *Harper's Weekly,* Oct. 24, 1874 **19** Library of Congress **21** The Kansas State Historical Society, Topeka **25** Library of Congress **32** Culver Pictures **56** Culver Pictures **64** Library of Congress **71** Culver Pictures **73** Library of Congress **82** Illinois Labor History Society **85** Historical Pictures Service **97, 106** Brown Brothers **119** Trustees of the Imperial War Museum, London **123** © JB&R Inc., *Old Life* **127** Culver Pictures **140** UPI **153** Culver Pictures **161** UPI **171** Dorothea Lange, The Oakland Museum **175** Brown Brothers **183** Austin History Center, Austin (Texas) Public Library **199** SF **213** Wide World **220** U.S. Army **227** U.S. Navy **230** UPI **251** Wayne Miller/Magnum Photos **261** Wide World **271** The Lester Glassner Collection **275** *The Chicago Tribune,* photo by Michael Budrys **282** Wide World **298** Culver Pictures **310** Susan Meiselas/Magnum Photos **319** Wide World **329** Peter Menzel/Stock, Boston

LIBRARY OF CONGRESS CATALOGING-IN-PUBLICATION DATA
American experiences/[edited by] Randy Roberts, James S. Olson.—
  2nd ed.
    p. cm.
  Includes bibliographies.
  Contents: v. 1. 1607-1877—v. 2. 1877 to the present.
  ISBN 0-673-38862-X (v. 1): $12.00.—ISBN 0-673-38863-8 (v. 2):
$12.00
  1. United States—History. I. Roberts, Randy
II. Olson, James Stuart
E178.6.A395 1990
973—dc20   89-10428
                                    CIP

Preface

American history instructors enjoy talking about the grand sweep of the American past. Many note the development of unique traditions such as the American political tradition and the American diplomatic tradition. They employ the article "the" so often that they depict history as a seamless garment and Americans as all cut from the same fabric. Nothing could be further from the truth. America is a diverse country, and its population is the most ethnically varied in the world—white and black, Indian and Chicano, rich and poor, male and female. No single tradition can encompass this variety. *American Experiences* shows the complexity and richness of the nation's past by focusing on the people themselves—how they coped with, adjusted to, or rebelled against America. The readings examine them as they worked and played, fought and made love, lived and died.

We designed *American Experiences* as a supplement to the standard textbooks used in college survey classes in American history. Unlike other readers, it covers ground not usually found in textbooks. For example, instead of an essay on the effect of the New Deal, it includes a selection on life in the Hill Country of Texas before rural electrification. Instead of a discussion of the political impact of the Populist Movement, it explores the Wizard of Oz as a Populist parable. In short, it presents different slants on standard and not-so-standard topics.

We have tested each essay in classrooms so that *American Experiences* reflects not only our interest in social history but student interests in American history in general. We selected essays that are readable, interesting, and help illuminate important aspects of America's past. For example, to show the nature of the class system in the South and to introduce the topic of southern values, we selected one essay on gambling and horse racing in the Old South and another on gouging matches in the southern backcountry. As an introduction to the conventional and medical view of women in the late nineteenth century, we selected an essay about Lizzie Borden. Each essay, then, serves at least two purposes: to tell a particular story well, and to help illuminate the social or political landscape of America.

This reader presents a balanced picture of the experiences of Americans. The characters in these volumes are not exclusively white males from the Northeast, whose eyes are continually focused on Boston, New York, and Washington. Although their stories are certainly important, so, too, are the stories of blacks adjusting with dignity to a barbarous labor system, Chicanos coming to terms with Anglo society, and women striving for increased opportunities in a sexually restrictive society. We have looked at all of these stories and, in doing so, we have assumed that Americans express themselves in a variety of ways, through work, sex, and games, as well as politics and diplomacy.

During the last three years, we have solicited a variety of opinions, from colleagues and students, about the selections for *American Experiences*. Based on that feedback we have made a number of changes in the Second Edition, always with the intention of selecting articles that undergraduate students will find interesting and informative. The new articles for this second volume of *American Experiences*, Second Edition, include Dee Brown's "Day of the Longhorns," Robert Maddox's "Teddy Roosevelt and the Rough Riders," a selection from Upton Sinclair's *The Jungle*, Estelle Freedman's " 'Uncontrolled Desires': The Response to the Sexual Psychopath, 1920–1960," David Burner's piece on John F. Kennedy and the civil rights movement, and Randy Roberts and James S. Olson's "Perfect Bodies, Eternal Youth."

Each volume of *American Experiences* is divided into standard chronological and topical parts. Each part is introduced by a brief discussion of the major themes of the period or topic. In turn, each individual selection is preceded by a short discussion of how it fits into the part's general theme. We employed this method to give students some guidance through the complexity of the experiences of Americans. At the conclusion of each selection is a series of study questions and a brief bibliographic essay. These are intended to further the usefulness of *American Experiences* for students as well as teachers.

Randy Roberts
James S. Olson

Contents

THE AGE OF CONSPIRACY AND CONFORMITY:
INVASION OF THE BODY SNATCHERS
Stuart Samuels
page 264

Part Seven

■■   COMING APART: ■■
1960–1990
page 274

JOHN F. KENNEDY AND THE BLACK REVOLUTION
David Burner
page 276

DR. STRANGELOVE (1964):
NIGHTMARE COMEDY AND THE
IDEOLOGY OF LIBERAL CONSENSUS
Charles Maland
page 290

THE WOUNDED GENERATION:
THE TWENTY-SEVEN MILLION MEN
OF VIETNAM
Lawrence M. Baskir and William A. Strauss
page 304

THE ELVIS PRESLEY PHENOMENON
Greil Marcus
page 312

PERFECT BODIES, ETERNAL YOUTH:
THE OBSESSION OF MODERN AMERICA
Randy Roberts and James S. Olson
page 322

Part One

RECONSTRUCTION
AND
THE WEST

Although the Civil War did not begin as a crusade against slavery, it ended that way. The Emancipation Proclamation and Thirteenth Amendment to the Constitution destroyed human bondage in the United States, and during Reconstruction Republicans worked diligently to extend full civil rights to southern blacks. Despite the concerted opposition of President Andrew Johnson, the Radical Republicans in Congress pushed through a strong legislative program. The Civil Rights Act of 1866 and the Fourteenth and Fifteenth Amendments to the Constitution were all basically designed to bring the emancipated slaves into the political arena and build a respectable Republican Party in the South. Both of those goals were stillborn. When Congress removed the troops from the last southern states in 1877, the old planter elite resumed its control of southern politics. They disfranchised and relegated blacks to second-class citizenship, and the South became solidly "Democratic." The South had indeed been brought back into the Union, but the grandiose hopes for a true reconstruction of southern life would not be realized for more than a century.

Genuine change in the southern social structure required more than most Northerners could accept. Confiscation and redistribution of the plantations among poor whites and former slaves was too brazen an assault on property rights; northern

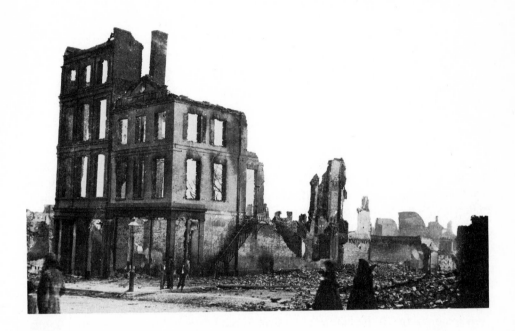

businessmen feared that someday their own workers might demand similar treatment. Nor were Northerners prepared for real social change. Advocating political rights for blacks was one thing; true social equality was quite another. Prejudice ran deep in the American psyche, too deep in the 1870s to allow for massive social change. Finally, most Americans were growing tired of the debate over civil rights and becoming preoccupied with business, money, and economic growth. Heavy industry in the East and vacant land in the West were absorbing their energies.

Just as Reconstruction was coming to an end, out west, ambitious farmers were rapidly settling the frontier, anxious to convert the land into an agricultural empire. Civilization was forever replacing a wilderness mentality with familiar political, economic, and social institutions. Already the "Old West" was becoming the stuff of which nostalgia is made. Normal, if somewhat eccentric, people were being transformed into larger than life heroes as American society tried to maintain its rural, individualistic roots. Back East, cities and factories were announcing a future of bureaucracies, interest groups, crowds, and enormous industrial production. America would never be the same again. The cult of Western heroes helped people forget the misery of the Civil War and vicariously preserve a disappearing way of life.

THE KNIGHTS OF THE RISING SUN

Allen W. Trelease

The Civil War, which started in 1861 and ended in 1865, was like a nightmare come true for most Americans. Four years later, the nightmare had come true. More than 600,000 young men were dead, countless others wounded and permanently maimed, and the South a prostrate ruin. For the next twelve years, northern Republicans tried to "reconstruct" the South in a chaotic crusade mixing retribution, corruption, and genuine idealism. Intent on punishing white southerners for their disloyalty, northern Republicans, especially the Radicals, also tried to extend full civil rights—through the Fourteenth and Fifteenth Amendments—to former slaves. For a variety of reasons, the attempt at giving equality to southern blacks failed, and by 1877 political power in the South reverted to the white elite.

A major factor in the failure of Radical Republicans to "reconstruct" the South was the rise of the Ku Klux Klan. Enraged at the very thought of black political power, Klansmen resorted to intimidation and violence, punishing southern blacks even suspected of sympathizing with Radicals' goals for the South. In "The Knights of the Rising Sun," historian Allen W. Trelease describes Klan activities in Texas during the late 1860s. Isolated from the main theaters of the Civil War, much of Texas remained unreconstructed, and the old white elite, along with their Klan allies, succeeded in destroying every vestige of black political activity and in eliminating the Republican Party from the political life of the state.

Large parts of Texas remained close to anarchy through 1868. Much of this was politically inspired despite the fact that the state was not yet reconstructed and took no part in the national election. In theory the Army was freer to take a direct hand in maintaining order than was true in the states which had been readmitted, but the shortage of troops available for this duty considerably lessened that advantage. At least twenty counties were involved in the Ku Klux terror, from Houston north to the Red River. In Houston itself Klan activity was limited to the holding of monthly meetings in a gymnasium and posting notices on lampposts, but in other places there was considerable violence.

By mid-September disguised bands had committed several murders in Trinity County, where two lawyers and both justices of the peace in the town of Sumter were well known as Klansmen. Not only did the crimes go unpunished, but Conservatives used them to force a majority of the Negroes to swear allegiance to the Democratic party; in return they received the familiar protection papers supposedly guaranteeing them against further outrage. "Any one in this community opposed to the Grand Cyclops and his imps is in danger of his life," wrote a local Republican in November. In Washington County the Klan sent warning notices to Republicans and committed at least one murder. As late as January 1869 masked parties were active around Palestine, shaving heads, whipping, and shooting among the black population, as well as burning down their houses. The military arrested five or six men for these offenses, but the Klan continued to make the rounds of Negroes' and Union men's houses, confiscating both guns and money. Early in November General J. J. Reynolds, military commander in the state, declared in a widely quoted report that "civil law east of

"Texas: The Knights of the Rising Sun" from *White Terror: The Ku Klux Klan Conspiracy and Southern Reconstruction* by Allen W. Trelease. Copyright © 1971 by Allen W. Trelease. Reprinted by permission of the author.

the Trinity river is almost a dead letter" by virtue of the activities of Ku Klux Klans and similar organizations. Republicans had been publicly slated for assassination and forced to flee their homes, while the murder of Negroes was too common to keep track of. These lawless bands, he said, were "evidently countenanced, or at least not discouraged, by a majority of the white people in the counties where [they] are most numerous. They could not otherwise exist." These statements did not endear the general to Conservative Texans, but they were substantially true.

The worst region of all, as to both Klan activity and general banditry, remained northeast Texas. A correspondent of the Cincinnati *Commercial* wrote from Sulphur Springs early in January 1869:

Armed bands of banditti, thieves, cut-throats and assassins infest the country; they prowl around houses, they call men out and shoot or hang them, they attack travellers upon the road, they seem almost everywhere present, and are ever intent upon mischief. You cannot pick up a paper without reading of murders, assassinations and robbery. . . . And yet not the fourth part of the truth has been told; not one act in ten is reported. Go where you will, and you will hear of fresh murders and violence. . . . The civil authority is powerless—the military insufficient in number, while hell has transferred its capital from pandemonium to Jefferson, and the devil is holding high carnival in Gilmer, Tyler, Canton, Quitman, Boston, Marshall and other places in Texas.

Judge Hardin Hart wrote Governor Pease in September to say that on account of "a regularly organized band which has overrun the country" he could not hold court in Grayson, Fannin, and Hunt counties without a military escort.

Much of this difficulty was attributable to outlaw gangs like those of Ben Bickerstaff and Cullen Baker, but even their activities were often racially and politically inspired, with Negroes and Union men the chief sufferers. Army officers and soldiers reported that most of the population at Sulphur Springs was organized into Ku Klux clubs affiliated with the Democratic party and some of the outlaws called themselves Ku Klux Rangers. At Clarksville a band of young men calling themselves Ku Klux broke up a Negro school and forced the teacher to flee the state.

White Conservatives around Paris at first took advantage of Klan depredations among Negroes by issuing protection papers to those who agreed to join the Democratic party. But the marauding reached such proportions that many freedmen fled their homes and jobs, leaving the crops untended. When a body of Klansmen came into town early in September, apparently to disarm more blacks, some of the leading citizens warned them to stop. The freedmen were not misbehaving, they said, and if they needed disarming at a later time the local people would take care of it themselves. Still the raiding continued, and after a sheriff's posse failed to catch the culprits the farmers in one neighborhood banded together to oppose them by force. (Since the Klan had become sacred among Democrats, these men claimed that the raiding was done by an unauthorized group using its name. They carefully denied any idea of opposing the Klan itself.) Even this tactic was ineffective so far as the county as a whole was concerned, and the terror continued at least into November. The Freedmen's Bureau agent, Colonel DeWitt C. Brown, was driven away from his own farm thirty miles from Paris and took refuge in town. There he was subjected to constant threats of assassination by Klansmen or their sympathizers. From where he stood the Klan seemed to be in almost total command.

The Bureau agent at Marshall (like his predecessor in the summer) suspected that the planters themselves were implicated in much of the terrorism. By driving Negroes from their homes just before harvest time the Klan enabled many landowners to collect the crop without having to pay the laborers' share.

Jefferson and Marion County remained the center of Ku Klux terrorism, as the Cincinnati

reporter pointed out. A garrison of twenty-six men under Major James Curtis did little to deter violence. Bands of hooded men continued to make nocturnal depredations on Negroes in the surrounding countryside during September and October as they had for weeks past. "Whipping the freedmen, robbing them of their arms, driving them off plantations, and murdering whole families are of daily, and nightly occurrence," wrote the local Bureau agent at the end of October, "all done by disguised parties whom no one can testify to. The civil authorities never budge an inch to try and discover these midnight marauders and apparently a perfect apathy exists throughout the whole community regarding the general state of society. Nothing but martial law can save this section as it is at present. . . ." Inside town, Republicans hardly dared go outdoors at night, and for several weeks the county judge, who was afraid to go home even in the daytime, slept at the Army post. The local Democratic newspapers, including the *Ultra Ku Klux*, encouraged the terror by vying with one another in the ferocity of their denunciations of Republicans.

Major Curtis confirmed this state of affairs in a report to General Reynolds:

Since my arrival at this Post . . . [in mid-September] I have carefully observed the temper of the people and studied their intentions. I am constrained to say that neither are pacific. The amount of unblushing fraud and outrage perpetrated upon the negroes is hardly to be believed unless witnessed. Citizens who are esteemed respectable do not hesitate to take every unfair advantage. My office is daily visited by large numbers of unfortunates who have had money owing them, which they have been unable to obtain. The moral sense of the community appears blunted and gray headed apologists for such men as Baker and Bickerstaff can be met on all the street corners. . . . The right of franchise in this section is a farce. Numbers of negroes have been killed for daring to be Radicals, and their houses have so often been broken into by their Ku Klux neighbors in search of arms that they are now pretty well defenceless. The civil officers cannot and will not punish these outrages. Cavalry armed with double barrelled shotguns would soon scour the country and these desperadoes be met on their own ground. They do not fear the arms that the troops now have, for they shoot from behind hedges and fences or at night and then run. No more notice is taken here of the death of a Radical negro than of a mad dog. A democratic negro however, who was shot the other day by another of his stripe, was followed to his grave through the streets of this city by a long procession in carriages, on horseback, and on foot. I saw some of the most aristocratic and respectable white men in this city in the procession.

On the same night that Curtis wrote, the new Grand Officers of the Knights of the Rising Sun were installed in the presence of a crowd of 1,200 or 1,500 persons. "The town was beautifully illuminated," a newspaper reported, "and the Seymour Knights and the Lone Star Club turned out in full uniform, with transparencies and burners, in honor of the occasion." Sworn in as Grand Commander for the ensuing twelve months was Colonel William P. Saufley, who doubled as chairman of the Marion County Democratic executive committee. Following the installation "able and patriotic speeches" were delivered by several notables, including a Democratic Negro.

As usual, the most hated Republican was the one who had the greatest Negro following. This was Captain George W. Smith, a young Union army veteran from New York who had settled in Jefferson as a merchant at the end of the war. His business failed, but the advent of Radical Reconstruction opened the prospect of a successful political career; at the age of twenty-four Smith was elected to the state constitutional convention by the suffrage of the Negro majority around Jefferson. At the convention, according to a perhaps overflattering posthumous account, he was recognized as one of the abler members. "In his daily life he was correct, almost austere. He nev-

er drank, smoked, chewed, nor used profane language." However, "he was odious as a negro leader, as a radical, as a man who could not be cowed, nor scared away." Smith may also have alienated his fellow townspeople by the strenuous efforts he made to collect debts they owed him. Even a few native Republicans like Judge Charles Caldwell, who was scarcely more popular with Conservatives, refused to speak from the same platform with him. As his admirer pointed out, Smith "was ostracized and his life often threatened. But he refused to be scared. He sued some of his debtors and went to live with colored people." One day, as he returned from a session of the convention, his carpetbag—perhaps symbolically—was stolen, its contents rifled, and a list of them published in a local newspaper.

The beginning of the end for Smith came on the night of October 3, after he and Anderson Wright, a Negro, had spoken at a Republican meeting. As he opened the door of a Negro cabin to enter, Smith was fired upon by four men outside including Colonel Richard P. Crump, one of Jefferson's leading gentry. Smith drew his revolver and returned the fire, wounding two of the assailants and driving them away. He then went to Major Curtis at the Army post. Here Crump, with the chief of police and others, soon arrived bearing a warrant for his arrest on a charge of assault. The attackers' original intention to kill Smith now assumed greater urgency because he and several Negroes present had recognized their assailants. Smith objected strenuously to their efforts to get custody of him, protesting that it was equivalent to signing his death warrant. Nevertheless Curtis turned him over to the civil authorities on their assurance of his safety. Smith was taken off to jail and a small civilian guard was posted around it. The major was uneasy, however, and requested reinforcements from his superior, but they were refused.

The next day there were signs in Jefferson of an assembling of the Knights of the Rising Sun. Hoping to head off a lynching, Curtis dispatched sixteen soldiers (the greater part of his com-

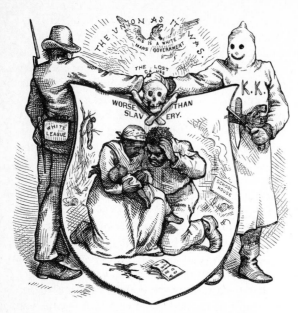

Terrorist activities by Ku Klux Klansmen, such as those related in this article, convinced many Republicans that conditions for southern blacks and their white supporters were "worse than slavery," as this cartoon from Harper's Weekly (October 26, 1874) graphically depicts.

mand) to help guard the jail. At 9 P.M., finally, a signal was sounded—a series of strokes on a bell at the place where the Knights held their meetings. About seventy members now mobilized under the command of Colonel Saufley and proceeded to march in formation toward the jail; they were in disguise and many carried torches. The jail building lay in an enclosed yard where at that time four black men were confined for a variety of petty offenses. One of the prisoners was Anderson Wright, and apparently the real reason for their being there was that they had witnessed the previous night's attempt to murder Smith; they may even have been fellow targets at that time. When the Knights reached this enclosure they burst through it with a shout and overpowered the guard, commanded by a young Army lieutenant. The invaders then turned to the Negro prisoners and dragged them into some adjoining woods. Wright and a second man,

Cornelius Turner, managed to escape from them, although Wright was wounded; the other two prisoners were shot nearly to pieces. As soon as Major Curtis heard the shooting and firing he came running with his remaining soldiers; but they too were quickly overpowered. Repeatedly the major himself tried to prevent the mob from entering the jail building in which Smith was confined, only to be dragged away from the door each time. They had no trouble unlocking the door, for city marshal Silas Nance, who possessed the key, was one of the conspirators.

At first Smith tried to hold the door shut against their entry. Eventually failing at this, he caught the foremost man, pulled him into the room, and somehow killed him. "It is common talk in Jefferson now," wrote a former Bureau agent some months later, "that Capt. Smith killed the first man who entered—that the Knights of the Rising Sun afterward buried him secretly with their funeral rites, and it was hushed up, he being a man from a distance. It is an established fact that one Gray, a strong man, who ventured into the open door, was so beaten by Capt. Smith that he cried, 'Pull me out! He's killing me!' and he was dragged out backward by the leg." All this took place in such darkness that the Knights could not see their victim. Some of them now went outside and held torches up to the small barred window of Smith's cell. By this light they were able to shoot him four times. "The door was burst open and the crowd surged in upon him as he fell, and then, man after man, as they filed around fired into the dying body. This refinement of barbarity was continued while he writhed and after his limbs had ceased to quiver, that each one might participate in the triumph."

Once the mob had finished its work at the jail it broke up into squads which began patrolling the town and searching for other Republican leaders. County Judge Campbell had anticipated trouble earlier in the evening and taken refuge as usual at Major Curtis' headquarters. Judge Caldwell was hated second only to Smith after his well-publicized report as chairman of the constitutional convention's committee on lawlessness. Hearing the shooting around the jail, he fled from his home into the woods. In a few moments twenty-five or thirty Knights appeared at the house, looking for him. Some of the party were for killing him, and they spent two hours vainly trying to learn his whereabouts from his fifteen-year-old son, who refused to tell. Another band went to the house of G. H. Slaughter, also a member of the convention, but he too escaped.

The next day the few remaining white Republicans in town were warned by friends of a widely expressed desire to make a "clean sweep" of them. Most of them stayed at the Haywood House hotel the following night under a military guard. Meanwhile the KRS scoured the city looking for dangerous Negroes, including those who knew too much about the preceding events for anyone's safety. When Major Curtis confessed that the only protection he could give the white Republicans was a military escort out of town, most of them decided to leave. At this point some civic leaders, alarmed at the probable effects to the town and themselves of such an exodus under these circumstances, urged them to stay and offered their protection. But the Republicans recalled the pledge to Smith and departed as quickly as they could, some openly and others furtively to avoid ambush.

White Conservatives saw these events—or at least their background and causes—in quite another light. They regarded Smith as "a dangerous, unprincipled carpet-bagger" who "lived almost entirely with negroes, on terms of perfect equality." Whether there was evidence for it or not, they found it easy to believe further that this "cohabitation" was accompanied by "the most unbridled and groveling licentiousness"; according to one account he walked the streets with Negroes in a state of near-nudity. For at least eighteen months he had thus "outraged the moral sentiment of the city of Jefferson," defying the whites to do anything about it and threatening a race war if they tried. This might have been

overlooked if he had not tried repeatedly to precipitate such a collision. As head of the Union League he delivered inflammatory speeches and organized the blacks into armed mobs who committed assaults and robberies and threatened to burn the town. When part of the city did go up in flames earlier in the year Smith was held responsible. Overlooking the well-attested white terrorism which had prevailed in the city and county for months, a Democratic newspaper claimed that all had been peace and quiet during Smith's absence at the constitutional convention. But on his return he resumed his incendiary course and made it necessary for the whites to arm in self-defense.

According to Conservatives the initial shooting affray on the night of October 3 was precipitated by a group of armed Negroes with Smith at their head. They opened fire on Crump and his friends while the latter were on their way to protect a white man whom Smith had threatened to attack. Democrats did not dwell overlong on the ensuing lynching, nor did they bother to explain the killing of the Negro prisoners. In fact the affair was made deliberately mysterious and a bit romantic in their telling. According to the Jefferson *Times*, both the soldiers and the civilians on guard at the jail characterized the lynch party as "entirely sober and apparently well disciplined." (One of the party later testified in court that at least some of them had put on their disguises while drinking at a local saloon.) "After the accomplishment of their object," the *Times* continued, "they all retired as quietly and mysteriously as they came—none knowing who they were or from whence they came." (This assertion, it turned out, was more hopeful than factual.)

The *Times* deplored such proceedings in general, it assured its readers, but in this case lynching "had become . . . an unavoidable necessity. The sanctity of home, the peace and safety of society, the prosperity of the country, and the security of life itself demanded the removal of so base a villain." A month later it declared: "Every community in the South will do well to relieve themselves [sic] of their surplus Geo. Smiths, and others of like ilk, as Jefferson rid herself of hers. This is not a healthy locality for such incendiaries, and no town in the South should be." Democratic papers made much of Judge Caldwell's refusal to appear publicly with Smith—which was probably inspired by his Negro associations. They claimed that Smith's fellow Republicans were also glad to have him out of the way, and noted that the local citizens had assured them of protection. But there was no mention of the riotous search and the threats upon their lives which produced that offer, nor of their flight from the city anyway.

The Smith affair raises problems of fact and interpretation which appeared in almost every Ku Klux raid across the South. Most were not so fully examined or reported as this, but even here it is impossible to know certainly where the truth lay. Republican and Democratic accounts differed diametrically on almost every particular, and both were colored by considerations of political and personal interest. But enough detailed and impartial evidence survives to sustain the Republican case on most counts. Negro and Republican testimony concerning the actual events in October is confirmed by members of the KRS who turned state's evidence when they were later brought to trial. Smith's prior activities and his personal character are less clear. Republicans all agreed later that he was almost puritanical in his moral code and that he was hated because of his unquestioned social associations and political influence with the blacks. He never counseled violence or issued threats to burn the town, they insisted; on the contrary, the only time he ever headed a Negro crowd was when he brought a number of them to help extinguish the fire which he was falsely accused of starting.

As elsewhere in the South, the logic of some of the charges against Smith is not convincing. Whites had a majority in the city and blacks in the county. Theoretically each could gain by racial violence, offsetting its minority status. But Conservatives always had the advantage in such confrontations. They were repeatedly guilty of intimidating the freedmen, and in case of an open collision everyone (including Republicans) knew they could win hands down. Democrats were certainly sincere in their personal and political detestation of Smith; almost as certainly they were sincere in their fears of his political activity and what it might lead to. From their viewpoint an open consorter with and leader of Negroes was capable of anything. It was easy therefore to believe the worst and attribute the basest motives without clear evidence. If some Negroes did threaten to burn the town—often this was a threat to retaliate for preceding white terrorism—it was easy to overlook the real cause and attribute the idea to Smith. The next step, involving hypocrisy and deliberate falsehood in some cases, was to charge him with specific expressions and activities which no other source substantiates and which the logic of the situation makes improbable. Men who practiced or condoned terrorism and murder in what they conceived to be a just cause would not shrink from character assassination in the same cause.

Interestingly enough, most of the character assassination—in Smith's case and generally—followed rather than preceded Ku Klux attacks. This did not arise primarily from a feeling of greater freedom or safety once the victim was no longer around to defend himself; some victims, unlike Smith, lived to speak out in their own behalf. Accusations after the fact were intended rather to rationalize and win public approval of the attack once it had occurred; since these raids were the product of at least semisecret conspiracy there was less need to win public approval beforehand. Sometimes such accusations were partially true, no doubt, and it was never easy for persons at a distance to judge them; often it is no easier now. Democrats tended to believe and Republicans to reject them as a matter of course. The *Daily Austin Republican* was typical of Radical papers in its reaction to Democratic newspaper slurs against Smith after his death: "We have read your lying sheets for the last *eighteen* months, and this is the first time you have made any such charges. . . ." It was surely justified in charging the Democratic editors of Texas with being accessories after the fact in Smith's murder.

The military authorities had done almost nothing to stop KRS terrorism among the Negroes before Smith's murder, and this violence continued for at least two months afterward. Similar conditions prevailed widely, and there were too few troops—especially cavalry—to patrol every lawless county. But the murder of a white man, particularly one of Smith's prominence and in such a fashion, aroused officials to unwonted activity. The Army recalled Major Curtis and sent Colonel H. G. Malloy to Jefferson as provisional mayor with orders to discover and bring to justice the murderers of Smith and the two freedmen killed with him. More troops were also sent, amounting ultimately to nine companies of infantry and four of cavalry. With their help Malloy arrested four of Jefferson's leading men on December 5. Colonel W. P. Saufley, whom witnesses identified as the organizer of the lynching, would have been a fifth, but he left town the day before on business, a Democratic newspaper explained, apparently unaware that he was wanted. (This business was to take him into the Cherokee Indian Nation and perhaps as far as New York, detaining him so long that the authorities never succeeded in apprehending him.) That night the KRS held an emergency meeting and about twenty men left town for parts unknown while others prepared to follow.

General George P. Buell arrived soon afterward as commandant, and under his direction the arrests continued for months, reaching thirty-seven by early April. They included by common repute some of the best as well as the worst citizens of Jefferson. Detectives were sent as far as New York to round up suspects who had scattered in all directions. One of the last to leave was General H. P. Mabry, a former judge and a KRS leader who was serving as one of the counsel for the defense. When a soldier revealed that one of the prisoners had turned state's evidence

and identified Mabry as a leader in the lynching, he abruptly fled to Canada.

The authorities took great pains to recover Anderson Wright and Cornelius Turner, the Negro survivors of the lynching, whose testimony would be vital in the forthcoming trials. After locating Wright, General Buell sent him with an Army officer to find Turner, who had escaped to New Orleans. They traveled part of the way by steamboat and at one point, when the officer was momentarily occupied elsewhere, Wright was set upon by four men. He saved himself by jumping overboard and made his way to a nearby Army post, whence he was brought back to Jefferson. Buell then sent a detective after Turner, who eventually was located, and both men later testified at the trial.

The intention of the authorities was to try the suspects before a military commission, as they were virtually sure of acquittal in the civil courts. Defense counsel (who consisted ultimately of eleven lawyers—nearly the whole Jefferson bar) made every effort to have the case transferred; two of them even went to Washington to appeal personally to Secretary of War Schofield, but he refused to interfere. R. W. Loughery, the editor of both the Jefferson *Times* and the *Texas Republican* in Marshall, appealed to the court of public opinion. His editorials screamed indignation at the "terrible and revolting ordeal through which a refined, hospitable, and intelligent people are passing, under radical rule," continually subject to the indignity and danger of midnight arrest. He also sent requests to Washington and to Northern newspapers for intercession against Jefferson's military despotism. The prisoners, he said, were subject to brutal and inhuman treatment. Loughery's *ex parte* statement of the facts created a momentary ripple but no reversal of policy. In reality the prisoners were treated quite adequately and were confined in two buildings enclosed by a stockade. Buell released a few of them on bond, but refused to do so in most cases for the obvious reason that they would have followed their brothers in flight. Although they seem to have been denied visitors at first, this rule was lifted and friends regularly brought them extra food and delicacies. The number of visitors had to be limited, however, because most of the white community regarded them as martyrs and crowded to the prison to show their support.

After many delays the members of the military commission arrived in May and the trial got under way; it continued into September. Although it proved somewhat more effective than the civil courts in punishing Ku Klux criminals, this tribunal was a far cry from the military despotism depicted by its hysterical opponents. The defense counsel presented their case fully and freely. Before long it was obvious that they would produce witnesses to swear alibis for most or all of the defendants. Given a general public conspiracy of this magnitude, and the oaths of KRS members to protect each other, this was easy to do; and given the dependence of the prosecution by contrast on Negro witnesses whose credibility white men (including Army officers) were accustomed to discounting, the tactic was all too effective. The results were mixed. At least fourteen persons arrested at one time or another never went on trial, either for lack of evidence or because they turned state's evidence. Seventeen others were tried and acquitted, apparently in most cases because of sworn statements by friends that they were not present at the time of the lynching. Only six were convicted. Three of these were sentenced to life terms, and three to a term of four years each in the Huntsville penitentiary. General Reynolds refused to accept the acquittal of Colonel Crump and three others, but they were released from custody anyway, and the matter was not raised again. Witnesses who had risked their lives by testifying against the terrorists were given help in leaving the state, while most of the defendants returned to their homes and occupations. The arrests and trials did bring peace to Jefferson, however. The Knights of the Rising Sun rode no more, and the new freedom for Radicals was symbolized in August by the appearance of a Republican newspaper.

Relative tranquillity came to northeast Texas generally during the early part of 1869. Some Republicans attributed this to the election of General Grant, but that event brought no such result to other parts of the South. Both Ben Bickerstaff and Cullen Baker were killed and their gangs dispersed, which certainly helped. The example of military action in Jefferson likely played a part; it was accompanied by an increase of military activity throughout the region as troops were shifted here from the frontier and other portions of the state. Immediately after the Smith lynching in October, General Reynolds ordered all civil and military officials to "arrest, on the spot any person wearing a mask or otherwise disguised." Arrests did increase, but it was probably owing less to this order than to the more efficient concentration of troops. In December the Bureau agent in Jefferson had cavalry (for a change) to send out after men accused of Ku Klux outrages in Upshur County. Between October 1868 and September 1869 fifty-nine cases were tried before military commissions in Texas, chiefly involving murder or aggravated assault; they resulted in twenty-nine convictions. This record was almost breathtaking by comparison with that of the civil courts.

The Texas crime rate remained high after 1868. Organized Ku Klux activity declined markedly, but it continued in sporadic fashion around the state for several years. A new state government was elected in November 1869 and organized early the next year under Republican Governor E. J. Davis. In his first annual message, in April 1870, Davis called attention to the depredations of disguised bands. To cope with them he asked the legislature to create both a state police and a militia, and to invest him with the power of martial law. In June and July the legislature responded affirmatively on each count. The state police consisted of a mounted force of fewer than 200 men under the state adjutant general; in addition, all county sheriffs and their deputies and all local marshals and constables were considered to be part of the state police and subject to its orders. In November 1871 a law against armed and disguised persons followed. Between July 1870 and December 1871 the state police arrested 4,580 persons, 829 of them for murder or attempted murder. Hundreds of other criminals probably fled the state to evade arrest. This activity, coupled with occasional use of the governor's martial law powers in troubled local-

ities, seems to have diminished lawlessness by early 1872. There still remained the usual problems of prosecuting or convicting Ku Klux offenders, however, and very few seem to have been punished legally.

■■■

STUDY QUESTIONS

1. Why was Klan terrorism so rampant in Texas? Did the federal government possess the means of preventing it?

2. What was the relationship between the Ku Klux Klan in Texas and the Democratic Party?

3. How did well-to-do white planters respond to the Ku Klux Klan?

4. What were the objectives of the Ku Klux Klan in Texas?

5. Who were the White Conservatives? How did they view Klan activities?

6. Why did the state government try to curtail Klan activities in the early 1870s? Did state officials succeed?

BIBLIOGRAPHY

The standard work on Reconstruction, one which created two generations of stereotypes by vindicating the South and indicting the North, is William A. Dunning, *Reconstruction, Political and Economic* (1907). The first major dissent from Dunning was W. E. B. Du Bois's classic work *Black Reconstruction* (1935). It was not until the social changes of the 1960s, triggered by the civil rights movement, that historians took a new look at Reconstruction. John Hope Franklin's *Reconstruction After the Civil War* (1961) first questioned the Dunning view, arguing that northern intentions toward the South were humanitarian as well as political. Kenneth Stampp's *The Era of Reconstruction* (1965) carried that argument further, restoring the reputation of "carpetbaggers" and "scalawags," describing the successes of black politicians, and criticizing the Ku Klux Klan. Also see Allen Trelease, *White Terror* (1967); Sarah Wiggins, *The Scalawag in Alabama Politics, 1865–1881* (1977); and L. N. Powell, *New Masters: Northern Planters During the Civil War and Reconstruction* (1980).

For studies of Andrew Johnson, see Howard K. Beale, *The Critical Year: A Study of Andrew Johnson and Reconstruction* (1930), which takes the traditional point of view. A very critical view is Eric McKitrick, *Andrew Johnson and Reconstruction* (1960). Also see Michael Benedict, *The Impeachment of Andrew Johnson* (1973).

DAY OF THE LONGHORNS

Dee Brown

The Texas Longhorn looked slightly unbalanced, as if it were about to fall over. Its body often appeared thin, and its horns stretched out like the curved balancing rod of a high-wire performer. And its face—only another Longhorn or a Texan could love it. Nevertheless, this rugged breed of steer was the focus of the long drives during the dusty, golden age of cowboys.

Ironically, this era of the cowboy was made possible by the westward push of railroad builders. After the Civil War, a three- or four-dollar Texas Longhorn could be sold in the upper Mississippi region for forty dollars. If Texas entrepreneurs could drive the steers to the railheads, they could earn a $100,000 profit from 3,000 head of cattle. And so the drive was on, first to Sedalia, Missouri, and later, as railways extended west, to the Kansas cowtowns of Newton, Abilene, Ellsworth, and Dodge City. During the late 1860s and 1870s, a total of over four million cattle survived the heat, dust, Indian attacks, and other problems and reached the Kansas railroads. Dee Brown describes the difficult journey and the Longhorns, and the cowboys who drove them to the railheads.

W hen Coronado marched northward from Mexico in 1540, searching for the mythical golden cities of Cibola, he brought with his expedition a number of Spanish cattle. These were the first of the breed to enter what is now the United States. Over the next century other Spanish explorers and missionaries followed, most of them bringing at least "a bull and a cow, a stallion and a mare." From these seed stocks, Longhorns and mustangs and cowboys and ranching slowly developed in the Southwest, the Spanish cattle mutating and evolving, the vaquero perfecting his costume and the tools of his trade.

The Longhorns, which also came to be known as Texas cattle, took their name from their wide-spreading horns which sometimes measured up to eight feet across, and there are legends of horn spreads even more extensive. From their mixed ancestry of blacks, browns, reds, duns, slates, and brindles the Longhorns were varicolored, the shadings and combinations of hues so differentiated that, as J. Frank Dobie pointed out, no two of these animals were ever alike in appearance. "For all his heroic stature," said Dobie, "the Texas steer stood with his body tucked up in the flanks, his high shoulder-top sometimes thin enough to split a hail stone, his ribs flat, his length frequently so extended that his back swayed."

Ungraceful though they were, the Longhorns showed more intelligence than domesticated cattle. They were curious, suspicious, fierce, and resourceful. After all, by the mid–19th century they were the survivors of several generations which had lived under wild or semiwild conditions. They possessed unusually keen senses of smell, sight, and hearing; their voices were powerful and penetrating; they could survive extreme heat or cold; they could exist on the sparest of vegetation and water; they could outwalk any other breed of cattle. It was this last attribute that brought the Texas Longhorns out of their native habitat and onto the pages of history to create the romantic era of the cowboys, the long drives, and riproaring trail towns of the Great Plains.

The drives began even before Texas became a state. A few enterprising adventurers occasionally would round up a herd out of the brush and drive them overland to Galveston or Shreveport where the animals were sold mainly for their hides and tallow. After the California gold rush of 1849 created a demand for meat, a few daring young Texans drove herds all the way to the Pacific coast. W. H. Snyder put together an outfit that moved out of Texas into New Mexico, and then crossed Colorado, Wyoming, Utah, and Nevada. After two years Snyder finally got his Longhorns to the miners. Captain Jack Cureton of the Texas Rangers followed a southern route across New Mexico and Arizona, dodging Apaches all the way, but from the meat-hungry goldseekers Cureton took a profit of $20,000, a considerable fortune in those days.

In the early 1850s a young English emigrant named Tom Candy Ponting probably established the record for the longest trail drive of Longhorns. Ponting was engaged in the livestock business in Illinois when he learned of the easy availability of Longhorns in Texas. Late in 1852 he and his partner traveled there on horseback, carrying a small bag of gold coins. They had no trouble assembling a herd of 700 bawling Longhorns at nine dollars or less a head. Early in 1853 they headed north for Illinois. It was a rainy spring and Ponting and his partner had to hire Cherokees to help swim the cattle across the Arkansas River. "I sat on my horse every night while we were crossing through the Indian country," said Ponting. "I was so afraid I could not sleep in the tent, but we had no stampede." Missouri was still thinly settled, and there was plenty of vegetation to keep the Longhorns from losing weight. At St. Louis the

Dee Brown, "Day of the Longhorns." From *American History Illustrated* 9 (January 1975), pp. 4–9, 42–48. Reprinted through the courtesy of Cowles Magazines, publisher of AMERICAN HISTORY ILLUSTRATED.

animals were ferried across the Mississippi, and on July 26, Ponting and his cattle reached Christian County, Illinois.

There through the winter months he fed them on corn, which cost him fifteen cents a bushel. He sold off a few scrubs to traveling cattle buyers, and then in the spring he cut out the best of the herd and started trail driving again, this time toward the East. At Muncie, Indiana, Ponting found that railroad cars were available for livestock transport to New York. "We made arrangements and put the cattle on the cars. We unloaded them at Cleveland, letting them jump out on the sand banks. We unloaded them next at Dunkirk, then at Harnesville, and then at Bergen Hill." On July 3, 1854, from Bergen Hill in New Jersey, Ponting ferried the much-traveled Longhorns across the Hudson to the New York cattle market, completing a two-year journey of 1,500 miles on foot and 600 miles by rail. They were the first Texas Longhorns to reach New York City.

"The cattle are rather long-legged though finehorned, with long taper horns, and something of a wild look," reported the New York *Tribune*. "The expense from Texas to Illinois was about two dollars a head, the owners camping all the way. From Illinois to New York, the expense was seventeen dollars a head." To the New York buyers the Longhorns were worth eighty dollars a head. Tom Ponting had more than doubled his investment.

About this same time another young adventurer from Illinois, Charles Goodnight, was trying to build up his own herd of Longhorns in the Brazos River country. As a young boy Goodnight had journeyed to Texas with his family, riding much of the way bareback. When he was 21, he and his stepbrother went to work for a rancher, keeping watch over 400 skittish Longhorns and branding the calves. Their pay for this work was one-fourth of the calves born during the year. "As the end of the first year's branding resulted in only thirty-two calves for our share," Goodnight recalled afterward, "and as the value was about three dollars per head, we figured out that we had made between us, not counting expenses, ninety-six dollars."

Goodnight and his partner persevered, however, and after four years of hard work they owned a herd of 4,000. Before they could convert many of their animals into cash, however, the Civil War began. Goodnight soon found himself scouting for a company of Confederate mounted riflemen and spent most of the war disputing control of the upper Brazos and Red River country with Comanches and Kiowas instead of with blue-coated Yankees. At the war's end his makeshift uniform was worn out, his Confederate money was worthless, and his Longhorn herd had virtually disappeared. "I suffered great loss," Goodnight said. "The Confederate authorities had taken many of my cattle without paying a cent. Indians had raided our herds and cattle thieves were branding them, to their own benefit without regard to our rights." He was 30 years old and financially destitute.

Almost every other Texan returning from the war found himself in the same situation. When rumors reached the cattle country early in the spring of 1866 that meat was in short supply in the North, hundreds of young Texans began rounding up Longhorns. Huge packing houses were being constructed in Northern cities, and on a 345-acre tract where nine railroads converged, the Chicago Union Stock Yards was opened for business. A Longhorn steer worth five dollars in useless Confederate money in Texas would bring forty dollars in good U.S. currency in the Chicago market.

From the brush country, the plains, and the coastal regions of Texas, mounted drivers turned herd after herd of cattle northward across Indian Territory. Their goal was the nearest railhead, Sedalia, in west-central Missouri. Following approximately the route used by Tom Ponting thirteen years earlier, the trail drivers forded Red River and moved on to Fort Gibson, where they had to cross the more formidable Arkansas. Plagued by unseasonable cold weather, stampedes, and flooded streams, they pushed their Longhorns on into southeastern Kansas.

Here they encountered real trouble. From Baxter Springs northward to Sedalia railhead, the country was being settled by small farmers, many of them recent battlefield enemies of the Texans. The settlers did not want their fences wrecked and their crops trampled, and they used force in stopping the Texans from driving cattle across their properties. By summer's end, over 100,000 stalled cattle were strung out between Baxter Springs and Sedalia. The grass died or was burned off by defiant farmers. Dishonest cattle buyers from the North bought herds with bad checks. The unsold cattle died or were abandoned, and the great drives of 1866 came to an end. For many of the Texans it had been a financial bust.

A less optimistic folk might have gone home defeated, but not the cattlemen of Texas. By the spring of 1867 many were ready to drive Longhorns north again. And in that year, thanks to an enterprising Yankee stockman, a convenient shipping point was waiting to welcome their coming. At the end of the Civil War, Joseph McCoy of Springfield, Illinois, had started a business of buying livestock for resale to the new packinghouses in Chicago. Appalled by the Baxter Springs–Sedalia debacle of 1866, McCoy was determined to find a railroad shipping point somewhere at the end of an open trail from Texas. He studied the maps of new railroads being built westward and chose a town in Kansas—Abilene, near the end of the Kansas Pacific Railroad.

"Abilene in 1867 was a very small, dead place," McCoy admitted. But it met all the requirements for a cattle-shipping town. It was west of the settled farming country; it had a railroad, a river full of water for thirsty steers, and a sea of grass for miles around for holding and fattening livestock at the end of the drives. And nearby was Fort Riley, offering protection from possible Indian raids.

Within sixty days McCoy managed to construct a shipping yard, a barn, an office, and a hotel. From the Kansas Pacific he wheedled railroad ties to build loading pens sturdy enough to hold wild Longhorns. Meanwhile, he had sent messengers southward to inform the cattlemen of Texas that Abilene was "a good safe place to drive to, where they could sell, or ship cattle unmolested to other markets."

Over what soon became known as the Chisholm Trail, thousands of Texas cattle began moving into Abilene. Although the 1867 season got off to a late start and rail shipments did not begin until September, 36,000 Longhorns were marketed that first year. In 1868 the number doubled, and in 1870 the Kansas Pacific could scarcely find enough cars to handle the 300,000 Longhorns sold to Northern packing houses. Abilene in the meantime had grown into a boom town of stores, hotels, saloons, and honkytonks where Texas cowboys celebrated the end of their trail drive and engendered the legends of gunmen, lawmen, shootouts, and exotic dance hall girls.

One Texas cowman who did not make the long drive north to Abilene was Charles Goodnight. Back in the spring of 1866 when most of his neighbors were driving herds across Indian Territory for the Sedalia railhead, Goodnight was still trying to round up his scattered Longhorns. By the time he was ready to move out, he suspected that there was going to be a glut of cattle in Kansas and Missouri. Instead of heading north, he combined his Longhorns with those of Oliver Loving and they started their herd of 2,000 west toward New Mexico. Cattle were reported to be in great demand there by government agents who bought them for distribution to reservation Indians.

To reach New Mexico, Goodnight and Loving followed the abandoned route of the Butterfield Overland Stage along which waterholes and wells had been dug by the stage company. For this arduous journey, Goodnight constructed what was probably the first chuckwagon. Obtaining an old military wagon, he rebuilt it with the toughest wood he knew, a wood used by Indians for fashioning their bows—Osage orange or *bois d'arc*. At the rear he built a chuckbox with a hinged lid to which a folding leg was attached so that when it was lowered it formed a cook's work table. Fastened securely in front of the wagon was a convenient spigot running through to a barrel of water. Beneath the driver's seat was a supply of necessary tools such as axes and spades, and below the wagon was a cowhide sling for transporting dry wood or buffalo chips to be used in making cooking fires. A generation of trail drivers would adopt Goodnight's chuckwagon for long drives and roundups, and variations of it are still in use today.

Goodnight's and Loving's first drive to New Mexico was uneventful until they began crossing the lower edge of the Staked Plains, where the water holes had gone dry. For three days the rangy Longhorns became almost unmanageable from thirst, and when they scented the waters of the Pecos they stampeded, piling into the river, some drowning under the onrush of those in the rear. The partners succeeded, however, in driving most of the herd into Fort Sumner, where several thousand Navajos confined in the Bosque Redondo were near starvation.

A government contractor took more than half the Longhorns, paying Goodnight and Loving $12,000 in gold. By the standards of that day they had suddenly become prosperous. While Loving drove the remainder of the cattle to the Colorado mining country, Goodnight returned to Texas to round up another herd of Longhorns.

In the years immediately following the disruptions of the Civil War, thousands of unbranded Longhorns roamed wild in the Texas brush country. The cowboys soon discovered that the easiest way to round up these cattle was to lure them out of the chaparral with tame decoys. James H. Cook, an early trail driver who later became a leading cattleman of the West, described such a wild Longhorn roundup:

"About sunrise we left the corral, taking with us the decoy herd, Longworth leading the way. After traveling a mile or more he led the herd into a dense clump of brush and motioned us to stop driving it. Then, telling two men to stay with the cattle he rode off, signaling the other men and myself to follow him . . . in the brush ahead I caught a glimpse of some cattle. A few minutes later I heard voices singing a peculiar melody without words. The sounds of these voices indicated that the singers were scattered in the form of a circle about the cattle. In a few moments some of the cattle came toward me, and I recognized a few of them as belonging to the herd which we had brought from our camp. In a few seconds more I saw that we had some wild ones, too. They whirled back when they saw me, only to find a rider wherever they might turn. The decoy cattle were fairly quiet, simply milling around through the thicket, and the wild ones were soon thoroughly mingled with them." Cook and the other cowboys now had little difficulty driving the combined tame and wild Longhorns into a corral where they were held until time to start an overland drive to market.

The work of rounding up Longhorns gradually developed into an organized routine directed by a man who came to be known as the range boss. During a roundup, his authority was as ironclad as that of a ship's captain. At the beginning of a "gather" the range boss would assemble an outfit of about twenty cowhands, a horse wrangler to look after the mounts and, most important of all, a camp cook. Roundups began very early in the spring because every cattleman was eager to be the first to hit the trail before the grass overgrazed along the route to Kansas.

On the first morning of a roundup the men would be up before sunrise to eat their breakfasts hurriedly at the chuckwagon; then in the gray light of dawn they would mount their best ponies and gather around the range boss for orders. As soon as he had outlined the limits of the day's roundup, the boss would send his cowhands riding out in various directions to sweep the range. When each rider reached a specified point, he turned back and herded all the cattle within his area back into the camp center.

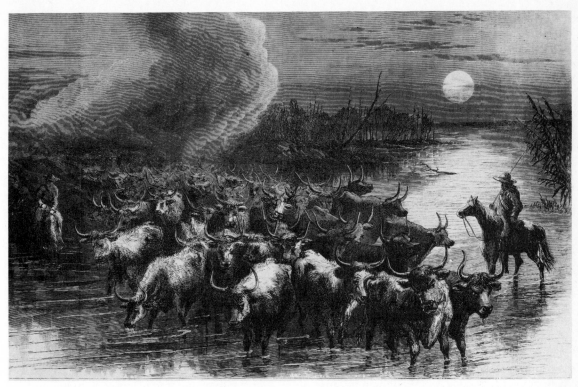

■ ■ *Texas Longhorns are herded across a stream during an 1867 cattle drive. Between 1867 and 1887, a total of 5.5 million head of Texas Longhorns were trailed north.*

After a herd was collected, the second operation of a roundup began. This next step was to separate the young stock which were to be branded for return to the range from the mature animals which were to be driven overland to market. "Cutting out" it was fittingly called, and this performance was, and still is, the highest art of the cowboy. Cutting out required a specially trained pony, one that could "turn on a dime," and a rider who had a sharp eye, good muscular reflexes, and who was an artist at handling a lariat. After selecting an animal to be separated from the herd, the rider and his horse would begin a quick-moving game of twisting and turning, of sudden stops and changes of pace.

Roping, the final act of the cutting out process, also required close cooperation between pony and rider. Forming an oval-shaped noose six or seven feet in diameter, the cowboy would spin it over his head with tremendous speed. A second before making the throw, he would draw his arm and shoulder back, then shoot his hand forward, aiming the noose sometimes for the animal's head, sometimes for its feet. As the lariat jerked tight, the rider instantly snubbed it around his saddle horn. At the same moment the pony had to be stopped short. The position of the pony at the moment of throw was important; a sudden jerk of a taut lariat could spill both horse and rider.

As soon as the unbranded animal was roped, it was immediately herded or dragged to the nearest bonfire where branding irons were kept heated to an orange red. In Texas, all branding was done in a corral, a legal requirement devised to prevent hasty and illegal branding by rustlers on the open range. The first brands in Texas were usually the initials of the owners, and if two cattlemen had the same initials, a bar or a circle distinguished one from the other. Law required that brands be publicly registered by counties in Texas; other Western states had state brand books. In the early years when ranches were unfenced and land boundaries poorly marked, friction over unbranded cattle caused many a gunfight. To discourage rustlers who could easily change a "C" to an "O," an "F" to an "E," a "V" to a "W," ranchers designed unusual brands, some of the more famous being the Stirrup, Andiron, Scissors, Frying Pan, and Dinner Bell.

As soon as the work of branding was completed, preparations for the trail drive began in earnest. The owner of the cattle was responsible for food and other supplies, but each cowboy assembled the personal gear he would need on the journey. Every item he wore or carried was designed for utility. Tents were seldom taken along, two blankets being considered sufficient shelter from the elements. If the weather was warm, the cowboys shed their coats, and if they wore vests they rarely buttoned them because of the rangeland belief that to do so would bring on a bad cold. Most wore leather chaps to protect their legs from underbrush and weather. They put high heels on their boots to keep their feet from slipping through the stirrups, and they wore heavy leather gloves because the toughest palms could be burned raw by the lariats they used constantly in their work. They paid good money for wide-brimmed hats because they served as roofs against rain, snow, and sun. They used bandannas for ear coverings, as dust masks, as strainers when drinking muddy water, for drying dishes, as bandages, towels, slings for broken arms, to tie hats on in very windy weather, and for countless other purposes.

Getting the average trail herd of about 3,000 cattle underway was as complicated an operation as starting a small army on a march across country. Each rider needed several spare mounts for the long journey, and this herd of horses accompanying a cow column was known as the remuda—from a Spanish word meaning re-

placement. A trail boss, sixteen to eighteen cowboys, a cook and chuckwagon, and a horse wrangler for the remuda made up the personnel of an average drive.

It was necessary to move slowly at first until the restive Longhorns grew accustomed to daily routines. To keep a herd in order a wise trail boss would search out a huge dominating animal and make it the lead steer. Charles Goodnight had one called Old Blue which he considered so valuable as a leader that after every long drive he brought the animal back to the home ranch. Two or three quiet days on the trail was usually long enough to calm a herd of Longhorns. After that the cattle would fall into place each morning like infantrymen on the march, each one keeping the same relative position in file as the herd moved along.

Cattleman John Clay left a classic description of an early trail herd in motion: "You see a steer's head and horns silhouetted against the skyline, and then another and another, till you realize it is a herd. On each flank is a horseman. Along come the leaders with a swinging gait, quickening as they smell the waters of the muddy river." The pattern of trail driving soon became as routinized as that of roundups—the trail boss a mile or two out in front, horse herd and chuckwagon following, then the point riders directing the lead steers, and strung along the widening flow of the herd the swing and flank riders, until at the rear came the drag riders in clouds of dust, keeping the weaker cattle moving.

Not many trail drivers had time to keep diaries, that of George Duffield being one of the rare survivors. From it a reader can feel the tensions and weariness, the constant threats of weather, the difficult river crossings, and dangers of stampedes.

May 1: Big stampede. Lost 200 head of Cattle.
May 2: Spent the day hunting & found but 25 Head. It has been Raining for three days. These are dark days for me.
May 3: Day spent in hunting Cattle. Found 23. Hard rain and wind. Lots of trouble.

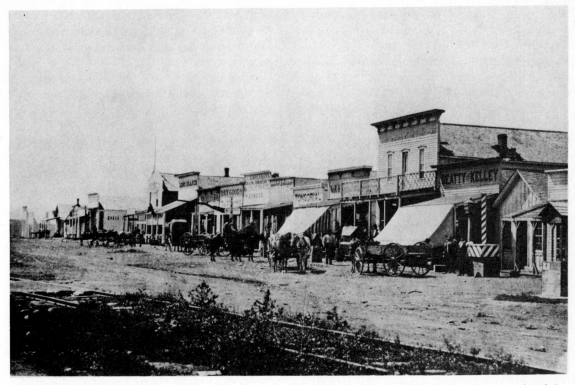

■ ■ *In 1878, Dodge City was the "king of the trail towns." Longhorns and cattlemen made the city what it was, but their day of glory ended during Dodge's long reign.*

May 8: Rain pouring down in torrents. Ran my horse into a ditch & got my Knee badly sprained—15 miles.

May 9: Still dark and gloomy. River up. Everything looks *Blue* to me.

May 14: Swam our cattle & Horses & built Raft & Rafted our provisions & blanket & covers. Lost Most of our Kitchen furniture such as camp Kittles Coffee Pots Cups Plates Canteens &c &c.

May 17: No Breakfast. Pack & off is the order.

May 31: Swimming Cattle is the order. We worked all day in the River & at dusk got the last Beefe over—I am now out of Texas—This day will long be remembered by me—There was one of our party Drowned today.

George Duffield made his drive along the eastern edge of Indian Territory in 1866. Ten years later the drives were still as wearisome and dangerous, but the trails had shifted much farther westward and there had been a swift succession of trail towns. A new railroad, the Sante Fe, pushed sixty-five miles south of Abilene in 1871, and Newton became the main cattle-shipping town. Newton's reign was brief, however; it was replaced by Ellsworth and Wichita. Although the advancing railroad tracks were a boon to cattlemen seeking shorter routes to markets, they also brought settlers west by the thousands. By 1876 the life of the Chisholm Trail was ending and the Western Trail, or Dodge City Trail, had taken its place.

Dodge City was the king of the trail towns, the "cowboy capital," a fabulous town of innumerable legends for a golden decade. The names survive in history: Long Branch Saloon, the Lady Gay, the Dodge Opera House, Delmonico's, Wyatt Earp, Doc Holliday, Boot Hill, Bat Masterson, Clay Allison, Luke Short, and Big Nose Kate. But it was Longhorns and cattlemen that made Dodge City, and it was during Dodge's long reign that the Longhorns came to the end of their day of glory.

One of the men responsible for the change was Charles Goodnight. In the year that Dodge opened as a cow town, 1875, Goodnight found himself financially destitute for the second time in his life. He had made a fortune with Texas cattle, bought a ranch in Colorado, become a banker, and then lost everything in the Panic of 1873. All he had left in 1875 was a small herd of unmarketable Longhorns, and he decided it was time to return to Texas and start all over again.

He chose an unlikely region, the Texas Panhandle, an area long shunned by cattlemen because it was supposed to be a desert. Goodnight, however, recalled the immense herds of buffalo which had roamed there for centuries, and he reasoned that wherever buffalo could thrive so could Longhorns. He found a partner, John Adair, to furnish the capital and drove his Longhorns into the heart of the Panhandle, to the Palo Duro Canyon, where he discovered plenty of water and grass. There he founded the JA Ranch. Soon after starting operations, Goodnight began introducing Herefords and shorthorns, cross-breeding them at first with Longhorns so that his cattle produced more and better beef, yet retained the ability to flourish on the open range and endure long drives to Dodge City.

Other ranchers soon followed his example, and "White Faces" instead of "Longhorns" gradually became the symbol of trail cattle. After a continuing flood of homesteaders, brought west by the proliferating railroads, made it necessary to close the trail to Dodge City, one more overland route—the National Trail to Wyoming and Montana—saw the last treks of the Longhorns.

As the 19th century came to an end, so did open range ranching and trail driving. There was no longer any place for rangy Longhorns. Until the day he died, however, Charles Goodnight kept a small herd of them to remind him of the old days. A few specimens survive today in wildlife refuges and on larger ranches as curiosities, or for occasional use in parades and Western movies. But most of these animals are descendants of crossbreds. The day of the genuine Texas Longhorn—with his body tucked up in the flanks, his high shoulder-top thin enough to split a hail stone, his ribs flat, his back swayed, his ability to outwalk any other breed of cattle—now belongs to history.

■ ■ ■

STUDY QUESTIONS

1. What were the origins of the Texas Longhorn? Why were they so well suited for the long drive?

2. How did the Civil War affect the cattle business?

3. Why did Joseph McCoy choose to drive cattle to Abilene?

4. What was life like on the long drive?

5. Why did the drives end?

BIBLIOGRAPHY

Ray Allen Billington's *The Far Western Frontier* (1963) and *Westward Expansion* (1974) are excellent introductions to the westward movement. Ernest S. Osgood, *The Day of the Cattlemen* (1929) is a classic work on the subject, and Lewis Atherton, *The Cattle Kings* (1961) is a more recent study. Gene M. Gressley, *Bankers and Cattlemen* (1966) deals with Eastern as well as Western interests. Wayne Gard, *The Chisholm Trail* (1954) is an outstanding study of the Long Drive, and J. Frank Dobie *The Longhorns* (1941) tells the story delightfully well. Robert R. Dykstra, *The Cattle Town* (1968) and Joe B. Frantz and J. E. Choate, *The American Cowboy* (1981) remove the myths that surround their subjects.

Part Two

THE GILDED
AGE

Change dominated the American scene during the last quarter of the nineteenth century. Noted throughout most of the century for its agricultural output, America suddenly became an industrial giant, and by 1900 it led the world in industrial production. Unfettered by governmental codes and regulations, industrialists created sprawling empires. In 1872, Scottish immigrant Andrew Carnegie built his first steel mill, and his holdings steadily expanded until, almost thirty years later, he sold his steel empire to J. Pierpont Morgan for close to a half-billion dollars. In oil, meat packing, and other industries, the pattern was the same—a handful of ruthless, efficient, and farsighted men dominated and directed America's industrial growth.

Just as important as the ambitious industrialists were the millions of men and women who provided the muscle that built the industries and ran the machines. Some came from the country's farmlands, victims of dropping agricultural prices or the loneliness and boredom of farm life. Others were immigrants who came to the United States to escape poverty and political oppression. Crowded into booming cities, the workers—native and immigrant alike—labored long and hard for meager rewards.

The changes wrought by industrial growth and urban expansion created an atmosphere characterized by excitement and confusion. Some people, like Andrew Carnegie and John D. Rockefeller, moved from relatively humble origins to fabulous wealth and impressive social standing. Each symbolized the possibility of rising

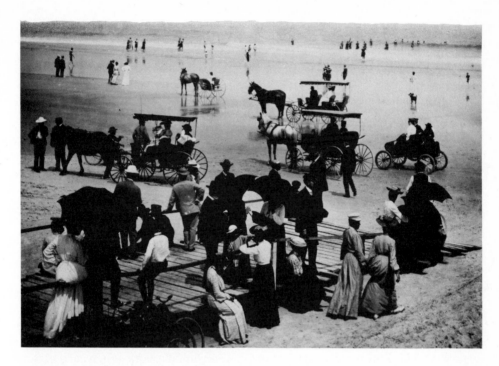

from rags to riches. New opportunities created new wealth, and the important older American families were forced to make room for the new. As a result, wealthy Americans went to extraordinary lengths to display their status. J. P. Morgan bought yachts and works of art while still other industrialists built mansions along the rocky shore of Newport, Rhode Island. Both the boats and houses marked the owners as men who had "arrived." The clubs, restaurants, and resorts of the late nineteenth century were part of the attempt to define the new American aristocracy.

Other people suffered during this time of change. For example, the social and economic position of farmers declined during the late nineteenth century. Once considered the "salt of the earth" and "the backbone of America," they were viewed now as ignorant rubes and country bumpkins. Outmatched by unpredictable weather, expanding railroads, and declining prices produced by overexpansion, they consistently tried to overcome their problems by working harder, organizing cooperatives, and forming political parties. They labored heroically, but most of their efforts and organizations ended in failure.

Minority and ethnic Americans similarly faced difficult battles. Most of them were locked out of the opportunities available to educated white male Americans. Nor could women easily improve their social and economic positions. They experienced the excitement of the period from a distance, but the pain and frustration they knew firsthand.

AMERICAN ASSASSIN: CHARLES J. GUITEAU

James W. Clarke

Abraham Lincoln, James Garfield, William McKinley, Huey Long, John Kennedy, Robert Kennedy, Martin Luther King, Jr.—our history has been too often altered by an assassin's bullet. Some of America's political assassins were clearly insane, others were motivated by political beliefs or dark personal desires. Normally it is difficult to determine where political partisanship ends and insanity begins. In ''American Assassin,'' James W. Clarke recounts the case of Charles J. Guiteau, a tireless self-promoter who shot President James A. Garfield on July 2, 1881. Guiteau was certainly unusual; part con man, part religious fanatic, he believed he was destined for some sort of greatness. But was he insane? And if so, was his insanity a legal defense for his actions? These and other questions had to be answered by the jurors who sat in judgment of Guiteau. In an age before Sigmund Freud's work, when each person was assumed to be responsible for his actions, these questions were difficult, if not impossible, to fully answer. Indeed, as the recent incident with John Hinckley demonstrates, these cases continue to perplex the American legal system.

W ith the single exception of Richard Lawrence, there has been no American assassin more obviously deranged than Charles Guiteau. Unlike Lawrence [who attempted to assassinate Andrew Jackson], however, who could be described as a paranoid schizophrenic, Guiteau was not paranoid. Indeed, he possessed a rather benign view of the world until shortly before he was hanged. On the gallows, he did lash out at the injustice of his persecutors, but even then his anger was tempered by a sense of martyrdom, glories anticipated in the next world, and a dying man's belief that in the future a contrite nation would erect monuments in his honor.

That Lawrence was confined in mental hospitals for the remainder of his life and Guiteau hanged can be attributed primarily to two facts: Jackson survived; Garfield did not. For certainly the symptoms of severe mental disturbance in Guiteau's case, although of a different sort, were as striking as in Lawrence's. As we will see, the convenient label and implied motive—"disappointed office-seeker"—that has been attached to Guiteau by writers and historians confuses symptoms with causes.

Religion, Law, and Politics

Charles Julius Guiteau was born on September 8, 1841 in Freeport, Illinois. His mother, a quiet, frail woman, died seven years and two deceased infants later of complications stemming from a mind-altering "brain fever" she had initially contracted during her pregnancy with Charles. In addition to Charles, she was survived by her husband, Luther, an intensely religious man and Charles' older brother and sister, John and Frances.

From the beginning, people noticed that little Julius, as he was called (until he dropped the

James W. Clarke, *American Assassins: The Darker Side of Politics.* Copyright © 1982 by Princeton University Press. Excerpt, pp. 198–214, reprinted with permission of Princeton University Press.

name in his late teens because "there was too much of the Negro about it"), was different. Luther Guiteau soon became exasperated with his inability to discipline his unruly and annoying youngest son and, as a result, Julius was largely raised by his older sister and her husband, George Scoville. Years later, in 1881, Scoville would be called to represent the accused assassin at his trial.

Although plagued by a speech impediment, for which he was whipped by his stern father, Guiteau was, in his fashion, a rather precocious youngster who learned to read quickly and write well. An annoying aversion to physical labor was observed early and remained with him the rest of his life. At the age of eighteen, Charles became interested in furthering his education and, against his father's will, used a small inheritance he had received from his grandfather to enter the University of Michigan.

His father, who was scornful of secular education, had urged his son to seek a scripture-based education at the utopian Oneida Community in New York. The curriculum there focused on study of the Bible. The elder Guiteau had hopes that his errant son might also acquire some self-discipline in a more authoritarian God-fearing environment.

After a couple of semesters at Ann Arbor, Charles, as he was now called, decided to heed his father's advice and transfer to Oneida where, in addition to religious instruction, he had recently learned that they practiced free love. With sex and the Lord on his mind, he enthusiastically entered the New York commune in June 1860. Like his father, Charles now believed that Oneida was the first stage in establishing the Kingdom of God on Earth.

Not long after his arrival, Charles came to believe that he had been divinely ordained to lead the community because, as he announced with a typical lack of humility, he alone possessed the ability. Since no one else had received this revelation, Charles soon found himself at odds with the community leadership. Moreover, the Oneida leaders believed that Charles' vigorously protested need of increasing periods for contemplative pursuits was merely evidence of the slothfulness his father had hoped they would correct.

Other tensions also began to build. Young Charles was becoming increasingly frustrated because the young women of the community were not responding to his amorous overtures. Convinced of his personal charm, this nervous, squirrel-like little man was annoyed because these objects of his intended affection were so unresponsive. Adding insult to injury they soon laughingly referred to him as Charles "Git-out."

As his position within the community continued to deteriorate, Charles became more isolated and alienated until, in April 1865, he left for New York City. He wrote to his father to explain his decision after arriving in Hoboken:

Dear Father:

I have left the community. The cause of my leaving was because I could not conscientiously and heartily accept their views on the labor question. They wanted to make a hard-working businessman of me, but I could not consent to that, and therefore deemed it expedient to quietly withdraw, which I did last Monday. . . .

I came to New York in obedience to what I believed to be the call of God for the purpose of pursuing an independent course of theological and historical investigation. With the Bible for my textbook and the Holy Ghost for my schoolmaster, I can pursue my studies without interference from human dictation. In the country [Oneida] my time was appropriated, *but now it is at my own* disposal, *a very favorable change. I have procured a small room, well furnished, in Hoboken, opposite the city, and intend to fruitfully pursue my studies during the next three years.*

Then he announced a new scheme:

And here it is proper to state that the energies of my life are now, and have been for months, pledged to God, *to do all that within me lies to extend the sovereignty of Jesus Christ by placing at*

his disposal a powerful daily paper. I am persuaded that theocratic presses are destined, in due time, to supersede to a great extent pulpit oratory. There are hundreds of thousands of ministers in the world but not a single daily theocratic press. It appears to me that there is a splendid chance for some one to do a big thing for God, for humanity and for himself.

With a new suit of clothes, a few books, and a hundred dollars in his pocket, he planned to publish his own religious newspaper that would, he was convinced, spearhead a national spiritual awakening.

In another lengthy letter to his father, Charles continued to detail his plans for the "Theocratic Daily" that would "entirely discard all muddy theology, brain philosophy and religious cant, and seek to turn the heart of men toward the living God." Buoyed with an ill-founded sense of well-being and enthusiasm, Charles went on euphorically: "I claim that I am in the employ of Jesus Christ and Co., the very ablest and strongest firm in the universe, and that what I can do is limited only by their power and purpose." And knowing full well that *he* would edit the paper, he announced confidently:

Whoever edits such a paper as I intend to establish will doubtless occupy the position of Target General to the Press, Pulpit, and Bench of the civilized world; and if God intends me for that place, I fear not, for I know that He will be "a wall of fire round me," and keep me from all harm.

Confidently expecting to promote the Kingdom of God without the restrictions of the Oneida Community and, not incidentally, also enjoy wealth and fame in the process, Guiteau sought financial backing for the paper in New York City. In a flurry of optimistic salesmanship, he scurried about presenting his proposal to prospective subscribers and advertisers; they, as it turned out, were not impressed with this odd little entrepreneur and his religious views. Soon finding himself short of money, somewhat discouraged, and tiring of a diet of dried beef, crackers, and lemonade that he ate in his dingy Hoboken room, Charles returned to Oneida after only three months in the big city.

But his return only confirmed his original reservations about the place, and he soon left again—this time more embittered by his experiences there than ever before. Again without money, Charles wrote to the Community requesting a $9,000 reimbursement—$1,500 a year for the six years he had spent there. When the Community refused to pay, Charles sued, threatening to make public the alleged sexual, as well as financial, exploitation employed by the Oneida leadership—especially its founder, John Humphrey Noyes.

Undoubtedly bitter about the rejection he had endured in this sexually permissive environment, Charles lashed out in an unintentionally amusing attack on both Noyes and the Oneida women. Charging that Noyes lusted after little girls, Guiteau angrily told a reporter: "All the girls that were born in the Community were forced to cohabit with Noyes at such an early period it dwarfed them. The result was that most of the Oneida women were small and thin and homely."

Obviously stung by such criticism, Noyes threatened to bring extortion charges against Guiteau. In a letter to Charles' father, who was mortified by his son's behavior, he advised that Charles had admitted to, among other sins, stealing money, frequenting brothels, and being treated for a venereal ailment. Noyes added that Charles also had apparently thrown in the towel, so to speak, in an uninspired battle with masturbation. Such appraisals confirmed his father's sad suspicion that Charles' real purpose in going to Oneida was "the free exercise of his unbridled lust." Charles' "most shameful and wicked attack" and subsequent episodes convinced Luther Guiteau that his prodigal son was "absolutely insane." In despair, he wrote to his oldest son John that, unless something stopped him, Charles would become "a fit subject for the lunatic asylum."

Having thus incurred his father's anger and

facing the prospects of a countersuit for extortion, Charles abandoned his legal claim and left New York for Chicago. There, given the standards of the day, he began to practice law, after a fashion. In 1869, he married a young woman he had met at the Y.M.C.A., a Miss Annie Bunn. After only one memorably incoherent attempt to argue a case, his practice of law was reduced to collecting delinquent bills for clients. By 1874, the law practice and marriage had both failed, the latter as a result of his adultery with a "high toned" prostitute and the occasional beatings he used to discipline his beleaguered wife.

When his marriage ended, Charles wandered back to New York. Continually borrowing small sums of money that he never repaid voluntarily, Guiteau soon found himself, as usual, in trouble with creditors. Resentful of such unseemly harassment, he wrote in indignant letter to his brother John addressing him as "Dear Sir." This and other letters reveal the unfounded arrogance and unintentional humor of a man with only the most tenuous grasp of the reality of his position:

Your letter from Eaton . . . dated Nov. 8, '72, received. I got the $75 on my supposed responsibility as a Chicago lawyer. I was introduced to Eaton by a gentleman I met at the Young Men's Christian Association, and it was only incidentally that your name was mentioned.

I wrote to Eaton several times while at Chicago, and he ought to have been satisfied, but he had the impertinence to write you and charge me with fraud, when he knew he let me have the money entirely upon my own name and position. Had he acted like a "white" man, I should have tried to pay it long ago. I hope you will drop him.

    Yours truly,
    CHARLES J. GUITEAU.

A few days after this letter was written, Charles' exasperated brother himself became the target of an angry response when he requested a repayment of a small loan:

J. W. GUITEAU: NEW YORK, March 13th, 1873 Find $7 enclosed. Stick it up your bung-hole

*and wipe your nose on it, and that will remind
you of the estimation in which you are held by*
                    CHARLES J. GUITEAU
*Sign and return the enclosed receipt and I will
send you $7, but not before, and that, I hope, will
end our acquaintance.*

Disdainful of the pettiness of such small lenders, Charles confidently launched another major venture in the publishing business: he wanted to purchase the Chicago *Inter-Ocean* newspaper. But businessmen and bankers, from whom he sought financial backing, were unimpressed and not a little skeptical about this seedy little man with a confidential manner. Frustrated but ever the undaunted optimist, Charles turned again to religion.

Impressed with the bountiful collection plates at the Chicago revival meetings of Dwight Moody where he served as an usher in the evening services, Charles decided to prepare himself for the ministry. After a short period of voracious reading in Chicago libraries, he soon had himself convinced that he alone had ascertained the "truth" on a number of pressing theological questions. With familiar enthusiasm, he launched his new career with pamphlets and newspaper advertisements. Adorned with sandwich board posters, Charles walked the streets inviting all who would listen to attend his sermons on the physical existence of hell, the Second-Coming, and so forth. The self-promotion campaign was repeated in one town after another as he roamed between Milwaukee, Chicago, New York, and Boston.

In handbills, Charles proclaimed himself "the Eloquent Chicago Lawyer." His performances, in fact, followed a quite different pattern: a bombastic introduction that soon deteriorated into a series of incoherent nonsequiturs, whereupon he would end inconclusively and abruptly dash from the building amid the jeers and laughter of his audiences—the whole episode lasting perhaps ten to fifteen minutes. With his dubious reputation as an evangelist growing, Charles darted from one town to another leaving in his path a growing accumulation of indignant audiences and unpaid bills. Often arrested, he was periodically jailed for short periods between 1877 and 1880 when he again turned his attention to politics.

The Garfield Connection

Describing himself as a "lawyer, theologian, and politician," Guiteau threw himself into the Stalwart faction's fight for the 1880 Republican presidential nomination in New York. When a third term was denied the Stalwart's choice, Ulysses S. Grant, the nomination went to a darkhorse, James A. Garfield. Guiteau quickly jumped on the Garfield bandwagon. In New York, he began to hang around the party headquarters and, as he was to remind people later, he did work on the "canvass" for the candidate. In his view, his most noteworthy contribution to the campaign and Garfield's subsequent election, however, was an obscure speech he wrote (and may have delivered once in Troy, New York) entitled, "Garfield vs. Hancock." A few weeks before, the same speech had been entitled "Grant vs. Hancock." Undeterred by the change in candidates, the speech, Guiteau later claimed, originated and developed the issue that won the election for Garfield. That issue, in brief, was the claim that if the Democrats gained the presidency it would mean a resumption of the Civil War because the Democrats had only sectional, rather than national, loyalties. In a personal note, dated March 11, 1881, to the newly appointed secretary of state, James G. Blaine, Guiteau explained his claim:

I think I have a right to claim your help on the strength of this speech. It was sent to our leading editors and orators in August. It was the first shot in the rebel war claim idea, and it was their idea that elected Garfield. . . . I will talk with you about this as soon as I can get a chance. There is nothing against me. I claim to be a gentleman and a Christian.

Indeed, from the moment the election results

were in, Guiteau had begun to press his claims in letters to Garfield and Blaine. He also became a familiar figure at the Republican party headquarters in New York, confident that he would be rewarded for his efforts with a consulship appointment; the only question remaining, he believed, was the location. Would it be Paris, Vienna, or some other post of prominence? With this in mind, he moved from New York to Washington on March 5, 1881, where he began to badger not only the President's staff but Blaine and the President himself in the corridors of the White House. Striking a posture of gallingly unwarranted familiarity with those he encountered, he also let loose a barrage of "personal" notes written in the same annoying style. Typical is the following:

[Private]

GEN'L GARFIELD:

From your looks yesterday I judge you did not quite understand what I meant by saying "I have not called for two or three weeks." I intended to express my sympathy for you on account of the pressure that has been on you since you came into office.

I think Mr. Blaine intends giving me the Paris consulship with your and Gen. Logan's approbation, and I am waiting for the break in the Senate.

I have practiced law in New York and Chicago, and presume I am well qualified for it.

I have been here since March 5, and expect to remain some little time, or until I get my commission.

Very respectfully,
CHARLES GUITEAU.

AP'L 8.

Shortly before he had written to the secretary of state to inquire whether President Hayes' appointments to foreign missions would expire in March 1881, as he expected. Learning that they would, Guiteau became more persistent in pressing his claims for an appointment to the missions of either Vienna, Paris, or possibly Liv-

erpool. Earlier he had written again to Garfield, whom he had never met, to advise him of his plans to wed a wealthy and cultured woman (whose acquaintance, also, he had not at that time, or ever, made). Such unknowingly ludicrous acts were intended, in the bizarre judgment of Charles J. Guiteau, to enhance his already eminent qualifications for a foreign ministry.

In the meantime, the newspapers were filled with the controversy that had developed between the new President and the boss-dominated Stalwart faction of the Republican party over patronage appointments in New York. Finally, on May 13, 1881, the two most powerful of the Stalwart bosses, Roscoe Conkling and Tom "Me Too" Platt of New York, resigned their Senate seats in protest over the President's failure to follow their preferences in his patronage appointments. In so doing, they discounted the fact that Garfield had accepted their man, "Chet" Arthur, as his running mate and vice-president. Angrily condemning the beleaguered Garfield's disloyalty and traitorous tactics, the resignations triggered numerous editorial attacks and denunciations of the President and his mentor Blaine, which were to continue until July 2, 1881.

On the same day the resignations were announced, Guiteau once again approached Blaine with his by now familiar blandishments, only to have the exasperated secretary roar, "Never bother me again about the Paris consulship as long as you live!" But Guiteau persisted. A week later, he wrote again to the President:

[Private]

General GARFIELD:

I have been trying to be your friend; I don't know whether you appreciate it or not, but I am moved to call your attention to the remarkable letter from Mr. Blaine which I have just noticed.

According to Mr. Farwell, of Chicago, Blaine is "a vindictive politician" and "an evil genius," and you will "have no peace till you get rid of him."

This letter shows Mr. Blaine is a wicked man, and you ought to demand his immediate resignation; otherwise you and the Republican party will come to grief. I will see you in the morning, if I can, and talk with you.

Very respectfully,
CHARLES GUITEAU.
May 23.

If past behavior is any clue to the future, at this point Guiteau would have begun to consider yet another occupational change, returning again perhaps with his typical enthusiastic optimism to theology or law. Previously, Guiteau had accepted failure with remarkable equanimity, sustained always by the exalted opinion he had of himself. As one scheme after another collapsed—his leadership aspirations at Oneida, his journalistic ventures, the law practice, and the evangelistic crusade—his bitterness and disappointment were short-lived as he moved on to other careers. His confidence in his own ability and the Horatio Alger-like opportunities that abounded in nineteenth-century America remained unshaken. Even his angry exchanges with the Oneida establishment possessed the tone of someone who enjoyed the battle as well as the spoils; certainly these exchanges reflected none of the desperation of the all-time loser that he, in fact, was. In Guiteau's delusional world, these frustrations were merely temporary setbacks in a career that was, he remained convinced, destined for wealth and fame.

Now, for the first time in his oddly chaotic life, Guiteau found himself sharing his outsider status with men he admired: Conkling and Platt and the other Stalwarts. And it was in this realization—not the denial of the various appointments he had sought—that his assassination scheme germinated. Indeed, a month later, on June 16, he wrote in his "Address to the American People":

I conceived of the idea of removing the President four weeks ago. Not a soul knew of my purpose. I conceived the idea myself. I read the newspapers carefully, for and against the administration, and

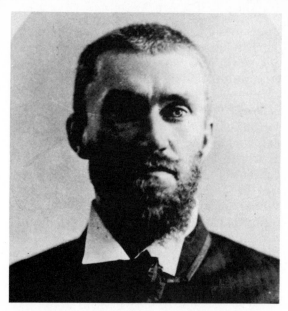

■ ■ *Charles J. Guiteau, assassin of President James Garfield (1881). Much of the public viewed his insanity plea as a "dodge," arguing that Guiteau's methodical planning and self-seeking motives could not be the product of a disordered mind.*

gradually the conviction settled on me that the President's removal was a political necessity, because he proved a traitor to the men who made him, and thereby imperiled the life of the Republic. At the late Presidential election, the Republican party carried every Northern State. Today, owing to the misconduct of the President and his Secretary of State, they could hardly carry ten Northern States. They certainly could not carry New York, and that is the pivotal State.

Ingratitude is the basest of crimes. That the President, under the manipulation of his Secretary of State, has been guilty of the basest ingratitude to the Stalwarts admits of no denial. . . . In the President's madness he has wrecked the once grand old Republican party; and for this he dies. . . .

I had no ill-will to the President.

This is not murder. It is a political necessity. It will make my friend Arthur President, and save the Republic. I have sacrificed only one. I shot the President as I would a rebel, if I saw him pulling down the American flag. I leave my justification to God and the American people.

I expect President Arthur and Senator Conkling will give the nation the finest administration it has ever had. They are honest and have plenty of brains and experience.

[signed] Charles Guiteau [Emphasis added.]

Later, on June 20, he added this even more bizarre postscript:

The President's nomination was an act of God. The President's election was an act of God. The President's removal is an act of God. I am clear in my purpose to remove the President. Two objects will be accomplished: It will unite the Republican party and save the Republic, and it will create a great demand for my book, "The Truth." This book was written to save souls and not for money, and the Lord wants to save souls by circulating the book.

Charles Guiteau

It is unlikely that Guiteau would have chosen the course of action he did without the sense that he was in good company—"a Stalwart of the Stalwarts," as he liked to describe himself. In his distorted mind, to "remove" the President, as he euphemistically described it, would provide the same status and recognition he had sought in a consulship appointment and, more importantly, in every hare-brained scheme he had botched since the time he first entered the Oneida Community to establish the Kingdom of God on Earth. In this last grandly deluded plan, his aspirations in theology, law, and politics were to culminate in a divinely inspired and just act "to unite the Republican party and save the Republic" and, not incidentally, launch a new career for Charles Guiteau not only as a lawyer, theologian, and politician, but as a national hero with presidential aspirations.

With this in mind, on June 8, Guiteau borrowed fifteen dollars and purchased a silver-mounted English revolver. He planned to have it, along with his papers, displayed after the assassination at the Library of the State Depart-

ment or the Army Medical Museum. To prepare for the big event, he began target practice on the banks of the Potomac. After stalking the President for several weeks and bypassing at least two opportunities to shoot him, Guiteau rose early on Saturday, July 2, 1881. He had rented a room a few days before at the Riggs House and, on this morning, began preparations to meet the President at the Baltimore and Potomac Railroad Station. The President was scheduled to leave that morning for a vacation trip. Downing a hearty breakfast, which he charged to his room, he pocketed the last of a series of bizarre explanations:

July 2, 1881

To the White House:

The President's tragic death was a sad necessity, but it will unite the Republican party and save the Republic. Life is a fleeting dream, and it matters little when one goes. A human life is of small value. During the war thousands of brave boys went down without a tear. I presume the President was a Christian, and that he will be happier in Paradise than here.

It will be no worse for Mrs. Garfield, dear soul, to part with her husband this way than by natural death. He is liable to go at any time anyway.

I had no ill-will towards the President. His death was a political necessity. I am a lawyer, a theologian, a politician. I am a Stalwart of the Stalwarts. I was with General Grant and the rest of our men in New York during the canvass. I have some papers for the press, which I shall leave with Byron Andrews and his co-journalists at 1440 N.Y. Ave., where all the reporters can see them.

I am going to jail.

[signed] Charles Guiteau

Guiteau then walked to the banks of the Potomac where after taking a few final practice shots he proceeded to the railroad station to await the President's arrival. Once at the station, he used the men's room, had his shoes shined, and, after estimating that his assignment would be completed shortly before the President's train was scheduled to leave, he reserved a hackman for an anticipated 9:30 arrest and departure to the District Prison. He had already checked the prison's security, lest in the emotion of the moment he might be attacked by crowds who had not had time to realize what a great patriotic service he had just rendered. He was convinced that after his explanation was published the wisdom and justice of his act would be appreciated. Until such time, however, he had taken a further precaution of drafting a letter requesting that General Sherman see to his safekeeping in jail. The letter, which fell from his pocket during the scuffle that followed the shooting, read as follows:

TO GENERAL SHERMAN:

I have just shot the President. I shot him several times, as I wished him to go as easily as possible. His death was a political necessity. I am a lawyer, theologian and politician. I am a Stalwart of the Stalwarts. I was with General Grant and the rest of our men in New York during the canvass. I am going to jail. Please order out your troops and take possession of the jail at once.

Very respectfully,
[signed] Charles Guiteau

So it was with this completely distorted view of reality that Charles Guiteau fired two shots into the President's back as he walked arm-in-arm with Secretary Blaine toward the waiting train. The President, failing to respond to treatment, lingered two and a half months before dying on September 19, 1881.

The Trial

Throughout his lengthy seventy-two-day trial, Guiteau's delusional state was apparent to anyone inclined to acknowledge it. His brother-in-law, George Scoville, represented him at the trial and entered a plea of insanity. In Scoville's opening statement for the defense, he described in some detail the history of mental illness in the Guiteau family: at least two uncles, one aunt, and two cousins, not to mention his mother who died of "brain fever" but was probably insane. He went on to mention the highly eccentric

behavior of his father that, at least one physician thought, properly qualified him for this category. It should also be noted that Guiteau's sister, Frances, the wife of George Scoville, behaved so strangely during her brother's trial that her probable insanity was noted by one participating physician who had had occasion to observe her closely. And indeed, her husband later had her declared insane and institutionalized in October 1882, after her brother's execution.

This seemingly overwhelming evidence of an hereditary affliction was ignored or discounted by expert witnesses and finally the jury. Also discounted were the defendant's own delusional symptoms evident in the past schemes, bizarre letters to prominent persons he had never met, and his distorted conception of reality, which was apparent in his remarks throughout the trial and to the day he was executed. Scoville's line of defense was rejected by the defendant himself and greatly resented by John W. Guiteau, Charles' older brother. In a letter to Scoville, dated October 20, 1881, shortly after the trial began, John denied the history of family insanity described by the defense. Rather than heredity, he argued indignantly, most of the cases Scoville cited could be explained by self-induced factors such as insobriety and "mesmerism"; the others, specifically his parents' symptoms, he categorically denied. Falling into line with previous diagnoses of the causes of Charles' problems, most notably that of leaders of the Oneida Community, John Guiteau wrote: "I have no doubt that masturbation and self-abuse is at the bottom of his [Charles'] mental imbecility."

As for Charles himself, thoroughly contemptuous of his brother-in-law's legal abilities, he drafted his own plea, which read as follows:

I plead not guilty to the indictment and my defense is threefold:

1. Insanity, in that it was God's act and not mine. The Divine pressure on me to remove the President was so enormous that it destroyed my free agency, and therefore I am not legally responsible for my act.

Throughout his trial, Guiteau would acknowledge only this interpretation of insanity; that is, he was insane only in the sense that he did something that was not his will but God's. He did not accept the idea that he was in any way mentally deficient. Typical of his remarks on this issue made throughout the trial is the following:

. . . the Lord interjected the idea [of the President's removal] into my brain and then let me work it out my own way. That is the way the Lord does. He doesn't employ fools to do his work; I am sure of that; he gets the best brains he can find.

His plea continued describing two rather novel circumstances that, he claimed, were the Lord's will just as the assassination:

2. The President died from malpractice. About three weeks after he was shot his physicians, after careful examination, decided he would recover. Two months after this official announcement he died. Therefore, I say he was not fatally shot. If he had been well treated he would have recovered.

The third circumstance had to do with the court's jurisdiction:

3. The President died in New Jersey and, therefore, beyond the jurisdiction of this Court. This malpractice and the President's death in New Jersey are special providences, and I am bound to avail myself of them in my trial in justice to the Lord and myself.

He went on to elaborate:

I undertake to say that the Lord is managing my case with eminent ability, and that he had a special object in allowing the President to die in New Jersey. His management of this case is worthy of Him as the Deity, and I have entire confidence in His disposition to protect me, and to send me forth to the world a free and innocent man.

The jury's guilty verdict notwithstanding, it was clear that Guiteau had no grasp of the reality of his situation. Almost to the last, he believed he would be acquitted, at which point, he planned to begin a lecture tour in Europe and later return to the United States in time to re-enter politics as a presidential contender in 1884. He was confident that the jury, like the great majority of Americans, would recognize that Garfield's "removal" was divinely ordained and that the Almighty himself was responsible. He was convinced they would recognize that he was only an instrument in the Master's hands.

Contrary to some assessments, there was no evidence of paranoia in his behavior. Buoyed by a delusion-based optimism, he mistook the crowds of curious on-lookers at the jail as evidence of respect and admiration: bogus checks for incredible sums of money and ludicrous marriage proposals that were sent to him by cranks were sincerely and gratefully acknowledged; and promotional schemes evolved in his distorted mind to market his ridiculous books and pamphlets—all this while anticipating a run for the presidency in 1884! Meanwhile, in high spirits, the poor wretch ate heartily and slept well in a small cell located both literally and figuratively in the shadow of the gallows.

The Execution

When at the very last he realized that there was no hope for survival, his anger was, considering the circumstances, tempered much as it had been during his dispute with the Oneida Community. There were warnings of divine retribution for the ungrateful new president, Chester Arthur, the unfair prosecuting attorneys, and the jury, but again his anger lacked the intensity and desperation of someone facing death. As the execution date approached, Charles, realizing failure once again, simply set his sights elsewhere as he had on many previous occasions. Eschewing politics, the presidency, the Stalwarts, and the law that had failed him, the lawyer and politician once again became the theologian. Anticipating an other-worldly position at the side of the Almighty, Charles walked serenely to the gallows. Earlier he had given the letter below to the chaplain who stood by him at the last:

Washington, D.C.
June 29, 1882

TO THE REV. WILLIAM W. HICKS:

I, Charles Guiteau, of the City of Washington, in the District of Columbia, now under sentence of death, which is to be carried into effect between the hours of twelve and two o'clock on the 30th day of June, A.D., 1882, in the United States jail in the said District, do hereby give and grant to you my body after such execution; provided, however, it shall not be used for any mercenary purposes.

And I hereby, for good and sufficient considerations, give, deliver and transfer to said Hicks my book entitled "The Truth and Removal" and copyright thereof to be used by him in writing a truthful history of my life and execution.

And I direct that such history be entitled "The Life and Work of Charles Guiteau"; and I hereby solemnly proclaim and announce to all the world that no person or persons shall ever in any manner use my body for any mercenary purpose whatsoever.

And if at any time hereafter any person or persons shall desire to honor my remains, they can do it by erecting a monument whereon shall be inscribed these words: "Here lies the body of Charles Guiteau, Patriot and Christian. His soul is in glory."

[signed] Charles Guiteau
Witnesses: Charles H. Reed
            James Woodward

Before the noose was placed around his neck, he was given permission to read his "last dying prayer" to the crowd of faces gazing up at him from the prison yard below. Comparing his situation to that of Christ at Calvary, Guiteau condemned President Arthur's ingratitude "to the man that made him and saved his party and land" and warned of divine retribution.

After completing his prayer, he again looked throughtfully out over the crowd before announcing in a loud clear voice:

I am now going to read some verses which are intended to indicate my feelings at the moment of leaving this world. If set to music they may be rendered effective. The idea is that of a child babbling to his mamma and his papa. I wrote it this morning about 10 o'clock.

Then with childlike mournfulness, Guiteau read:

I am going to the Lordy. I am so glad.
I am going to the Lordy. I am so glad.
I am going to the Lordy. Glory, hallelujah;
    glory hallelujah.
I am going to the Lordy;
I love the Lordy with all my soul; glory,
    hallelujah.
And that is the reason I am going to the Lord.
Glory, hallelujah; glory, hallelujah. I am going
    to the Lord.
I saved my party and my land; glory, hallelujah.
But they have murdered me for it, and that is the
    reason
I am going to the Lordy.
Glory, hallelujah; glory, hallelujah. I am going
    to the Lordy.
I wonder what I will do when I get to the Lordy;
I guess that I will weep no more when I get to the
    Lordy.
Glory, hallelujah!
I wonder what I will see when I get to the Lordy,
I expect to see most splendid things, beyond all
    earthly conception.

As he neared completion, he raised his voice to a very high pitch and concluded with

When I am with the Lordy, glory, hallelujah!
Glory, hallelujah! I am with the Lord.

Whereupon attendants strapped his legs, adjusted the noose, and placed a black hood over his head as Rev. Hicks prayed, "God the Father be with thee and give thee peace evermore." Guiteau, according to his own request, signaled the hangman by dropping a slip of paper from his fingers. As the trap sprung, Charles Guiteau slipped confidently into eternity with "Glory, Glory, Glory" on his lips.

Conclusions

Although the debate on the true state of Guiteau's mental condition was to continue among physicians for some years afterward, a brief article in the *Medical News* a day after the execution seems to have been representative of the prevailing view of the medical profession. While conceding that the neurologists who testified to the assassin's obvious insanity may have been correct, society would still be better, the editors reasoned, for having rid itself of such persons. As a further practical matter, it is unlikely that in 1881 any jury in the country would have acquitted the President's assassin whatever his mental condition.

■ ■ ■

STUDY QUESTIONS

1. Was Guiteau's life before the assassination consistent with his plea of insanity?

2. What were the political motivations for Guiteau's actions?

3. What were the problems with evaluating the evidence presented by the experts on insanity? Did Guiteau, according to the author, actually suffer from paranoia?

4. How would you describe Guiteau's religious beliefs? In your opinion, did those values inhibit his ability to interpret reality?

5. Was the verdict of the jury just? Could any other verdict have been reasonably justified?

BIBLIOGRAPHY

The most thoughtful and thought-provoking exploration of the Guiteau episode is Charles E. Rosenberg, *The Trial of the Assassin Guiteau* (1968). However, some of the contemporary articles also make interesting reading. John P. Gray, a leading late nineteenth-century American expert on insanity and an important witness in the Guiteau trial, presented his conclusions in ''The United States vs. Charles J. Guiteau,'' *American Journal of Insanity,* 38 (1882). Edward C. Spitzka, the other major expert in the case, offered his opinion in ''A Contribution to the Question on the Mental Status of Guiteau and the History of His Trial,'' *Alienist and Neurologist,* 4 (1883).

The most recent work on American political assassinations is James W. Clarke, *American Assassins: The Darker Side of Politics* (1982). Clarke provides a good general bibliography on the subject. For the politics of the period see H. Wayne Morgan, *From Hayes to McKinley: National Party Politics, 1877–1896* (1969) and John M. Taylor, *Garfield of Ohio: The Available Man* (1970).

THE WIZARD OF OZ: PARABLE ON POPULISM

Henry M. Littlefield

The late nineteenth century was not a period known for its social justice. Angry and exploited workers found little sympathy in the halls of government. Consistently during strikes, federal authorities intervened on the side of management rather than labor, even though strikes were usually responses to wage cuts. In the 1894 Pullman strike, for example, President Grover Cleveland sided with the rights of property over the rights of labor and crushed the strike. Thus the newly formed unions won few concessions for their members. At the end of the century, the work week for the "average" industrial worker was almost 60 hours. The average skilled worker earned twenty cents an hour, twice as much as the average unskilled worker.

Life on the farms in the Midwest and South was probably even worse than life in the northern industries. Technological innovations and scientific farming techniques led to increased production, which in turn sent prices spiraling downward. Discriminatory railroad rates and the government's tight money policies further weakened the economic positions of farmers. As a result, farmers faced an economic depression which cost many their farms. Returning to his midwestern home in 1889, writer Hamlin Garland noted, "Nature was as bountiful as ever . . . but no splendor of cloud, no grace of sunset could conceal the poverty of these people; on the contrary, they brought out, with a more intolerable poignancy, the gracelessness of these homes, and the sordid quality of the mechanical routine of these lives." In the following essay, Henry M. Littlefield takes a fascinating look at Lyman Frank Baum's *The Wonderful Wizard of Oz* and the light it shed on the workers' and farmers' plight in the late nineteenth century.

On the deserts of North Africa in 1941 two tough Australian brigades went to battle singing,

Have you heard of the wonderful wizard,
The wonderful Wizard of Oz,
And he is a wonderful wizard,
If ever a wizard there was.

It was a song they had brought with them from Australia and would soon spread to England. Forever afterward it reminded Winston Churchill of those "buoyant days." Churchill's nostalgia is only one symptom of the world-wide delight found in American fairy-tale about a little girl and her odyssey in the strange land of Oz. The song he reflects upon came from a classic 1939 Hollywood production of the story, which introduced millions of people not only to the land of Oz, but to a talented young lady named Judy Garland as well.

Ever since its publication in 1900 Lyman Frank Baum's *The Wonderful Wizard of Oz* has been immensely popular, providing the basis for a profitable musical comedy, three movies and a number of plays. It is an indigenous creation, curiously warm and touching, although no one really knows why. For despite wholehearted acceptance by generations of readers, Baum's tale has been accorded neither critical acclaim, nor extended critical examination. Interested scholars, such as Russell B. Nye and Martin Gardiner, look upon *The Wizard of Oz* as the first in a long and delightful series of Oz stories, and understandably base their appreciation of Baum's talent on the totality of his works.

The Wizard of Oz is an entity unto itself, however, and was not originally written with a sequel in mind. Baum informed his readers in 1904 that he had produced *The Marvelous Land of Oz* reluctantly and only in answer to well over a thousand letters demanding that he create another Oz tale. His original effort remains unique and to some degree separate from the books which follow. But its uniqueness does not rest alone on its peculiar and transcendent popularity.

Professor Nye finds a "strain of moralism" in the Oz books, as well as "a well-developed sense of satire," and Baum stories often include searching parodies on the contradictions in human nature. The second book in the series, *The Marvelous Land of Oz,* is a blatant satire on feminism and the suffragette movement. In it Baum attempted to duplicate the format used so successfully in *The Wizard,* yet no one has noted a similar play on contemporary movements in the latter work. Nevertheless, one does exist, and it reflects to an astonishing degree the world of political reality which surrounded Baum in 1900. In order to understand the relationship of *The Wizard* to turn-of-the-century America, it is necessary first to know something of Baum's background.

Born near Syracuse in 1856, Baum was brought up in a wealthy home and early became interested in the theater. He wrote some plays which enjoyed brief success and then, with his wife and two sons, journeyed to Aberdeen, South Dakota, in 1887. Aberdeen was a little prairie town and there Baum edited the local weekly until it failed in 1891.

For many years Western farmers had been in a state of loud, though unsuccessful, revolt. While Baum was living in South Dakota not only was the frontier a thing of the past, but the Romantic view of benign nature had disappeared as well. The stark reality of the dry, open plains and the acceptance of man's Darwinian subservience to his environment served to crush Romantic idealism.

Hamlin Garland's visit to Iowa and South

Dakota coincided with Baum's arrival. Henry Nash Smith observes,

Garland's success as a portrayer of hardship and suffering on Northwestern farms was due in part to the fact that his personal experience happened to parallel the shock which the entire West received in the later 1880's from the combined effects of low prices, . . . grasshoppers, drought, the terrible blizzards of the winter of 1886–1887, and the juggling of freight rates. . . .

As we shall see, Baum's prairie experience was no less deeply etched, although he did not employ naturalism to express it.

Baum's stay in South Dakota also covered the period of the formation of the Populist party, which Professor Nye likens to a fanatic "crusade." Western farmers had for a long time sought governmental aid in the form of economic panaceas, but to no avail. The Populist movement symbolized a desperate attempt to use the power of the ballot. In 1891 Baum moved to Chicago where he was surrounded by those dynamic elements of reform which made the city so notable during the 1890s.

In Chicago Baum certainly saw the results of the frightful depression which had closed down upon the nation in 1893. Moreover, he took part in the pivotal election of 1896, marching in "torch-light parades for William Jennings Bryan." Martin Gardiner notes besides, that he "consistently voted as a democrat . . . and his sympathies seem always to have been on the side of the laboring classes." No one who marched in even a few such parades could have been unaffected by Bryan's campaign. Putting all the farmers' hopes in a basket labeled "free coinage of silver," Bryan's platform rested mainly on the issue of adding silver to the nation's gold standard. Though he lost, he did at least bring the plight of the little man into national focus.

Between 1896 and 1900, while Baum worked and wrote in Chicago, the great depression faded away and the war with Spain thrust the United States into world prominence. Bryan maintained Midwestern control over the Demo-

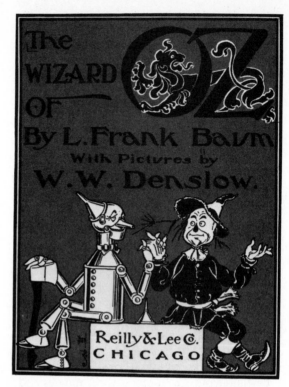

■ ■ ■ *Original title page of Frank Baum's populist classic (1900). The spectacularly successful 1939 film based on the Wizard of Oz came out during another Great Depression and prefigured happiness in "Somewhere Over the Rainbow."*

cratic party, and often spoke out against American policies toward Cuba and the Philippines. By 1900 it was evident that Bryan would run again, although now imperialism and not silver seemed the issue of primary concern. In order to promote greater enthusiasm, however, Bryan felt compelled once more to sound the silver leitmotif in his campaign. Bryan's second futile attempt at the presidency culminated in November 1900. The previous winter Baum had attempted unsuccessfully to sell a rather original volume of children's fantasy, but that April, George M. Hill, a small Chicago publisher, finally agreed to print *The Wonderful Wizard of Oz*.

Baum's allegiance to the cause of Democratic Populsim must be balanced against the fact that he was not a political activist. Martin Gardiner finds through all of his writings "a theme of tolerance, with many episodes that poke fun at narrow nationalism and ethnocentrism." Nevertheless, Professor Nye quotes Baum as having a desire to write stories that would "bear the stamp of our times and depict the progressive fairies of today."

The Wizard of Oz has neither the mature religious appeal of a *Pilgrim's Progress,* nor the philosophic depth of a *Candide.* Baum's most thoughtful devotees see in it only a warm, cleverly written fairy tale. Yet the original Oz book conceals an unsuspected depth, and it is the purpose of this study to demonstrate that Baum's immortal American fantasy encompasses more than heretofore believed. For Baum created a children's story with a symbolic allegory implicit within its story line and characterizations. The allegory always remains in a minor key, subordinated to the major theme and readily abandoned whenever it threatens to distort the appeal of the fantasy. But through it, in the form of a subtle parable, Baum delineated a Midwesterner's vibrant and ironic portrait of this country as it entered the twentieth century.

We are introduced to both Dorothy and Kansas at the same time:

Dorothy lived in the midst of the great Kansas prairies, with Uncle Henry, who was a farmer, and Aunt Em, who was the farmer's wife. Their house was small, for the lumber to build it had to be carried by wagon many miles. There were four walls, a floor and a roof, which made one room; and this room contained a rusty-looking cooking stove, a cupboard for the dishes, a table, three or four chairs, and the beds.

When Dorothy stood in the doorway and looked around, she could see nothing but the great gray prairie on every side. Not a tree nor a house broke the broad sweep of flat country that reached to the edge of the sky in all directions. The sun had baked the plowed land into a gray mass, with little cracks running through it. Even the grass was not green, for the sun had burned the tops of the long blades until they were the same gray color to be seen everywhere. Once the house had been painted, but the sun blistered the paint and the rains washed it away, and now the house was as dull and gray as everything else.

When Aunt Em came there to live she was a young, pretty wife. The sun and wind had changed her, too. They had taken the sparkle from her eyes and left them a sober gray; they had taken the red from her cheeks and lips, and they were gray also. She was thin and gaunt, and never smiled now. When Dorothy, who was an orphan, first came to her, Aunt Em had been so startled by the child's laughter that she would scream and press her hand upon her heart whenever Dorothy's merry voice reached her ears; and she still looked at the little girl with wonder that she could find anything to laugh at.

Uncle Henry never laughed. He worked hard from morning till night and did not know what joy was. He was gray also, from his long beard to his rough boots, and he looked stern and solemn, and rarely spoke.

It was Toto that made Dorothy laugh, and saved her from growing as gray as her other surroundings. Toto was not gray; he was a little black dog, with long silky hair and small black eyes that twinkled merrily on either side of his funny, wee nose. Toto played all day long, and Dorothy played with him, and loved him dearly.

Hector St. John de Crèvecoeur would not have recognized Uncle Henry's farm; it is straight out of Hamlin Garland. On it a deadly environment dominates everyone and everything except Dorothy and her pet. The setting is Old Testament and nature seems grayly impersonal and even angry. Yet it is a fearsome cyclone that lifts Dorothy and Toto in their house and deposits them "very gently—for a cyclone—in the midst of a country of marvelous beauty." We immediately sense the contrast between Oz and Kansas. Here there are "stately trees bearing rich and luscious fruits . . . gorgeous flowers . . . and birds with . . . brilliant plumage" sing in the trees. In Oz "a small brook rushing and sparkling along" mur-

murs "in a voice very grateful to a little girl who had lived so long on the dry, gray prairies."

Trouble intrudes. Dorothy's house has come down on the wicked Witch of the East, killing her. Nature, by sheer accident, can provide benefits, for indirectly the cyclone has disposed of one of the two truly bad influences in the Land of Oz. Notice that evil ruled in both the East and the West; after Dorothy's coming it rules only in the West.

The wicked Witch of the East had kept the little Munchkin people "in bondage for many years, making them slave for her night and day." Just what this slavery entailed is not immediately clear, but Baum later gives us a specific example. The Tin Woodman, whom Dorothy meets on her way to the Emerald City, had been put under a spell by the Witch of the East. Once an independent and hard working human being, the Woodman found that each time he swung his axe it chopped off a different part of his body. Knowing no other trade he "worked harder than ever," for luckily in Oz tinsmiths can repair such things. Soon the Woodman was all tin. In this way Eastern witchcraft dehumanized a simple laborer so that the faster and better he worked the more quickly he became a kind of machine. Here is a Populist view of evil Eastern influences on honest labor which could hardly be more pointed.

There is one thing seriously wrong with being made of tin; when it rains rust sets in. Tin Woodman had been standing in the same position for a year without moving before Dorothy came along and oiled his joints. The Tin Woodman's situation has an obvious parallel in the condition of many Eastern workers after the depression of 1893. While Tin Woodman is standing still, rusted solid, he deludes himself into thinking he is no longer capable of that most human of sentiments, love. Hate does not fill the void, a constant lesson in the Oz books, and Tin Woodman feels that only a heart will make him sensitive again. So he accompanies Dorothy to see if the Wizard will give him one.

Oz itself is a magic oasis surrounded by impassable deserts, and the country is divided in a very orderly fashion. In the North and South the people are ruled by good witches, who are not quite as powerful as the wicked ones of the East and West. In the center of the land rises the magnificent Emerald City ruled by the Wizard of Oz, a successful humbug whom even the witches mistakenly feel "is more powerful than all the rest of us together." Despite these forces, the mark of goodness, placed on Dorothy's forehead by the Witch of the North, serves as protection for Dorothy throughout her travels. Goodness and innocence prevail even over the powers of evil and delusion in Oz. Perhaps it is this basic and beautiful optimism that makes Baum's tale so characteristically American—and Midwestern.

Dorothy is Baum's Miss Everyman. She is one of us, levelheaded and human, and she has a real problem. Young readers can understand her quandary as readily as can adults. She is good, not precious, and she thinks quite naturally about others. For all of the attractions of Oz Dorothy desires only to return to the gray plains and Aunt Em and Uncle Henry. She is directed toward the Emerald City by the good Witch of the North, since the Wizard will surely be able to solve the problem of the impassable deserts. Dorothy sets out on the Yellow Brick Road wearing the Witch of the East's magic Silver Shoes. Silver shoes walking on a golden road; henceforth Dorothy becomes the innocent agent of Baum's ironic view of the Silver issue. Remember, neither Dorothy, nor the good Witch of the North, nor the Munchkins understand the power of these shoes. The allegory is abundantly clear. On the next to last page of the book Baum has Glinda, Witch of the South, tell Dorothy, "Your Silver Shoes will carry you over the desert. . . . If you had known their power you could have gone back to your Aunt Em the very first day you came to this country." Glinda explains, "All you have to do is to knock the heels together three times and command the shoes to carry you wherever you wish to go." William Jennings

Bryan never outlined the advantages of the silver standard any more effectively.

Not understanding the magic of the Silver Shoes, Dorothy walks the mundane—and dangerous—Yellow Brick Road. The first person she meets is a Scarecrow. After escaping from his wooden perch, the Scarecrow displays a terrible sense of inferiority and self doubt, for he has determined that he needs real brains to replace the common straw in his head. William Allen White wrote an article in 1896 entitled "What's the Matter with Kansas?" In it he accused Kansas farmers of ignorance, irrationality and general muddle-headedness. What's wrong with Kansas are the people, said Mr. White. Baum's character seems to have read White's angry characterization. But Baum never takes White seriously and so the Scarecrow soon emerges as innately a very shrewd and very capable individual.

The Scarecrow and the Tin Woodman accompany Dorothy along the Yellow Brick Road, one seeking brains, the other a heart. They meet next the Cowardly Lion. As King of Beasts he explains, "I learned that if I roared very loudly every living thing was frightened and got out of my way." Born a coward, he sobs, "Whenever there is danger my heart begins to beat fast." "Perhaps you have heart disease," suggests Tin Woodman, who always worries about hearts. But the Lion desires only courage and so he joins the party to ask help from the Wizard.

The Lion represents Bryan himself. In the election of 1896 Bryan lost the vote of Eastern labor, though he tried hard to gain their support. In Baum's story the Lion, on meeting the little group, "struck at the Tin Woodman with his sharp claws." But, to his surprise, "he could make no impression on the tin, although the Woodman fell over in the road and lay still." Baum here refers to the fact that in 1896 workers were often pressured into voting for McKinley and gold by their employers. Amazed, the Lion says, "he nearly blunted my claws," and he adds even more appropriately, "When they scratched against the tin it made a cold shiver run down my back." The King of Beasts is not after all very

cowardly, and Bryan, although a pacifist and an anti-imperialist in a time of national expansion, is not either. The magic Silver Shoes belong to Dorothy, however. Silver's potent charm, which had come to mean so much to so many in the Midwest, could not be entrusted to a political symbol. Baum delivers Dorothy from the world of adventure and fantasy to the real world of heartbreak and desolation through the power of Silver. It represents a real force in a land of illusion, and neither the Cowardly Lion nor Bryan truly needs or understands its use.

All together now the small party moves toward the Emerald City. Coxey's Army of tramps and indigents, marching to ask President Cleveland for work in 1894, appears no more naively innocent than this group of four characters going to see a humbug Wizard, to request favors that only the little girl among them deserves.

Those who enter the Emerald City must wear green glasses. Dorothy later discovers that the greenness of dresses and ribbons disappears on leaving, and everything becomes a bland white. Perhaps the magic of any city is thus self imposed. But the Wizard dwells here and so the Emerald City represents the national Capitol. The Wizard, a little bumbling old man, hiding behind a facade of papier mâché and noise, might be any President from Grant to McKinley. He comes straight from the fair grounds in Omaha, Nebraska, and he symbolizes the American criterion for leadership—he is able to be everything to everybody.

As each of our heroes enters the throne room to ask a favor the Wizard assumes different shapes, representing different views toward national leadership. To Dorothy, he appears as an enormous head, "bigger than the head of the biggest giant." An apt image for a naive and innocent little citizen. To the Scarecrow he appears to be a lovely, gossamer fairy, a most appropriate form for an idealistic Kansas farmer. The Woodman sees a horrible beast, as would any exploited Eastern laborer after the trouble of the 1890s. But the Cowardly Lion, like W. J.

Bryan, sees a "Ball of Fire, so fierce and glowing he could scarcely bear to gaze upon it." Baum then provides an additional analogy, for when the Lion "tried to go nearer he singed his whiskers and he crept back tremblingly to a spot nearer the door."

The Wizard has asked them all to kill the Witch of the West. The golden road does not go in that direction and so they must follow the sun, as have many pioneers in the past. The land they now pass through is "rougher and hillier, for there were no farms nor houses in the country of the West and the ground was untilled." The Witch of the West uses natural forces to achieve her ends; she is Baum's version of sentient and malign nature.

Finding Dorothy and her friends in the West, the Witch sends forty wolves against them, then forty vicious crows and finally a great swarm of black bees. But it is through the power of a magic golden cap that she summons the flying monkeys. They capture the little girl and dispose of her companions. Baum makes these Winged Monkeys into an Oz substitute for the plains Indians. Their leader says, "Once . . . we were a free people, living happily in the great forest, flying from tree to tree, eating nuts and fruit, and doing just as we pleased without calling anybody master." "This," he explains, "was many years ago, long before Oz came out of the clouds to rule over this land." But like many Indian tribes Baum's monkeys are not inherently bad; their actions depend wholly upon the bidding of others. Under the control of an evil influence, they do evil. Under the control of goodness and innocence, as personified by Dorothy, the monkeys are helpful and kind, although unable to take her to Kansas. Says the Monkey King, "We belong to this country alone, and cannot leave it." The same could be said with equal truth of the first Americans.

Dorothy presents a special problem to the Witch. Seeing the mark on Dorothy's forehead and the Silver Shoes on her feet, the Witch begins "to tremble with fear, for she knew what

a powerful charm belonged to them." Then "she happened to look into the child's eyes and saw how simple the soul behind them was, and that the little girl did not know of the wonderful power the Silver Shoes gave her." Here Baum again uses the Silver allegory to state the blunt homily that while goodness affords a people ultimate protection against evil, ignorance of their capabilities allows evil to impose itself upon them. The Witch assumes the proportions of a kind of western Mark Hanna or Banker Boss, who, through natural malevolence, manipulates the people and holds them prisoner by cynically taking advantage of their innate innocence.

Enslaved in the West, "Dorothy went to work meekly, with her mind made up to work as hard as she could; for she was glad the Wicked Witch had decided not to kill her." Many Western farmers have held these same grim thoughts in less mystical terms. If the Witch of the West is a diabolical force of Darwinian or Spencerian nature, then another contravening force may be counted upon to dispose of her. Dorothy destroys the evil Witch by angrily dousing her with a bucket of water. Water, that precious commodity which the drought-ridden farmers on the great plains needed so badly, and which if correctly used could create an agricultural paradise, or at least dissolve a wicked witch. Plain water brings an end to malign nature in the West.

When Dorothy and her companions return to the Emerald City they soon discover that the Wizard is really nothing more than "a little man, with a bald head and a wrinkled face." Can this be the ruler of the land?

Our friends looked at him in surprise and dismay.

"I thought Oz was a great Head," said Dorothy. . . . "And I thought Oz was a terrible Beast," said the Tin Woodman. "And I thought Oz was a Ball of Fire," exclaimed the Lion. "No; you are all wrong," said the little man meekly. "I have been making believe."

Dorothy asks if he is truly a great Wizard. He

confides, "Not a bit of it, my dear; I'm just a common man." Scarecrow adds, "You're more than that . . . you're a humbug."

The Wizard's deception is of long standing in Oz and even the Witches were taken in. How was it accomplished? "It was a great mistake my ever letting you into the Throne Room," the Wizard complains. "Usually I will not see even my subjects, and so they believe I am something terrible." What a wonderful lesson for youngsters of the decade when Benjamin Harrison, Grover Cleveland and William McKinley were hiding in the White House. Formerly the Wizard was a mimic, a ventriloquist and a circus balloonist. The latter trade involved going "up in a balloon on circus day, so as to draw a crowd of people together and get them to pay to see the circus." Such skills are as admirably adapted to success in late-nineteenth-century politics as they are to the humbug wizardry of Baum's story. A pointed comment on Midwestern political ideals is the fact that our little Wizard comes from Omaha, Nebraska, a center of Populist agitation. "Why that isn't very far from Kansas," cries Dorothy. Nor, indeed, are any of the characters in the wonderful land of Oz.

The Wizard, of course, can provide the objects of self-delusion desired by Tin Woodman, Scarecrow and Lion. But Dorothy's hope of going home fades when the Wizard's balloon leaves too soon. Understand this: Dorothy wishes to leave a green and fabulous land, from which all evil has disappeared, to go back to the gray desolation of the Kansas prairies. Dorothy is an orphan, Aunt Em and Uncle Henry are her only family. Reality is never far from Dorothy's consciousness and in the most heartrending terms she explains her reasoning to the Good Witch Glinda,

Aunt Em will surely think something dreadful has happened to me, and that will make her put on mourning; and unless the crops are better this year than were last I am sure Uncle Henry cannot afford it.

The Silver Shoes furnish Dorothy with a magic means of travel. But when she arrives back in Kansas she finds, "The Silver Shoes had fallen off in her flight through the air, and were lost forever in the desert." Were the "her" to refer to America in 1900, Baum's statement could hardly be contradicted.

Current historiography tends to criticize the Populist movement for its "delusions, myths and foibles," Professor C. Vann Woodward observed recently. Yet *The Wonderful Wizard of Oz* has provided unknowing generations with a gentle and friendly Midwestern critique of the Populist rationale on these very same grounds. Led by naive innocence and protected by good will, the farmer, the laborer and the politician approach the mystic holder of national power to ask for personal fulfillment. Their desires, as well as the Wizard's cleverness in answering them, are all self-delusion. Each of these characters carries within him the solution to his own problem, were he only to view himself objectively. The fearsome Wizard turns out to be nothing more than a common man, capable of shrewd but mundane answers to these self-induced needs. Like any good politician he gives the people what they want. Throughout the story Baum poses a central thought; the American desire for symbols of fulfillment is illusory. Real needs lie elsewhere.

Thus the Wizard cannot help Dorothy, for of all the characters only she has a wish that is selfless, and only she has a direct connection to honest, hopeless human beings. Dorothy supplies real fulfillment when she returns to her aunt and uncle, using the Silver Shoes, and cures some of their misery and heartache. In this way Baum tells us that the Silver crusade at least brought back Dorothy's lovely spirit to the disconsolate plains farmer. Her laughter, love and good will are no small addition to that gray land, although the magic of Silver has been lost forever as a result.

Noteworthy too is Baum's prophetic placement of leadership in Oz after Dorothy's departure. The Scarecrow reigns over the Emerald City, the Tin Woodman rules in the West and the

Lion protects smaller beasts in "a grand old forest." Thereby farm interests achieve national importance, industrialism moves West and Bryan commands only a forest full of lesser politicians.

Baum's fantasy succeeds in bridging the gap between what children want and what they should have. It is an admirable example of the way in which an imaginative writer can teach goodness and morality without producing the almost inevitable side effect of nausea. Today's children's books are either saccharine and empty, or boring and pedantic. Baum's first Oz tale—and those which succeed it—are immortal not so much because the "heart-aches and nightmares are left out" as that "the wonderment and joy" are retained.

Baum declares, "The story of 'the Wonderful Wizard of Oz' was written solely to pleasure children of today." In 1963 there are very few children who have never heard of the Scarecrow, the Tin Woodman or the Cowardly Lion, and whether they know W. W. Denslow's original illustrations of Dorothy, or Judy Garland's whimsical characterization, is immaterial. *The Wizard* has become a genuine piece of American folklore because, knowing his audience, Baum never allowed the consistency of the allegory to take precedence over the theme of youthful entertainment. Yet once discovered, the author's allegorical intent seems clear, and it gives depth and lasting interest even to children who only sense something else beneath the surface of the story. Consider the fun in picturing turn-of-the-century America, a difficult era at best, using these ready-made symbols provided by Baum. The relationships and analogies outlined above are admittedly theoretical, but they are far too consistent to be coincidental, and they furnish a teaching mechanism which is guaranteed to reach any level of student.

The Wizard of Oz says so much about so many things that it is hard not to imagine a satisfied and mischievous gleam in Lyman Frank Baum's eye as he had Dorothy say, "And oh, Aunt Em! I'm so glad to be at home again!"

■ ■ ■

STUDY QUESTIONS

1. Why was Lyman Frank Baum in a good position to understand the problems of workers in the late nineteenth century?

2. What sort of picture does *The Wonderful Wizard of Oz* paint of farm life? What was the effect of agrarian labor on the farmers themselves?

3. How does the story detail the complexities of the silver issue? Does Baum seem to feel that the gold standard was the major problem facing the farmers?

4. How does the Tin Woodman dramatize the plight of the northern industrial worker? How does the Scarecrow symbolize the plight of the farmers?

5. In what ways is the Cowardly Lion similar to William Jennings Bryan?

6. What roles do the good and bad witches play in the story?

7. Is *The Wondeful Wizard of Oz* an effective parable?

BIBLIOGRAPHY

Martin Gardiner and Russell B. Nye, *The Wizard of Oz and Who He Was* (1957) examine Baum and his works. The best studies of the Populist movement are John D. Hicks, *The Populist Revolt* (1931); C. Vann Woodward, *Tom Watson: Agrarian Rebel* (1938); Lawrence Goodwyn, *Democratic Promise: The Populist Movement in America* (1976); Robert C. McMath, Jr., *Populist Vanguard: A History of the Southern Farmers' Alliance* (1975); and Stanley B. Parsons, *The Populist Context: Rural Versus Urban Power on a Great Plains Frontier* (1973). Paul W. Glad, *McKinley, Bryan, and the People* (1964) and Robert F. Durden, *The Climax of Populism: The Election of 1896* (1965) examine the crucial election of 1896. For industrial working conditions in the late nineteenth century see Herbert G. Gutman, *Work, Class, and Society in Industrializing America* (1976); David Brody, *Steelworkers in America: The Nonunion Era* (1960); and Albert Rees, *Real Wages in Manufacturing, 1890–1914* (1961).

SHE COULDN'T HAVE DONE IT, EVEN IF SHE DID

Kathryn Allamong Jacob

There is something infinitely compelling and fascinating about an unsolved murder. England has Jack the Ripper, and although it has been almost one hundred years since the last Ripper murder was committed, historians of the crimes still speculate on the identity of the murderer. The American equivalent to Jack the Ripper is Lizzie Borden, who very likely killed her father and stepmother on August 2, 1892. Although she was judged innocent of the murders, strong circumstantial evidence points toward her guilt. However, in a larger sense the jury was more concerned with the physical and psychological nature of upper-class womanhood than with the actual crimes. As Kathryn Allamong Jacob writes, during the summer of 1893 "the entire Victorian conception of womanhood was on trial for its life." The question most commonly asked that summer was to the point: How could a well-bred woman, who by her very nature was innocent, childlike, and moral, commit such a horrible crime? The answer of most well-bred men, and of all twelve of the prosperous, Yankee jurors, was that she could not. An examination of the case thus illuminates an entire cultural landscape, casting light especially on American attitudes toward women. Were women, as a writer for *Scribner's* believed, "merely large babies . . . shortsighted, frivolous, and [occupying] an intermediate stage between children and men. . . ."? Or was there something more to the issue?

During the summer of 1893, Americans riveted their attention on the town of New Bedford, Massachusetts, where Lizzie Andrew Bordon was being tried for the gruesome ax murder of her father and stepmother. All other news paled in comparison, for here, in southeastern Massachusetts, not only a particular woman, but the entire Victorian conception of womanhood, was on trial for its life.

The drama began in August of 1892 at Number 92 Second Street in Fall River, Massachusetts, the home of Andrew Jackson Borden, whose family coat of arms prophetically bore a lion holding a battle-ax. The household consisted of Andrew, seventy; Abby Gray Borden, sixty-five, his wife; his two daughters, Lizzie Andrew and Emma Lenora, aged thirty-two and forty-two; and Bridget Sullivan, twenty-six, an Irish servant who had been with the family for nearly three years.

Andrew Borden began his business career as an undertaker. It was rumored that he had cut the feet off corpses to make them fit into undersized coffins, but however ill-gotten his initial profits, Borden invested them wisely. By 1892 he was worth nearly half a million dollars, served as a director of several banks and as a board member of three woolen mills, and had built the imposing A. J. Borden Building on Main Street as a testimony to his business acumen. To keep his fortunes increasing, Borden foreclosed, undercut, overcharged, and hoarded without flinching.

Borden's first wife, Sarah, had died in 1862 after bearing him three daughters, only two of whom survived past infancy. Two years later, he married Abby Gray, a thirty-eight-year-old spinster. Nothing suggests that Abby was anything but kind to the two little girls whose stepmother she became, but they never returned her affection. After her marriage, Abby became a compulsive eater. Only a little over five feet tall, by 1892 she weighed more than two hundred pounds.

Emma, the older daughter, still lived at home at age forty-two. By all accounts, she was dowdy and narrow-minded. Lizzie Borden, ten years younger, also lived at home. Otherwise tightfisted, Andrew Borden doted on his younger daughter: over the years he lavished on Lizzie expensive gifts—a diamond ring, a sealskin cape, even a Grand Tour of Europe. Lizzie worshiped her father in return, and even gave him her high school ring to wear as a token of her affection.

Like her sister, Lizzie had evidently given up hope of marriage, but she led a more active life, centered around good works and the Central Congregational Church, where she taught a Sunday-school class of Chinese children, the sons and daughters of Fall River laundrymen. Though she loathed doing housework, she enthusiastically helped cook the church's annual Christmas dinner for local newsboys. In addition to being secretary-treasurer of the Christian Endeavor, Lizzie was active in the Ladies' Fruit and Flower Mission, the Women's Christian Temperance Union, and the Good Samaritan Charity Hospital.

Lizzie's Christian charity did not extend to her own home. The Borden family was not happy. While Emma tolerated her stepmother, Lizzie openly disliked her. Ill feelings increased in 1887, when Andrew gave Abby a house for the use of her sister. Seeking peace, Andrew gave his daughters a house of greater value to rent out, but they were not placated. A dressmaker later remembered making the mistake of referring to Abby as Lizzie's "mother," causing Lizzie to snap, "Don't call her that to me. She is a mean thing and we hate her."

Even the house Lizzie lived in vexed her. Its Grant-era furnishings contrasted sharply with her stylish clothes. There was no bath and no electricity, though such conveniences were common elsewhere in town. Beside the water closet in the basement stood a pile of old newspapers

"She Couldn't Have Done It, Even If She Did" by Kathryn Allamong Jacob, from *American Heritage 29* (February/March, 1978). Reprinted by permission.

for sanitary purposes. No interior space was wasted on hallways. Rooms simply opened into one another, making it difficult for anyone to pass through unnoticed. Lizzie longed to live "on the hill," Fall River's most elegant neighborhood and the symbol of the social prominence she craved. While her father's wealth entitled her to live there, Andrew insisted on living on déclassé Second Street.

On Tuesday, August 2, 1892, strange things began to happen in the Borden house. Mr. and Mrs. Borden and Bridget suffered severe vomiting; Lizzie later claimed she felt queasy the next day. Emma, on vacation in Fairhaven, was spared. Over Andrew's objections, Abby waddled across the street to Dr. Bowen's to tell him she feared they had been poisoned. When he learned that the previous night's dinner had been warmed-over fish, the doctor laughingly sent her home.

The next day, Uncle John Morse, brother of the first Mrs. Borden, arrived unexpectedly on business. Like Andrew, Morse was single-minded in his pursuit of wealth, and the two men had remained friends. That evening, Lizzie visited Miss Alice Russell, a friend of Emma's. Miss Russell later testified that their conversation had been unsettling. Lizzie had spoken of burglary attempts on the Borden home, of threats against her father from unknown enemies. "I feel as if something was hanging over me that I cannot throw off. . . ," she said. "Father has so much trouble. . . ." Though Miss Russell tried to reassure her, Lizzie left on an ominous, but prescient, note: "I am afraid somebody will do something."

On Thursday morning, August 4, Bridget rose about six and lit the breakfast fire. Around seven, the elder Bordens and their guest sat down to eat in the dining room. Lizzie did not appear downstairs till nine. By then, Mrs. Borden had begun dusting the downstairs and Morse had left the house to visit relatives across town. Lizzie told Bridget she did not feel well enough to eat breakfast, but sat in the kitchen sipping coffee. About twenty after nine, Andrew, too, left the

house, setting off downtown to oversee his investments. Perhaps ten minutes later, Abby Borden went upstairs to tidy the guest room, and Bridget went outside to begin washing the downstairs windows. Only Lizzie and Abby remained in the house; Abby was never seen alive again.

Perhaps because of the oppressive heat, Andrew broke his long-established routine by coming home for lunch at a quarter of eleven, an hour and a half early. Bridget later testified that she had just begun scrubbing the inside of the windows when she heard him struggling with the front-door lock and let him in. Lizzie, by her own admission, was coming down the stairs from the second floor where Abby's body lay. (At the Borden trial the following year, the prosecution would produce witnesses who testified that Abby's body, lying on the guest-room floor, was clearly visible from the staircase, while the defense claimed it was almost completely obscured by a bed.) Andrew asked Lizzie about Abby's whereabouts, according to Bridget, and Lizzie told him that Abby had received a note asking her to attend a sick friend.

Bridget finished her windows and climbed the back stairs to her attic room to rest at about eleven. Andrew lay down on the parlor sofa to nap. On the guest-room floor above him lay Abby's bleeding corpse. The house was hot and silent. Within minutes, Bridget recalled, she was awakened by Lizzie calling, "Come down quick; father's dead; somebody came in and killed him."

Little was left of Andrew's face. Half an eye hung from its socket. Doctors testified that a single ax blow had killed him; nine others had been gratuitous. Shortly after the police arrived, Bridget and a neighbor ventured upstairs for a sheet to cover the hideous sight, and there they found Abby. Her plump body lay face down in a pool of blood, her head and neck a bloody mass. Those first on the scene noted that Lizzie remained remarkably calm throughout the ordeal. While one woman claimed that there were tears in her eyes, several others testified that Lizzie's eyes were dry and her hands steady.

News traveled fast from neighbor to neighbor, and even before the evening presses rolled, everyone in Fall River seemed to know of the horrifying incident. A local reporter recalled that "The cry of murder swept through the city like a typhoon . . . murder committed under the very glare of the midday sun within three minutes walk of the City Hall. . . ." By the next day, the story was front-page news throughout the country and when, after two days, no crazed ax-wielder was produced, newspapers which had praised the police began to question their competence. Trial transcripts suggest that the police did err on the side of caution. If the victims had not been so prominent, matters would have been simpler. The *New York Times* appreciated this fact, and on August 6 noted that "The police are acting slowly and carefully in the affair giving way, no doubt, to feelings of sentiment because of the high social standing of the parties involved." No systematic search of the Borden house was conducted until thirty-two hours after the murders. Out of deference to the bereaved daughters, neither Lizzie nor Emma, who had been summoned home from her vacation, was closely questioned for nearly three days.

Yet, by Saturday, the day of the funerals, the police felt that they had little choice but to arrest Lizzie. She alone, they felt, had had the opportunity to commit the murders. They found it hard to believe that anyone could have passed through the house unseen by Lizzie, who claimed to have been on the first floor while Abby was being murdered above. It also strained credibility to assert, as Lizzie did, that Abby's 210-pound body had crashed to the floor without a sound. Furthermore, despite a reward offered by the Borden sisters, no sender of the note that Lizzie claimed had called Abby to town could be found.

Lizzie's own contradictory answers to the first questions put to her by police were highly damaging. When asked her whereabouts when her father was killed, she gave different answers to different interrogators: "In the back yard"; ". . . in the loft getting a piece of iron for sinkers"; ". . . up in the loft eating pears." The closed barn loft would have been so insufferably hot that day that few would have visited it voluntarily, much less lingered to eat pears. Furthermore, an officer who claimed to have been the first to examine the loft after the crimes testified that the dust on the floor was undisturbed by footprints or trailing skirts.

In Lizzie's favor was the fact that she had been neat and clean when first seen after the murders. The police were certain that the murderer would have been covered with blood. (Medical experts would later examine the trajectories of the spurting blood and argue otherwise, but belief in a blood-drenched killer persisted.)

Though puzzled by Lizzie's cleanliness, police were certain that they had found the murder weapon. Lying in a box of dusty tools, stored high on a chimney jog in the basement, was a hatchet head. It was neither rusty nor old, though it had been freshly rubbed in ashes, perhaps to make it appear so. Moreover, its wooden handle, from which blood would have been difficult to remove, had been broken off near the head.

When the news broke that Lizzie was under suspicion, newspaper readers were horrified—not over the possibility that Lizzie might have murdered her parents, but that the police would harbor such horrid thoughts. The Boston *Globe* expressed its readers' indignation: "The only person that the government can catch is one whose innocence placed her in its power; the poor, defenseless child, who ought to have claimed by very helplessness their protection."

Angry letters denouncing the police flooded newspaper offices from New York to Chicage. Editorials appeared castigating the brutish officers who would suspect a grieving daughter of such a crime. Americans were certain that well-brought-up daughters could not commit murder with a hatchet on sunny summer mornings. And their reaction was not entirely without rationale.

Throughout the 1890's, nearly every issue of *Forum, Arena, Scribner's, North America Review, Popular Science Monthly,* and *Harper's* (one of Lizzie's favorites) carried at least one article attesting to the gentleness, physical frailty, and docility of the well-bred American woman. Many of these articles were written in response to the growing number of women who were demanding equal rights, and were written with the intention of proving women hopelessly unable to handle the sacred privileges of men. After having read many such articles written by "learned gentlemen"—and antifeminist women—by the summer of 1892, men and women, regardless of how they stood on women's rights, felt certain that Lizzie Borden could not have hacked her parents to death. Physical and psychological frailties simply made it impossible.

Popular theories about women's physiological and psychological make-up took on new importance to followers of the Borden case. After detailed anatomical analysis, scientists confidently declared that the women of their era differed little from their prehistoric sisters. They spoke with assurance of women's arrested evolution. The fault, they agreed, lay in her reproductive capacity, which sapped vital powers that in men contributed to ever-improving physique and intellect.

The defects of the female anatomy included sloping shoulders, broad hips, underdeveloped muscles, short arms and legs, and poor coordination. To those who believed Lizzie innocent, evidence was abundant that no short-armed, uncoordinated, weakling of a woman could swing an ax with enough force to crash through hair and bone almost two dozen times.

But there was more to it than that. Having already noted woman's smaller frame, anatomists should hardly have been surprised to find her skull proportionately smaller than man's, yet they held up this revelation, too, as further proof of her inferiority. Rather than follow intellectual pursuits, for which they were woefully ill-equipped, women were advised to accept their intended roles as wives and mothers. After all, they were reminded, "Woman is only womanly when she sets herself to man 'like perfect music unto noble works.' "

Spinsters like Lizzie were, as one author charitably put it, "deplorable accidents," but they were not wholly useless. The nation's old maids were urged to devote themselves to Christian charities and to teaching—a "reproductive calling." Lizzie's devotion to good works and the church followed this prescription precisely. Compelling indeed was the image of this pious daughter serving steaming bowls of soup to indigent newsboys and diligently trying to bring the gospel to the heathen Chinese of Fall River.

While anatomists studied the size of woman's skull, psychologists examined its contents. Among the qualities found to be essentially female were spiritual sensitivity, a good memory for minutiae, and a great capacity for "ennobling love." These positive attributes, however, could not obscure the psychologists' basic premise: women were illogical, inconsistent, and incapable of independent thought.

It is no accident that these traits bore striking resemblance to those attributed to children. As on psychologist pointed out in *Scribner's:* "Women are merely large babies. They are shortsighted, frivolous and occupy an intermediate stage between children and men. . . ."

Several authors manfully chuckled over woman's inability to plan and think things through. Clearly the murderer of the Bordens had planned things quite well. Not only had "he" managed to murder two people and elude the police, but "he" had shown remarkable tenacity by hiding for more than an hour after murdering Abby in order to do the same to Andrew.

Woman was considered man's superior in one area only: the moral sphere. She was thought to possess more "natural refinement," "diviner instincts," and stronger "spiritual sensibility" than man. She was inherently gentle, and abhorred cruelty—hardly the virtues of an ax murderer. Woman was also truthful, though some authors attributed her inability to lie to a lack of intelligence rather than to innate goodness. When reporters interviewed Lizzie's friends, the young women repeatedly mentioned her honesty.

Lizzie benefited greatly from the prevailing stereotypes of feminine delicacy and docility: her cause was also served by the widely accepted stereotype of the female criminal. Ironically, the same periodicals which carried articles about women's gentle nature also carried enough sordid stories of crimes committed by them to cast considerable doubt on their moral superiority. But writers did not find the situation paradoxical. To them, there were clearly two types of women: the genteel ladies of their own class and those women beneath them. Gentlemen authors believed that the womanly instincts of gentleness and love were the monopoly of upper-class women.

Scientists could hardly charge women of their own class with propensities toward violence without casting doubt on their own good breeding. For lower-class women with whom they had no intimate ties (at least none to which they would admit), the situation was quite different. These writers made it very clear that no woman servant, housekeeper, prostitute, nurse, washerwoman, barmaid, or factory girl could be above suspicion.

Several authors even believed that the female criminal had to look the part. In an article in *North American Review*, August, 1895, one criminologist thoughtfully provided the following description: "[She] has coarse black hair and a good deal of it. . . . She has often a long face, a receding forehead, overjutting brows, prominent cheek-bones, an exaggerated frontal angle as seen in monkeys and savage races, and nearly always square jaws."

She could also be marked by deep wrinkles, a tendency toward baldness, and numerous moles. Other authors noted her long middle fingers, projecting ears, and overlapping teeth. While Lizzie had a massive jaw, her hair was red, her teeth were straight, and her ears flat. Perhaps fortunately for Bridget, a member of the suspect servant class, she was mole-free and brown-haired, and she did not have protruding middle fingers.

Criminal women supposedly exhibited neither the aversion to evil not the love of mankind which ennobled their upper-class sisters. Among their vices were said to be great cruelty, passionate temper, a craving for revenge, cunning greed, rapacity, contempt for truth, and vulgarity. Such women were thought to be "erotic," but incapable of devoted love. Certainly the Bordens' murderer had been exceedingly cruel. But, while Lizzie was admittedly fond of money and volunteered her dislike of her stepmother, few would have called her rapacious or vengeful, and erotic was hardly an adjective one would have applied to the chaste treasurer of the Fruit and Flower Mission.

The ferocity of the criminal woman fascinated many authors. A favorite murderess was Catherine Hayes, who, in 1890, stabbed her husband to death, cut off his head with a penknife, and boiled it. But then, Mrs. Hayes was a mill worker. One writer did admit that murders might be committed by well-bred women; their weapon would be poison, however, rather than a penknife or an ax, because its passivity appealed to their nature.

Lizzie's attorneys skillfully exploited these two stereotypes—the genteel young woman and the wart-ridden murderess—to their client's advantage throughout the Borden trial. Even before the case reached court, the press had firmly implanted in the public mind a clear picuture of Lizzie as bereaved daughter. The image-making began with the very first—and entirely false—story about Lizzie printed in the Boston *Globe* on the day after the murders; "The young woman, with her customary cheery disposition, evidenced her feelings in the tuneful melody from *Il Trovatore*, her favorite opera, which she was singing as she returned to the house. . . . One glance into the living room changed her from a buoyant-spirited young woman into a nervous wreck, every fiber of her being palpitating with the fearful effects of that look. . . ."

In the dozens of articles that followed, Lizzie

became the embodiment of genteel young womanhood. A reporter who interviewed her friends found "not one unmaidenly nor a single deliberately unkind act." Voicing the belief of many, he concluded, "Miss Borden, without a word from herself in her own defense, is a strong argument in her own favor."

The attributes of womanliness which vindicated Lizzie did not apply to Bridget. A servant, semiliterate, nearly friendless, Catholic and Irish, Bridget was the perfect target for suspicion. To the dismay of many, no evidence or motive ever could be found to implicate her in the deaths of her employers. Nevertheless, the police received dozens of letters urging her arrest. One man wrote demanding that Bridget and "her Confessor"—that is, her priest—be thrown into prison until she admitted her guilt.

The inquest began in Fall River on August 9. Two pharmacists from Smith's Drug Store testified that Lizzie had been shopping for poison on the afternoon before the murders. She had not asked for arsenic, which was sold over the counter, they said, but for the more lethal prussic acid, claiming she needed it to clean her sealskin cape. On the stand, Lizzie steadfastly denied the pharmacists' story, even denied knowing where Smith's Drug Store was, though it had been there for fourteen years on a street not five minutes from the house in which she had lived since childhood.

Lizzie's own testimony was full of contradictions. Discrepancies in her story might have been explained by hysteria or grief, but she had displayed neither. On August 5, a reporter at the murder scene for the Providence *Journal* noted: "She wasn't the least bit scared or worried. Most women would faint at seeing their father dead, for I never saw a more horrible sight. . . . She is a woman of remarkable nerve and self-control."

Such self-control seemed unnatural in an age when women were expected to swoon, and many pepole were alarmed by it. The Reverend Mr. Buck, Lizzie's minister, reassured her champions that "her calmness is the calmness of inno-

cence." Her lawyer, Mr. Jennings, sought to explain away her inconsistent answers by noting that "she was having her monthly illness" on the day of the murders, thereby evoking embarrassed nods of understanding.

Public sentiment on Lizzie's behalf rose to extraordinary heights. In full agreement with their pastor, her church declared her innocent. Ecclesiastical supporters were joined by several noted feminists. Mary Livermore, Susan Fessenden (president of the Women's Christian Temperance Union), and Lucy Stone took up the cudgels on Lizzie's behalf. Livermore declared her arrest to be another outrage perpetrated by "the tyrant man." Lizzie became the sacrificial lamb, the simple, warmhearted girl offered up by corrupt police to the altar of a power-hungry district attorney.

Nonetheless, the judge ordered her arrest at the inquest's end.

Reporters found Lizzie disappointingly composed after the indictment. With no tears to report, they concentrated on her cherry-trimmed hat and the two ministers on whose arms she leaned as she went off to jail in Taunton, the county seat. The horrible cell that awaited her was described in detail. In fact, Lizzie was not confined to a cell, but spent much of her time in the matron's room. Little mention was made of the flowers that graced the prison's window sill, or the lace-edged pillow slips brought by Emma, or of the meals which Lizzie had sent over from Taunton's best hotel.

When the preliminary hearing before Judge Blaisdell began in late November, reporters from more than forty out-of-town newspapers attended. Police held back huge crowds while ladies and gentlemen from Fall River's elite filed into the courtroom to claim the best seats.

A new piece of evidence, damaging to Lizzie's cause, was introduced. She had turned over to the police a spotlessly clean, fancy, blue bengaline dress that she swore she had worn on the day of the murders. Women in New England were surprised. No one wore party dresses of bengaline, a partly woolen fabric, around the house in the August heat. While witnesses swore that Lizzie was indeed wearing blue that day, none could swear that this dress was the one they had seen. To confound the problem, Alice Russell reluctantly admitted that she had seen Lizzie burn a blue cotton dress in the kitchen stove three days after the murders. The dress was soiled, she said Lizzie had told her, with brown paint—a color, noted the prosecutor, not unlike that of dried blood.

Except for rubbing her shoe buttons together, Lizzie sat quietly and displayed little interest. On the very last day, however, she broke into sobs as she heard her lawyer declare that no "person could have committed that crime unless his heart was black as hell." Delighted newspaper artists sketched a tearful Lizzie listening to Mr. Jennings as he asked: "Would it be the stranger, or would it be the one bound to the murdered man by ties of love? . . . what does it mean when we say the youngest daughter? The last one whose baby fingers have been lovingly entwined about her father's brow? Is there nothing in the ties of love and affection?"

Judge Blaidell listened to all the evidence. It was no stranger who sat before him, but the daughter of a family he knew well. Jennings' image of the twining baby fingers was compelling, but so was the evidence prosecutor Hosea Knowlton produced. The judge finally began to speak: "Suppose for a single moment that *a man* was standing there. He was found close by that guestchamber which to Mrs. Borden was a chamber of death. Suppose that *a man* had been found in the vicinity of Mr. Borden and the only account he could give of himself was the unreasonable one that he was out in the barn looking for sinkers, that he was in the yard. . . . Would there be any question in the minds of men what should be done with such a man?" The judge's voice broke, but he continued: ". . . the judgment of the court is that you are probably guilty and you are ordered to wait the action of the Superior Court."

The trial began in New Bedford, Massachusetts, on June 5, 1893. Reporters from all over the East Coast converged on the town. Every hotel room within miles was reserved. Fences had to be erected around the courthouse to control the crowds.

Lizzie's newly inherited fortune of several hundred thousand dollars bought her excellent counsel. George Robinson, former governor of the state, was a masterful orator with a politician's shrewd sense of public opinion: at his suggestion, Lizzie went into mourning for the first time since the murders. Laboring against him were District Attorneys Hosea Knowlton and William Moody (a future U.S. Supreme Court justice), as able as Robinson, but with a distaste for flamboyance. Among the three judges who would hear Lizzie's case was Justice Justin Dewey, whom Robinson had elevated to the bench while governor.

One hundred and forty-eight men awaited jury selection. It was assumed that all had formed opinions; they were asked only if their minds were still open enough to judge the evidence fairly. The first man called claimed he could never convict a woman of a capital offense and was dismissed. Of the final twelve, the foreman was a real estate broker and sometime politician, two were manufacturers, three were mechanics, and six were farmers with considerable acreage. Not one foreign-sounding name was among them. Nearly all were over fifty: all were good Yankees.

The first blow to the prosecution came when Judge Dewey ruled Lizzie's damaging inquest testimony inadmissible and barred evidence regarding the alleged attempt to buy poison. While these rulings made Knowlton's task more difficult, his biggest worry was that jury men believed, as did the Boston *Globe,* in the "moral improbability that a woman of refinement and gentle training. . . could have conceived and executed so bloody a butchery." As he repeatedly reminded the jury, "We must face this case as men, not gallants."

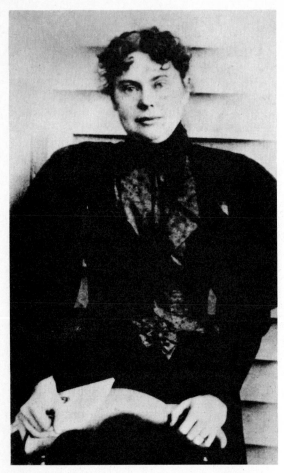

■ ■ *Lizzie Borden, accused of the ax murders of her father and stepmother in Fall River, Massachusetts (August 1892) was aquitted by an all male jury that refused to believe a well-bred woman could be capable of such an act.*

Knowlton produced medical experts from Harvard who testified that any average-sized woman could have swung an ax with force enough to commit the murders, and that the trajectory of blood would have been away from the assailant: Lizzie's tidy appearance minutes after the crimes had no bearing on her guilt or innocence. Robinson blithely discounted their testimony by asking the jurymen whether they put more store in Harvard scientists than in their own New England common sense.

Though Lizzie later professed to be shocked at his bill of $25,000, Robinson was worth every penny. As she sat before the jury, a Sunday-school teacher and loving youngest daughter, the jurymen, nearly all of whom were fathers themselves, heard Robinson conclude: "If the little sparrow does not fall unnoticed, then indeed in God's great providence, this woman has not been alone in this courtroom."

The jury was sent off to deliberate with what one reporter called Judge Dewey's "plea for the innocent." The other two judges were said to have been stunned by his lack of objectivity. Though Dewey was indeed grateful to Robinson for his judgeship, a more compelling reason for his unswerving belief in Lizzie's innocence may have been the three daughters he had at home, the eldest of whom was Lizzie's age.

The jurors who filed out with Dewey's plea ringing in their ears were bewhiskered, respectable, family men. If they could believe that a gentlewoman could pick up a hatchet such as surely lay in their own basements, and by murdering her parents become an heiress, what could they think next time they looked into their own girls' eyes?

They returned in one hour. The *New York Times* reported that Lizzie's "face became livid, her lips were compressed as she tottered to her feet to hear the verdict!" Before the clerk could finish asking for it, the foreman cried, "Not guilty!" Lizzie dropped to her seat as an enormous cheer went up from the spectators who climbed onto the benches, waving hats and handkerchiefs and weeping.

It would have been difficult for any jury to convict "beyond all reasonable doubt" on the circumstantial evidence presented. However, in the nearby bar to which the jurors dashed, a reporter learned that there had been no debate at all among the twelve. All exhibits were ignored. Their vote had been immediate and unanimous. It was only to avoid the impression that their minds had been made up in advance that they sat and chatted for an hour before returning with their verdict.

The following morning, Americans found reflected in the headlines their own joy that the jury had been so wise. Lizzie and Emma returned to Second Street.

Fall River society, which had defended her throughout her ordeal, fell away thereafter, and Lizzie was left pretty much alone. Undaunted, she determined to have all the things she had missed in her youth. With what some considered indiscreet haste, she bought a large house on the hill and named it Maplecroft. She also asked to be called Lisbeth and stopped going to the church whose parishioners had defended her so energetically. Matters were not improved when townspeople learned that she had bought and destroyed every available copy of local reporter Edwin Porter's *The Fall River Tragedy*, which had included portions of her inquest testimony.

Lizzie sealed her isolation in 1904 by striking up a friendship with Nance O'Neil, a Boston actress. The following year, to her neighbors' horror, Lizzie gave a party—complete with caterers and potted palms—for Miss O'Neil and her troupe. That night, Emma quietly moved out and never spoke to or saw Lizzie again.

Lizzie continued to live at Maplecroft in increasing isolation. Undoubtedly, she heard the nasty rhyme children began to sing to the tune of "Ta-Ra-Ra Boom-De-Ay!":

Lizzie Borden took an ax
And gave her mother forty whacks;
When she saw what she had done,
She gave her father forty-one!

Lizzie Borden died on June 1, 1927, at the age of sixty-six in Fall River. Emma died ten days later in New Hampshire. Few gravestones conceal a puzzle more intricate than that sealed away by the imposing Borden monument in Oak Grove Cemetery. The truth about the events on Second Street lies buried there along with Andrew, Abby, Emma, and Lizzie, but back then, in the summer of 1893, most Americans knew in their hearts that no young lady like Lizzie could have murdered her parents with an ax. Reputable authors in respectable magazines assured them their intuition was correct. They did not even want to think that it could be otherwise.

■ ■ ■

STUDY QUESTIONS

1. How did Lizzie Borden's class and social standing influence the way she was treated by legal authorities?

2. What were the physical, psychological, intellectual, and moral characteristics that popular magazines in the late nineteenth century attributed to well-bred women? How closely did Lizzie conform to these expectations?

3. What did late nineteenth-century writers mean by such concepts as "arrested evolution" and "deplorable accidents"? How do these concepts indicate a sexually biased society?

4. In what area were women considered superior to men? Why was this so?

5. How did popular attitudes toward upper-class and lower-class women differ? Why were many people more inclined to suspect Bridget Sullivan than Lizzie Borden of the crime?

6. How was Lizzie's behavior during the entire episode interpreted?

7. Why was the trial politically and symbolically significant?

BIBLIOGRAPHY

The Borden murder case has been examined and reexamined. Victoria Lincoln, *Lizzie Borden, a Private Disgrace* (1967) and Robert Sullivan, *Goodbye Lizzie Borden* (1974) argue that she was indeed guilty of the crimes. Edward D. Radin, *Lizzie Borden: The Untold Story* (1961) views the case from a different perspective.

Recent historical scholarship has only begun to explore the complexities of American attitudes toward women. Lois W. Banner, *Women in Modern America: A Brief History* (1974, second edition 1984) presents a fine introduction to the topic and a good bibliography. Other useful studies on women in the late nineteenth century include John S. Haller, Jr., and Robin M. Haller, *The Physician and Sexuality in Victorian America* (1974); G. J. Barker-Benfield, *The Horrors of the Half-Known Life: Male Attitudes Toward Women and Sexuality in Nineteenth-Century America* (1976); Linda Gordon, *Woman's Body, Woman's Right: A Social History of Birth Control in America* (1976); and Lois Banner, *American Beauty* (1983).

Two other books present different views of the role of women in America. Kate Chopin, *The Awakening* (1980) is a wonderful novel written with depth and sensitivity. Questions of isolation and alienation in a small American town are touched upon in Michael Lesy, *Wisconsin Death Trip* (1973).

THE QUEST FOR SUBCOMMUNITIES AND THE RISE OF AMERICAN SPORT

Benjamin G. Rader

Sports, their supporters claim, both aid society and the individual participant. They promote good health, exorcise pent-up aggressions, and satisfy people's desires for entertainment and spectacle. Perhaps most important of all, they provide a sense of community for millions of Americans. In an age of geographic mobility, rapid urbanization, and bureaucratic impersonalization, sports teams permit people from different backgrounds and different occupations to form bonds of loyalty and community. Sports also help cement ties between people of similar backgrounds and similar economic conditions.

Given this social function, it is not surprising that the "rise of sports" occurred during the years when America was changing from a rural agrarian country to an urban industrial nation. This process was rapid and complex, and all too often the people who experienced the remarkable changes were left with feelings of loneliness and loss. The sporting clubs and athletic teams of the period helped ease the pain of the difficult transition. As historian Benjamin G. Rader notes, "Sports clubs . . . became one of the basic means by which certain groups sought to establish subcommunities within the larger society." It is important to recognize, however, that sporting organizations function on several social levels. Some seek to preserve group identity by excluding outsiders. Others try to promote solidarity between different groups and classes. The difference is often the difference between the nineteenth- and the twentieth-century sporting experience.

One of the most intriguing problems for the sport historian is to account for the relationship between the American social structure and the "take-off" stage of organized sport in the United States. We still know little about why sport arose in the latter half of the nineteenth century. Equally obscure are the relationships of sport to groups and individuals within American society. What social functions, either latent or manifest, did sport perform during the take-off stage? This essay contends that a quest for subcommunities in the nineteenth century furnishes an important key to understanding the rise of American sport. As earlier communities based on small geographic areas—typically agricultural villages—declined or were undermined, Americans turned to new forms of community. Sport clubs, as one type of voluntary association, became one of the basic means by which certain groups sought to establish subcommunities within the larger society.

As early as the 1830s voluntary associations had become a striking feature of American society. Tocqueville observed that "In no country in the world has the principle of association been more successfully used or applied to a greater multitude of objects than in America. . . ." A contemporary of Tocqueville believed that since Americans had destroyed "classes, and corporate bodies of every kind, and come to simple direct individualism," the vacuum had been filled by the "production of voluntary associations to an immense extent." Although many of the organizations of the 1830s were temporary, designed to accomplish only a specific purpose, they provided a "noble and expansive feeling which identifies self with community." Max Weber summed up the transcendent importance of voluntary organizations to American society.

"In the past and up to the very present," wrote Weber, "it has been a characteristic precisely of the specifically American democracy that it did not constitute a formless sand heap of individuals, but rather a buzzing complex of strictly exclusive, yet voluntary associations." The clubs could sort out persons according to any criteria they chose: it might be common interests, sex, ethnicity, occupation, religion, status, or a combination thereof. Like-minded men found in voluntary organizations a milieu in which they could counter the impersonality of the burgeoning cities.

The voluntary association became one of several means by which Americans sought to replace the old village community with new subcommunities. In addition to voluntary societies, important considerations for determining the membership of a subcommunity could be living in a particular neighborhood, belonging to a certain religious denomination, and attending specific educational institutions. For example, essential to becoming a member of a high status community might be living in a section of the city with others of a similar income range, sharing a common ethnicity and religious preference (native-born American and Protestant Episcopal), and attending the "right" schools (a New England boarding school and an Ivy League college). Birth into an old family continued to provide a person with advantages in obtaining membership in a status community, but less so than it had in the eighteenth century.

Of special interest for the rise of sport was the quest for two types of subcommunities: ethnic and status. (When prefaced by "status" or "ethnic," the use of the term "subcommunity" is redundant and thus community will be substituted.) The ethnic community usually arose from contradictory forces of acceptance and rejection of the immigrant by the majority society. The status community, by contrast, was a product of status equals who wanted to close their ranks from those they considered inferior. Several tests can be applied to determine whether a sport club was integral to the quest for ethnic

"The Quest for Subcommunities and the Rise of American Sport" by Benjamin G. Rader, from *American Quarterly, XXIX* (Fall, 1977). Published by the American Studies Association. Copyright © 1977. Reprinted by permission of American Quarterly and the author.

or status communities: the adoption of exclusionary membership policies, the promotion of other activities besides sport, the development of appropriate symbols which facilitated communication between members, and the belief, either implicit or explicit, that sport participation was useful in socializing youth.

Since sport per se was not threatening to deeply held personal beliefs and yet provided a milieu for fellowship and common purpose, the sport club was an attractive alternative to other forms of voluntary associations. Athletic activity, which is necessarily subordinated to rules, encouraged a temporary equality between members. The equality of play strengthened the bonds between members who might be divided by personal values. The sport club could be easily transformed into a multifaceted social agency. It could also be an instrument for social exclusion, for the socialization of youth, and for disciplining the behavior of its members. In short the sport club assumed some of the traditional functions of the church, the state, and the geographic community. Almost incidentally the sport club of the nineteenth century provided a tremendous impetus to the growth of American sport.

The need of immigrant groups to form separate ethnic communities depended upon a host of variables including their nationality, religious beliefs, language, and status. The majority society of native-born Americans (hereafter referred to as native-Americans) was less likely to discriminate against immigrants who were most like themselves. Immigrants from England, Scotland, and Wales tended to assimilate more rapidly than those from other parts of Europe. The history of nineteenth-century sport clubs reflected the process of acculturation by distinctive ethnic groups. The Scottish Caledonian clubs, for example, functioned briefly as an ethnic community. But as Scottish immigration declined and the Scots adopted the native-American culture, the need for an ethnic community subsided. The German Turner societies began as ethnic communities, and as the club members

assimilated they sometimes became status communities.

The Scottish Caledonian clubs may have been the most significant ethnic community in encouraging the growth of nineteenth-century American sport. Extending back into the mists of Scottish history, rural communities had held annual track and field games. Beginning in the 1850s these games began to provide one of the bases for organizing Caledonian clubs in America. Wherever a few Scots settled, they usually founded a Caledonian club; eventually they formed well over 100 clubs. In 1887, for example, the *Scottish-American Journal* reported that "A Caledonian Club has been organized at Great Falls, Montana, with a membership of 37 enthusiastic Scots." The clubs restricted membership to persons of Scottish birth or descent.

Although the evidence is not conclusive, it appears that the Caledonian clubs functioned as a major agency for the formation of a Scottish ethnic community in many American cities. The purposes of the clubs, as one of the founders of the Boston organization put it, was to perpetuate "the manners and customs, literature, the Highland costume and the athletic games of Scotland, as practiced by our forefathers." Apart from sport, the clubs sponsored extensive social activities such as dinners, dancing, and bagpipe playing. In short the clubs provided a sense of community in a strange society.

Native-born Americans exhibited an unexpected enthusiasm for the annual Caledonian games. Huge crowds, upwards to 20,000 in New York City, turned out to view competition in footracing, tug o'war, hurdling, jumping, pole vaulting, hammer throwing, and shot-putting. The clubs quickly recognized the potential for financial gain. They opened competition to all athletes regardless of nationality or race, charged admission, and offered lucrative prizes to winners. From the 1850s to the mid-1870s the Caledonians were the mot important promoters of track and field in the country. The success of the games helped to stimulate the formation of the native-American athletic clubs (in this era "athletic" was synonymous with track and field) and the growth of intercollegiate track and field. In fact, by the 1880s the wealthy native-American clubs had seized basic control of American track and field from the Caledonians. The Caledonians then began to decline rapidly as promoters of sport, but they coninued to serve as the focal point of Scottish communities. With the slackening of Scottish immigration and the rapid assimilation of Scots into American society, most of the clubs disappeared by the turn of the twentieth century. Most of the Scots no longer felt a compelling need for a distinctive ethnic community.

Unlike the Scottish Caledonian clubs, the Turner societies had first been organized in their native land. In reaction to the rule of Napoleon, the power of the German aristocracy, and the disunity of the German states, Friederick Ludwig Jahn formed the first Turner society in Berlin in 1811. From the start, the Turners had a strong ideological cast. By establishing universal education and a systematic program of gymnastics (the latter modeled after the ancient Greeks), Jahn hoped to create a united Germany ruled by the people. Young men of the middle class—petty officials, intellectuals, journalists, and students—flocked to Jahn's new society. The Revolution of 1848 brought disaster for the Turners in Germany; many of them emigrated to the United States.

The Turner immigrants faced a different challenge in America, since the Americans had already achieved several of the Turner goals. The United States had no hereditary aristocracy to combat, and a representative democracy was accepted as the ideal political form. Yet the Turners were utopian, free-thinking, and socialistic. They sought an organic community. American individualism ran counter to their deepest social instincts. They also arrived during the heyday of the Know-Nothing movement. Though the nativists directed their energies primarily at the Catholic Church and Irish immigrants, the Turners bore the brunt of mob action in several American cities. Perhaps even more crucial in

driving the Turners together was the fierce antagonism they experienced from the "church" Germans. The haughty anticlericalism and superior cultural achievements of the Turners made it impossible for them to find refuge in the larger German ethnic communities. Consequently, the Turner societies formed distinctive subcommunities in many American cities sharply separated from those Germans whose lives centered around the churches.

Even prior to the immigration of the Forty-Eighters, the Turners had begun to influence American thinking about the human body and the relationship of the body to the rest of man's being. The Turners initiated America's first physical training programs. In 1826, Carl Follen, who was called to teach German literature at Harvard, organized the first college gymnasium modeled after the Jahn system. A year earlier Francis Lieber, the famous encyclopedist, was appointed as the first director of the Tremont Gymnasium in Boston. And Carl Beck, a Latin teacher, founded a gymnastics program at Round Hill School.

Shortly after their arrival in the New World the Forty-Eighters began to organize Turner societies. Friedrich Hecker, a hero of the Revolution in Baden, erected a gymnasium in Cincinnati in 1849 to cultivate "rational training, both physical and intellectual." The Turner halls provided a complete social center with lectures, libraries, and usually a bar. Here the Turners tried to preserve the speech, songs, and customs of the Fatherland, often forming separate militia companies. In 1851 the Turners held a national gymnastics festival in Philadelphia. This competitive event became an annual affair, with gymnasts from over 150 societies participating. After the Civil War the Turners abandoned most of their radical political program and assimilated rapidly into the host society, but they continued to agitate for their physical training program. One of the striking features of the Chicago World's Fair of 1893 was a mass exercise performed by 4,000 German-American members of the national *Turnerbund*. In 1898 the United

States Commissioner of Education declared that the introduction of school gymnastics in Chicago, Kansas City, Cleveland, Denver, Indianapolis, St. Louis, Milwaukee, Cincinnati, St. Paul, and San Francisco was due to the Turners and that "the directors of physical education [in these cities] are graduates of the Seminary or Normal School of the North American Turnerbund."

The examples of the Caledonian clubs and the Turner societies by no means exhaust the involvement of ethnic communities in sport. Both the Irish parishes and Irish volunteer fire departments sponsored and promoted athletics. Ironically, as late as the 1920s a French-Canadian faction in Woonsocket, Rhode Island "resorted to the archetypical American game [baseball]" as a means of preserving their community from the forces of assimilation. While sport should not be considered a necessary precondition for the existence of any of the nineteenth-century ethnic communities, it often helped coalesce and preserve traditional cultural patterns. Sport seemed to assist in blurring economic and ideological differences within the community. In turn, of course, the ethnic communities encouraged the rise of sport. In the cases of both the Caledonians and the Turners, native-Americans eventually took over the immigrants' sports and transformed them to meet their own needs.

Many native-American groups in the nineteenth century tried to cope with the new urban-industrial society by forming subcommunities based on status. The socially exclusive club became the main agency of status ascription. As automatic social deference declined in the nineteenth century, the number of private clubs ballooned. These clubs capitalized on the indefinite social differentiations of American society; they tried to promote a specific style of life that would exclude outsiders. The style usually included a code of honor, a proper mode of dress and speech, education at the "right" schools, pursuit of the appropriate sports, and a host of in-group behavioral nuances. The exclusive club, then, provided "an intricate web of primary group milieux which [gave] . . . form and structure to an otherwise impersonal urban society composed of secondary groups."

The private clubs served as accurate barometers of different levels of nineteenth-century status communities. At the apex of the status structure in large American cities were the metropolitan men's clubs, such as the Philadelphia Club founded in 1835, the Union (1836) and the Century Clubs (1847) in New York, and the Somerset in Boston (1851). The members of these clubs came to dominate the social and economic life of their respective cities. Usually composed of older men, these clubs did not promote sport. After the Civil War the Union Leagues, centers of Republican respectability, and the University clubs, composed of the graduates of prestigious colleges, ranked slightly below the patrician metropolitan clubs. Neither the University clubs nor Union Leagues considered sport an important part of club life. On the third rung of the upper status layer of the American club structure were the athletic clubs organized in the late nineteenth century. These clubs originated with younger men who shared a common interest in sports. In due time the athletic, cricket (in Philadelphia), racquet, and yacht clubs became important instruments of status ascription and sometimes served as stepping stones to membership in the metropolitan clubs.

Yacht clubs were one of the first voluntary sport organizations to be formed by an upper-status group. John C. Stevens, scion of a wealthy New York family and former president of the prestigious Union Club, founded the New York Yacht Club in 1844. A "succession of gentlemen ranking high in the social and financial circles" of the city soon joined the club. Among then was William R. Travers, later the leading promoter of the New York Athletic Club. The club erected an elaborate facility at the Elysian Fields, a part of Stevens' estate at Hoboken, New Jersey. Each year the clubs sponsored a regatta off the clubhouse promontory. Apart from owning plush

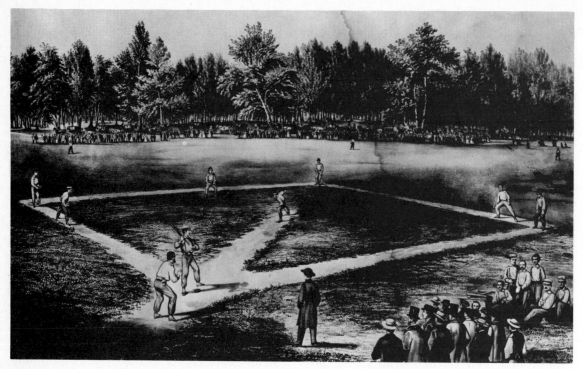

■ ■ *The 1868 Grand Match for the championship of the National Game of Base Ball, played at the Elysian Fields in Hoboken, New Jersey (Currier & Ives).*

yachts, club members had to pay dues of $40 the first year and $25 thereafter. The club prescribed expensive uniforms for members and sponsored regular balls and social cruises to Newport, Rhode Island, Bar Harbor, Maine, and other nearby wealthy summer resorts. In 1851 Stevens, with his yacht *America,* defeated 18 British yachts at the Isle of Wight, to win a coveted cup donated by the Royal Yacht Squadron; in 1857 he gave the cup to the New York Yacht Club on the condition that it would be "a perpetual challenge cup for friendly competition between foreign countries." By 1893 six international matches had been held for the America's Cup, all incidentally won by American yachts. By the 1890s every major eastern seaboard city had its exclusive yacht club.

The first baseball clubs occupied a position somewhere near the bottom of the upper status structure, ranking below the status achieved by the yacht clubs or the metropolitan athletic clubs. The membership of the New York Knickerbocker baseball club, organized in 1845, included young professionals, merchants, and white collar workers. As Harold Seymour noted, they were not simply interested in playing baseball. "They were primarily a social club with a distinctly exclusive flavor—somewhat similar to what country clubs represented in the 1920s and 1930s. . . ." Membership was limited to forty, applicants could be blackballed, and the club insisted on strict rules of proper conduct. Since the club held contests every Monday and Thursday, those without a substantial amount of leisure time were automatically excluded. Players who failed to appear for the contests could be fined. The club held a large banquet after each game and sponsored festive social affairs in the off season. Club members, Seymour wrote, "were more expert with the knife and fork at post-game banquets than with bat and ball on the diamond." The Knickerbocker baseball club provided both a means by which its members could distinguish themselves from the urban masses and a setting for close interpersonal relations between men of similar tastes and social standing.

The early clubs which imitated the Knickerbockers tried to prevent baseball from becoming a mass commercial spectacle. In 1858 they organized the National Association of Baseball Players to stop the creeping commercialism which was invading the sport. By 1860 about 60 clubs had joined the Association, which "clung to the notion that baseball ought to be a gentleman's game. For this reason amateurism was applauded, and participants were expected to be persons of means and local standing." The clubs scheduled outside contests only with teams that enjoyed equal social stature. Influenced by the English notion that sport should be an exclusive prerogative of gentlemen, club members were supposed to be magnanimous in victory and friendly in defeat. After contests the home club usually gave a large banquet for the visitors.

Baseball clubs survived only briefly as effective agencies of status communities. Since baseball could be played relatively quickly in any open space, and since it required inexpensive equipment, from the 1850s on it became a favorite sport of the lower and middle classes. Seymour found that in the decade of the 1850s in New York City there were clubs composed exclusively of fire companies, policemen, barkeepers, dairymen, school teachers, physicians, and even clergymen. The social decorum of the game changed dramatically. The clubs began to charge admission and divide the receipts among their best players. Betting, cheering, and general rowdyism (sometimes leading to riots) became commonplace. The "founding" clubs either folded or sometimes took up another sport. Baseball would never again be suited for the needs of those who were striving to form high

status communities. The sport did, however, serve as a mechanism for the perpetuation of occupational identities.

Organized in the post–Civil War era, the metropolitan athletic clubs were far more socially prestigious than the early baseball clubs. The founders of the athletic clubs were usually wealthy young men who enjoyed track and field competition. At first they did not conceive of their clubs in terms of social exclusiveness but in terms of the common congeniality and sporting interests of the members. Professional athletes, gamblers, and "rowdies" tended to dominate the existing world of track and field. Drawing upon the English sporting heritage, the clubs began to draw rigid distinctions between amateur and professional athletes by the mid-1880s. By becoming champions of the amateur code of athletics, they, in effect, were able to bar lower-income persons from participation in the track and field competition which they sponsored.

The athletic clubs provided the major stimulus to the growth of amateur athletics. The New York Athletic Club (NYAC), the first and most prestigious of the clubs, began sponsoring open track and field meets in 1868. By special invitation the New York Caledonian Club participated, allegedly making it an "international match— America against Scotland." In the 1870s NYAC expanded its activities by building the first cinder track in the country at Mott Haven and sponsoring the first national amateur championships in track and field (1876), swimming (1877), boxing (1878), and wrestling (1878). In 1879, eight of the exclusive clubs formed the National Association of Amateur Athletes of America, to which NYAC transferred the annual track and field championships. By 1883 there were some 150 athletic clubs in the United States and each usually held at least one annual competition. In 1888 the National Association foundered on attempts to define and enforce the amateur code. A few of the affiliated clubs formed the Amateur Athletic Union. Composed of the most exclusive clubs, the union claimed jurisdiction over more than 40 sports and rigorously enforced the amateur code in the contests that it sponsored. Until the formation of the National Collegiate Athletic Association in 1905, the union and its collegiate affiliates dominated all amateur sport of championship quality.

Metropolitan athletic clubs became an important link in a web of associations that constituted elite status communities. For example, William R. Travers, long-time president of the New York Athletic Club, belonged to 27 social clubs including New York's two most prestigious men's clubs. The athletic clubs excluded from membership all except those near the top of the social hierarchy. Ironically, as the clubs became more effective agencies of community formation, they tended to lose their emphasis on sport. Usually they opened their doors to the entire family, they built special facilities for women, and they began to sponsor dazzling balls and banquets. By the 1880s and 1890s only a few of the members were top-flight athletes; most of the members either were too old to play, were occasional athletes, or did not engage in competition at all. Frederick W. Janssen, a member of the Staten Island Athletic Club and an active athlete, rued the tendency of the clubs to become social centers:

The social element in clubs is like 'dry rot' and eats into the vitals of athletic clubs, and soon causes them to fail in the purpose for which they were organized. . . . Palatial club houses are erected at great cost and money is spent in adorning them that, if used to beautify athletic grounds and improve tracks, would cause a wide-spread interest in athletic sports and further the development of the wind and muscles of American youth.

The tendency noted by Janssen was irreversible, for the social functions performed by the clubs had become more important to the members than athletic competition.

The metropolitan athletic clubs were forerunners of the great country club movement of the twentieth century. Unlike athletic clubs, country clubs became havens for those seeking to estab-

lish status communities in the suburbs and smaller cities. While golf was not the initial reason for forming the first country clubs, it became the most potent agency for the spread of the clubs throughout the nation. Beginning in 1888 with the formation of the St. Andrews Golf Club of Yonkers, New York, golf slowly invaded the wealthy suburban areas of New York, Boston, Philadelphia, and Chicago. In 1894 both St. Andrews and the Newport Golf Club scheduled national amateur championships; the formation of the Amateur Golf Association of the United States in 1894 eliminated the confusion. With but few exceptions, a reporter wrote in 1898, golf "is a sport restricted to the richer classes in this country." Until the 1920s golf continued to have a highly select following.

Sport clubs, such as the country clubs, were far less significant as constituents of status communities in England than in the United States. The contrasts between the functions of the clubs were sharply drawn by George Birmingham, an Englishman:

There are also all over England clubs especially devoted to particular objects, golf clubs, yacht clubs, and so forth. In these the members are drawn together by their interest in a common pursuit, and are forced into some kind of acquaintanceship. But these are very different in spirit and intention from the American country club. It exists as a kind of center of the social life of the neighborhood. Sport is encouraged by these clubs for the sake of general sociability. In England sociability is a by-product of an interest in sport.

The country club at Tuxedo [New York] is not perhaps the oldest, but it is one of the oldest institutions of its kind in America. At the proper time of year there are dances, and a debutante acquires, I believe, a certain prestige by 'coming out' at one of them. But the club exists primarily as a social center of Tuxedo. It is in one way the ideal, the perfect country club. It not only fosters, it regulates and governs the social life of the place.

In addition to the early baseball, yacht, metropolitan athletic, and country clubs, several other voluntary sport organizations served as instruments of status communities. The Philadelphia cricket clubs and the racquet clubs of the large cities were as socially prestigious as the metropolitan athletic clubs. The history of these clubs followed a pattern similar to the athletic clubs. Cricket as a sport in Philadelphia, for example, declined when the clubs assumed larger social functions. For a time, several of the Philadelphia cricket clubs became major centers of lawn tennis. But in the 1920s, when lawn tennis began to move out of the network of the exclusive clubs, the cricket clubs no longer furnished players of championship quality.

Lawn tennis first flourished in Newport, Rhode Island, a summer resort of the very rich. In Newport, the nation's wealthiest families constructed huge palaces of stone for summer homes and entertained each other lavishly. Dixon Wector has written that "Other than social consciousness, the only bond which drew this summer colony together was sport—which might consist of sailing around Block Island, or having cocktails upon one's steam yacht reached by motor-boat from the landing of the New York Yacht Club, or bathing at Bailey's Beach or the Gooseberry Island Club, or tennis on the Casino courts." The posh Newport Casino Club, built by James Gordon Bennett, Jr., publisher of the New York *Herald*, became the home of the United States National Lawn Tennis Association (1881) and was the site of the national championships until 1913 when the tournament was moved to Forest Hills, New York. Lawn tennis long remained a sport dominated by clubs of impeccably high status aspirations.

The sponsorship of tennis and golf by the elite clubs expanded the opportunities for women to participate in sport. Many of the first tennis courts were built specifically for the wives and daughters of club members. During the first decades of the development of American tennis, many observers believed that tennis would remain primarily a sport for women. In the early

years the women preferred doubles to singles, possibly because they were encumbered by bustles and full-length skirts. Women held a few tournaments as early as 1881 and in 1887 they scheduled the first women's national tennis championships. The task of breaking the sex barrier in golf was more difficult. In the closing years of the nineteenth century the golf clubs along the Atlantic Coast began reluctantly to set aside the links on certain afternoons for female players. Only 13 women participated in the first national tournament held on the Meadowbrook course on Long Island in 1895. In 1898, H. L. Fitz Patrick announced probably prematurely, that "the American golf girl has arrived!" Golfing women helped initiate a more liberated stlye of dress; by 1898 a few brave ladies were playing without hats and with elbow-length sleeves. But, compared to men, the number of women athletes remained exceedling small. Most of the women engaged only in the social life of the clubs.

Within a limited context and for a short time the collegiate athletic associations represented a quest for subcommunities. In the 1880s, as newly enriched groups sought a college education as a means of achieving a social position commensurate with their wealth, college enrollments spurted upwards. The academic degree, particularly from an Ivy League school, was a passport to polite society. But the new students found themselves confronted with a large number of strangers, often a boring curriculum and uninspired teaching, and few opportunities for social intercourse except through sedate literary and oratorical societies. In response to this unexciting, impersonal academic setting, they formed a vast array of clubs, fraternities, and athletic associations. Athletic associations usually opened their doors to any student who was athletically talented. Because of this membership policy, the associations probably served as less satisfactory subcommunity agencies than did the other collegiate social clubs. At any rate, in the 1890s the associations began to collapse as independent student-run clubs. Colleges hired professional coaches, seized control of athletics from the students, and transformed intercollegiate sports into commercial ventures.

This essay has focused on voluntary sport organizations which tended to be central to the formation of either ethnic or status communities. Neighborhoods and persons with common occupations or religious preferences formed a host of smaller sport clubs in the nineteenth century. Since these clubs rarely had elaborate athletic facilities nor seemed to be concerned about social activities other than sport, they were apparently not as important as agencies of community formation. Yet they should not be neglected as a dimension of the general nineteenth-century quest for communities. Sport could supplement other institutions or associations that were more vital to the existence of communities. Some of the churches, for example, apparently found that sponsoring an athletic team bound their membership closer together and reinforced common values. Some skilled craftsmen found in sport a means by which they could distinguish themselves more clearly from ordinary workingmen. School sports, particularly in the twentieth century, helped give an identity and common purpose to many neighborhoods, towns, and cities which were otherwise divided by class, race, ethnicity, and religious differences. In a larger, less tangible sense, mass sporting spectacles may have been an aspect of a search for city-wide, regional, or even national communities.

■ ■ ■

STUDY QUESTIONS

1. Why did Americans so readily join voluntary associations? What need did the voluntary associations fill in their lives?

2. How did sports help to preserve ethnic and status identities?

3. How were the Caledonian clubs and Turner societies similar or different?

4. What were the different levels of sporting clubs? How did the clubs serve as valuable subcommunities?

5. What was the origin of the distinction between professionals and amateurs? How did the division serve class ends?

6. What was the role of women in the exclusive clubs?

7. What role did sports play in college life in the late nineteenth century?

BIBLIOGRAPHY

Benjamin G. Rader further develops his thesis of the development of subcommunities in *American Sports: From the Age of Folk Games to the Age of Spectators* (1983). Frederick L. Pavon's "The Rise of Sport," *Mississippi Valley Historical Review*, IV (1917) presents an early examination of the social value of sports. John R. Betts,

American Sporting Heritage, 1850–1950 (1974) details the role that industrialization and urbanization played in the rise of sports. Paul Hoch, *Rip Off the Big Game: The Exploitation of Sports by the the Power Elite* (1972) presents a neo-Marxist appraisal of the social uses of sports. Gerald Redmond, *The Caledonian Games in Nineteenth-Century America* (1971) and A. E. Zucker, ed., *The Forty-Eighters: Political Refugees of the German Revolution of 1848* (1950) study two important ethnic subcommunities. Harold Seymour, *Baseball: The Early Years* (1960) and David Q. Voight, *American Baseball: From Gentlemen's Sport to the Commissioner System* (1966) discuss the emergence of baseball as the national game. The best study of sports in an individual city is Dale A. Somers, *The Rise of Sports in New Orleans, 1850–1900* (1971).

Part Three

WAR AND PEACE
IN A
NEW CENTURY

The years between the assassination of William McKinley in 1901 and America's entry into the Great War in 1917 has been labeled as the Progressive Era. In character and tone the years mirrored the first Progressive president, Theodore Roosevelt. Animated and energetic, T. R. used the presidency as a "bully pulpit," readily giving his opinion on a variety of subjects, ranging from literature and politics to football and divorce. Roosevelt believed that America's greatness was the result of its Anglo-Saxon heritage. Although he hoped to bring a "Square Deal" to all Americans, his reforming impulse was conservative in nature; he maintained that only through moderate reform could America preserve its traditional social, economic, and political structure. He had no sympathy for such "radical fanatics" as socialists or anarchists; nor did he trust the masses of American people who lacked his breeding and education. His answer for any sort of mob action was "taking ten or a dozen of their leaders out, standing . . . them against a wall, and shooting them dead."

Despite their ethnocentricity and self-righteousness, Roosevelt and the next two Progressive presidents—William Howard Taft and Woodrow Wilson—did attempt to curb some of the worst abuses of the urban-industrial society. They saw legislation through Congress that limited the number of hours that women and children could work and enacted the Pure Food and Drug Act (1906) and the Meat Inspection Act (1906). However, other Progressives, often with the support of the president, supported prohibition and antidivorce legislation, thereby seeking to regulate the private lives of millions of Americans.

A major shortcoming of the Progressive Movement was the general reluctance to support minority and ethnic groups. Such Progressives as James K. Vardaman

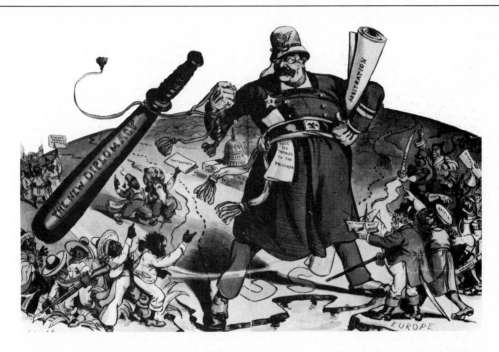

and Theodore G. Bilbo, both from Mississippi, supported forward-looking legislation for whites but were violent race-baiters. Progressives rarely attacked the Jim Crow system in the South or introduced antilynching legislation in Congress. Segregation within the federal government expanded under Woodrow Wilson.

Similarly, vocal and independent labor unions and women's rights organizations seldom found support among influential Progressives. Margaret Sanger's birth control movement met strong opposition from middle-class men and women who saw it as a threat to family and morality. Such radical working-class organizations as the Industrial Workers of the World (the IWW, or "Wobblies") were not embraced by the mainstream of the Progressive Movement.

The Progressive Movement, however, did not really survive World War I. As a result of the Spanish-American War of 1898, the United States had acquired new territories in the distant Pacific, requiring a two-ocean navy and leaving Americans with global responsibilities. Those responsibilities eventually complicated and compromised the reform spirit. The Great War of 1914–18 damaged the reform impulses of Progressivism. It inspired skepticism, pessimism, and ultimately cynicism, and in the death-filled trenches of Western Europe, the Progressive Movement met its demise.

The following essays deal with different characteristics of the Progressive Movement. Confronted by the powerful forces of urbanization and industrialization, Americans attempted—sometimes successfully, often unsuccessfully—to come to terms with their changing society. Amidst that attempt, World War I complicated Progressivist dreams with the reality of horror, stupidity, and mass death.

TEDDY ROOSEVELT AND THE ROUGH RIDERS

Robert J. Maddox

Aboard the *Yucatan*, anchored off the coast of Cuba, Theodore Roosevelt received the news on the evening of June 21, 1898. He and his men, a volunteer cavalry regiment dubbed the Rough Riders, had received their orders to disembark from the safety of the ship and join the fighting ashore. It was a welcomed invitation, celebrated with cheers, war dances, songs, boasts, and toasts. "To the officers— may they get killed, wounded, or promoted," urged one toast that captured the mood aboard ship.

Who were these Rough Riders who seemed so bent on winning glory? As one of them told Roosevelt, "Who would not risk his life for a star?" And who was Theodore Roosevelt, the energetic rich kid who lusted after fame and perhaps had his eyes—albeit nearsighted—focused on the presidency? Robert J. Maddox retells the story of Theodore Roosevelt, the Rough Riders, and America's "splendid little war" with Spain. In the process he tells a great deal about the future President and the nation that made him its hero.

The war against Spain in 1898 was one of the more popular conflicts in American history. Victory came easily, there were relatively few casualties, and the cause seemed just in the minds of most people. From it the United States acquired the Philippine Islands, Puerto Rico, Guam, and a virtual protectorate over Cuba. The nation acquired several heroes as well, Admiral Dewey to name one, but none more colorful than the flamboyant Teddy Roosevelt. His exploits in Cuba, at the head of his Rough Riders, made him a legend in his own lifetime and helped make him President of the United States.

Roosevelt was in the prime of his life when the war broke out. Not yet forty years old, he possessed an imposing if somewhat overweight physique which he kept fit by almost daily exercise. In this regard he was a self-made man. Spindly and a trifle owlish as a youngster, Roosevelt, through what one of his biographers termed the "Cult of Strenuosity," had built up his body by relentless physical activity. Only one of his faculties had failed to respond—his eyesight. Cursed from boyhood with extreme nearsightedness, which grew worse over the years, Roosevelt was very self-conscious about this weakness in an otherwise healthy organism. During the war he was so worried it would betray him in combat that he had at least a half-dozen pairs of spectacles sewn into various parts of his uniform as insurance.

Mentally, Roosevelt was a complex individual. Exceedingly bright, he read voraciously, and penned his own books and articles without the help of a ghostwriter. He was, or would become, friendly with some of the leading intellectuals of the era. One side of him, however, remained boyish until the day he died. "You must always remember," a British diplomat wrote a friend some years later, "that the Pres-

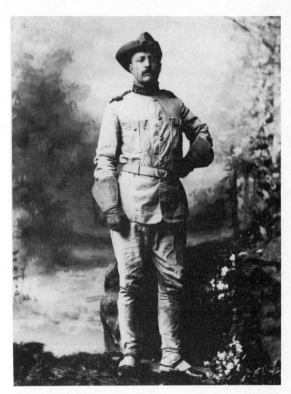

■ ■ *An 1898 photo shows Teddy Roosevelt as colonel of the Rough Riders. Teddy's uniforms, which had extra spectacles sewn into them, were tailored by Brooks Brothers to ensure a proper fit.*

ident [Roosevelt] is about six." Without in any way belittling his patriotism, it seems safe to say that Teddy's enthusiasm for fighting the Spaniards stemmed at least as much from his desire to have a "bully" time doing it.

No one ever accused Roosevelt of being a pacifist. During the 1880s and 1890s the United States had gotten into a number of scrapes with other nations over issues large and small. Almost invariably T.R. had called for the most militant actions in response to these situations, and had denounced those who urged caution. War to him was not a catastrophe to be avoided; it could be a tonic to the nation's bloodstream. A country too long at peace, he believed, tended to grow soft and effeminate, while war encouraged "manliness," a characteristic he prized above all else.

Robert J. Maddox, "Teddy Roosevelt and the Rough Riders." From *American History Illustrated* 12 (November 1977), pp. 8–15, 18–19. Reprinted through the courtesy of Cowles Magazines, publisher of AMERICAN HISTORY ILLUSTRATED.

Before 1897 Roosevelt had held no office which dealt directly with military or foreign affairs. He had served in the New York state legislature as federal Civil Service Commissioner, and as a commissioner of the New York City Police Department. Despite having held such prestigious jobs for a man of his years, Roosevelt's political future was clouded by his tendency to alienate some of those who could help him and by the strident views on foreign policy which he never hesitated to voice — often to the great embarrassment of his own party. When, as a reward for his services in the election of 1896, T.R.'s friends began pushing for his appointment as Assistant Secretary of the Navy in the new Republican administration, they encountered stiff opposition. The President-elect himself had reservations about Teddy, but named him anyway. "I hope he has no preconceived plans," McKinley said wistfully, "which he would wish to drive through the moment he got in."

McKinley hoped in vain. Within two months of his appointment, Roosevelt wrote the well-known naval expert, Captain Alfred Thayer Mahan, that:

If I had my way, we would annex those islands [Hawaii] tomorrow. If that is impossible, I would establish a protectorate. . . . I believe we should build the Nicaraguan Canal at once, and should build a dozen new battleships, half of them on the Pacific Coast. I am fully alive to the danger from Japan.

These and similar sentiments clearly demonstrated that T.R. had no intention of vanishing into the bureaucracy. Nor did he. A short time later, when Secretary of the Navy John D. Long went on vacation, one newspaper reported that Roosevelt soon had "the whole Navy bordering on a war footing. It remains only to sand down the decks and pipe to quarters for action." Teddy did not try to conceal his delight in being left to mind the store. "The Secretary is away," he wrote in one letter, "and I am having immense fun running the Navy." One story had it that

when asked about his Assistant Secretary, Long dourly responded "Why 'Assistant'?"

Sticking pins in maps and running around on inspection tours must have amused him, but Roosevelt wanted some real action. Spain provided the most likely source. Once the possessor of a world empire, Spain by this time was a minor power clinging grimly to its few remaining territories. One of these, Cuba, lay less than 100 miles from American shores, and for several years had smouldered with insurrection against Spanish domination. Though he refrained from speaking out publicly, Roosevelt, in private talks and correspondence, recommended war against Spain almost from the day he became Assistant Secretary. American honor demanded it, he said, and a brief war would help rekindle martial instincts which had flagged through years of peace. There would be an additional dividend, he wrote on one occasion, that being "the benefit done our military forces by trying both the Army and Navy in actual practise."

Roosevelt did not bring on the war with Spain, of course, however much he tried. Cuban propaganda, sensationalist American newspapers, and jingoes in and outside Congress, combined to keep talk of war before the public. Still, through 1897, President McKinley refused to be stampeded, and the Spanish Government (which very much wished to avoid war) repeatedly gave in to American demands over the treatment of Cuba.

Then, early in 1898, two events occurred which made war virtually inevitable. First, a letter critical of McKinley, written by the Spanish minister in Washington, was stolen from the mails and reprinted in the American press. Trivial in itself, this blunder enraged many Americans. More important, the warship, *Maine* blew up in a Cuban harbor with the loss of more than 200 sailors. Though not a shred of evidence has ever emerged to indicate that the Spanish were responsible, most Americans (abetted by much of the press) assumed that they were and demanded revenge. McKinley simply was not strong enough to stand against this pressure. On

April 10 he asked Congress for what amounted to a declaration of war.

Well before the war began Roosevelt had told others that if it came he would not be content to remain in Washington. He was true to his word. By March he was beseeching New York state officials to permit him to raise a regiment of volunteers, which unit, he promised, would be "jim-dandy." That he had never served in the military, let alone seen combat, fazed Teddy not at all. He was greatly miffed when his generous offer was spurned.

Roosevelt, as usual, had other irons in the fire. Due to the minuscule size of the Regular Army, Congress had authorized the recruitment of three volunteer cavalry regiments from the Southwest. Because of his political connections, which he used to the utmost, Roosevelt was offered the command of one of these units. Modesty suddenly descended upon him. Estimating that it might take him a month or so to familiarize himself thoroughly with military procedures and tactics, T.R. asked that his friend, Captain Leonard Wood (at that time a military surgeon), be promoted to colonel and given command of the regiment. He would be satisfied with a mere lieutenant-colonelcy and would serve under Wood. Roosevelt's light could not be hidden, however, and from the start the First Volunteer Cavalry was known as "Roosevelt's Rough Riders."

Teddy was eager to get going. Quickly ordering the appropriate uniforms from Brooks Brothers (to ensure a proper fit), he began complaining that the war might be over before he could get into it—"it will be awful if we miss the fun." At last, in early May, he set out for San Antonio, Texas, where the First Volunteers were undergoing preliminary training. He arrived to the welcome of a brass band and "his boys."

And what a group it was. "Mingling among the cowboys and momentarily reformed bad men from the West," Henry Pringle has written, "were polo players and steeplechase riders from the Harvard, Yale and Princeton clubs of New York City." Though from time to time Roosevelt protested against the carnival atmosphere which pervaded the camp, he enjoyed himself hugely. After one period of mounted drill, for instance, he told his men to "drink all the beer they want, which I will pay for" and had a few himself. Colonel Wood admonished Teddy for this kind of behavior, which the latter admitted was out of place. "Sir," Roosevelt replied, "I consider myself the damnedest ass within ten miles of this camp."

Two weeks after Teddy arrived in San Antonio, the Rough Riders were ordered to report to the Tampa, Florida staging area for the expedition against Cuba. By this time they had been transformed from an undisciplined group in civilian clothes to an undisciplined group in uniform. Tampa was, if possible, even more chaotic than San Antonio had been. Units of Regulars, National Guard, and volunteers milled about with little over-all direction and inadequate facilities. Some units were without arms, others had arms but no ammunition, still others lacked uniforms, bedding, or tents. It was a mess. "No head," Roosevelt wrote angrily in his diary, "a breakdown of both the railroad and military system of the country."

With an aroused public clamoring for action, the War Department ordered the expedition to sail despite its obvious lack of preparation. At this point the Rough Riders had what amounted to their first engagement of the war—against other American soldiers. Port Tampa lay about nine miles from Tampa, where the troops were quartered, with only a single track railway connecting them. The orders sent to individual regiments included no scheduling, so it was up to each unit to get to the port as best it could. A mad scramble ensued to commandeer whatever rolling stock was available: The Rough Riders were lucky enough to come upon an engine with some coal cars which they promptly seized. But the excitement was not yet over. Arriving at the port, Roosevelt and Wood found that the ship allotted to them was also designated for two other regiments and there was not enough space for all three. As Teddy later re-counted the episode:

Accordingly, I ran at full speed to our train; and leaving a strong guard with the baggage I double-quicked the rest of the regiment up to the boat just in time to board her as she came into the quay and then to hold her against the 2d Regulars and the 71st, who had arrived a little too late. . . . There was a good deal of expostulation, but we had possession.

It was a false alarm. On the eve of departure, another message arrived from the War Department. "Wait until you get further orders before you sail," it read. "Answer quick." As things turned out the officers and men of the expeditionary force spent almost two weeks sweating and cursing in the tightly packed ships at anchor under the Florida sun. At last, on June 14, thirty-two steamers moved out of Port Tampa heading slowly toward Cuba. The Fifth Army Corps, as it was designated, consisted of two divisions and an independent brigade of infantry, a division of dismounted cavalry, four batteries of field artillery, and some auxiliary troops. The Rough Riders were aboard, of course, but like the other cavalry units they had nothing to ride. Because of the lack of space, the only animals brought along were horses for the officers and mules for carrying supplies.

Eventually the flotilla reached Cuba and landings were made virtually unopposed in several places. The debarkations resembled the disorder which had reigned at Tampa Bay. The men and equipment were brought ashore in helter-skelter fashion by an assortment of launches and other small boats. The animals were even less fortunate: They were driven off the sides of ships and left to fend for themselves. Some reached shore safely, others swam to watery graves. Once again, Teddy was unwilling to trust luck. Recognizing the captain of a small vessel which drew alongside as a man he had known in the Navy Department, Roosevelt directed that the ship be used solely for getting the Rough Riders ashore as

quickly as possible. After spending weeks aboard what they referred to as "prison hulks," the men must have appreciated the initiative of their second-in-command.

The course of the Cuban campaign cannot be recounted in detail here. The most charitable single word to describe it is "muddled." The commander of the Fifth Corps was General William R. Shafter, a rather lethargic man who weighed well over 300 pounds. Suffering from the heat since arriving in Florida, Shafter, during the latter part of the fighting, had to be transported reclining on a barn door. His immediate subordinates were three other general officers, who seemed at least as much concerned with outdoing one another as with fighting the Spaniards. One of them, "Fighting Joe" Wheeler, had last seen combat as a Confederate officer during the Civil War. During moments of stress, it was reported, he became confused as to who his opponents were and several times referred to them as "those Yankees." Fortunately for the Americans, the Spanish were in even worse shape. Although some individual Spanish troops and units fought well, they were badly led and defeatism permeated the defending forces.

Once a semblance of order was created on the beach, preparations were made for the expedition's advance against the main target, the harbor city of Santiago, less than twenty miles west along the coastline. The only available overland route, however, swung inland through jungles which provided excellent concealment for defenders. The movement took place in fits and starts and was not without incident — and losses. The Spanish fought a brief rearguard action at a place called Las Guásimas, for instance, during which sixteen Americans were killed and another fifty wounded. The Rough Riders took part in this engagement, as did some regular units, and there is evidence to indicate that Wood and Roosevelt led their men into an ambush. In later years Roosevelt indignantly denied any such thing and claimed that "every one of the officers had full knowledge of where he would find the enemy." In any event, Teddy boasted, ". . . we wanted the first whack at the Spaniards and we got it.''

Finally, by the end of June, American forces were within striking distance of Santiago. Their way was blocked by a series of fortifications and trenches located on a chain of hills surrounding the city — the most prominent of which was San Juan Hill. The difficulty in moving up supplies and ammunition by pack animal along narrow jungle trails caused the troops to remain before Santiago for several days. The plan of attack was simple. One division would move several miles north to attack a stronghold at El Caney, the rest of the units would march head-on against the San Juan and nearby hills. Both assaults began on the morning of July 1.

From where they had grouped, American troops had to push through several miles of jungle and ford a stream before reaching clear ground in front of the hills. They began taking losses while still in the jungle. There were only two trails they could use and Spanish artillery had these zeroed in. One column had at its head an observation balloon pulled along by men holding guy ropes. It proved to be of little help to the Americans, but showed Spanish artillery-men exactly where the enemy was. Fortunately for the men underneath it, the bag was pierced several times and settled gently to the ground before it could cause even greater damage.

The jungle ended abruptly at a stream which ran along its edge roughly parallel to the Spanish lines on the ridges. Across the stream there were several hundred yards of meadowlands before reaching the slopes. As the troops emerged from the jungle, therefore, they were exposed to withering Spanish rifle fire from above. What little order there was broke down as the advancing columns began clogging up at the jungle's edge. Some units refused to cross the stream, others became disorganized as they tried to move through and get into position. The situation presented a cruel dilemma to American commanders. To attack with insufficient numbers of men would be to risk defeat. To wait until all units were deployed would mean exposing those who crossed the stream first to an extended period under the crippling fire. Finally, a little past noon and before elements in the rear had left the jungle, the assault began.

San Juan Hill was the main objective. Somewhat to the right and much closer to American lines lay Kettle Hill, assigned to the dismounted cavalry. Since Colonel Wood earlier had taken command of a brigade, Roosevelt now led the Rough Riders. This was what he had been waiting for, and he would not be found wanting. Showing complete disdain for enemy bullets, Teddy galloped around on his horse, Little Texas, exhorting his men to form up for attack. They were joined by elements from several other regiments, including black troopers from the 10th Cavalry. Roosevelt waved his hat and the men moved forward. "By this time we were all in the spirit of the thing and greatly excited by the charge," he wrote later, "the men cheering and running forward between shots. . . . I . . . galloped toward the hill. . . ."

According to his own account Roosevelt quickly moved ahead of the men, preceded only by his orderly, Henry Bardshar, "who had run ahead very fast in order to get better shots at the Spaniards. . . ." About forty yards from the crest Teddy encountered a wire fence and jumped off Little Texas, letting the horse run free. Almost immediately he saw Bardshar shoot down two Spaniards who emerged from the trenches. Soon Roosevelt and Bardshar were surrounded by the rest of the men as they swarmed over the hill, capturing or killing the few Spanish troops who had not retreated. The charge up Kettle Hill was over.

From their newly won position, Roosevelt and his men had an excellent view of the assault against San Juan Hill. Earlier artillery barrages had failed to cause much damage to the breast-works, and the black powder used in American guns produced smoke which drew Spanish counterfire. Now, however, three Gatling guns opened up with good effect. "They went b-r-r-r, like a lawn mower cutting grass over our trenches,'' a Spanish officer said later. ''We could not stick a finger up when you fired without getting it cut off.'' Still the Spaniards held their positions as the ragged blue lines moved forward. Despite heavy losses, the Americans pushed doggedly up the hill. At last, just before they reached the top, the Spanish defenders fired a last volley and fled.

Beyond Kettle Hill and to the right of San Juan lay another ridge from which the enemy kept shooting. Rallying his men again, Roosevelt led them down the far side of Kettle, across the intervening valley, and up the slopes. ''I was with Henry Bardshar, running up at the double,'' Teddy later recalled, ''and two Spaniards leaped from the trenches and fired at us, not ten yards away. As they turned to run I closed in and fired twice, missing the first and killing the second. My revolver was from the sunken battleship *Maine*.'' Again the Americans drove the Spanish before them. When they took possession of these crests, ''we found ourselves overlooking Santiago.''

Although the Americans had won the day, the battle for Santiago was not yet over. The Spanish had about 16,000 men to defend the city, the Americans an equal number to take it. The latter were exhausted from their attacks and lacked reserves, food, and ammunition. By July 3, two days after the initial assaults, the Americans had lost 224 men killed and 1,370 wounded. The result was a stand-off. Spanish units did not attempt to break out of the ring; the Americans were in no shape to move against the city's defenses. ''Tell the President for Heaven's sake to send us every regiment and above all every battery possible,'' Roosevelt wrote a friend. ''We have won so far at a heavy cost, but the Spaniards fight very hard and charging these intrenchments against modern rifles is terrible. . . . We *must* have help—thousands of men, batteries, and *food* and ammunition.'' Fortunately, the Spanish launched no major counterattacks.

While the men dug themselves into the hills, the battle for Santiago was decided by another engagement—at sea. A Spanish fleet had been bottled up in Santiago Harbor for some time: Shafter's expedition was supposed to take the city, thereby forcing the Spanish ships to leave the harbor or surrender. At 9:30 A.M. on July 3, Spanish ships began coming out singly under the guns of the blockaders. It was a courageous but futile effort. Despite some bungling on the part of the U.S. Navy, all the opposing ships were sunk or disabled. After two weeks of negotiation Shafter received the surrender of Santiago, and less than a month after that the Spanish Government sued for peace.

Although the war had ended in complete victory for the United States, it came in for a great deal of criticism in the period following. Charges of incompetence were leveled against the top echelons, there were undignified exchanges between generals and admirals over who deserved credit for which victory, and the condition of the men returning from Cuba caused a public outcry. Many troops died from tropical illnesses, and still others from food poisoning caused by tainted meat.

It was probably for these reasons that Roosevelt's star came to shine so brightly. He had performed heroically, after all, and he was sufficiently subordinate in rank to escape any blame about the war's mismanagement.

Teddy himself was not loath to accept the limelight; indeed, he eagerly sought it. Almost immediately he began campaigning for the governorship of New York state and, lest anyone forget his exploits, kept the Rough Rider bugler at his side during his speeches. Roosevelt had other assets, of course, but being the ''Hero of San Juan Hill'' (he was not disposed to argue about which hill he had climbed) did him no harm. He had become fixed in the national mind as Colonel Teddy Roosevelt of the Rough Riders.

''I would honestly rather have my position of colonel,'' Roosevelt had told his men at their mustering-out ceremony, ''than any other position on earth.'' No doubt he meant it at the time. As governor of New York, and later as President of the United States, he looked back fondly on his days in Cuba and the men who had served with him. In both positions he tried to accommodate as many as possible of the former Rough Riders who petitioned him for a job. His loyalty, if not his judgment, could scarcely be questioned. In one case he tried to have appointed as territorial marshal a man who, it was found, was serving time in prison for homicide. Undaunted, Teddy later tried to have the person installed as warden of the very prison in which he had been confined. "When I told this to John Hay," Roosevelt said, "he remarked (with a brutal absence of feeling) that he believed the proverb ran, 'Set a Rough Rider to catch a thief.'"

For once in his life, Teddy was at a loss for a reply.

■ ■ ■

STUDY QUESTIONS

1. What character traits inclined Roosevelt toward war? What events led the United States to war with Spain?

2. What sorts of men joined the Rough Riders?

3. What problems did the United States have mobilizing for war?

4. What role did the Battles of Kettle Hill and San Juan Hill play in the war in Cuba?

5. How did Roosevelt capitalize on his newly won fame?

BIBLIOGRAPHY

The best overview of the Spanish–American War is David Trask, *The War with Spain in 1898* (1981). Shorter, but still useful is Frank Freidel, *The Splendid Little War* (1958). Theodore Roosevelt's own account of his moments of glory is *The Rough Riders* (1899). Among the more readable biographies of Roosevelt are Edmund Morris, *The Rise of Theodore Roosevelt* (1979) and David McCullough, *Mornings on Horseback* (1981). More scholarly biographies are G. Wallace Chessman, *Theodore Roosevelt and the Politics of Power* (1969) and Howard K. Beals, *Theodore Roosevelt and the Rise of America to World Power* (1956). On the war also see Gerald F. Linderman, *The Mirror of War: American Society and the Spanish–American War* (1974) and H. Wayne Morgan, *America's Road to Empire* (1965).

LIVING AND DYING IN PACKINGTOWN, CHICAGO
from *The Jungle*

Upton Sinclair

In the late fall of 1904 Upton Sinclair, a young ambitious novelist imbued with a zealous sense of socialism, traveled to Chicago to gather information about the horrors and abuses of the meatpacking industry. For the next seven weeks, as a cold fall gave way to a brutal winter, Sinclair lived in the workers' ghetto of Packingtown, talked with workers, and studied the meatpacking industry.

On Christmas Day of 1904 he began writing *The Jungle*, the story of Jurgis Rudkus. A Lithuanian immigrant of great strength, Rudkus came to America full of hope—only to be used, abused, and discarded by the unfeeling powers of Packingtown. Sinclair wrote frantically for three months, stopping only occasionally to eat or sleep. He poured all his emotions into Rudkus's story, hoping to show Americans how evil the industry—and by extension, capitalism—had become. He recorded the stench and unhealthy conditions of Packingtown and the dangers of working in the packinghouses. Of the work, one historian wrote, "Each job had its own dangers: the dampness and cold of the packing rooms and hide cellar, the sharp blade of the beef boner's knife, the noxious dust of the wood department and fertilizer plant, the wild charge of a half-crazed steer on the killing floor." The following selection from *The Jungle* describes some of the working and living conditions in Packingtown.

During this time that Jurgis was looking for work occurred the death of little Kristoforas, one of the children of Teta Elzbieta. Both Kristoforas and his brother, Juozapas, were cripples, the latter having lost one leg by having it run over, and Kristoforas having congenital dislocation of the hip, which made it impossible for him ever to walk. He was the last of Teta Elzbieta's children, and perhaps he had been intended by nature to let her know that she had had enough. At any rate he was wretchedly sick and undersized; he had the rickets, and though he was over three years old, he was no bigger than an ordinary child of one. All day long he would crawl around the floor in a filthy little dress, whining and fretting; because the floor was full of draughts he was always catching cold, and snuffling because his nose ran. This made him a nuisance, and a source of endless trouble in the family. For his mother, with unnatural perversity, loved him best of all her children, and made a perpetual fuss over him—would let him do anything undisturbed, and would burst into tears when his fretting drove Jurgis wild.

And now he died. Perhaps it was the smoked sausage he had eaten that morning—which may have been made out of some of the tubercular pork that was condemned as unfit for export. At any rate, an hour after eating it, the child had begun to cry with pain, and in another hour he was rolling about on the floor in convulsions. Little Kotrina, who was all alone with him, ran out screaming for help, and after a while a doctor came, but not until Kristoforas had howled his last howl. No one was really sorry about this except poor Elzbieta, who was inconsolable. Jurgis announced that so far as he was concerned the child would have to be buried by the city, since they had no money for a funeral; and at this the poor woman almost went out of her senses, wringing her hands and screaming with grief and despair. Her child to be buried in a pauper's grave! And her stepdaughter to stand by and hear it said without protesting! It was enough to make Ona's father rise up out of his grave to rebuke her! If it had come to this, they might as well give up at once, and be buried all of them together! . . . In the end Marija said that she would help with ten dollars; and Jurgis being still obdurate, Elzbieta went in tears and begged the money from the neighbors, and so little Kristoforas had a mass and a hearse with white plumes on it, and a tiny plot in a graveyard with a wooden cross to mark the place. The poor mother was not the same for months after that; the mere sight of the floor where little Kristoforas had crawled about would make her weep. He had never had a fair chance, poor little fellow, she would say. He had been handicapped from his birth. If only she had heard about it in time, so that she might have had that great doctor to cure him of his lameness! . . . Some time ago, Elzbieta was told, a Chicago billionaire had paid a fortune to bring a great European surgeon over to cure his little daughter of the same disease from which Kristoforas had suffered. And because this surgeon had to have bodies to demonstrate upon, he announced that he would treat the children of the poor, a piece of magnanimity over which the papers became quite eloquent. Elzbieta, alas, did not read the papers, and no one had told her; but perhaps it was as well, for just then they would not have had the car-fare to spare to go every day to wait upon the surgeon, nor for that matter anybody with the time to take the child.

All this while that he was seeking for work, there was a dark shadow hanging over Jurgis; as if a savage beast were lurking somewhere in the pathway of his life, and he knew it, and yet could not help approaching the place. There are all stages of being out of work in Packingtown, and he faced in dread the prospect of reaching the lowest. There is a place that waits for the lowest man—the fertilizer-plant!

The men would talk about it in awe-stricken whispers. Not more than one in ten had ever

Upton Sinclair, "Living and Dying in Packingtown, Chicago." From Upton Sinclair, *The Jungle*. Chicago, 1905.

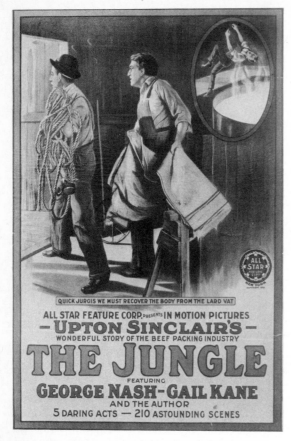

QUICK JURGIS WE MUST RECOVER THE BODY FROM THE LARD VAT

ALL STAR FEATURE CORP. presents IN MOTION PICTURES
—UPTON SINCLAIR'S—
WONDERFUL STORY OF THE BEEF PACKING INDUSTRY
THE JUNGLE
FEATURING
GEORGE NASH · GAIL KANE
AND THE AUTHOR
5 DARING ACTS — 210 ASTOUNDING SCENES

■ ■ *The drama and emotion of Upton Sinclair's 1905 novel held great appeal for the fledgling motion picture industry. This poster for the 1913 film highlights one of the novel's gruesome details.*

really tried it; the other nine had contented themselves with hearsay evidence and a peep through the door. There were some things worse than even starving to death. They would ask Jurgis if he had worked there yet, and if he meant to; and Jurgis would debate the matter with himself. As poor as they were and making all the sacrifices that they were, would he dare to refuse any sort of work that was offered to him, be it as horrible as ever it could? Would he dare to go home and eat bread that had been earned by Ona, weak and complaining as she was, knowing that he had been given a chance, and had not had the nerve to take it?—And yet he

might argue that way with himself all day, and one glimpse into the fertilizer-works would send him away again shuddering. He was a man, and he would do his duty; he went and made application—but surely he was not also required to hope for success.

The fertilizer-works of Durham's lay away from the rest of the plant. Few visitors ever saw them, and the few who did would come out looking like Dante, of whom the peasants declared that he had been into hell. To this part of the yards came all the "tankage" and waste products of all sorts; here they dried out the bones—and in suffocating cellars where the daylight never came you might see men and women and children bending over whirling machines and sawing bits of bone into all sorts of shapes, breathing their lungs full of the fine dust, and doomed to die, every one of them, within a certain definite time. Here they made the blood into albumen, and made other foul-smelling things into things still more foul-smelling. In the corridors and caverns where it was done you might lose yourself as in the great caves of Kentucky. In the dust and the steam the electric lights would shine like far-off twinkling stars—red and blue, green and purple stars, according to the color of the mist and the brew from which it came. For the odors in these ghastly charnel-houses there may be words in Lithuanian, but there are none in English. The person entering would have to summon his courage as for a cold-water plunge. He would go on like a man swimming under water; he would put his handkerchief over his face, and begin to cough and choke; and then, if he were still obstinate, he would find his head beginning to ring, and the veins in his forehead to throb, until finally he would be assailed by an overpowering blast of ammonia fumes, and would turn and run for his life, and come out half-dazed.

On top of this were the rooms where they dried the "tankage," the mass of brown stringy stuff that was left after the waste portions of the carcasses had had the lard and tallow tried out of them. This dried material they would then grind to a fine powder, and after they had mixed it up well with a mysterious but inoffensive brown rock which they brought in and ground up by the hundreds of carloads for that purpose, the substance was ready to be put into bags and sent out to the world as any one of a hundred different brands of standard bone-phosphate. And then the farmer in Maine or California or Texas would buy this, at say twenty-five dollars a ton, and plant it with his corn; and for several days after the operation the fields would have a strong odor, and the farmer and his wagon and the very horses that had hauled it would all have it too. In Packingtown the fertilizer is pure, instead of being a flavoring, and instead of a ton or so spread on several acres under the open sky, there are hundreds and thousands of tons of it in one building, heaped here and there in haystack piles, covering the floor several inches deep, and filling the air with a choking dust that becomes a blinding sand-storm when the wind stirs.

It was to this building that Jurgis came daily, as if dragged by an unseen hand. The month of May was an exceptionally cool one, and his secret prayers were granted; but early in June there came a record-breaking hot spell, and after that there were men wanted in the fertilizer-mill.

The boss of the grinding room had come to know Jurgis by this time, and had marked him for a likely man; and so when he came to the door about two o'clock this breathless hot day, he felt a sudden spasm of pain shoot through him—the boss beckoned to him! In ten minutes more Jurgis had pulled off his coat and over-shirt, and set his teeth together and gone to work. Here was one more difficulty for him to meet and conquer!

His labor took him about one minute to learn. Before him was one of the vents of the mill in which the fertilizer was being ground—rushing forth in a great brown river, with a spray of the finest dust flung forth in clouds. Jurgis was given a shovel, and along with half a dozen others it was his task to shovel this fertilizer into carts. That others were at work he knew by the sound,

and by the fact that he sometimes collided with them; otherwise they might as well not have been there, for in the blinding dust-storm a man could not see six feet in front of his face. When he had filled one cart he had to grope around him until another came, and if there was none on hand he continued to grope till one arrived. In five minutes he was, of course, a mass of fertilizer from head to feet; they gave him a sponge to tie over his mouth, so that he could breathe, but the sponge did not prevent his lips and eyelids from caking up with it and his ears from filling solid. He looked like a brown ghost at twilight—from hair to shoes he became the color of the building and of everything in it, and for that matter a hundred yards outside it. The building had to be left open, and when the wind blew Durham and Company lost a great deal of fertilizer.

Working in his shirt-sleeves, and with the thermometer at over a hundred, the phosphates soaked in through every pore of Jurgis's skin, and in five minutes he had a headache, and in fifteen was almost dazed. The blood was pounding his brain like an engine's throbbing; there was a frightful pain in the top of his skull, and he could hardly control his hands. Still, with the memory of his four months' siege behind him, he fought on, in a frenzy of determination; and half an hour later he began to vomit—he vomited until it seemed as if his inwards must be torn to shreds. A man could get used to the fertilizer-mill, the boss had said, if he would only make up his mind to it; but Jurgis now began to see that it was a question of making up his stomach.

At the end of that day of horror, he could scarcely stand. He had to catch himself now and then, and lean against a building and get his bearings. Most of the men, when they came out, made straight for a saloon—they seem to place fertilizer and rattlesnake poison in one class. But Jurgis was too ill to think of drinking—he could only make his way to the street and stagger on to a car. He had a sense of humor, and later on, when he became an old hand, he used to think it fun to board a street-car and see what happened. Now, however, he was too ill to notice it—how the people in the car began to gasp and sputter, to put their handkerchiefs to their noses, and transfix him with furious glances. Jurgis only knew that a man in front of him immediately got up and gave him a seat; and that half a minute later the two people on each side of him got up; and that in a full minute the crowded car was nearly empty—those passengers who could not get room on the platform having gotten out to walk.

Of course Jurgis had made his home a miniature fertilizer-mill a minute after entering. The stuff was half an inch deep in his skin—his whole system was full of it, and it would have taken a week not merely of scrubbing, but of vigorous exercise, to get it out of him. As it was, he could be compared with nothing known to men, save that newest discovery of the savants, a substance which emits energy for an unlimited time, without being itself in the least diminished in power. He smelt so that he made all food at the table taste, and set the whole family to vomiting; for himself it was three days before he could keep anything upon his stomach—he might wash his hands, and use a knife and fork, but were not his mouth and throat filled with the poison?

And still Jurgis stuck it out! In spite of splitting headaches he would stagger down to the plant and take up his stand once more, and begin to shovel in the blinding clouds of dust. And so at the end of the week he was a fertilizer-man for life—he was able to eat again, and though his head never stopped aching, it ceased to be so bad that he could not work.

So there passed another summer. It was a summer of prosperity, all over the country, and the country ate generously of packing-house products, and there was plenty of work for all the family, in spite of the packers' efforts to keep a superfluity of labor. They were again able to pay their debts and to begin to save a little sum; but there were one or two sacrifices they considered too heavy to be made for long—it was too bad that the boys should have to sell papers at their age. It was utterly useless to caution them and plead with them; quite without knowing it, they were taking on the tone of their new environment. They were learning to swear in voluble English; they were learning to pick up cigar-stumps and smoke them, to pass hours of their time gambling with pennies and dice and cigarette-cards; they were learning the location of all the houses of prostitution on the "Levée," and the names of the "madames" who kept them, and the days when they gave their state banquets, which the police captains and the big politicians all attended. If a visiting "country-customer" were to ask them, they could show him which was "Hinkydink's" famous saloon, and could even point out to him by name the different gamblers and thugs and "hold-up men" who made the place their headquarters. And worse yet, the boys were getting out of the habit of coming home at night. What was the use, they would ask, of wasting time and energy and a possible car-fare riding out to the stockyards every night when the weather was pleasant and they could crawl under a truck or into an empty doorway and sleep exactly as well? So long as they brought home a half dollar for each day, what mattered it when they brought it? But Jurgis declared that from this to ceasing to come at all would not be a very long step, and so it was decided that Vilimas and Nikalojus should return to school in the fall, and that instead Elzbieta should go out and get some work, her place at home being taken by her younger daughter.

Little Kotrina was like most children of the poor, prematurely made old; she had to take care of her little brother, who was a cripple, and also of the baby; she had to cook the meals and wash the dishes and clean house, and have supper ready when the workers came home in the evening. She was only thirteen, and small for her age, but she did all this without a murmur; and her mother went out, and after trudging a couple of days about the yards, settled down as a servant of a "sausage-machine."

Elzbieta was used to working, but she found

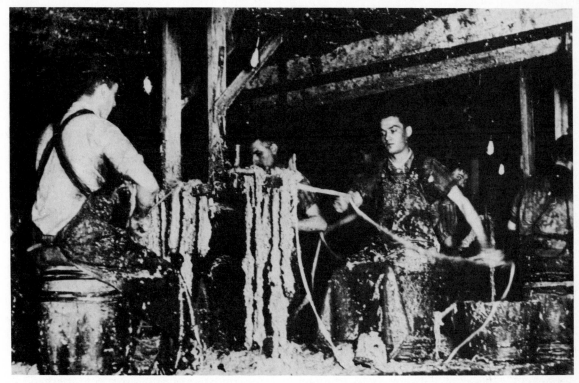

■ ■ *Chicago's meatpacking industry grew up with little or no governmental control. These sausagemakers at Armour & Co. worked in extreme temperatures and without adequate ventilation, causing many to faint or to vomit from the stench.*

this change a hard one, for the reason that she had to stand motionless upon her feet from seven o'clock in the morning till half-past twelve, and again from one till half-past five. For the first days it seemed to her that she could not stand it—she suffered almost as much as Jurgis had from the fertilizer—and would come out at sundown with her head fairly reeling. Besides this, she was working in one of the dark holes, by electric light, and the dampness, too, was deadly—there were always puddles of water on the floor, and a sickening odor of moist flesh in the room. The people who worked here followed the ancient custom of nature, whereby the ptarmigan is the color of dead leaves in the fall and of snow in winter, and the chameleon, who is black when he lies upon a stump and turns green when he moves to a leaf. The men

and women who worked in this department were precisely the color of the "fresh country sausage" they made.

The sausage-room was an interesting place to visit, for two or three minutes, and provided that you did not look at the people; the machines were perhaps the most wonderful things in the entire plant. Presumably sausages were once chopped and stuffed by hand, and if so it would be interesting to know how many workers had been displaced by these inventions. On one side of the room were the hoppers, into which men shovelled loads of meat and wheelbarrows full of spices; in these great bowls were whirling knives that made two thousand revolutions a minute, and when the meat was ground fine and adulterated with potato-flour, and well mixed with water, it was forced to the stuffing-machines on the other side of the room. The latter were tended by women; there was a sort of spout, like the nozzle of a hose, and one of the women would take a long string of "casing" and put the end over the nozzle and then work the whole thing on, as one works on the finger of a tight glove. This string would be twenty or thirty feet long, but the woman would have it all on in a jiffy; and when she had several on, she would press a lever, and a stream of sausage-meat would be shot out, taking the casing with it as it came. Thus one might stand and see appear, miraculously born from the machine, a wriggling snake of sausage of incredible length. In front was a big pan which caught these creatures, and two more women who seized them as fast as they appeared and twisted them into links. This was for the uninitiated the most perplexing work of all; for all that the woman had to give was a single turn of the wrist; and in some way she contrived to give it so that instead of an endless chain of sausages, one after another, there grew under her hands a bunch of strings, all dangling from a single centre. It was quite like the feat of a prestidigitator—for the woman worked so fast that the eye could literally not follow her, and there was only a mist of motion, and tangle after tangle of sausages appearing. In the midst of the mist, however, the visitor would suddenly notice the tense set face, with the two wrinkles graven in the forehead, and the ghastly pallor of the cheeks; and then he would suddenly recollect that it was time he was going on. The woman did not go on; she stayed right there—hour after hour, day after day, year after year, twisting sausage-links and racing with death. It was piece-work, and she was apt to have a family to keep alive; and stern and ruthless economic laws had arranged it that she could only do this by working just as she did, with all her soul upon her work, and with never an instant for a glance at the well-dressed ladies and gentlemen who came to stare at her, as at some wild beast in a menagerie.

With one member trimming beef in a cannery, and another working in a sausage factory, the family had a first-hand knowledge of the great majority of Packingtown swindles. For it was the custom, as they found, whenever meat was so spoiled that it could not be used for anything else, either to can it or else to chop it up into sausage. With what had been told them by Jonas, who had worked in the pickle-rooms, they could now study the whole of the spoiled-meat industry on the inside, and read a new and grim meaning into that old Packingtown jest—that they use everything of the pig except the squeal.

Jonas had told them how the meat that was taken out of pickle would often be found sour, and how they would rub it up with soda to take away the smell, and sell it to be eaten on free-lunch counters; also of all the miracles of chemistry which they performed, giving to any sort of meat, fresh or salted, whole or chopped, any color and any flavor and any odor they chose. In the pickling of hams they had an ingenious apparatus, by which they saved time and increased the capacity of the plant—a machine consisting of a hollow needle attached to a pump; by plunging this needle into the meat and working with his foot, a man could fill a ham with pickle in a few seconds. And yet, in spite of this, there would be hams found spoiled, some of them with an odor so bad that a man could hardly bear to be in the room with them. To pump into these the packers had a second and much stronger pickle which destroyed the odor—a process known to the workers as "giving them thirty percent." Also, after the hams had been smoked, there would be found some that had gone to the bad. Formerly these had been sold as "Number Three Grade," but later on some ingenious person had hit upon a new device, and now they would extract the bone, about which the bad part generally lay, and insert in the hole a white-hot iron. After this invention there was no longer Number One, Two, and Three Grade—there was only Number One Grade. The packers were always originating such schemes—they had what they called "boneless hams," which were all the odds and ends of pork stuffed into casings; and "California hams," which were the shoulders, with big knuckle-joints, and nearly all the meat cut out; and fancy "skinned hams," which were made of the oldest hogs, whose skins were so heavy and coarse that no one would buy them—that is, until they had been cooked and chopped fine and labelled "head cheese"!

It was only when the whole ham was spoiled that it came into the department of Elzbieta. Cut up by the two-thousand-revolutions-a-minute flyers, and mixed with half a ton of other meat, no odor that ever was in a ham could make any difference. There was never the least attention paid to what was cut up for sausage; there would come all the way back from Europe old sausage that had been rejected, and that was mouldy and white—it would be dosed with borax and glycerine, and dumped into the hoppers, and made over again for home consumption. There would be meat that had tumbled out on the floor, in the dirt and sawdust, where the workers had tramped and spit uncounted billions of consumption germs. There would be meat stored in great piles in rooms; and the water from leaky roofs would drip over it, and thousands of rats would race about on it. It was too dark in these storage places to see well, but a man could run his hand over these piles of meat and sweep off handfuls of the dried dung of rats. These rats were nuisances, and the packers would put poisoned bread out for them; they would die, and then rats, bread, and meat would go into the hoppers together. This is no fairy story and no joke; the meat would be shovelled into carts, and the man who did the shovelling would not trouble to lift out a rat even when he saw one—there were things that went into the sausage in comparison with which a poisoned rat was a tidbit. There was no place for the men to wash their hands before they ate their dinner, and so they made a practice of washing them in the water that was to be ladled into the sausage. There were the butt-ends of smoked meat, and the scraps of corned beef, and

all the odds and ends of the waste of the plants, that would be dumped into old barrels in the cellar and left there. Under the system of rigid economy which the packers enforced, there were some jobs that it only paid to do once in a long time, and among these was the cleaning out of the waste-barrels. Every spring they did it; and in the barrels would be dirt and rust and old nails and stale water—and cart load after cart load of it would be taken up and dumped into the hoppers with fresh meat, and sent out to the public's breakfast. Some of it they would make into "smoked" sausage—but as the smoking took time, and was therefore expensive, they would call upon their chemistry department, and preserve it with borax and color it with gelatine to make it brown. All of their sausage came out of the same bowl, but when they came to wrap it they would stamp some of it "special," and for this they would charge two cents more a pound.

Such were the new surroundings in which Elzbieta was placed, and such was the work she was compelled to do. It was stupefying, brutalizing work; it left her no time to think, no strength for anything. She was part of the machine she tended, and every faculty that was not needed for the machine was doomed to be crushed out of existence. There was only one mercy about the cruel grind—that it gave her the gift of insensibility. Little by little she sank into a torpor—she fell silent. She would meet Jurgis and Ona in the evening, and the three would walk home together, often without saying a word. Ona, too, was falling into the habit of silence—Ona, who had once gone about singing like a bird. She was sick and miserable, and often she would barely have strength enough to drag herself home. And there they would eat what they had to eat, and afterwards, because there was only their misery to talk of, they would crawl into bed and fall into a stupor and never stir until it was time to get up again, and dress by candlelight, and go back to the machines. They were so numbed that they did not even suffer much from hunger, now; only the children continued to fret when the food ran short.

Yet the soul of Ona was not dead—the souls of none of them were dead, but only sleeping; and now and then they would waken, and these were cruel times. The gates of memory would roll open—old joys would stretch out their arms to them, old hopes and dreams would call to them, and they would stir beneath the burden that lay upon them, and feel its forever immeasurable weight. They could not even cry out beneath it; but anguish would seize them, more dreadful than the agony of death. It was a thing scarcely to be spoken—a thing never spoken by all the world, that will not know its own defeat.

They were beaten; they had lost the game, they were swept aside. It was not less tragic because it was so sordid, because that it had to do with wages and grocery bills and rents. They had dreamed of freedom; of a chance to look about them and learn something; to be decent and clean, to see their child grow up to be strong. And now it was all gone—it would never be! They had played the game and they had lost. Six years more of toil they had to face before they could expect the least respite, the cessation of the payments upon the house; and how cruelly certain it was that they could never stand six years of such a life as they were living! They were lost, they were going down—and there was no deliverance for them, no hope; for all the help it gave them the vast city in which they lived might have been an ocean waste, a wilderness, a desert, a tomb. So often this mood would come to Ona, in the night-time, when something wakened her; she would lie, afraid of the beating of her own heart, fronting the blood-red eyes of the old primeval terror of life. Once she cried aloud, and woke Jurgis, who was tired and cross. After that she learned to weep silently—their moods so seldom came together now! It was as if their hopes were buried in separate graves.

Jurgis, being a man, had troubles of his own. There was another spectre following him. He had never spoken of it, nor would he allow any one else to speak of it—he had never acknowledged its existence to himself. Yet the battle with it took all the manhood that he had—and once or twice, alas, a little more. Jurgis had discovered drink.

He was working in the steaming pit of hell; day after day, week after week—until now there was not an organ of his body that did its work without pain, until the sound of ocean breakers echoed in his head day and night, and the buildings swayed and danced before him as he went down the street. And from all the unending horror of this there was a respite, a deliverance—he could drink! He could forget the pain, he could slip off the burden; he would see clearly again, he would be master of his brain, of his thoughts, of his will. His dead self would stir in him, and he would find himself laughing and cracking jokes with his companions—he would be a man again, and master of his life.

It was not an easy thing for Jurgis to take more than two or three drinks. With the first drink he could eat a meal, and he could persuade himself that that was economy; with the second he could eat another meal—but there would come a time when he could eat no more, and then to pay for a drink was an unthinkable extravagance, a defiance of the age-long instincts of his hunger-haunted class. One day, however, he took the plunge, and drank up all that he had in his pockets, and went home half "piped," as the men phrase it. He was happier than he had been in a year; and yet, because he knew that the happiness would not last, he was savage, too—with those who would wreck it, and with the world, and with his life; and then again, beneath this, he was sick with the shame of himself. Afterward, when he saw the despair of his family, and reckoned up the money he had spent, the tears came into his eyes, and he began the long battle with the spectre.

It was a battle that had no end, that never could have one. But Jurgis did not realize that very clearly; he was not given much time for reflection. He simply knew that he was always fighting. Steeped in misery and despair as he was, merely to walk down the street was to be put upon the rack. There was surely a saloon on the corner—perhaps on all four corners, and some in the middle of the block as well; and each one stretched out a hand to him—each one had a personality of its own, allurements unlike any other. Going and coming—before sunrise and after dark—there was warmth and a glow of light, and the steam of hot food, and perhaps music, or a friendly face, and a word of good cheer. Jurgis developed a fondness for having Ona on his arm whenever he went out on the street, and he would hold her tightly, and walk fast. It was pitiful to have Ona know of this—it drove him wild to think of it; the thing was not fair, for Ona had never tasted drink, and so could not understand. Sometimes, in desperate hours, he would find himself wishing that she might learn what it was, so that he need not be ashamed in her presence. They might drink together, and escape from the horror—escape for a while, come what would.

So there came a time when nearly all the conscious life of Jurgis consisted of a struggle with the craving for liquor. He would have ugly moods, when he hated Ona and the whole family, because they stood in his way. He was a fool to have married; he had tied himself down, and made himself a slave. It was all because he was a married man that he was compelled to stay in the yards; if it had not been for that he might have gone off like Jonas, and to hell with the packers. There were few single men in the fertilizer-mill—and those few were working only for a chance to escape. Meantime, too, they had something to think about while they worked—they had the memory of the last time they had been drunk, and the hope of the time when they would be drunk again. As for Jurgis, he was expected to bring home every penny; he could not even go with the men at noon-time—he was supposed to sit down and eat his dinner on a pile of fertilizer dust.

This was not always his mood, of course; he still loved his family. But just now was a time

of trial. Poor little Antanas, for instance—who had never failed to win him with a smile—little Antanas was not smiling just now, being a mass of fiery red pimples. He had had all the diseases that babies are heir to, in quick succession—scarlet fever, mumps, and whooping-cough in the first year, and now he was down with the measles. There was no one to attend him but Kotrina; there was no doctor to help him, because they were too poor, and children did not die of the measles—at least not often. Now and then Kotrina would find time to sob over his woes, but for the greater part of the time he had to be left alone, barricaded upon the bed. The floor was full of draughts, and if he caught cold he would die. At night he was tied down, lest he should kick the covers off him, while the family lay in their stupor of exhaustion. He would lie and scream for hours, almost in convulsions; and then when he was worn out, he would lie whimpering and wailing in his torment. He was burning up with fever, and his eyes were running sores; in the daytime he was a thing uncanny and impish to behold, a plaster of pimples and sweat, a great purple lump of misery.

Yet all this was not really as cruel as it sounds, for, sick as he was, little Antanas was the least unfortunate member of that family. He was quite able to bear his sufferings—it was as if he had all these complaints to show what a prodigy of health he was. He was the child of his parents' youth and joy; he grew up like the conjurer's rose bush, and all the world was his oyster. In general, he toddled around the kitchen all day with a lean and hungry look—the portion of the family's allowance that fell to him was not enough, and he was unrestrainable in his demand for more. Antanas was but little over a year old, and already no one but his father could manage him.

It seemed as if he had taken all of his mother's strength—had left nothing for those that might come after him. Ona was with child again now, and it was a dreadful thing to contemplate; even Jurgis, dumb and despairing as he was, could not but understand that yet other agonies were on the way, and shudder at the thought of them.

For Ona was visibly going to pieces. In the first place she was developing a cough, like the one that had killed old Dede Antanas. She had had a trace of it ever since that fatal morning when the greedy street-car corporation had turned her out into the rain; but now it was beginning to grow serious, and to wake her up at night. Even worse than that was the fearful nervousness from which she suffered; she would have frightful headaches and fits of aimless weeping; and sometimes she would come home at night shuddering and moaning, and would fling herself down upon the bed and burst into tears. Several times she was quite beside herself and hysterical; and then Jurgis would go half mad with fright. Elzbieta would explain to him that it could not be helped, that woman was subject to such things when she was pregnant; but he was hardly to be persuaded, and would

beg and plead to know what had happened. She had never been like this before, he would argue—it was monstrous and unthinkable. It was the life she had to live, the accursed work she had to do, that was killing her by inches. She was not fitted for it—no woman was fitted for it, no woman ought to be allowed to do such work; if the world could not keep them alive any other way it ought to kill them at once and be done with it. They ought not to marry, to have children; no working-man ought to marry—if he, Jurgis, had known what a woman was like, he would have had his eyes torn out first. So he would carry on, becoming half hysterical himself, which was an unbearable thing to see in a big man; Ona would pull herself together and fling herself into his arms, begging him to stop, to be still, that she would be better, it would be all right. So she would lie and sob out her grief upon his shoulder, while he gazed at her, as helpless as a wounded animal, the target of unseen enemies.

■ ■ ■

STUDY QUESTIONS

1. What was health care like for children in Packingtown?

2. What sort of men worked in the fertilizer plants? What were the hazards of the job?

3. How did the constant demand for money affect families?

4. What were the abuses of the "spoiled-meat" industry?

5. What response was Upton Sinclair hoping to achieve with The Jungle?

BIBLIOGRAPHY

On the life of Upton Sinclair see Floyd Dell, Upton Sinclair: A Study in Social Protest (1927); Jon Yoder, Upton Sinclair (1975); Leon Harris, Upton Sinclair, American Rebel (1975); and his own The Autobiography of Upton Sinclair (1962). Three good books on the literature of the period are Daniel Aaron, Writers of the Left (1969); James Burkhart Gilbert, Writers and Partisans: A History of Literary Radicalism in

America (1968); and Larzer Ziff, *The American 1890s: Life and Times of a Lost Generation* (1966). On the meatpacking industry, Packingtown, and the lives of the workers, consult Louis Carroll Wade, *Chicago's Pride: The Stockyards, Packingtown, and Environs in the Nineteenth Century* (1987) and James R. Barrett, *Work and Community in the Jungle: Chicago's Packinghouse Workers* (1988).

ROSE SCHNEIDERMAN AND THE TRIANGLE SHIRTWAIST FIRE

Bonnie Mitelman

The progress Americans made during the Progressive Era depended upon one's perspective. For middle-class Americans, progress was everywhere visible. Real income rose and the government worked to insure order and efficiency in the industrial world. For their part, most large industrialists cooperated with the government's effort to impose order, which often resulted in the elimination of bothersome competition. For example, leading meatpackers supported the Meat Inspection Act of 1906. The act raised inspection standards, thereby driving out small competitors and guaranteeing the quality of American meat on the competitive world market.

America's working class, however, had reason to question the nature of the "progress" that was being made. The men and women who labored in industrial America often performed uncreative, repetitive tasks at a pace set by machines. Possibly worse than the monotony of industrial life was the danger of it. Machines were blind and uncaring; they showed no sympathy for tired or bored workers who allowed their fingers to move too close to moving cogs. Injuries were common, and far too often industrialists were as unsympathetic as their machines. And for most unskilled workers, labor unions were weak and unrecognized by leading industrialists and manufacturers. In the following essay, Bonnie Mitelman discusses the 1911 Triangle Waist Company fire, a tragedy which saw 146 workers die. The fire and its results raise serious questions about the extent and nature of progress during the early twentieth century.

On Saturday afternoon, March 25, 1911, in New York City's Greenwich Village, a small fire broke out in the Triangle Waist Company, just as the 500 shirtwaist employees were quitting for the day. People rushed about, trying to get out, but they found exits blocked and windows to the fire escape rusted shut. They panicked.

As the fire spread and more and more were trapped, some began to jump, their hair and clothing afire, from the eighth and ninth floor windows. Nets that firemen held for them tore apart at the impact of the falling bodies. By the time it was over, 146 workers had died, most of them young Jewish women.

A United Press reporter, William Shepherd, witnessed the tragedy and reported, "I looked upon the heap of dead bodies and I remembered these girls were the shirtwaist makers. I remembered their great strike of last year in which these same girls had demanded more sanitary conditions and more safety precautions in the shops. These dead bodies were the answer."

The horror of that fire touched the entire Lower East Side ghetto community, and there was a profuse outpouring of sympathy. But it was Rose Schneiderman, an immigrant worker with a spirit of social justice and a powerful way with words, who is largely credited with translating the ghetto's emotional reaction into meaningful, widespread action. Six weeks following the tragedy, and after years of solid groundwork, with one brilliant, well-timed speech, she was able to inspire the support of wealthy uptown New Yorkers and to swing public opinion to the side of the labor movement, enabling concerned civic, religious, and labor leaders to mobilize their efforts for desperately needed safety and industrial reforms.

"Rose Schneiderman and the Triangle Fire" by Bonnie Mitelman, from *American History Illustrated* (July, 1981). Copyright © 1981 by Historical Times, Inc. Reprinted through the courtesy of Historical Times, Inc., publishers of *American History Illustrated*.

The Triangle fire, and the deaths of so many helpless workers, seemed to trigger in Rose Schneiderman an intense realization that there was absolutely nothing or no one to help working women except a strong union movement. With fierce determination, and the dedication, influence, and funding of many other people as well, she battled to regulate hours, wages, and safety standards and to abolish the sweatshop system. In so doing, she brought dignity and human rights to all workers.

The dramatic "uprising of the 20,000" of 1909–10, in which thousands of immigrant girls and women in the shirtwaist industry had endured three long winter months of a general strike to protest deplorable working conditions, had produced some immediate gains for working women. There had been agreements for shorter working hours, increased wages, and even safety reforms, but there had not been formal recognition of their union. At Triangle, for example, the girls had gained a 52 hour week, a 12–15 percent wage increase, and promises to end the grueling subcontracting system. But they had not gained the only instrument on which they could depend for lasting change: a viable trade union. This was to have disastrous results, for in spite of the few gains that they seemed to have made, the workers won no rights or bargaining power at all. In fact, "The company dealt only with its contractors. It felt no responsibility for the girls."

There were groups as well as individuals who realized the workers impotence, but their attempts to change the situation accomplished little despite long years of hard work. The Women's Trade Union League and the International Ladies' Garment Workers' Union, through the efforts of Mary Dreier, Helen Marot, Leonora O'Reilly, Pauline Newman, and Rose Schneiderman had struggled unsuccessfully for improved conditions: the futility that the union organizers were feeling in late 1910 is reflected in the WTUL minutes of December 5 of that year.

A scant eight months after their historic waist-makers' strike, and three months before the deadly Triangle fire, a Mrs. Malkiel (no doubt Theresa Serber Malkiel, who wrote the legendary account of the strike, *The Diary of a Shirtwaist Striker: A Story of the Shirtwaist Makers' Strike in New York*) is reported to have come before the League to urge action after a devastating fire in Newark, New Jersey killed twenty-five working women. Mrs. Malkiel attributed their loss to the greed and negligence of the owners and the proper authorities. The WTUL subsequently demanded an investigation of all factory buildings and it elected an investigation committee from the League to cooperate with similar committees from other organizations.

The files of the WTUL contain complaint after complaint about unsafe factory conditions; many were filled out by workers afraid to sign their names for fear of being fired had their employers seen the forms. They describe factories with locked doors, no fire escapes, and barred windows. The New York *Times* carried an article which reported that fourteen factories were found to have no fire escapes, twenty-three that had locked doors, and seventy-eight that had obstructed fire escapes. In all, according to the article, 99 percent of the factories investigated in New York were found to have serious fire hazards.

Yet no action was taken.

It was the Triangle fire that emphasized, spectacularly and tragically, the deplorable safety and sanitary conditions of the garment workers. The tragedy focused attention upon the ghastly factories in which most immigrants worked; there was no longer any question about what the strikers had meant when they talked about safety and sanitary reform, and about social and economic justice.

The grief and frustration of the shirtwaist strikers were expressed by one of them, Rose Safran, after the fire: "If the union had won we would have been safe. Two of our demands were for adequate fire escapes and for open doors from the factories to the street. But the bosses defeated us and we didn't get the open doors or the better fire escapes. So our friends are dead."

The families of the fire victims were heartbroken and hysterical, the ghetto's *Jewish Daily Forward* was understandably melodramatic, and the immigrant community was completely enraged. Their Jewish heritage had taught them an emphasis on individual human life and worth; their shared background in the *shtetl* and common experiences in the ghetto had given them a sense of fellowship. They were, in a sense, a family—and some of the most helpless among them had died needlessly.

The senseless deaths of so many young Jewish women sparked within these Eastern Europeans a new determination and dedication. The fire had made reform absolutely essential. Workers' rights were no longer just socialist jargon: They were a matter of life and death.

The Triangle Waist Company was located on the three floors of the Asch Building, a 10-story, 135-foot-high structure at the corner of Greene Street and Washington Place in Greenwich Village. One of the largest shirtwaist manufacturers, Triangle employed up to 900 people at times, but on the day of the fire, only about 500 were working.

Leon Stein's brilliant and fascinating account of the fire, entitled simply *The Triangle Fire*, develops and documents the way in which the physical facilities, company procedures, and human behavior interacted to cause this great tragedy. Much of what occurred was ironic, some was cruel, some stupid, some pathetic. It is a dramatic portrayal of the eternal confrontation of the "haves" and the "havenots," told in large part by those who survived.

Fire broke out at the Triangle Company at approximately 4:45 P.M. (because time clocks were reportedly set back to stretch the day, and because other records give differing times of the first fire alarm, it is uncertain exactly what time the fire started), just after pay envelopes had been distributed and employees were leaving their work posts. It was a small fire at first, and there was a calm, controlled effort to extinguish it. But the fire began to spread, jumping from one pile of debris to another, engulfing the combustible shirtwaist fabric. It became obvious that the fire could not be snuffed out, and workers tried to reach the elevators or stairway. Those who reached the one open stairway raced down eight flights of stairs to safety; those who managed to climb onto the available passenger elevators also got out. But not everyone could reach the available exits. Some tried to open the door to a stairway and found it locked. Others were trapped between long working tables or behind the hordes of people trying to get into the elevators or out through the one open door.

Under the work tables, rags were burning; the wooden floors, trim, and window frames were also afire. Frantically, workers fought their way to the elevators, to the fire escape, and to the windows—to any place that might lead to safety.

Fire whistles and bells sounded as the fire department raced to the building. But equipment proved inadequate, as the fire ladders reached only to the seventh floor. And by the time the firemen connected their hoses to douse the flames, the crowded eighth floor was completely ablaze.

For those who reached the windows, there seemed to be a chance for safety. The New York *World* describes people balancing on window sills, nine stories up, with flames scorching them from behind, until firemen arrived: "The nets were spread below with all promptness. Citizens were commandeered into service, as the firemen necessarily gave their attention to the one engine and hose of the force that first arrived. The catapult force that the bodies gathered in the long plunges made the nets utterly without avail. Screaming girls and men, as they fell, tore the nets from the grasp of the holders, and the bodies struck the sidewalks and lay just as they fell. Some of the bodies ripped big holes through the life nets."

One reporter who witnessed the fire remembered how,

A young man helped a girl to the window sill on the ninth floor. Then he held her out deliberately, away from the building, and let her drop. He held out a second girl the same way and let her drop. He held out a third girl who did not resist. They were all as unresisting as if he were helping them into a street car instead of into eternity. He saw that a terrible death awaited them in the flames and his was only a terrible chivalry. He brought around another girl to the window. I saw her put her arms around him and kiss him. Then he held her into space—and dropped her. Quick as a flash, he was on the window sill himself. His coat fluttered upwards—the air filled his trouser legs as he came down. I could see he wore tan shoes.

Those who had rushed to the fire escape found the window openings rusted shut. Several precious minutes were lost in releasing them. The fire escape itself ended at the second floor, in an airshaft between the Asch Building and the building next door. But too frantic to notice where it ended, workers climbed on to the fire escape, one after another until, in one terrifying moment, it collapsed from the weight, pitching the workers to their death.

Those who had made their way to the elevators found crowds pushing to get into the cars. When it became obvious that the elevators could no longer run, workers jumped down the elevator shaft, landing on the top of the cars, or grabbing for cables to ease their descent. Several died, but incredibly, some did manage to save themselves in this way. One man was found, hours after the fire, beneath an elevator car in the basement of the building, nearly drowned by the rapidly rising water from the firemen's hoses.

Several people, among them Triangle's two owners, raced to the roof, and from there were led to safety. Others never had that chance. "When Fire Chief Croker could make his way into the [top] three floors," states one account of the fire, "he found sights that utterly staggered him . . . he saw as the smoke drifted away bodies burned to bare bones. There were skeletons bending over sewing machines.''

The day after the fire, the New York *Times* announced that ''the building was fireproof. It shows hardly any signs of the disaster that overtook it. The walls are as good as ever, as are the floors: nothing is worse for the fire except the furniture and 14 [*sic*] of the 600 men and girls that were employed in its upper three stories.''

The building *was* fireproof. But there had never been a fire drill in the factory, even though the management had been warned about the possible hazard of fire on the top three floors. Owners Max Blanck and Isaac Harris had chosen to ignore these warnings in spite of the fact that many of their employees were immigrants who could barely speak English, which would surely mean panic in the event of a crisis.

The New York *Times* also noted that Leonora O'Reilly of the League had reported Max Blanck's visit to the WTUL during the shirtwaist strike, and his plea that the girls return to work. He claimed a business reputaton to maintain and told the Union leaders he would make the necessary improvements right away. Because he was the largest manufacturer in the business, the League reported, they trusted him and let the girls return.

But the improvements were never made. And there was nothing that anybody could or would do about it. Factory doors continued to open in instead of out, in violation of fire regulations. The doors remained bolted during working hours, apparently to prevent workers from getting past the inspectors with stolen merchandise. Triangle had only two staircases where there should have been three, and those two were very narrow. Despite the fact that the building was deemed fireproof, it had wooden window frames, floors, and trim. There was no sprinkler system. It was not legally required.

These were the same kinds of conditions which existed in factories throughout the garment industry; they had been cited repeatedly in the complaints filed with the WTUL. They were not unusual nor restricted to Triangle; in fact, Triangle was not as bad as many other factories.

But it was at Triangle that the fire took place.

The *Jewish Daily Forward* mourned the dead with sorrowful stories, and its headlines talked of ''funerals instead of weddings'' for the dead young girls. The entire Jewish immigrant community was affected, for it seemed there was scarcely a person who was not in some way touched by the fire. Nearly everyone had either been employed at Triangle themselves, or had a friend or relative who had worked there at some time or another. Most worked in factories with similar conditions, and so everyone identified with the victims and their families.

Many of the dead, burned beyond recognition, remained unidentified for days, as searching family members returned again and again to wait in long lines to look for their loved ones. Many survivors were unable to identify their mothers, sisters, or wives; the confusion of handling so many victims and so many survivors who did not understand what was happening to them and to their dead led to even more anguish for the community. Some of the victims were identified by the names on the pay envelopes handed to them at quitting time and stuffed deeply into pockets or stockings just before the fire. But many bodies remained unclaimed for days, with bewildered and bereaved survivors wandering among them, trying to find some identifying mark.

Charges of first- and second-degree manslaughter were brought against the two men who owned Triangle, and Leon Stein's book artfully depicts the subtle psychological and sociological implications of the powerful against the oppressed, and of the Westernized, German-Jewish immigrants against those still living their old-world, Eastern European heritage. Ultimately, Triangle owners Blanck and Harris were acquitted of the charges against them, and in due time they collected their rather sizable insurance.

The shirtwaist, popularized by Gibson girls,

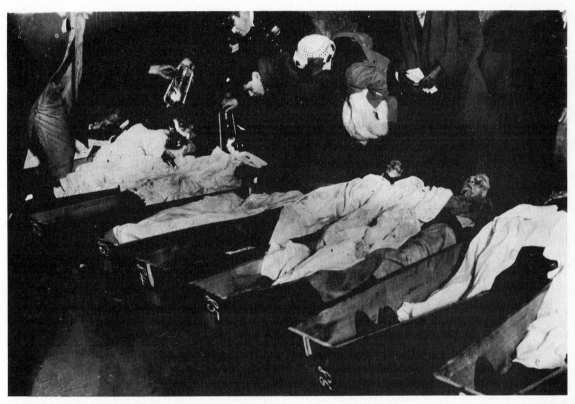

■■■ *A few days after the holocaust in 1911 at the Triangle Shirtwaist Company in New York City, eighty thousand people marched in the rain in a funeral procession up Fifth Avenue. A quarter million spectators stood witness.*

had come to represent the new-found freedom of females in America. After the fire, it symbolized death. The reaction of the grief-sticken Lower East Side was articulated by socialist lawyer Morris Hillquit:

The girls who went on strike last year were trying to readjust the conditions under which they were obliged to work. I wonder if there is not some connection between the fire and that strike. I wonder if the magistrates who sent to jail the girls who did picket duty in front of the Triangle shop realized last Sunday that some of the responsibility may be theirs. Had the strike been successful, these girls might have been alive today and the citizenry of New York would have less of a burden upon its conscience.

For the first time in the history of New York's garment industry there were indications that the public was beginning to accept responsibility for the exploitation of the immigrants. For the first time, the establishment seemed to understand that these were human beings asking for their rights, not merely trouble-making anarchists.

The day after the Triangle fire a protest meeting was held at the Women's Trade Union League, with representatives from twenty leading labor and civic organizations. They formed "a relief committee to cooperate with the Red Cross in its work among the families of the victims, and another committee . . . to broaden the investigation and research on fire hazards in New York factories which was already being carried on by the League."

The minutes of the League recount the deep indignation that members felt at the indifference of a public which had ignored their pleas for safety after the Newark fire. In an attempt to translate their anger into constructive action, the League drew up a list of forceful resolutions that included a plan to gather delegates from all of the city's unions to make a concerted effort to force safety changes in factories. In addition, the League called upon all workers to inspect factories and then report any violations to the proper city authorities and to the WTUL. They called upon the city to immediately appoint organized workers as unofficial inspectors. They resolved to submit the following fire regulations suggestions: compulsory fire drills, fireproof exits, unlocked doors, fire alarms, automatic sprinklers, and regular inspections. The League called upon the legislature to create the Bureau of Fire Protection and finally, the League underscored the absolute need for all workers to organize themselves at once into trade unions so that they would never again be powerless.

The League also voted to participate in the funeral procession for the unidentified dead of the Triangle fire.

The city held a funeral for the dead who were unclaimed. "More than 120,000 of us were in the funeral procession that miserable rainy April day," remembered Rose Schneiderman. "From ten in the morning until four in the afternoon we of the Women's Trade Union League marched in the procession with other trade-union men and women, all of us filled with anguish and regret that we had never been able to organize the Triangle workers."

Schneiderman, along with many others, was absolutely determined that this kind of tragedy would never happen again. With single-minded dedication, they devoted themselves to unionizing the workers. The searing example of the Triangle fire provided them with the impetus they needed to gain public support for their efforts.

They dramatized and emphasized and capitalized on the scandalous working conditions of the immigrants. From all segments of the community came cries for labor reform. Stephen S. Wise, the prestigious reform rabbi, called for the formation of a citizens' committee. Jacob H. Schiff, Bishop David H. Greer, Governor John A. Dix, Anne Morgan (of *the* Morgans) and other leading civic and religious leaders collaborated in a mass meeting at the Metropolitan Opera House on May 2 to protest factory conditions and to show support for the workers.

Several people spoke at that meeting on May 2, and many in the audience began to grow restless and antagonistic. Finally, 29-year-old Rose Schneiderman stepped up to the podium.

In a whisper barely audible, she began to address the crowd.

I would be a traitor to these poor burned bodies, if I came here to talk good fellowship. We have tried you good people of the public and we have found you wanting. The old Inquisition had its rack and its thumbscrews and its instruments of torture with iron teeth. We know what these things are today: the iron teeth are our necessities, the thumbscrews the high-powered and swift machinery close to which we must work, and the rack is here in the fireproof structures that will destroy us the minute they catch on fire.

This is not the first time girls have burned alive in the city. Every week I must learn of the untimely death of one of my sister workers. Every year thousands of us are maimed. The life of men and women is so cheap and property is so sacred. There are so many of us for one job it matters little if 140-odd are burned to death.

We have tried you, citizens, we are trying you now, and you have a couple of dollars for the sorrowing mothers and daughters and sisters by way of a charity gift. But every time the workers come out in the only way they know to protest against conditions which are unbearable, the strong hand of the law is allowed to press down heavily upon us.

Public officials have only words of warning to us—warning that we must be intensely orderly

*and must be intensely peaceable, and they have the
workhouse just back of all their warnings. The
strong hand of the law beats us back when we rise
into the conditions that make life bearable.*

*I can't talk fellowship to you who are gathered
here. Too much blood has been spilled. I know
from my experience it is up to the working people
to save themselves. The only way they can save
themselves is by a strong working-class movement.*

Her speech has become a classic. It is more
than just an emotional picture of persecution; it
reflects the pervasive sadness and profound
understanding that comes from knowing, finally, the cruel realities of life, the perspective of
history, and the nature of human beings.

The devastation of that fire and the futility of
the seemingly successful strike that had preceded
it seemed to impart an undeniable truth to Rose
Schneiderman: they could not fail again. The
events of 1911 seemed to have made her, and
many others, more keenly aware than they had
ever been that the workers' fight for reform was
absolutely essential. If they did not do it, it
would not be done.

In a sense, the fire touched off in Schneiderman an awareness of her own responsiblility in
the battle for industrial reform. This fiery socialist worker had been transformed into a highly
effective labor leader.

The influential speech she gave did help
swing public opinion to the side of the trade
unions, and the fire itself had made the workers
more aware of the crucial need to unionize.
Widespread support for labor reform and union-
ization emerged. Pressure from individuals, such
as Rose Schneiderman, as well as from groups
like the Women's Trade Union League and the
International Ladies' Garment Workers' Union,
helped form the New York State Factory Investigating Commission, the New York Citizens'
Committee on Safety, and other regulatory and
investigatory bodies. The League and Local 25
(the Shirtwaist Makers' Union of the ILGWU)
were especially instrumental in attaining a new
Industrial Code for New York State, which
became "the most outstanding instrument for
safeguarding the lives, health, and welfare of the
millions of wage earners in New York State and .
. . in the nation at large."

It took years for these changes to occur, and
labor reform did not rise majestically, Phoenix-
like, from the ashes of the Triangle fire. But that
fire, and Rose Schneiderman's whispered plea
for a strong working-class movement, had
indeed become the loud, clear call for action.

■■■

STUDY QUESTIONS

1. How successful had workers at the Triangle Waist Company been in gaining
better working conditions before the fire? What had been their major successes and
failures?

2. What were the major labor concerns of the immigrant women workers? How
had their Jewish heritage influenced their outlook on life and work?

3. Why did the fire lead to so many deaths? How did the design of the building
contribute to the tragedy?

4. What was the reaction to the fire in the Jewish community? How did the funeral help unify reform-minded people in New York City?

5. What role did Rose Schneiderman play in the aftermath of the tragedy? How did the fire influence the American labor movement?

BIBLIOGRAPHY

As Mitelman indicates, the best treatment of the tragedy is Leon Stein, *The Triangle Fire* (1962). Leslie Woodcock Tentler, *Wage-Earning Women: Industrial Work and Family Life in the United States, 1900–1930* (1979), treats the difficulties faced by working women. Useful treatments of the same theme are Susan Estabrook Kennedy, *If All We Did Was To Weep At Home: A History of White Working Class Women in America* (1979), and Barbara Mayer Wertheimer, *We Were There: The Story of Working Women in America* (1977). Two excellent introductions to general issues that concerned workers are Herbert Gutman, *Work, Culture and Society in Industrializing America* (1977), and David Montgomery, *Workers' Control in America: Studies in the History of Work, Technology, and Labor Struggles* (1979). Moses Rischin, *The Promised City: New York's Jews, 1870–1940* (1970); Arthur S. Goren, *New York Jews and the Quest for Community: The Kehillah Experiment, 1908–1922* (1970); and Irving Howe, *World of Our Fathers: The Journey of the Eastern European Jews to America and the LIfe They Found and Made* (1976), treat the Jewish experience in America.

JACK JOHNSON WINS THE HEAVYWEIGHT CHAMPIONSHIP

Randy Roberts

For the most part, the Progressive Movement was a for-whites-only affair. During the first twenty years of the twentieth century, Asian and black Americans faced open and violent discrimination. On the West Coast, Japanese and Chinese immigrants confronted a humiliating series of discriminatory laws, while in the South and even North blacks were equally hardpressed. Neither presidents Theodore Roosevelt nor Woodrow Wilson made any attempt to alter the social structure of the Jim Crow South, where the lives of the blacks were unequal to the lives of the whites. Although blacks retained some political and civil rights in the North, they still suffered from social and economic discrimination.

Some blacks responded to the injustice. Booker T. Washington was willing to forego social and political equality for economic opportunities. W. E. B. Du Bois demanded more; he worked for full equality. Other blacks lodged less articulate protests through their actions. They refused to live within the narrow borders proscribed for them by white society. Often these blacks were labeled "bad niggers." White authorities hated and punished them, but in black communities they were regarded as heroes and legends. The most famous of these real-life renegades was Jack Johnson, the first black heavyweight champion. He defeated white boxers, married white women, enraged white authorities, and lived by his own laws. In the following selection, historian Randy Roberts uses Johnson's fight with Tommy Burns as an opportunity to examine the racial attitudes of the early twentieth century.

Afterwards concerned whites said it should never have taken place. John L. Sullivan, who by 1908 had quit drinking and become a moral crusader, said, "Shame on the money-mad Champion! Shame on the man who upsets good American precedents because there are Dollars, Dollars, Dollars in it." A dejected sports columnist wrote, "Never before in the history of the prize ring has such a crisis arisen as that which faces the followers of the game tonight." The sadness these men felt could only be expressed in superlatives—greatest tragedy, deepest gloom, saddest day, darkest night. The race war had been fought. Armageddon was over. The Caucasian race had lost. Twenty years after the event, and after a few more such Armageddons, Alva Johnston tried to explain the mood of the day: "The morale of the Caucasian race had been at a low ebb long before the great blow fell in 1908. The Kaiser had been growing hysterical over the Yellow Peril. Africa was still celebrating the victory of Emperor Menelik of Abyssinia over the Italians. Dixie was still in ferment because Booker T. Washington . . . had had a meal at the White House. Then . . . Jack Johnson won the World Heavyweight Championship from Tommy Burns. The Nordics had not been so scared since the days of Tamerlane."

Black ghetto dwellers and sharecroppers rejoiced. In cities from New York to Omaha, blacks smiled with delight. "Today is the zenith of Negro sports," observed a *Colored American Magazine* editor. Other black publications felt such qualifications were too conservative. The *Richmond Planet* reported that "no event in forty years has given more genuine satisfaction to the colored people of this country than has the signal victory of Jack Johnson." Joy and pride spilled over into arrogance, or so some whites believed. The cotton-buying firm of Logan and Bryan predicted that Johnson's victory would encourage

other blacks to enter boxing, thereby creating a shortage of field labor. Independent of Logan and Bryan's report, the black writer Jim Nasium counseled black youths to consider seriously a boxing career—where else could they face whites on an equal footing? In that last week of 1908 social change seemed close at hand. The implication of most reports was that Jack Johnson had started a revolution.

How had it all come about? When Burns arrived in Perth in August 1908, the world did not seem in any immediate danger. He was treated like a conquering hero. From Perth to Sydney he was cheered and fêted. Mayors and members of Parliament courted Burns as if he were visiting royalty. When the train made its normal 6 A.M. stop at Abury, men stood shivering in the cold to greet Burns. And at Sydney, at a more civilized hour, more than 8,000 people cheered the champion. Speeches were made and applause modestly received. An Australian politician, Colonel Ryrie, extolled the virtues of boxing, telling the gathering that the sport produced sturdy young men needed for battle, "not those milksops who cry out against it."

At these august occasions Burns was frequently asked about Johnson. Would he fight the black champion? If so, where? When? Burns patiently answered the questions like a saint repeating a litany. He would fight Johnson when the right purse was offered. The place was not important. In fact, Australia was as good as —if not better than—any other place. As Burns told a Melbourne reporter: "There are a lot of newspaper stories that I don't want to fight Johnson. I do want to fight him, but I want to give the white boys a chance first." And since the early English settlers had exterminated the Tasmanians, there were a lot of white boys in Australia.

Listening to Burns was an ambitious promoter. Hugh D. "Huge Deal" McIntosh was an American success story with an Australian setting. As a boy he worked in the Broken Hill mines and as a rural laborer, but early in life he realized that a man could make more money

Reprinted with permission of The Free Press, a Division of Macmillan, Inc. from *PAPA JACK: Jack Johnson and the Era of White Hopes* by Randy Roberts. Copyright © 1983 by The Free Press.

using his brain than his back. His fortune was made as a pie salesman in Australian parks and sporting events, but his career included tours as a racing cyclist, a boxer, a waiter, a newspaper publisher, a member of parliament, a theatrical impresario, and other assorted jobs. All these stints equipped him with enough gab and gall to become a first-rate boxing promoter. It was McIntosh who had invited Burns to Australia to defend his title against Aussie boxers. A student of maps and calendars, he knew that when Teddy Roosevelt's Great White Fleet, then cruising about the Pacific, dropped anchor in Australia a heavyweight championship fight would prove a good draw. With this in mind, he rented a market garden at Rushcutter's Bay, on the outskirts of Sydney, and built an open-air stadium on it. By midsummer he was ready for Burns.

In June he matched Burns against Bill Squires, whom the champion had already knocked out twice, once in the United States and once in France. In defense of Squires, however, it was noted by the press that in his second fight with Burns he had lasted eight rounds, seven longer than the first fight. On his home continent Squires did even better. He was not knocked out until the thirteenth round. Though the fight was not particularly good, the overflowing stadium pleased McIntosh mightily. More than 40,000 people showed up for the fight, including American sailors from the Great White Fleet, but only 15,000 could be seated in the stadium. The 25,000 others milled about outside, listening to the noise made by lucky spectators watching the fight.

Less than two weeks later Burns again defended his title, this time against Bill Lang in Melbourne before 19,000 spectators. Like the stadium at Rushcutter's Bay, South Melbourne Stadium had been hurriedly constructed on McIntosh's orders—it was built in twelve days—and the result had been worth the effort. In the two fights Burns made more than $20,000 and McIntosh grossed about $100,000, half of which was clear profit. In addition, both fights had been filmed, and revenue from this pioneering effort

was much greater than anticipated. Burns, McIntosh, and the Australian boxing public were all exceedingly pleased.

In late October Johnson arrived, and the pulse of Australia picked up a beat. The fight had already been arranged. McIntosh guaranteed Burns $30,000. Before such a sum the color line faded. Therefore, when Johnson landed at Perth he was in an accommodating mood. "How does Burns want it? Does he want it fast and willing? I'm his man in that case. Does he want it flat footed? Goodness, if he does, why I'm his man again. Anything to suit; but fast or slow, I'm going to win." After eight years of trying Johnson was about to get his chance to fight for the heavyweight title.

Short of money, Johnson and Fitzpatrick set up their training quarters in the inexpensive Sir Joseph Banks Hotel in Botany, far less plush than the Hydro Majestic Hotel at Medlow Bath, where Burns trained. Yet Johnson, like Burns, trained in earnest. Johnson looked relaxed—he joked, smiled, made speeches, and played the double bass—but the men and women who watched him train failed to notice that he was also working very hard. Each morning he ran; each afternoon he exercised and sparred with Bill Lang, who imitated Burns's style. Johnson knew that Burns—short, inclined toward fatness, addicted to cigars and strong drink—was nonetheless a very good boxer. In Bohum Lynch's opinion, Burns was a "decidedly good boxer" who, though unorthodox, had a loose and easy style. And in the weeks before the fight Johnson showed by his training that he did not take Burns lightly.

Nor did he disregard the power of Australian racism. He feared that in the emotionally charged atmosphere of an interracial championship fight he might not be given an even break. His concern was not unfounded. An editorial in Sydney's *Illustrated Sporting and Dramatic News* correctly indicated the racial temper of Australian boxing fans: "Citizens who have never prayed before are supplicating Providence to give the white man a strong right arm with which to belt the coon into oblivion." But of more concern to Johnson than white men's prayers were his suspicions of McIntosh as promoter and self-named referee. Several times the two quarreled in public, and they nearly came to blows when Johnson greeted the promoter with "How do, Mr. McIntosh? How do you drag yourself away from Tahmy?" McIntosh, a big, burly, muscular man, thereafter began carrying a lead pipe wrapped in sheet music. As he told his friend Norman Lindsay, it was in case "that black bastard" ever "tries any funny business."

As the bout drew closer, the racial overtones destroyed the holiday atmosphere. It seemed as if all Australia were edgy. In the name of civilization, Protestant reformers spoke words that fell on deaf ears. The fight, said the Sydney Anglican Synod, with "its inherent brutality and dangerous nature" would surely "corrupt the moral tone of the community." But the community was worried less about being corrupted than about the implication of a Johnson victory. Lindsay, whom McIntosh hired to draw posters to advertise the fight, visually portrayed the great fear. Across Sydney could be seen his poster showing a towering black and a much smaller white. As Richard Broome has suggested, "This must have evoked the deepest feelings Australians held about the symbols of blackness and whiteness and evoked the emotiveness of a big man versus a small man and the populous coloured races versus the numerically smaller white race." Clearly, the *Australian Star* editors had this in mind when they printed a cartoon showing the fight being watched by representatives of the white and black races. Underneath was a letter that predicted that "this battle may in the future be looked back upon as the first great battle of an inevitable race war. . . . There is more in this fight to be considered than the mere title of pugilistic champion of the world."

Racial tension was nothing new to Australia. Race had mattered since the colony's founding. Partly it was an English heritage, passed down from the conquerors of Ireland, Scotland, and Wales—an absolute belief in the inferiority of everything and everyone non-English. In Australia, however, it had developed its own unique characteristics. There common English prejudices had been carried to extremes, and when confronted with dark-skinned natives, the Australians did not shrink from the notion of genocide. The most shocking example of racial relations was the case of the small island of Tasmania off the southeast coast of Australia. When the English first settled the island there were perhaps a few thousand Tasmanians. Short but long-legged, these red-brown people were described as uncommonly friendly natives. But the friendliness soon died, as British colonists hunted, raped, enslaved, abducted, or killed the Tasmanians. Slowly the race died off, until in 1876 Truganini, the very last survivor, died. Her passing struck many Australians as sad—but inevitable. As a correspondent for the *Hobart Mercury* wrote, "I regret the death of the last of the Tasmanian aborigines, but I know that it is the result of the *fiat* that the black shall everywhere give place to the white."

For Australia the problem was that other darker races had not given way fast enough in the generation after the death of Truganini. Though Social Darwinists preached the virtues of the light-skinned, by 1909 Australians felt threatened by the "lower" races. Increasingly after 1900 Australians demonstrated anxiety over their Oriental neighbors. Immigration restrictions aimed at keeping the country white were proposed and adopted. So bitter had the struggle become that in 1908, the year of the Johnson-Burns fight, the *Australia Bulletin* changed its banner from "Australia for Australians" to "Australia for the white men."

Johnson and Burns became both an example of and a contribution to the fears of white Australians. Small, white Burns became the symbol of small, white Australia, nobly battling against the odds. Burn's defense was his brain and pluck, his desire to stave off defeat through intelligence and force of will. Johnson became the large, vulgar, corrupt, and sensual enemy.

Reports said that he ignored training and instead wenched and drank. He had strength and size but lacked heart—in fact, he *should* win but probably would not. This last report gave rise to the rumor that the fight was fixed. Even the *New York Times* endorsed this view, as did the betting line that made Burns a 7 to 4 favorite.

Cool rains washed Sydney on Christmas night, the eve of the fight. To allow filming, the fight was not scheduled to begin until 11 A.M., but by 6 A.M. an orderly crowd of more than 5,000 was waiting at the gate. The stadium would be filled to capacity; yet interest was much more widespread. Throughout Australia men milled around newspaper offices hoping to hear a word about the progress of the fight. Inside the stadium at Rushcutter's Bay all Christmas cheer had vanished. The mood and tone of the day, from the gray, overcast sky to the uneasy quiet of the spectators, was eulogistic.

Johnson entered the ring first. Despite his dull gray robe his mood was almost carefree. There were a few cheers—though not many—as he slipped under the upper strand of the ropes, but calls of "coon" and "nigger" were more common. He smiled, bowed grandly, and threw kisses in every direction. He liked to strut the stage, and the vicious insults did not outwardly affect him. If anything, his smile became broader as he was more abused. In a country exhilarated by the discovery of gold, Johnson's gold-toothed smile ironically attracted only hate. Satisfied that he was not the crowd's favorite, he retired to his corner, where Sam Fitzpatrick massaged his shoulders and whispered words of assurance into an unlistening ear.

By contrast, when Burns climbed into the ring, the stadium was filled with sound. Burns did not seem to notice. For a time it looked as if he had come into the ring expecting something other than a fight. He was dressed in a worn blue suit, more appropriate for a shoe salesman than the heavyweight champion. Methodically he removed the suit, folded it neatly, and put it in a battered wicker suitcase. Yet even in his short,

tight boxing trunks he looked out of place. Jack London, covering the fight for the *New York Herald*, wrote that Burns looked "pale and sallow, as if he had not slept all night, or as if he had just pulled through a bout with fever." Pacing nervously in his corner, he avoided looking across the ring at Johnson.

Burns examined the bandages on Johnson's hands. He did this carefully, looking for hard tape or other unnatural objects. Satisfied, he returned to his corner. Johnson, however, was upset by the tape on Burns's elbows. He asked Burns to remove it. Burns refused. Johnson—suddenly serious—said he would not fight until the tape was removed. Still Burns refused. McIntosh tried to calm the two fighters. He was unsuccessful. The crowd, sensing an unexpected confrontation but not aware of the finer details, sided with Burns and used the moment as a pretext to shout more insults at Johnson, who smiled as if complimented on a new necktie but still refused to alter his protest. Finally, Burns removed the tape. Johnson nodded, satisfied.

McIntosh called the fighters to the center of the ring. He went over the do's and don'ts and the business of what punches would or would not be allowed. Then he announced that in the event that the police stopped the fight, he would render a decision based on who was winning at the time. The unpopular " no decision" verdict would not be given. Both Johnson and Burns had earlier agreed to this procedure. The fighters returned to their corners. A few moments later the bell rang. The color line in championship fights was erased.

Watching films of Johnson boxing is like listening to a 1900 recording of Enrico Caruso played on a 1910 gramophone. When Johnson fought Burns, film was still in its early days, not yet capable of capturing the subtleties of movement. Nuance is lost in the furious and stilted actions of the figures, which move about the screen in a Chaplinesque manner, as if some drunken cutter had arbitrarily removed three of every four frames. When we watch fighters of

Johnson's day on film, we wonder how they could have been considered even good. That some of them were champions strains credulity. They look like large children, wrestling and cuffing each other, but not actually fighting like real boxers, not at all like Ali captured in zoom-lensed, slow-motion, technological grace. But the film misleads.

It was no Charlie Chaplin that shuffled out of his corner in round one to meet Tommy Burns. It was a great boxer who at age thirty was in his physical prime. No longer thin, Johnson was well-muscled, with a broad chest and thick arms and legs. His head was shaved in the style of the eighteenth-century bare-knuckle fighters, and his high cheekbones gave his face a rounded appearance. Although he had fought often, his superb defensive skills had kept his face largely unmarked. Like his mother he had a broad, flat nose and full lips, but his eyes were small and oddly Oriental when he smiled. He was famous for his clowning, but this stereotype of a black man obscured the more serious reality. He was often somber, and even when he smiled and acted like a black-faced minstrel, he could be serious. What he thought, he believed, was his own affair. His feelings could not be easily read on his face.

Both boxers began cautiously. Johnson flicked out a few probing jabs, designed more to test distance than to do any physical damage. Although Burns was much smaller than Johnson, he was considered a strong man with a powerful punch. Johnson clinched, tested Burns's strength, then shifted to long-range sparring. He allowed Burns to force the action, content to parry punches openhanded. Burns tried to hit Johnson with long left hooks, which fell short. Johnson feinted a long left of his own, but in the same motion he lowered his right shoulder, pivoted from the waist, stepped forward with his right foot, and delievered a perfect right uppercut. It was Johnson's finest weapon, and some ring authorities claim there never has been a fighter who could throw the punch as well as Johnson. Burns was caught flatfooted,

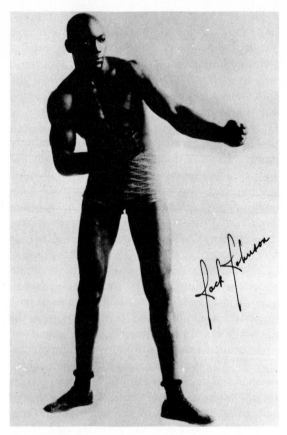

■ ■ *The first black man to gain the heavyweight boxing championship of the world was Afro-American Jack Johnson, who held the title from 1908 to 1915.*

leaning into the punch. His momentum was stopped and he fell backward. His head hit heavily on the floor. He lay still. The referee started to count.

"The fight," Jack London wrote only hours after it ended, "there was no fight. No Armenian massacre could compare with the hopeless slaughter that took place in the Sydney stadium today." From the opening seconds of the first round it was clear who would win. At least it was clear to London. It was a fight between a "colossus and a toy automation," between a "playful Ethiopian and a small and futile white man," between a "grown man and a naughty child." And through it all, London and the 20,000 white supporters of Burns watched in horror as their worst fears materialized.

"Hit the coon in his stomach." Burns needed no reminder. After surviving the first-round knockdown, he shifted to a different strategy, one he had thought about before. In the days before the fight, when reporters asked about his battle plan, he had smiled knowingly at his white chroniclers and said he would move in close and hit the black fighter where all black fighters were weak—in the stomach. This theory was hardly novel; it had long been considered axiomatic that black boxers had weak stomachs and hard heads. So thoroughly was the view accepted that black boxers took it for granted that white fighters would attack the body. Peter Jackson once told Fred Dartnell, "They are all after my body. Hit a nigger in the stomach and you'll settle him, they say, but it never seems to occur to them that a white man might just as quickly be beaten by a wallop in the same region." Sam Langford agreed: blacks hated to be hit by a hard punch to the stomach, but so too did whites.

Boxing was not immune to the scientific explanations of the day. Polygenists believed—and Darwinists did not deny—that the black race was an "incipient species." Therefore, whites maintained, physically blacks and whites were very different. Burns, for example, assumed that Johnson not only had a weak stomach but lacked physical endurance. So he believed that the longer the fight lasted the better were his chances. Behind these stereotypes rested the science of the day. Writing only a year before in the *North American Review,* Charles F. Woodruff claimed that athletes raised in Southern climates lacked endurance: "The excessive light prods the nervous system to do more than it should, and in time such constant stimulation is followed by irritability and finally by exhaustion." Only athletes from the colder Northern latitudes had enough stamina to remain strong during the course of a long boxing match. There-

fore, Burns, a Canadian, had reason to remain hopeful. By contrast, Johnson, raised about as far south as one could travel in the United States and only a generation or two removed from Africa, had to win quickly or not at all. At least, this was what Burns and his white supporters hoped.

Burns's strategy was thus founded on the racist belief that scientists, armed with physiological and climatological evidence, had proved that blacks were either inferior to whites, or—as in the case of harder heads—superior because of some greater physiological inferiority; that is to say, blacks had thicker skulls because they had smaller brains. Burns never questioned that his abdominal strength and his endurance were superior to Johnson's. Nor did he doubt that his white skin meant that his desire to win and willingness to accept pain were greater than Johnson's. But above all, he was convinced that as a white he could outthink Johnson, that he could solve the problems of defense and offense more quickly than his black opponent. Burns's faith, in short, rested ultimately on the color of his skin.

Burns forgot, however, that he was facing a boxer liberated from the myths of his day. Johnson's stomach was not weak, and, more important, he knew it was not. As the fight progressed, he exposed the fallacy of Burns's theory. He started to taunt Burns. "Go on, Tommy, hit me here," Johnson said pointing to his stomach. When Burns responded with a blow to Johnson's midsection, Jack laughed and said to try again. "Is that all the better you can do, Tommy?" Another punch. "Come on, Tommy, you can hit harder than that, can't you?" And so it continued; Johnson physically and verbally was destroying the white man's myths.

Burns fought gamely, but without success. Johnson did not try for a knockout; he was content to allow the fight to last until the later rounds. Partly his decision was based on economics. The bout was being filmed, and few boxing fans in America would pay to watch pictures of pressmen, seconds, and other boxers for five minutes as a build-up for a fight that lasted only half a minute. But more important was Johnson's desire for revenge. He hated Burns and wanted to punish him. And he did. By the second round Burn's right eye was discolored and his mouth was bloody. By the middle rounds Burns was bleeding from a dozen minor facial cuts. Blood ran over his shoulders and stained the canvas ring. Before the white audience, Johnson badly punished Burns. And he enjoyed every second of it.

But punishment was not enough. Johnson wanted also to humiliate Burns. He did this verbally. From the very first round Johnson insulted Burns, speaking with an affected English accent, so that "Tommy" became "Tahmy." Mostly what Johnson said was banal: "Poor little Tahmy, who told you you were a fighter?" Or, "Say little Tahmy, you're not fighting. Can't you? I'll have to show you how." Occasionally, when Burns landed a punch, Johnson complimented him: "Good boy, Tommy; good boy, Tommy." In almost every taunt Johnson referred to Burns in the diminutive. It was always "Tommy Boy'; or "little Tommy." And always a derisive smile accompanied the words.

Sometimes Johnson sought to emasculate Burns verbally. Referring to Burns's wife, Johnson said, "Poor little boy, Jewel won't know you when she gets you back from this fight." Once when Burns landed what looked to be an effective punch, Johnson laughed: "Poor, poor Tommy. Who taught you to hit? Your mother? You a woman?" Crude, often vulgar and mean, Johnson's verbal warfare was nevertheless effective.

Burns responded in kind. Bohum Lynch, who was a great fan of Burns, admitted that his champion's ring histrionics included baleful glaring, foot stomping, and mouth fighting. He often called Johnson a "cur" or a "big dog." At other times, when he was hurt or frustrated, he said, "Come on and fight, nigger. Fight like a white man." Burns's comments, however, were self-defeating. When Johnson insulted Burns, the champion lost control and fought recklessly. But

Burns's taunts pleased Johnson, who responded by fighting in an even more controlled way than before. Johnson gained particular strength from Burns's racist statements. It was like playing the Dozens, where accepting abuse with an even smile and concealing one's true emotions were the sign of a sure winner.

When Johnson was not insulting Burns, he was talking to ringsiders. Usually he just joked about how easy the fight was and what he would do with the money he won from betting on the bout. That the ringsiders hated Johnson and screamed racial insults did not seem to bother him. Only rarely did Johnson show his disgust with the white audience. Once as he moved from his corner at the start of a round he spat a mouthful of water toward the press row, but such actions were unusual. More common was the smile—wide, detached, inscrutable. In describing the grin, Jack London came closest to the truth: it was "the fight epitomized." It was the smile of a man who has mastered the rules to a slightly absurd game.

After a few rounds the only question that remained unanswered was not who would win but how much punishment Burns could take. By the middle rounds that too was evident—he could survive great amounts of punishment. His eyes were bruised and discolored, his mouth hung open, his jaw was swollen and looked broken, and his body was splotched with his own blood. In the corner between rounds his seconds sponged his face with champagne, which was popularly believed to help revive hurt fighters. It did not help Burns. Yet at the bell he always arose to face more punishment and insults. For the white spectators, Burns's fortitude was itself inspiring. As Bohum Lynch wrote, "To take a beating any time, even from your best friend, is hard work. But to take a beating from a man you abhor, belonging to a race you despise, to know that he is hurting you and humiliating you with the closest attention to detail, and the coldest deliberation . . . this requires pluck."

By the thirteenth round everyone but Burns

and Johnson was surfeited with the carnage. Spectators, left with nothing and nobody to cheer, now yelled for the fight to be stopped. After the thirteenth round police entered the ring. They talked with McIntosh, then with Burns. The white champion refused to concede. He insisted that he could win. But in the fourteenth Burns was again severely punished. A hard right cross knocked him to the canvas. He arose at the count of eight but was wobbly. Again policemen climbed into the ring, only this time there was no talking. The fight was stopped, although Burns—dazed, covered with blood, but still game—screamed at the police to give him another chance.

Everywhere was a stunned silence as the spectators accepted that the inevitable was now the actual. It had happened. A black man now wore the crown that had once belonged to Sullivan, Corbett, and Jeffries. As far as Australia was concerned, an "archetypal darkness" had replaced sweetness and light; the barbarian had defeated the civilized man. As the *Daily Telegraph* observed in doggerel:

And yet for all we know and feel,
For Christ and Shakespeare, knowledge, love,
We watch a white man bleeding reel,
We cheer a black with bloodied glove.

The imagery in which the fight was reported clearly reflects the white Australian attitude toward Johnson. He was portrayed as a destructive beast. *Fairplay,* the liquor trades weekly, called Johnson "a huge primordial ape," and the *Bulletin's* cartoons likened him to a shaven-headed reptile. He was the discontented black and yellow masses that haunted the Australian mind. Journalist Randolph Bedford, perhaps the most unabashedly racist reporter at the fight, depicted it in ominous terms: "Yet the white beauty faced the black unloveliness, forcing the fight, bearing the punishment as if it were none . . . weight and reach were ebbing against intrepidity, intelligence and lightness. . . . His courage still shone in his eyes; his face was disfigured and swollen and bloodied. He was still beauty by

contrast—beautiful but to be beaten; clean sunlight fighting darkness and losing."

In America the fight was not viewed in quite so maudlin a manner. Certainly the white American press was not pleased by the result, but it generally tried to dismiss it in a light-hearted mood. Perhaps, reporters reasoned, all was not lost. "Br'er Johnson is an American anyway," commented a reporter for the *Omaha Sunday Bee.* Then, too, boxing had declined so much in recent years that some experts wondered if the fight meant anything at all. Though John L. Sullivan criticized Burns for fighting Johnson, he added that "present day bouts cannot truly be styled prize fights, but only boxing matches." A fine distinction, but Sullivan believed it was enough to invalidate Johnson's claim as heavyweight champion. And certainly even if Johnson were the champion, reporters all agreed that he was far below the likes of Sullivan, Corbett, or Jeffries.

Though the mood had not yet reached a crisis stage, the fight's portent was still most unsettling to American whites. This was especially true about the manner in which blacks celebrated Johnson's victory. It was reported that the Manassas Club, a Chicago organization of wealthy blacks who had white wives, hired white waiters to serve the food at their banquet. And one of their members said that "Johnson's victory demonstrates the physical superiority of the black over the Caucasian. The basis of mental superiority in most men is physical superiority. If the negro can raise his mental standard to his physical eminence, some day he will be a leader among men." In other parts of the country blacks were reported as acting rude to whites and being swelled by false price.

Johnson's actions in Australia did little to calm Caucasian fears. Turning against the sportsmanlike tradition of praising one's opponent, Johnson openly said that Burns was a worthless boxer: "He is the easiest man I ever met. I could have put him away quicker, but I wanted to punish him. I had my revenge." Nor was Johnson discreet about the company with whom he was seen in public. Hattie McClay, his companion who had remained in the background during the weeks before the fight, was now prominently on display. Dressed in silk and furs, she seemed as prized a possession of Johnson's as his gold-capped teeth.

Johnson now seemed more apt to emphasize racial issues that irritated whites. Interviewed during the days after the fight, he told reporters that he had the greatest admiration for the aboriginal Australians. Commenting on their weapons, he said, "Your central Australian natives must have been men of genius to have turned out such artistic and ideal weapons." Nor, he hinted, was he any less a genius. He understood human nature: because he defeated Burns he could expect to be hated by all whites. But, he added, he could find solace in his favorite books—*Paradise Lost, Pilgrim's Progress* and *Titus Andronicus.* His comments achieved their purpose; everywhere white Australians snorted in disgust. But his choice of books certainly did not reflect his own attitude. Unlike Milton's Adam, Johnson did not practice the standard Christian virtues.

Burns left Australia soon after the fight. A richer man by some $30,000, he nevertheless was bitter and filled with hatred. Johnson, however, decided to stay for a while in Australia. His side of the purse, a mere $5,000, was hardly enough to make the venture profitable. He hoped instead to capitalize on his fame by touring Australia as a vaudeville performer. It was common for any famous boxer to make such tours. In 1908 he had toured in America and Canada with the Reilly and Woods Big Show and had enjoyed the experience. He loved the limelight and, unlike other boxers, put on a good show. He demonstrated a few boxing moves, sang several songs, danced, and played the base fiddle. During his Australian tour he actually made more money than he had in his fight with Burns. Not until mid-February was he ready to go home.

He had changed. The Johnson who left Australia in February was not the same man who had arrived in October. Inwardly, perhaps, he was much the same. But outwardly he was different. He was more open about his beliefs and his pleasures, less likely to follow the advice of white promoters and managers. Undoubtedly he believed the title of world champion set him apart from others of his race. And in this he was right. He would never be viewed as just another black boxer. But he was wrong in his assumption that the crown carried with it some sort of immunity against the dictates of whites and traditions of white society. Now more than ever Johnson was expected to conform. And now more than ever Johnson felt he did not have to. The collision course was set.

■ ■ ■

STUDY QUESTIONS

1. How did the promoters of the Johnson-Burns fight use racism to build up the gate? How did the racial attitudes of white Australians compare with those of white Americans?

2. How did Burns demonstrate racial stereotypes by the manner in which he fought Johnson?

3. What was the reaction of white Australians and Americans to Johnson's victory?

4. What was Johnson's attitude toward white society?

5. How else might one use sports or popular culture to demonstrate racial attitudes?

BIBLIOGRAPHY

The above selection is taken from Randy Roberts, *Papa Jack: Jack Johnson and the Era of White Hopes* (1983). Finis Farr, *Black Champion: The Life and Times of Jack Johnson* (1965), provides a readable popular history of the boxer, and Al-Tony Gilmore, *Bad Nigger! The National Impact of Jack Johnson* (1975), traces the newspaper reaction to Johnson. Johnson's image in black folklore is treated by William Wiggins, "Jack Johnson as Bad Nigger: The Folklore of His Life," *Black Scholar* (1969), and Lawrence W. Levine, *Black Culture and Black Consciousness: Afro-American Folk Thought from Slavery to Freedom* (1977). A number of books trace the evolution of white attitudes toward blacks. Among the best are George M. Fredrickson, *The Black Image in the White Mind: The Debate on Afro-American Character and Destiny, 1817–1914* (1971); Thomas F. Gossett, *Race: The History of an Idea in America* (1965); and John S. Haller, Jr., *Outcasts from Evolution: Scientific Attitudes of Racial Inferiority, 1859–1900* (1971).

THE TRENCH SCENE

Paul Fussell

For the generation which fought it, World War I was the Great War. It came after almost one hundred years of general European peace, and it shattered not only nations and people but also a system of thought, a world view. Before the Great War, intellectuals talked seriously and earnestly about the progress of mankind and the perfectability of societies and individuals. Men and women, they agreed, were reasonable creatures, fully capable of ordering their lives and environment. The terrible slaughter of Verdun and the Somme, the mud and lice and rats of the trenches, the horrors of poison gases and bullet-torn bodies draped over barbed-wire barriers—these unspeakable barbarities silenced talk of progress. Ernest Hemingway spoke for his generation when he wrote about the impact of the Great War: "I was always embarrassed by the words *sacred*, *glorious*, and *sacrifice* and the expression *in vain* . . . I had seen nothing sacred, and the things that were glorious had no glory and the sacrifices were like the stockyards at Chicago if nothing was done with the meat except to bury it. There were many words that you could not stand to hear and finally only the names of places had dignity. . . . Abstract words such as *glory*, *honor*, *courage*, or *hallow* were obscene beside the concrete names of villages, the numbers of roads, the names of rivers, the numbers of regiments and the dates."

In the following essay literary historian Paul Fussell discusses the Great War as experienced by millions of soldiers who served time in the trenches of the Western Front. In these ditches some 7,000 British soldiers were killed or wounded daily between 1914 and 1918. Though not in such horrendous numbers, Americans too died in the trenches of France, and the experience of mass death transformed American society. The United States went into the war to "make the world safe for democracy" but emerged from the war pessimistic, cynical, and discouraged. As Fussell observes, "To be in the trenches was to experience an unreal, unforgettable enclosure and constraint, as well as a sense of being unoriented and lost." This was the aspect of the Great War that changed the temper of Western culture.

The idea of "the trenches" has been assimilated so successfully by metaphor and myth ("Georgian complacency died in the trenches") that it is not easy now to recover a feeling for the actualities. *Entrenched*, in an expression like *entrenched power*, has been a dead metaphor so long that we must bestir ourselves to recover its literal sense. It is time to take a tour.

From the winter of 1914 until the spring of 1918 the trench system was fixed, moving here and there a few hundred yards, moving on great occasions as much as a few miles. London stationers purveying maps felt secure in stocking "sheets of 'The Western Front' with a thick wavy black line drawn from North to South alongside which was printed 'British Line.' " If one could have gotten high enough to look down at the whole line at once, one would have seen a series of multiple parallel excavations running for 400 miles down through Belgium and France, roughly in the shape of an *S* flattened at the sides and tipped to the left. From the North Sea coast of Belgium the line wandered southward, bulging out to contain Ypres, then dropping down to protect Béthune, Arras, and Albert. It continued south in front of Montidier, Compiégne, Soissons, Reims, Verdun, St. Mihiel, and Nancy, and finally attached its southernmost end to the Swiss border at Beurnevisin, in Alsace. The top forty miles—the part north of Ypres—was held by the Belgians; the next ninety miles, down to the river Ancre, were British; the French held the rest, to the south.

Henri Barbusse estimates that the French front alone contained about 6250 miles of trenches. Since the French occupied a little more than half the line, the total length of the numerous trenches occupied by the British must come to about 6000 miles. We thus find over 12,000 miles of trenches on the Allied side alone. When

From *The Great War and Modern Memory* by Paul Fussell. Copyright © 1975 by Oxford University Press, Inc. Reprinted by permission.

we add the trenches of the Central Powers, we arrive at a figure of about 25,000 miles, equal to a trench sufficient to circle the earth. Theoretically it would have been possible to walk from Belgium to Switzerland entirely below ground, but although the lines were "continuous," they were not entirely seamless: occasionally mere shell holes or fortified strong-points would serve as a connecting link. Not a few survivors have performed the heady imaginative exercise of envisioning the whole line at once. Stanley Casson is one who, imagining the whole line from his position on the ground, implicitly submits the whole preposterous conception to the criterion of the "normally" rational and intelligible. As he remembers, looking back from 1935.

Our trenches stood on a faint slope, just overlooking German ground, with a vista of vague plainland below. Away to right and left stretched the great lines of defense as far as eye and imagination could stretch them. I used to wonder how long it would take for me to walk from the beaches of the North Sea to that curious end of all fighting against the Swiss boundary; to try to guess what each end looked like; to imagine what would happen if I passed a verbal message, in the manner of the parlor game, along to the next man on my right to be delivered to the end man of all up against the Alps. Would anything intelligible at all emerge?

Another imagination has contemplated a similar absurd transmission of sound all the way from north to south. Alexander Aitken remembers the Germans opposite him celebrating some happy public event in early June, 1916, presumably either the (ambiguous) German success at the naval battle of Jutland (May 31-June 1) or the drowning of Lord Kitchener, lost on June 5 when the cruiser *Hampshire* struck a mine and sank off the Orkney Islands. Aitken writes, "There had been a morning in early June when a tremendous tin-canning and beating of shell-gongs had begun in the north and run south down their lines to end, without doubt, at Belfort and Mulhausen on the Swiss frontier."

Impossible to believe, really, but in this mad setting, somehow plausible.

The British part of the line was normally populated by about 800 battalions of 1000 men each. They were concentrated in the two main sectors of the British effort: the Ypres Salient in Flanders and the Somme area in Picardy. Memory has given these two sectors the appearance of two distinguishable worlds. The Salient, at its largest point about nine miles wide and projecting some four miles into the German line, was notable for its terrors of concentrated, accurate artillery fire. Every part of it could be covered from three sides, and at night one saw oneself almost surrounded by the circle of white and colored Very lights set up by the Germans to illuminate the ground in front of their trenches or to signal to the artillery behind them. The "rear area" at Ypres was the battered city itself, where the troops harbored in cellars or in the old fortifications built by Vauban in the seventeenth century. It was eminently available to the German guns, and by the end of the war Ypres was flattened to the ground, its name a byword for a city totally destroyed. Another war later, in 1940, Colin Perry—who was not born until four years after the Great War—could look at the ruins of London and speak of "the Ypres effect of Holborn." If the character of the Ypres sector was concentration and enclosure, inducing claustrophobia even above ground, the Somme was known—at least until July 1, 1916—for its greater amplitude and security. German fire came generally from only one direction; and troops at rest could move further back. But then there was the Somme mud; although the argument about whether the mud wasn't really worse at Ypres was never settled.

Each of these two sectors had its symbolic piece of ruined public architecture. At Ypres it was the famous Cloth Hall, once a masterpiece of medieval Flemish civic building. Its gradual destruction by artillery and its pathetic final dissolution were witnessed by hundreds of thousands, who never forgot this eloquent emblem of what happens when war collides with art. In the Somme the memorable ruined work of architecture, connoting this time the collision of the war with religion and the old pieties, was the battered Basilica in the town of Albert, or "Bert," as the troops called it. The grand if rather vulgar red and white brick edifice had been built a few years before the war, the result of a local ecclesiastic's enthusiasm. Together with his townsmen he hoped that Albert might become another Lourdes. Before the war 80,000 used to come on pilgrimages to Albert every year. The object of veneration inside the church was a statue of the Virgin, said to have been found in the Middle Ages by a local shepherd. But the statue of the Virgin never forgotten by the hordes of soldiers who passed through Albert was the colossal gilded one on top of the battered tall tower of the Basilica. This figure, called Notre Dame des Brebiéres, originally held the infant Christ in outstretched arms above her; but now the whole statue was bent down below the horizontal, giving the effect of a mother about to throw her child—in disgust? in sacrifice?—into the debris-littered street below. To Colonel Sir Maurice Hankey, Secretary of the War Committee, it was "a most pathetic sight." Some said that the statue had been bent down by French engineers to prevent the Germans from using it to aim at. But most—John Masefield among them—preferred to think it a victim of German artillery. Its obvious symbolic potential (which I will deal with later) impressed itself even on men who found they could refer to it only facetiously, as "The Lady of the Limp."

The two main British sectors duplicated each other also in their almost symbolic road systems. Each had a staging town behind: for Ypres it was Poperinghe (to the men, "Pop"); for the Somme, Amiens. From these towns troops proceeded with augmenting but usually well-concealed terror up a sinister road to the town of operations, either Ypres itself or Albert. And running into the enemy lines out of Ypres and Albert were the most sinister roads of all, one leading to Menin, the other to Bapaume, both in enemy territory. These roads defined the direction of ultimate attack and the hoped-for breakout. They were the goals of the bizarre inverse quest on which the soldiers were ironically embarked.

But most of the time they were not questing. They were sitting or lying or squatting in place below the level of the ground. "When all is said and done," Sassoon notes, "the war was mainly a matter of holes and ditches." And in these holes and ditches extending for ninety miles, continually, even in the quietest times, some 7000 British men and officers were killed and wounded daily, just as a matter of course. "Wastage," the Staff called it.

There were normally three lines of trenches. The front-line trench was anywhere from fifty yards or so to a mile from its enemy counterpart. Several hundred yards behind it was the support trench line. And several hundred yards behind that was the reserve line. There were three kinds of trenches: firing trenches, like these; communication trenches, running roughly perpendicular to the line and connecting the three lines; and "saps," shallower ditches thrust out into No Man's Land, providing access to forward observation posts, listening posts, grenade-throwing posts, and machine gun positions. The end of a sap was usually not manned all the time: night was the favorite time for going out. Coming up from the rear, one reached the trenches by following a communication trench sometimes a mile or more long. It often began in a town and gradually deepened. By the time pedestrians reached the reserve line, they were well below ground level.

A firing trench was supposed to be six to eight feet deep and four or five feet wide. On the enemy side a parapet of earth or sandbags rose about two or three feet above the ground. A corresponding "parados" a foot or so high was often found on top of the friendly side. Into the sides of trenches were dug one- or two-man holes ("funk-holes"), and there were deeper dugouts, reached by dirt stairs, for use as command posts and officers' quarters. On the enemy side of a trench was a fire-step two feet high on which the defenders were supposed to stand, firing and

throwing grenades, when repelling attack. A well-built trench did not run straight for any distance: that would have been to invite enfilade fire. Every few yards a good trench zig-zagged. It had frequent traverses designed to contain damage within a limited space. Moving along a trench thus involved a great deal of weaving and turning. The floor of a proper trench was covered with wooden duckboards, beneath which were sumps a few feet deep designed to collect water. The walls, perpetually crumbling, were supported by sandbags, corrugated iron, or bundles of sticks or rushes. Except at night and in half-light, there was of course no looking over the top except through periscopes, which could be purchased in the "Trench Requisites" section of the main London department stores. The few snipers on duty during the day observed No Man's Land through loopholes cut in sheets of armor plate.

The entanglements of barbed wire had to be positioned far enough out in front of the trench to keep the enemy from sneaking up to grenade-throwing distance. Interestingly, the two novelties that contributed most to the personal menace of the war could be said to be American inventions. Barbed wire had first appeared on the American frontier in the late nineteenth century for use in restraining animals. And the machine gun was the brainchild of Hiram Stevens Maxim (1840–1916), an American who, disillusioned with native patent law, established his Maxim Gun Company in England and began manufacturing his guns in 1889. He was finally knighted for his efforts. At first the British regard for barbed wire was on a par with Sir Douglas Haig's understanding of the machine gun. In the autumn of 1914, the first wire Private Frank Richards saw emplaced before the British positions was a single strand of agricultural wire found in the vicinity. Only later did the manufactured article begin to arrive from England in sufficient quantity to create the thickets of mock-organic rusty brown that helped give a look of eternal autumn to the front.

The whole British line was numbered by sections, neatly, from right to left. A section, normally occupied by a company, was roughly 300 yards wide. One might be occupying front-line trench section 51; or support trench S 51, behind it; or reserve trench SS 51, behind both. But a less formal way of identifying sections of trench was by place or street names with a distinctly London flavor. *Piccadilly* was a favorite; popular also were *Regent Street* and *Strand;* junctions were *Hyde Park Corner* and *Marble Arch.* Greater wit—and deeper homesickness—sometimes surfaced in the naming of the German trenches opposite. Sassoon remembers ''Durley'' 's account of the attack at Delville Wood in September, 1916: ''Our objective was Pint Trench, taking Bitter and Beer and clearing Ale and Vat, and also Pilsen Lane.'' Directional and traffic control signs were everywhere in the trenches, giving the whole system the air of a parody modern city, although one literally ''underground.''

The trenches I have described are more or less ideal, although not so ideal as the famous exhibition trenches dug in Kensington Gardens for the edification of the home front. These were clean, dry, and well furnished, with straight sides and sandbags neatly aligned. R. E. Vernède writes his wife from the real trenches that a friend of his has just returned from viewing the set of ideal ones. He ''found he had never seen anything at all like it before.'' And Wilfred Owen calls the Kensington Gardens trenches ''the laughing stock of the army.'' Explaining military routines to civilian readers, Ian Hay labors to give the impression that the real trenches are identical to the exhibition ones and that they are properly described in the language of normal domesticity a bit archly deployed:

The firing-trench is our place of business—our office in the city, so to speak. The supporting trench is our suburban residence, whither the weary toiler may betake himself periodically (or, more correctly, in relays) for purposes of refreshment and repose.

The reality was different. The British trenches were wet, cold, smelly, and thoroughly squalid. Compared with the precise and thorough German works, they were decidedly amateur,

reflecting a complacency about the British genius for improvisation. Since defense offered little opportunity for the display of pluck or swank, it was by implication derogated in the officers' *Field Service Pocket Book.* One reason the British trench system was so haphazard and ramshackle was that it had originally taken form in accord with the official injunction: ''The choice of a [defensive] position and its preparation must be made with a view to economizing the power expended on defense in order that the power of offense may be increased.'' And it was considered really useless to build solid fortifications anyway: ''An occasional shell may strike and penetrate the parapet, but in the case of shrapnel the damage to the parapet will be trifling, while in the case of a shell filled with high explosive, the effect will be no worse on a thin parapet than on a thick one. It is, therefore, useless to spend time and labor on making a thick parapet simply to keep out shell.'' The repeatedly revived hopes for a general breakout and pursuit were another reason why the British trenches were so shabby. A typical soldier's view is George Coppard's:

The whole conduct of our trench warfare seemed to be based on the concept that we, the British, were not stopping in the trenches for long, but were tarrying awhile on the way to Berlin and that very soon we would be chasing Jerry across country.
The result, in the long term, meant that we lived a mean and impoverished sort of existence in lousy scratch holes.

In contrast, the German trenches, as the British discovered during the attack on the Somme, were deep, clean, elaborate, and sometimes even comfortable. As Coppard found on the Somme, ''Some of the [German] dugouts were thirty feet deep, with as many as sixteen bunk-beds, as well as door bells, water tanks with taps, and cupboards and mirrors.'' They also had boarded walls, floors, and ceilings; finished wooden staircases; electric light; real kitchens; and wallpaper and overstuffed furniture, the whole protected by steel outer doors.

Foreign to the British style was a German dugout of the sort recalled by Ernst Jünger:

At Monchy . . . I was master of an underground dwelling approached by forty steps hewn in the solid chalk, so that even the heaviest shells at this depth made no more than a pleasant rumble when we sat there over an interminable game of cards. In one wall I had a bed hewn out. . . . . At its head hung an electric light so that I could read in comfort till I was sleepy. . . . The whole was shut off from the outer world by a dark-red curtain with rod and rings. . . .

As these example suggest, there were ''national styles'' in trenches as in other things. The French trenches were nasty, cynical, efficient, and temporary. Kipling remembered the smell of delicious cooking emanating from some in Alsace. The English were amateur, vague, *ad hoc,* and temporary. The German were efficient, clean, pedantic, and permanent. Their occupants proposed to stay where they were.

Normally the British troops rotated trench duty. After a week of ''rest'' behind the lines, a unit would move up—at night—to relieve a unit in the front-line trench. After three days to a week or more in that position, the unit would move back for a similar length of time to the support trench, and finally back to the reserve. Then it was time for a week of rest again. In the three lines of trenches the main business of the soldier was to exercise self-control while being shelled. As the poet Louis Simpson has accurately remembered:

Being shelled is the main work of an infantry soldier, which no one talks about. Everyone has his own way of going about it. In general, it means lying face down and contracting your body into as small a space as possible. In novels [The Naked and the Dead is an example] you read about soldiers, at such moments, fouling themselves. The opposite is true. As all your parts are contracting, you are more likely to be constipated.

Simpson is recalling the Second War, but he might be recalling the First. While being shelled, the soldier either harbored in a dugout and hoped for something other than a direct hit or made himself as small as possible in a funk-hole. An unlucky sentry or two was supposed to be out in the open trench in all but the worst bombardments, watching through a periscope or loophole for signs of an attack. When only light shelling was in progress, people moved about the trenches freely, and we can get an idea of what life there was like if we posit a typical twenty-four hours in a front-line trench.

The day began about an hour before first light, which often meant at about 4:30. This was the moment for the invariable ritual of morning stand-to (short for the archaic formal command for repelling attack, ''Stand to Arms''). Since dawn was the favorite time for launching attacks, at the order to stand-to everyone, officers, men, forward artillery observers, visitors, mounted the fire-step, weapon ready, and peered toward the German line. When it was almost full light and clear that the Germans were not going to attack that morning, everyone ''stood down'' and began preparing breakfast in small groups. The rations of tea, bread, and bacon, brought up in sandbags during the night, were broken out. The bacon was fried in mess-tin lids over small, and if possible smokeless, fires. If the men were lucky enough to be in a division whose commanding general permitted the issue of the dark and strong government rum, it was doled out from a jar with the traditional iron spoon, each man receiving about two tablespoonsful. Some put it into their tea, but most swallowed it straight. It was a precious thing, and serving it out was almost like a religious ceremonial, as David Jones recalls in *In Parenthesis,* where a corporal is performing the rite:

O have a care—don't spill the precious
O don't jog his hand—ministering;
do take care.
O please—give the poor bugger elbow room.

Larger quantities might be issued to stimulate troops for an assault, and one soldier remembers what the air smelled like during a British attack:

"Pervading the air was the smell of rum and blood." In 1922 one medical officer deposed before a parliamentary committee investigating the phenomenon of "shell shock": "Had it not been for the rum ration I do not think we should have won the war.

During the day the men cleaned weapons and repaired those parts of the trench damaged during the night. Or they wrote letters, deloused themselves, or slept. The officers inspected, encouraged, and strolled about looking nonchalant to inspirit the men. They censored the men's letters and dealt with the quantities of official inquiries brought them daily by runner. How many pipe-fitters had they in their company? Reply immediately. How many hairdressers, chiropodists, bicycle repairmen? Daily "returns" of the amount of ammunition and the quantity of trench stores had to be made. Reports of the nightly casualties had to be sent back. And letters of condolence, which as the war went on became form-letters of condolence, had to be written to the relatives of the killed and wounded. Men went to and fro on sentry duty or working parties, but no one showed himself above the trench. After evening stand-to, the real work began.

Most of it was above ground. Wiring parties repaired the wire in front of the position. Digging parties extended saps toward the enemy. Carrying parties brought up not just rations and mail but the heavy engineering materials needed for the constant repair and improvement of the trenches: timbers, A-frames, duckboards, stakes and wire, corrugated iron, sandbags, tarpaulins, pumping equipment. Bombs and ammunition and flares were carried forward. All this ant-work was illuminated brightly from time to time by German flares and interrupted very frequently by machine gun or arillery fire. Meanwhile night patrols and raiding parties were busy in No Man's Land. As morning approached, there was a nervous bustle to get the jobs done in time, to finish fitting the timers, filling the sandbags, pounding in the stakes, and then returning mauls and picks and shovels to the Quartermaster Sergeant. By the time of stand-to, nothing human was visible above ground anywhere, but every day each side scrutinized the look of the other's line for significant changes wrought by night.

Flanders and Picardy have always been notorious for dampness. It is not the least of the ironies of the war for the British that their trenches should have been dug where the water-table was the highest and the annual rainfall the most copious. Their trenches were always wet and often flooded several feet deep. Thigh-boots or waders were issued as standard articles of uniform. Wilfred Owen writes his mother from the Somme at the beginning of 1917: "The waders are of course indispensable. In 2½ miles of trench which I waded yesterday there was not one inch of dry ground. There is a mean depth of two feet of water." Pumps worked day and night but to little effect. Rumor held that the Germans not only could make it rain when they wanted it to—that is, all the time—but had contrived some shrewd technical method for conducting the water in their lines into the British positions—perhaps piping it underground. Ultimately there was no defense against the water but humor. "Water knee deep and up to the waist in places," one soldier notes in his diary. "Rumors of being relieved by the Grand Fleet." One doesn't want to dwell excessively on such discomforts, but here it will do no harm to try to imagine what, in these conditions, going to the latrine was like.

The men were not the only live things in the line. They were accompanied everywhere by their lice, which the professional delousers in rest positions behind the lines, with their steam vats for clothes and hot baths for troops, could do little to eliminate. The entry *lousy* in Eric Partridge's *Dictionary of Slang and Unconventional English* speaks volumes: "Contemptible; mean; filthy. . . . Standard English till 20th C, when, especially after the Great War, colloquial and used as a mere pejorative." *Lousy with*, meaning *full of*, was "originally military" and entered the colloquial word-hoard around 1915: "That ridge is lousy with Fritz."

The famous rats also gave constant trouble.

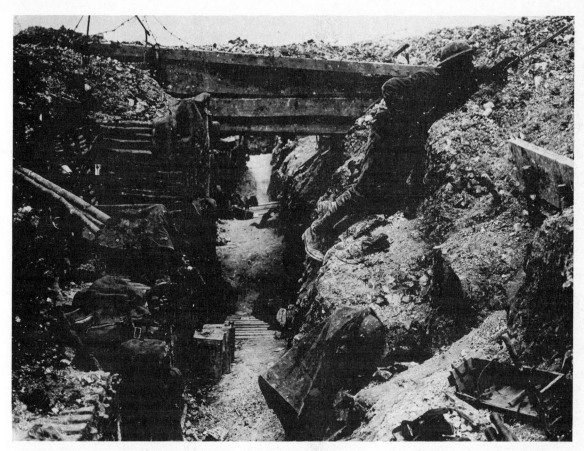

■ ■ *Front-line trenches in World War I. At some points on the front, a scant 1500 yards separated the Allied and the German lines.*

They were big and black, with wet, muddy hair. They fed largely on the flesh of cadavers and on dead horses. One shot them with revolvers or coshed them to death with pick-handles. Their hunger, vigor, intelligence, and courage are recalled in numerous anecdotes. One officer notes from the Ypres Salient: "We are fairly plagued with rats. They have eaten nearly everything in the mess, including the table-cloth and the operations orders! We borrowed a large cat and shut it up at night to exterminate them, and found the place empty next morning. The rats must have eaten it up, bones, fur, and all, and dragged it to their holes."

One can understand rats eating heartily there. It is harder to understand men doing so. The

stench of rotten flesh was over everything, hardly repressed by the chloride of lime sprinkled on particularly offensive sites. Dead horses and dead men—and parts of both—were sometimes not buried for months and often simply became an element of parapets and trench walls. You could smell the front line miles before you could see it. Lingering pockets of gas added to the unappetizing atmosphere. Yet men ate three times a day, although what they ate reflected the usual gulf between the ideal and the actual. The propagandist George Adam announced with satisfaction that "the food of the army is based upon the conclusions of a committee, upon which sat several eminent scientists." The result, he asserted, is that the troops are "better fed than they are at home.'' Officially, each man got daily: 1¼ pounds fresh meat (or 1 pound preserved meat), 1¼ pounds bread, 4 ounces bacon, 3 ounces cheese, ½ pound fresh vegetables (or 2 ounces dried), together with small amounts of tea, sugar, and jam. But in the trenches there was very seldom fresh meat, not for eating, anyway; instead there was ''Bully'' (tinned corned-beef) or ''Maconochie'' (ma-coń-o-chie), a tinned meat-and-vegetable stew named after its manufacturer. If they did tend to grow tedious in the long run, both products were surprisingly good. The troops seemed to like the Maconochie best, but the Germans favored the British corned beef, seldom returning from a raid on the British lines without taking back as much as they could carry. On trench duty the British had as little fresh bread as fresh meat. ''Pearl Biscuits'' were the substitute. They reminded the men of dog biscuits, although, together with the Bully beef, they were popular with the French and Belgian urchins, who ran (or more often strolled) alongside the railway trains bringing troops up to the front, soliciting gifts by shouting, ''Tommee! Bull-ee! Bee-skee!'' When a company was out of the line, it fed better. It was then serviced by its company cookers—stoves on wheels—and often got something approaching the official ration, as it might also in a particularly somnolent part of the line, when hot food might come up at night in the large covered containers known as Dixies.

Clothing and equipment improved as the war went on, although at the outset there was a terrible dearth and improvisation. During the retreat from Mons, as Frank Richards testifies, ''A lot of us had no caps: I was wearing a handkerchief knotted at the four corners—the only headgear I was to wear for some time.'' Crucial supplies had been omitted: ''We had plenty of small-arm ammunition but no rifle-oil or rifle-rag to clean our rifles with. We used to cut pieces off our shirts . . . and some of us who had bought small tins of vaseline . . . for use on sore heels or chafed legs, used to grease our rifles with that.'' At the beginning line officers dressed very differently from the men. They wore riding-boots or

leather puttees; melodramatically cut riding breeches; and flare-skirted tunics with Sam Browne belts. Discovering that this costume made them special targets in attacks (German gunners were instructed to fire first at the people with the thin knees), by the end they were dressing like the troops, wearing wrap puttees; straight trousers bloused below the knee; Other Ranks' tunics with inconspicuous insignia, no longer on the cuffs but on the shoulders; and Other Ranks' web belts and haversacks. In 1914 both officers and men wore peaked caps, and it was rakish for officers to remove the grommet for a ''Gorblimey'' effect. Steel helmets were introduced at the end of 1915, giving the troops, as Sassoon observed, ''a Chinese look.'' Herbert Read found the helmets ''the only poetic thing in the British Army, for they are primeval in design and effect, like iron mushrooms.'' A perceptive observer could date corpses and skeletons lying on disused battlefields by their evolving dress. A month before the end of the war, Major P. H. Pilditch recalls, he

spent some time in the old No Man's Land of four years' duration. . . . It was a morbid but intensely interesting occupation tracing the various battles amongst the hundreds of skulls, bones and remains scattered thickly about. The progress of our successive attacks could be clearly seen from the types of equipment on the skeletons, soft cloth caps denoting the 1914 and early 1915 fighting, then respirators, then steel helmets marking attack in 1916. Also Australian slouch hats, used in the costly and abortive attack in 1916.

To be in the trenches was to experience an unreal, unforgettable enclosure and constraint, as well as a sense of being unoriented and lost. One saw two things only: the walls of an unlocalized, undifferentiated earth and the sky above. Fourteen years after the war J. R. Ackerley was wandering through an unfrequented part of a town in India. ''The streets became narrower and narrower as I turned and turned,'' he writes, ''until I felt I was back in the trenches, the houses upon either side being so much of the same color and substance as the rough ground between." That lost feeling is what struck Major Frank Isherwood, who writes his wife in December, 1914: "The trenches are a labyrinth, I have already lost myself repeatedly. . . . you can't get out of them and walk about the country or see anything at all but two muddy walls on each side of you." What a survivor of the Salient remembers fifty years later are the walls of dirt and the ceiling of sky, and his eloquent optative cry rises as if he were still imprisoned there: "To be out of this present, everpresent, eternally present misery, this stinking world of sticky, trickling earth ceilinged by a strip of threatening sky." As the only visible theater of variety, the sky becomes all-important. It was the sight of the sky, almost alone, that had the power to persuade a man that he was not already lost in a common grave.

■ ■ ■

STUDY QUESTIONS

1. What was the effect of World War I on the landscape of Europe?

2. In theory, how were the trenches supposed to be constructed? What was life supposed to be like in the ideal trench? How did reality differ from theory?

3. What national differences were there in the construction and maintenance of trenches? What do the differences tell us about the different national characters and war aims?

4. Describe the sights, sounds, and smell of life in the trenches. How did trench life affect the soldiers?

5. What does Fussell mean when he describes the experience as "unreal"? How did trench life breed "a sense of being unoriented and lost"?

BIBLIOGRAPHY

The above selection is taken from Fussell's award-winning *The Great War and Modern Memory* (1975), the best discussion of the impact of the war on modern culture. Robert Wohl, *The Generation of 1914* (1979), recreates the experiences of the men who fought and wrote about the war. Three good military overviews of the war are James L. Stokesbury, *A Short History of World War I* (1981); B. H. Liddell Hart, *The Real War, 1914–1918* (1930); and Cyril Falls, *The Great War* (1959). S. B. Fay, *The Origins of World War* (2 vols., 1928–1930); L. Albertini, *The Origins of the War of 1914* (3 vols., 1952–1957); and Fritz Fischer, *Germany's Aims in the First World War* (1967), discuss the complex origins of the war. The best studies of America's entry into the war are E. R. May, *The First World War and American Isolation* (1957); P. Devlin, *Too Proud to Fight: Woodrow Wilsons' Neutrality* (1975); and Barbara Tuchman, *The Zimmerman Telegram* (1958). Military studies that give the reader a sense of the problems faced by the typical soldier include Martin Middlebrooks, *The First Day on the Somme* (1971); Alister Horne, *The Price of Glory: Verdun, 1916* (1962); Leon Wolff, *In Flanders Field* (1958); Barrie Pitt, *The Last Act* (1962); and John Keegan, *The Face of Battle: A Study of Agincourt, Waterloo, and the Somme* (1976).

Part Four

HEROES AND SOCIETY
IN THE 1920s

The year 1920 ushered in a decade that historians steadfastly refuse to discuss in anything less than superlative terms. The decade brings to mind Charles Dickens' description of the revolutionary years of the eighteenth century in his novel, *A Tale of Two Cities:* "It was the best of times, it was the worst of times . . . it was the season of Light, it was the season of Darkness, it was the spring of hope, it was the winter of despair, we had everything before us, we had nothing before us." If a decade may be said to have a personality, then the 1920s had the personality of a child; sometimes laughing and playful, at other times brooding, brutal, and ugly.

The first and perhaps most widely read book about the decade was Frederick Lewis Allen's *Only Yesterday: An Informal History of the 1920s.* Published in 1931 during the midst of the Great Depression, *Only Yesterday* describes a carefree decade that began with the end of the Great War and ended with the Stock Market Crash. Allen paints a decade that roars with excitement, a decade brimming with bathtub gin, bootleg liquor, and bubbling champaign. Gangsters, movie sex goddesses, athletic heroes, and fabulous moneymakers seem to come alive on the pages of *Only Yesterday.* In sweeping terms, Allen examines the "revolution in manners and morals," the "aching disillusionment" of intellectuals, and the crass materialism of millions of Americans.

Allen was not necessarily wrong. The sexual mores of the youth were changing, and there was evidence of intellectual disillusionment and crass materialism. The

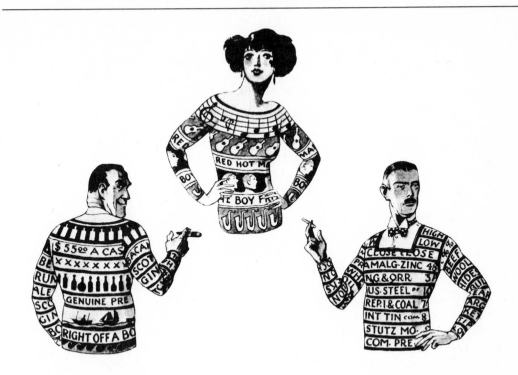

problem with the book is that its sweeping generalizations are simply too sweeping. In addition, too much of the activity of the decade is left out of *Only Yesterday*. The economic plight of rural Americans, the rise of the Ku Klux Klan, urban-rural tensions, racial injustice, nativism, and religious revivalism are just a few of the subjects that Allen does not treat. As a result, *Only Yesterday* is a flawed and unbalanced classic.

In recent years, historians have explored the areas where Allen did not venture. And they have presented a different view of the 1920s, viewing the decade as a period of transition where older rural and newer urban attitudes uneasily coexisted. Although the country was becoming increasingly urban and bureaucratic, many Americans clung tightly to the more traditional values of their parents and grandparents. In an effort to preserve these values, they supported a variety of movements such as the Society for the Preservation of New England Antiquities, the Ku Klux Klan, and the National Origins Act of 1924.

If rural America resisted change, most of urban America accepted it. Spectators filled movie theaters and athletic stadiums to watch others perform, and entertainment became a product that was packaged and marketed by business executives. Millions of Americans worshipped at the altar of business efficiency and organization. Even crime became more organized and efficient. By 1929 the debate between rural and urban America was decided. The future belonged to the cities.

THE REVOLUTION IN MANNERS AND MORALS

Frederick Lewis Allen

In 1934, Henry Seidel Canby, a noted literary critic and editor, published *The Age of Confidence,* a memoir that spoke frankly about the changes in American society. In the book Canby graphically described the Victorian code which ruled social behavior during most of his life. It was a code that emphasized the values of hard work, sobriety, thrift, and order. It was enforced by laws that prohibited drinking, gambling, and ribald behavior. As for sexual activity, Canby wrote, "except in sin or the reticence of marriage, sexual drives did not exist." Men channeled their energies into useful production, and women emphasized the superiority of the spirit over the body. Writing about the role of the Victorian woman, Canby noted, "one hint of the sexual made her 'common,' which was only one word above 'vulgar.'"

By 1934 Canby believed that a new, more permissive code had gained control of social behavior. He maintained that standards had been relaxed and that self-denial had been replaced by consumption. Other people of his generation agreed with Canby. In the following selection, Frederick Lewis Allen examines what he termed "the revolution in manners and morals." Certainly attitudes were changing, but the grip of Victorianism was perhaps stronger than either Canby or Allen realized. As recent studies have demonstrated, the "revolution" may not have been as all-encompassing as Allen believed. Nevertheless, Allen's discussion of the topic still provides insights into the changing patterns of American behavior.

A first-class revolt against the accepted American order was certainly taking place during those early years of the Post-war Decade, but it was one with which Nikolai Lenin had nothing whatever to do. The shock troops of the rebellion were not alien agitators, but the sons and daughters of well-to-do American families, who knew little about Bolshevism and cared distinctly less, and their defiance was expressed not in obscure radical publications or in soap-box speeches, but right across the family breakfast table into the horrified ears of conservative fathers and mothers. Men and women were still shivering at the Red Menace when they awoke to the no less alarming Problem of the Younger Generation, and realized that if the Constitution were not in danger, the moral code of the country certainly was.

This code, as it currently concerned young people, might have been roughly summarized as follows: Women were the guardians of morality; they were made of finer stuff than men and were expected to act accordingly. Young girls must look forward in innocence (tempered perhaps with a modicum of physiological instruction) to a romantic love match which would lead them to the altar and to living-happily-ever-after; and until the "right man" came along they must allow no male to kiss them. It was expected that some men would succumb to the temptations of sex, but only with a special class of outlawed women; girls of respectable families were supposed to have no such temptations. Boys and girls were permitted large freedom to work and play together, with decreasing and well-nigh nominal chaperonage, but only because the code worked so well on the whole that a sort of honor system was supplanting supervision by their elders; it was taken for granted that if they had been well brought up they would never take

advantage of this freedom. And although the attitude toward smoking and drinking by girls differed widely in different strata of society and different parts of the country, majority opinion held that it was morally wrong for them to smoke and could hardly imagine them showing the effects of alcohol.

The war had not long been over when cries of alarm from parents, teachers, and moral preceptors began to rend the air. For the boys and girls just growing out of adolescence were making mincemeat of this code.

The dresses that the girls—and for that matter most of the older women—were wearing seemed alarming enough. In July, 1920, a fashion-writer reported in the *New York Times* that "the American woman . . . has lifted her skirts far beyond any modest limitation," which was another way of saying that the hem was now all of nine inches above the ground. It was freely predicted that skirts would come down again in the winter of 1920–21, but instead they climbed a few scandalous inches farther. The flappers wore thin dresses, short-sleeved and occasionally (in the evening) sleeveless; some of the wilder young things rolled their stockings below their knees, revealing to the shocked eyes of virtue a fleeting glance of shin-bones and knee-cap; and many of them were visibly using cosmetics. "The intoxication of rouge," earnestly explained Dorothy Speare in *Dancers in the Dark*, "is an insidious vintage known to more girls than mere man can ever believe." Useless for frantic parents to insist that no lady did such things; the answer was that the daughters of ladies were doing it, and even retouching their masterpieces in public. Some of them, furthermore, were abandoning their corsets. "The men won't dance with you if you wear a corset," they were quoted as saying.

The current mode in dancing created still more consternation. Not the romantic violin but the barbaric saxophone now dominated the orchestra, and to its passionate crooning and wailing the fox-trotters moved in what the editor of the Hobart College *Herald* disgustedly called a "syncopated embrace." No longer did even an inch of space separate them; they danced as if glued together, body to body, cheek to cheek. Cried the *Catholic Telegraph* of Cincinnati in righteous indignation, "The music is sensuous, the embracing of partners—the female only half dressed—is absolutely indecent; and the motions—they are such as may not be described, with any respect for propriety, in a family newspaper. Suffice it to say that there are certain houses appropriate for such dances; but those houses have been closed by law."

Supposedly "nice" girls were smoking cigarettes—openly and defiantly, if often rather awkwardly and self-consciously. They were drinking—somewhat less openly but often all too efficaciously. There were stories of daughters of the most exemplary parents getting drunk—"blotto," as their companions cheerfully put it—on the contents of the hip-flasks of the new prohibition régime, and going out joyriding with men at four in the morning. And worst of all, even at well-regulated dances they were said to retire where the eye of the most sharp-sighted chaperon could not follow, and in darkened rooms or in parked cars to engage in the unspeakable practice of petting and necking.

It was not until F. Scott Fitzgerald, who had hardly graduated from Princeton and ought to know what his generation were doing, brought out *This Side of Paradise* in April, 1920, that fathers and mothers realized fully what was afoot and how long it had been going on. Apparently the "petting party" had been current as early as 1916, and was now widely established as an indoor sport. "None of the Victorian mothers—and most of the mothers were Victorian—had any idea how casually their daughters were accustomed to be kissed," wrote Mr. Fitzgerald. ". . . Amory saw girls doing things that even in his memory would have been impossible: eating three-o'clock, after-dance suppers in impossible cafés, talking of every side of life with an air half of earnestness, half of mockery, yet with a furtive excitement that Amory considered stood for a real moral let-down. But he never realized how widespread it was until he saw the cities

between New York and Chicago as one vast juvenile intrigue." The book caused a shudder to run down the national spine; did not Mr. Fitzgerald represent one of his well-nurtured heroines as brazenly confessing, "I've kissed dozens of men. I suppose I'll kiss dozens more"; and another heroine as saying to a young man *(to a young man!)*, "Oh, just one person in fifty has any glimmer of what sex is. I'm hipped on Freud and all that, but it's rotten that every bit of real love in the world is ninety-nine per cent passion and one little *soupçon* of jealousy"?

It was incredible. It was abominable. What did it all mean? Was every decent standard being thrown over? Mothers read the scarlet words and wondered if they themselves "had any idea how often their daughters were accustomed to be kissed." . . . But no, this must be an exaggerated account of the misconduct of some especially depraved group. Nice girls couldn't behave like that and talk openly about passion. But in due course other books appeared to substantiate the findings of Mr. Fitzgerald: *Dancers in the Dark, The Plastic Age, Flaming Youth*. Magazine articles and newspapers reiterated the scandal. To be sure, there were plenty of communities where nice girls did not, in actual fact, "behave like that"; and even in the more sophisticated urban centers there were plenty of girls who did not. Nevertheless, there was enough fire beneath the smoke of these sensational revelations to make the Problem of the Younger Generation a topic of anxious discussion from coast to coast.

The forces of morality rallied to the attack. Dr. Francis E. Clark, the founder and president of the Christian Endeavor Society, declared that the modern "indecent dance" was "an offense against womanly purity, the very fountainhead of our family and civil life." The new style of dancing was denounced in religious journals as "impure, polluting, corrupting, debasing, destroying spirituality, increasing carnality," and the mothers and sisters and church members of the land were called upon to admonish and instruct and raise the spiritual tone of these dreadful young people. President Murphree of the University of Florida cried out with true

Southern warmth, "The low-cut gowns, the rolled hose and short skirts are born of the Devil and his angels, and are carrying the present and future generations to chaos and destruction." A group of Episcopal church-women in New York, speaking with the authority of wealth and social position (for they included Mrs. J. Pierpont Morgan, Mrs. Borden Harriman, Mrs. Henry Phipps, Mrs. James Roosevelt, and Mrs. E. H. Harriman), proposed an organization to discourage fashions involving an "excess of nudity" and "improper ways of dancing." The Y. W. C. A. conducted a national campaign against immodest dress among high-school girls, supplying newspapers with printed matter carrying headlines such as "Working Girls Responsive to Modesty Appeal" and "High Heels Losing Ground Even in France." In Philadelphia a Dress Reform Committee of prominent citizens sent a questionnaire to over a thousand clergymen to ask them what would be their idea of a proper dress, and although the gentlemen of the cloth showed a distressing variety of opinion, the committee proceeded to design a "moral gown" which was endorsed by ministers of fifteen denominations. The distinguishing characteristics of this moral gown were that it was very loose-fitting, that the sleeves reached just below the elbows, and that the hem came within seven and a half inches of the floor.

Not content with example and reproof, legislators in several states introduced bills to reform feminine dress once and for all. The *New York American* reported in 1921 that a bill was pending in Utah providing fine and imprisonment for those who wore on the streets "skirts higher than three inches above the ankle." A bill was laid before the Virginia legislature which would forbid any woman from wearing shirtwaists or evening gowns which displayed "more than three inches of her throat." In Ohio the proposed limit of decolletage was two inches; the bill introduced in the Ohio legislature aimed also to prevent the sale of any "garment which unduly displays or accentuates the lines of the female figure," and to prohibit any "female over fourteen years of age" from wearing "a skirt which

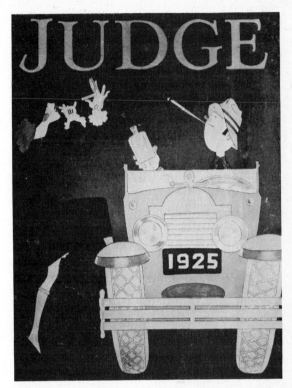

A popular, though overdrawn, image of the 1920s was "six-cylinder love," set in a flashy roadster and featuring a flapper with rolled stockings and a callow collegian sporting a long cigarette holder and a hipflask.

does not reach to that part of the foot known as the instep."

Meanwhile innumerable families were torn with dissension over cigarettes and gin and all-night automobile rides. Fathers and mothers lay awake asking themselves whether their children were not utterly lost; sons and daughters evaded questions, lied miserably and unhappily, or flared up to reply rudely that at least they were not dirty-minded hypocrites, that they saw no harm in what they were doing and proposed to go right on doing it. From those liberal clergymen and teachers who prided themselves on keeping step with all that was new, came a chorus of reassurance: these young people were at least franker and more honest than their elders had been; having experimented for themselves, would they not soon find out which standards were outworn and which represented the accumulated moral wisdom of the race? Hearing such hopeful words, many good people took heart again. Perhaps this flare-up of youthful passion was a flash in the pan, after all. Perhaps in another year or two the boys and girls would come to their senses and everything would be all right again.

They were wrong, however. For the revolt of the younger generation was only the beginning of a revolution in manners and morals that was already beginning to affect men and women of every age in every part of the country.

A number of forces were working together and interacting upon one another to make this revolution inevitable.

First of all was the state of mind brought about by the war and its conclusion. A whole generation had been infected by the eat-drink-and-be-merry-for-tomorrow-we-die spirit which accompanied the departure of the soldiers to the training camps and the fighting front. There had been an epidemic not only of abrupt war marriages, but of less conventional liaisons. In France, two million men had found themselves very close to filth and annihilation and very far from the American moral code and its defenders; prostitution had followed the flag and willing mademoiselles from Armentières had been plentiful; American girls sent over as nurses and war workers had come under the influence of continental manners and standards without being subject to the rigid protections thrown about their continental sisters of the respectable classes; and there had been a very widespread and very natural breakdown of traditional restraints and reticences and taboos. It was impossible for this generation to return unchanged when the ordeal was over. Some of them had acquired under the pressure of wartime conditions a new code which seemed to them quite defensible; millions of them had been provided with an emotional stimulant from which it was not easy to taper off. Their torn

nerves craved the anodynes of speed, excitement, and passion. They found themselves expected to settle down into the humdrum routine of American life as if nothing had happened, to accept the moral dicta of elders who seemed to them still to be living in a Pollyanna land of rosy ideals which the war had killed for them. They couldn't do it, and they very disrespectfully said so.

"The older generation had certainly pretty well ruined this world before passing it on to us," wrote one of them (John F. Carter in the *Atlantic Monthly,* September, 1920), expressing accurately the sentiments of innumerable contemporaries. "They give us this thing, knocked to pieces, leaky, red-hot, threatening to blow up; and then they are surprised that we don't accept it with the same attitude of pretty, decorous enthusiasm with which they received it, way back in the 'eighties."

The middle generation was not so immediately affected by the war neurosis. They had had time enough, before 1917, to build up habits of conformity not easily broken down. But they, too, as the let-down of 1919 followed the war, found themselves restless and discontented, in a mood to question everything that had once seemed to them true and worthy and of good report. They too had spent themselves and wanted a good time. They saw their juniors exploring the approaches to the forbidden land of sex, and presently they began to play with the idea of doing a little experimenting of their own. The same disillusion which had defeated Woodrow Wilson and had caused strikes and riots and the Big Red Scare furnished a culture in which the germs of the new freedom could grow and multiply.

The revolution was accelerated also by the growing independence of the American woman. She won the suffrage in 1920. She seemed, it is true, to be very little interested in it once she had it; she voted, but mostly as the unregenerate men about her did, despite the efforts of women's clubs and the League of Women Voters to awaken her to womanhood's civic opportunity; feminine candidates for office were few, and some of them—such as Governor Ma Ferguson of Texas—scarcely seemed to represent the starry-eyed spiritual influence which, it had been promised, would presently ennoble public life. Few of the younger women could rouse themselves to even a passing interest in politics: to them it was a sordid and futile business, without flavor and without hope. Nevertheless, the winning of the suffrage had its effect. It consolidated woman's position as man's equal.

Even more marked was the effect of woman's growing independence of the drudgeries of housekeeping. Smaller houses were being built, and they were easier to look after. Families were moving into apartments, and these made even less claim upon the housekeeper's time and energy. Women were learning how to make lighter work of the preparation of meals. Sales of canned foods were growing, the number of delicatessen stores had increased three times as fast as the population during the decade 1910–20, the output of bakeries increased by 60 per cent during the decade 1914–24. Much of what had once been housework was now either moving out of the home entirely or being simplified by machinery. The use of commercial laundries, for instance, increased by 57 per cent between 1914 and 1924. Electric washing-machines and electric irons were coming to the aid of those who still did their washing at home; the manager of the local electric power company at "Middletown," a typical small American city, estimated in 1924 that nearly 90 per cent of the homes in the city already had electric irons. The housewife was learning to telephone her shopping orders, to get her clothes ready-made and spare herself the rigors of dress-making, to buy a vacuum cleaner and emulate the lovely carefree girls in the magazine advertisements who banished dust with such delicate fingers. Women were slowly becoming emancipated from routine to "live their own lives."

And what were these "own lives" of theirs to be like? Well, for one thing, they could take jobs. Up to this time girls of the middle classes who had wanted to "do something" had been largely restricted to school-teaching, social-service work, nursing, stenography, and clerical work in business houses. But now they poured out of the schools and colleges into all manner of new occupations. They besieged the offices of publishers and advertisers; they went into tea-room management until there threatened to be more purveyors than consumers of chicken patties and cinnamon toast; they sold antiques, sold real estate, opened smart little shops, and finally invaded the department stores. In 1920 the department store was in the mind of the average college girl a rather bourgeois institution which employed "poor shop girls"; by the end of the decade college girls were standing in line for openings in the misses' sports-wear department and even selling behind the counter in the hope that some day fortune might smile upon them and make them buyers or stylists. Small-town girls who once would have been contented to stay in Sauk Center all their days were now borrowing from father to go to New York or Chicago to seek their fortunes—in Best's or Macy's or Marshall Field's. Married women who were encumbered with children and could not seek jobs consoled themselves with the thought that home-making and child-rearing were really "professions," after all. No topic was so furiously discussed at luncheon tables from one end of the country to the other as the question whether the married woman should take a job, and whether the mother had a right to. And as for the unmarried woman, she no longer had to explain why she worked in a shop or an office; it was idleness, nowadays, that had to be defended.

With the job—or at least the sense that the job was a possibility—came a feeling of comparative economic independence. With the feeling of economic independence came a slackening of husbandly and parental authority. Maiden aunts and unmarried daughters were leaving the shelter of the family roof to install themselves in kitchenette apartments of their own. For city-dwellers the home was steadily becoming less of a shrine, more of a dormitory—a place of casual shelter where one stopped overnight on the way from the restaurant and the movie theater to the office. Yet even the job did not provide the American woman with that complete satisfaction which the management of a mechanized home no longer furnished. She still had energies and emotions to burn; she was ready for the revolution.

Like all revolutions, this one was stimulated by foreign propaganda. It came, however, not from Moscow, but from Vienna. Sigmund Freud had published his first book on psychoanalysis at the end of the nineteenth century, and he and Jung had lectured to American psychologists as early as 1909, but it was not until after the war that the Freudian gospel began to circulate to a marked extent among the American lay public. The one great intellectual force which had not suffered disrepute as a result of the war was science; the more-or-less educated public was now absorbing a quantity of popularized information about biology and anthropology which gave a general impression that men and women were merely animals of a rather intricate variety, and that moral codes had no universal validity and were often based on curious superstitions. A fertile ground was ready for the seeds of Freudianism, and presently one began to hear even from the lips of flappers that "science taught" new and disturbing things about sex. Sex, it appeared, was the central and pervasive force which moved mankind. Almost every human motive was attributable to it: if you were patriotic or liked the violin, you were in the grip of sex—in a sublimated form. The first requirement of mental health was to have an uninhibited sex life. If you would be well and happy, you must obey your libido. Such was the Freudian gospel as it imbedded itself in the American mind after being filtered through the successive minds of interpreters and popularizers and guileless readers and people who had heard guileless readers talk about it. New words and phrases began to be bandied about the cocktail-tray and the mah jong table—inferiority complex, sadism, masochism, Œdipus complex. Intellectual ladies went to Europe to be analyzed; analysts plied their new trade in American cities, conscien-

tiously transferring the affections of their fair patients to themselves; and clergymen who preached about the virtue of self-control were reminded by outspoken critics that self-control was out-of-date and really dangerous.

The principal remaining forces which accelerated the revolution in manners and morals were all 100 per cent American. They were prohibition, the automobile, the confession and sex magazines, and the movies.

When the Eighteenth Amendment was ratified, prohibition seemed, as we have already noted, to have an almost united country behind it. Evasion of the law began immediately, however, and strenuous and sincere opposition to it—especially in the large cities of the North and East—quickly gathered force. The results were the bootlegger, the speakeasy, and a spirit of deliberate revolt which in many communities made drinking "the thing to do." From these facts in turn flowed further results: the increased popularity of distilled as against fermented liquors, the use of the hip-flask, the cocktail party, and the general transformation of drinking from a masculine prerogative to one shared by both sexes together. The old-time saloon had been overwhelmingly masculine; the speakeasy usually catered to both men and women. As Elmer Davis put it, "The old days when father spent his evenings at Cassidy's bar with the rest of the boys are gone, and probably gone forever; Cassidy may still be in business at the old stand and father may still go down there of evenings, but since prohibition mother goes down with him." Under the new régime not only the drinks were mixed, but the company as well.

Meanwhile a new sort of freedom was being made possible by the enormous increase in the use of the automobile, and particularly of the closed car. (In 1919 hardly more than 10 per cent of the cars produced in the United States were closed; by 1924 the percentage had jumped to 43, by 1927 it had reached 82.8.) The automobile offered an almost universally available means of escaping temporarily from the supervision of parents and chaperones, or from the influence of neighborhood opinion. Boys and girls now thought nothing, as the Lynds pointed out in *Middletown*, of jumping into a car and driving off at a moment's notice—without asking anybody's permission—to a dance in another town twenty miles away, where they were strangers and enjoyed a freedom impossible among their neighbors. The closed car, moreover, was in effect a room protected from the weather which could be occupied at any time of the day or night and could be moved at will into a darkened byway or a country lane. The Lynds quoted the judge of the juvenile court in "Middletown" as declaring that the automobile had become a "house of prostitution on wheels," and cited the fact that of thirty girls brought before his court in a year on charges of sex crimes, for whom the place where the offense had occurred was recorded, nineteen were listed as having committed it in an automobile.

Finally, as the revolution began, its influence fertilized a bumper crop of sex magazines, confession magazines, and lurid motion pictures, and these in turn had their effect on a class of readers and movie-goers who had never heard and never would hear of Freud and the libido. The publishers of the sex adventure magazines, offering stories with such titles as "What I Told My Daughter the Night Before Her Marriage," "Indolent Kisses," and "Watch Your Step-Ins," learned to a nicety the gentle art of arousing the reader without arousing the censor. The publishers of the confession magazines, while always instructing their authors to provide a moral ending and to utter pious sentiments, concentrated on the description of what they euphemistically called "missteps." Most of their fiction was faked to order by hack writers who could write one day "The Confessions of a Chorus Girl" and the next day recount, again in the first person, the temptations which made it easy for the taxi-driver to go wrong. Both classes of magazines became astonishingly numerous and successful. Bernarr McFadden's *True-Story*, launched as late as 1919, had over 300,000 readers by 1923; 848,000 by 1924; over a million and a half by 1925; and almost two million by 1926—a record of rapid growth probably unparalleled in magazine publishing.

Crowding the news stands along with the sex and confession magazines were motion-picture magazines which depicted "seven movie kisses" with such captions as "Do you recognize your little friend, Mae Busch? She's had lots of kisses, but she never seems to grow *blasé*. At least you'll agree that she's giving a good imitation of a person enjoying this one." The movies themselves, drawing millions to their doors every day and every night, played incessantly upon the same lucrative theme. The producers of one picture advertised "brilliant men, beautiful jazz babies, champagne baths, midnight revels, petting parties in the purple dawn, all ending in one terrific smashing climax that makes you gasp"; the venders of another promised "neckers, petters, white kisses, red kisses, pleasure-mad daughters, sensation-craving mothers, . . . the truth—bold, naked, sensational." Seldom did the films offer as much as these advertisements promised, but there was enough in some of them to cause a sixteen-year-old girl (quoted by Alice Miller Mitchell) to testify, "Those pictures with hot love-making in them, they make girls and boys sitting together want to get up and walk out, go off somewhere, you know. Once I walked out with a boy before the picture was even over. We took a ride. But my friend, she all the time had to get up and go out with her boy friend."

A storm of criticism from church organizations led the motion-picture producers, early in the decade, to install Will H. Hays, President Harding's Postmaster-General, as their arbiter of morals and taste, and Mr. Hays promised that all would be well. "This industry must have," said he before the Los Angeles Chamber of Commerce, "toward that sacred thing, the mind of a child, toward that clean virgin thing, that unmarked slate, the same responsibility, the same care about the impressions made upon it, that the best clergyman or the most inspired teacher of youth would have." The result of Mr. Hays's labors in behalf of the unmarked slate was to make the moral ending as obligatory as in the confession magazines, to smear over sexy pictures with pious platitudes, and to blacklist for motion-picture production many a fine novel and play which, because of its very honesty, might be construed as seriously or intelligently questioning the traditional sex ethics of the small town. Mr. Hays, being something of a genius, managed to keep the churchmen at bay. Whenever the threats of censorship began to become ominous he would promulgate a new series of moral commandments for the producers to follow. Yet of the practical effects of his supervision it is perhaps enough to say that the quotations given above all date from the period of his dicta-

torship. Giving lip-service to the old code, the movies diligently and with consummate vulgarity publicized the new.

Each of these diverse influences—the post-war disillusion, the new status of women, the Freudian gospel, the automobile, prohibition, the sex and confession magazines, and the movies—had its part in bringing about the revolution. Each of them, as an influence, was played upon by all the others; none of them could alone have changed to any great degree the folkways of America; together their force was irresistible.

■■■

STUDY QUESTIONS

1. What evidence does Allen offer to demonstrate that a "revolution in manners and morals" was taking place during the 1920s? Does the evidence warrant his conclusions? Is Allen writing about all Americans, or is he referring to a particular class?

2. How did various state legislators try to plug the tide of change? Were they successful? Why or why not?

3. What were the European forces which contributed to the "revolution"?

4. What were the American forces which accelerated the "revolution"?

5. Do you find Allen's argument convincing? Why or why not?

BIBLIOGRAPHY

The best treatments of the 1920s are Roderick Nash, *The Nervous Generation: American Thought, 1917–1930* (1970); William E. Leuchtenburg, *The Perils of Prosperity, 1914–1932* (1958); Paul Carter, *The Twenties in America* (1968), and *Another Part of the Twenties* (1976); and Geoffrey Perrett, *America in the Twenties* (1982). All five books either modify or challenge the conclusions Allen reached. The best study of the changing sexual attitudes of college-educated youth is Paul S. Fass, *The Damned and the Beautiful: American Youth in the 1920s* (1977). Gilman Ostrander, *America in the First Machine Age, 1890–1940* (1970), emphasizes the role of modern technology and consumption on the development of a youth culture. Lary May, *Screening Out the Past: The Birth of Mass Culture and the Motion Picture Industry* (1980), and Lewis A. Erenberg, *Steppin' Out: New York Nightlife and the Transformation of American Culture, 1890–1930* (1981), also discuss changing American attitudes toward sex during the 1920s.

THE MOOD
OF THE PEOPLE

Roderick Nash

No decade in American history has been more studded with heroes and idols as the 1920s. Such athletic heroes as Babe Ruth, Jack Dempsey, Red Grange, Bill Tilden, and Bobby Jones are still household names. In Hollywood, they were rivaled by stars such as Rudolph Valentino, Mary Pickford, Douglas Fairbanks, Clara Bow, and Charlie Chaplin. Heroes even came from the worlds of business, finance, and government. Herbert Hoover and Edward Bok demonstrated the appeal of self-made millionaires. The greatest hero, however, was Charles Lindbergh, who captured the public's imagination in 1927 by making the first solo flight across the Atlantic.

Nor has there been a decade that has been more acclaimed for its literary output. Novelists F. Scott Fitzgerald and Ernest Hemingway and poets E. E. Cummings, T. S. Eliot, and Edna St. Vincent Millay are among the most talented America ever produced. More people, however, read the stories of such popular novelists as Gene Stratton-Porter, Harold Bell Wright, Zane Grey, and Edgar Rice Burroughs.

In the following essay historian Roderick Nash probes the meaning behind the heroes people chose and the novels they read. Heroes, Nash claimed, reflect the "mood of the people"; they mirror the aspirations, longings, and fears of millions of unheralded Americans. Similarly, popular novelists' success depends on their ability to interpret and tap the mood of the nation. That mood, Nash feels, was not bold and carefree, as Frederick Lewis Allen believed, but rather timid and nervous. Americans chose heroes and read novels that glorified their rural past and eased their minds concerning their urban future.

Heroes abounded in the American 1920s. Their names, especially in sports, have been ticked off so frequently they have become clichés. Less often have commentators paused to probe for explanations. Why were the twenties ripe for heroism? And why did the heroics follow a predictable pattern? Such questions lead to an understanding of the mood of the people, because heroism concerns the public as well as the individual. It depends on achievement but even more on recognition. In the final analysis the hopes and fears of everyday Americans create national heroes.

The nervousness of the post-World War I generation provided fertile soil for the growth of a particular kind of heroism. Many Americans felt uneasy as they experienced the transforming effects of population growth, urbanization, and economic change. On the one hand, these developments were welcome as steps in the direction of progress. Yet they also raised vague fears about the passing of frontier conditions, the loss of national vigor, and the eclipse of the individual in a mass society. Frederick Jackson Turner and Theodore Roosevelt, among others, had pointed to the liabilities of the transformation at the turn of the century. World War I underscored the misgivings and doubts. By the 1920s the sense of change had penetrated to the roots of popular thought. Scarcely an American was unaware that the frontier had vanished and that pioneering, in the traditional sense, was a thing of the past. Physical changes in the nation were undeniable. They occurred faster, however, than intellectual adjustment. Although Americans, in general, lived in a densely populated, urban-industrial civilization, a large part of their values remained rooted in the frontier, farm, and village. Exposure of this discrepancy only served to increase the tightness with which insecure people clung to the old certainties. Old-style pio-

neering was impossible, but Americans proved ingenious in finding equivalents. The upshot in the twenties was the cult of the hero—the man who provided living testimony of the power of courage, strength, and honor and of the efficacy of the self-reliant, rugged individual who seemed on the verge of becoming as irrelevant as the covered wagon.

Sports and the star athlete were the immediate beneficiaries of this frame of mind. The American sports fan regarded the playing field as a surrogate frontier; the athletic hero was the twentieth-century equivalent of the pathfinder or pioneer. In athletic competition, as on the frontier, people believed, men confronted tangible obstacles and overcame them with talent and determination. The action in each case was clean and direct; the goals, whether clearing forests or clearing the bases, easily perceived and immensely satisfying. Victory was the result of superior ability. The sports arena like the frontier was pregnant with opportunity for the individual. The start was equal and the best man won. Merit was rewarded. True or not, such a credo was almost instinctive with Americans. They packed the stadiums of the 1920s in a salute to time-honored virtues. With so much else about America changing rapidly, it was comforting to find in sports a ritualistic celebration of the major components of the national faith.

Writing in the *North American Review* for October 1929, A. A. Brill, a leading American psychologist of the Freudian school, took a closer look at the meaning of athletics. Why, he wondered, do men play and why do they select the particular kinds of play they do? Brill was also interested in the reasons spectators came to games. His main point was that sports were not idle diversions but intensely serious endeavors rooted in the values and traditions of a civilization. "The ancestry of sport," Brill declared, "is written very plainly in the fact that the first games among all nations were simple imitations of the typical acts of warriors and huntsmen." The primary motivation of play, according to Brill, was the "mastery impulse"—an inherent aggressiveness in man stemming from the Darwinian struggle for existence. Modern man had largely transcended direct physical struggle, but the need for it persisted in the human psyche. Sports were contrived as substitutes for actual fighting, mock struggles that satisfied the urge to conquer. Brill did not suggest a relationship between American sports and the American frontier, but his argument suggested one. So did the fact that the rise of mass spectator sports and the decline of the frontier were simultaneous in the United States.

By the 1920s the nation went sports crazy. It seemed to many that a golden age of sport had arrived in America. Football received a large portion of the limelight. As they had in the declining days of Rome, fans thronged the stadiums to witness contact, violence, bloodshed, man pitted against man, strength against strength. The vicarious element was invariably present. For a brief, glorious moment the nobody in the bleachers *was* the halfback crashing into the end zone with the winning touchdown. For a moment he shared the thrill of individual success and fought off the specter of being swallowed up in mass society.

Big-time professional football began on September 17, 1920, when the American Football Association was organized with the great Indian athlete Jim Thorpe as its first president. When the Green Bay Packers joined the Association in 1921, the saga of pro football was solidly launched. Attendance rose dramatically. On November 21, 1925, the presence on the playing field of the fabled Harold "Red" Grange helped draw 36,000 spectators to a game. A week later 68,000 jammed the Polo Grounds in New York to watch Grange in action. The names of the pro teams were suggestive. As on the frontier of old, it was cowboys versus Indians, or giants versus bears—with the names of cities prefixed.

The twenties was also the time of the emergence of college football on an unprecedented scale. Heroes appeared in good supply: Red Grange at Illinois, Knute Rockne's "Four Horsemen" at Notre Dame in 1924, Harold "Brick"

Muller who began a dynasty at California that extended through fifty consecutive victories in the seasons 1919 through 1925. Hundreds of thousands attended the Saturday games, an estimated twenty million during the season. Millions more followed the action over their radios and made a Sunday morning ritual of devouring the newspaper accounts of the games of the previous day. To accommodate the crowds colleges and universities built huge new stadiums. Yale's and California's seated eighty thousand; Illinois, Ohio State, and Michigan were not far behind. The number of Americans who attended games doubled between 1921 and 1930. A *Harper's* writer caught the spirit of college football in 1928: "it is at present a religion, sometimes it seems to be almost our national religion." So, once, had been westward expansion.

Despite its popularity, football tended to obscure the heroic individual. It was, after all, a team sport. Even Red Grange received an occasional block on his long runs. But in sports pitting man against man or against the clock the heroism latent in competition achieved its purest expression. Americans in the 1920s had a glittering array of well-publicized individuals from which to choose their idol. In golf Robert T. "Bobby" Jones, Walter Hagen, and Gene Sarazen were the dominant figures. Tennis had "Big" Bill Tilden and "Little" Bill Johnson whose epic duels on the center court at Forest Hills filled the stands. The competition was even more direct in boxing with its "knock out," the symbol of complete conquest. During the twenties promoters like Tex Rickard built boxing into a big business. Jack Dempsey and Gene Tunney proved so attractive to the sporting public that a ticket sale of a million dollars for a single fight became a reality. By the end of the decade the figure was two million. Fifty bouts in the twenties had gates of more than $100,000. More than 100,000 fans came to Soldiers' Field in Chicago on September 22, 1927, to see the second Dempsey-Tunney fight with its controversial "long count" that helped Tunney retain the championship and earn $990,000 for thirty minutes of work. In a nation not oblivious to the approach of middle age, it was comforting to count the heavyweight champion of the world among the citizenry. Here was evidence, many reasoned, that the nation remained strong, young, and fit to survive in a Darwinian universe. Record-breaking served the same purpose, and in Johnny Weismuller, premier swimmer, and Paavo Nurmi, Finnish-born track star, the United States had athletes who set world marks almost every time they competed. Gertrude Ederle chose a longer course when she swam the English Channel in 1926, but she too set a record and was treated to one of New York's legendary ticker-tape parades.

And there was the Babe. No sports hero of the twenties and few of any decade had the reputation of George Herman Ruth. Baseball was generally acknowledged to be the national game, and Ruth played with a superb supporting cast of New York Yankees, but when he faced a pitcher Babe Ruth stood as an individual. His home runs (particularly the 59 in 1921 and the 60 in 1927) gave him a heroic stature comparable to that of legendary demigods like Odysseus, Beowulf, or Daniel Boone. Ruth's unsavory background and boorish personal habits were nicely overlooked by talented sportswriters anxious to give the twenties the kind of hero it craved. The payoff was public adulation of the Babe and of baseball.

The twenties also saw the public exposure of corruption in baseball and confronted Americans with the necessity of reviewing their entire hero complex. On September 28, 1920, three members of the Chicago White Sox appeared before a grand jury to confess that they and five other players had agreed to throw the 1919 World Series to Cincinnati for a financial consideration. Gradually the unhappy story of the "Black Sox" unfolded. Big-time gamblers had persuaded selected players to make sure that a bet on the underdog Cincinnati team would pay off. Some of the greatest names in the game were involved, preeminently that of "Shoeless" Joe Jackson. An illiterate farm boy from South Car-

olina, Jackson's natural batting eye helped him compile a .356 average in ten seasons as a major leaguer. In the process he became one of the most idolized players in baseball. It was Jackson's exit from the grand jury chamber on September 28 that allegedly precipitated the agonized plea from a group of boys: "Say it ain't so, Joe!" According to the newspapers, Jackson, shuffling, head down, replied, "Yes, boys, I'm afraid it is."

Reaction to the Black Sox testified to the importance baseball had for many Americans. One school of thought condemned the "fix" in the strongest terms and agitated for the restoration of integrity to the game. It was a serious matter. The Philadelphia *Bulletin* compared the eight players with "the soldier or sailor who would sell out his country and its flag in time of war." Suggesting the link between sports and the national character, the *New York Times* declared that bribing a ballplayer was an offense "which strikes at the very heart of this nation." If baseball fell from grace, what could be honest in America? The question haunted journalists and cartoonists. *Outlook* for October 13, 1920, carried a drawing of a crumpled statue of a ballplayer whose torn side revealed a stuffing of dollar bills. The statue bore the inscription "The National Game." A small boy wept in the foreground; the caption to the cartoon read "His Idol."

Baseball officials and club owners were similarly dismayed at the revelation of corruption and determined to clean up the game. Charles A. Comiskey, owner of the Chicago White Sox, led the way with a public statement that no man involved in the fix would ever wear the uniform of his club again. Other owners followed suit until all organized baseball, even the minor leagues, was closed to the Black Sox. On November 12, 1920, Kenesaw Mountain Landis, a former federal judge, was appointed commissioner of baseball with full control over the game and a charge to safeguard its integrity.

The everyday fans' response to the fix differed sharply from that of the sportswriters and owners. Many Americans seemed determined to deny the entire affair; more precisely, they didn't *want* to believe anything could be wrong with something as close to the national ideal as baseball. Like the boys of the "say it ain't so" episode, they begged for evidence that the old standards and values still applied. Especially in 1920 in the United States sports heroes were needed as evidence of the virtues of competition, fair play, and the self-reliant individual. Consequently, when confronted with the scandal, the average American simply closed his eyes and pretended nothing was wrong. The heroes remained heroes. When the Black Sox formed an exhibition team, it received enthusiastic support. Petitions were circulated in the major league cities to reinstate the players in organized baseball. But the most remarkable demonstration of the public's feeling came at the conclusion of the Black Sox trial on August 2, 1921. After deliberating two hours and forty-seven minutes, the jury returned a verdict of *not* guilty. According to the *New York Times* reporter at the scene, the packed courtroom rose as one man at the good news, cheering wildly. Hats sailed and papers were thrown about in the delirium. Men shouted "hooray for the clean sox." The bailiffs pounded for order until, as the *Times* reported, they "finally noticed Judge Friend's smiles, and then joined in the whistling and cheering." Finally the jury picked up the acquitted ballplayers and carried them out of the courtroom on their shoulders!

Baseball officials and journalists regarded the acquittal of the Black Sox as a technical verdict secured by the lenient interpretation of the Illinois statute involved. The fans in the courtroom, however, and, presumably, many elsewhere were on the side of the players regardless, and viewed the verdict as a vindication. They were not prepared to believe that baseball or its heroes could become tarnished. The game was too important to the national ego. Following baseball gave Americans an opportunity to pay tribute to what many believed was the best part of their heritage. The game was a sacred rite undertaken not merely to determine the winner of league championships but to celebrate the values

of a civilization. As one newspaper account of the scandal put it, to learn that "Shoeless" Joe Jackson had sold out the world series was like discovering that "Daniel Boone had been bought by the Indians to lose his fights in Kentucky."

In the gallery of popular heroes in the United States the only rival of the frontiersman and his athletic surrogate was the self-made man. In the 1920s the archtype was Herbert Hoover, a hero-President hewn out of the traditional rags-to-riches mold. Left an orphan in 1884 at the age of ten, Hoover launched an international career in mining that made him rich. During World War I he became famous, heading the American Relief Commission abroad and the Food Administration at home. A genius in matters of large-scale efficiency, Hoover neatly executed apparent miracles. After the decline of Woodrow Wilson in the wake of the Versailles Treaty, Hoover was easily the foremost American beneficiary of war-caused popularity. In 1922, while Secretary of Commerce under Warren G. Harding, he set forth his creed in a slender book entitled *American Individualism.* Apparently oblivious of the doubts that beset intellectuals at the time, Hoover professed his "abiding faith in the intelligence, the initiative, the character, the courage, and the divine touch in the individual." But he also believed that individuals differed greatly in energy, ability, and ambition. Some men inevitably rose to the top of the heap, and for Hoover this was entirely right and proper. It was necessary, moreover, if society were to progress. Hoover's philosophy was the old American one of rugged individualism and free enterprise that the Social Darwinists had decorated with scientific tinsel after the Civil War. Intellectually, Hoover was a bedfellow with Benjamin Franklin and William Graham Sumner.

Hoover's social, political, and economic ideas followed from these assumptions. He staunchly defended the unregulated profit system. Society and government owed the people only three things: "liberty, justice, and equality of opportunity." Competition took care of the rest, carrying the deserving to their just rewards and the failures to deserved defeat. Any interference, such as philanthropy to the poor or favoritism to the rich, only dulled *"the emery wheel of competition."* To be sure, Hoover paid lip service to restricting the strong in the interest of the society, but the main thrust of his thought awarded the victors their spoils. Critics were disarmed with three words—"equality of opportunity." The state should interfere to preserve it; otherwise, hands off! An exponent of the gospel of efficiency in economic affairs, Hoover believed that the road to the good life lay in the direction of more and better production. His mind equated material success with progress.

In the concluding chapter of *American Individualism,* Hoover drew the connection between his philosophy and the frontier. "The American pioneer," he declared, "is the epic expression of . . . individualism and the pioneer spirit is the response to the challenge of opportunity, to the challenge of nature, to the challenge of life, to the call of the frontier." Undismayed by the ending of the geographical frontier in the United States, Hoover declared that "there will always be a frontier to conquer or to hold to as long as men think, plan, and dare. . . . The days of the pioneer are not over."

When Hoover was elected President in 1928, these ideals were accorded the nation's highest accolade. They dominated popular thought as they had for three centuries of American history. In fact, all the men who occupied the Presidency from 1917 to 1930 were distinctly old-fashioned in their beliefs and in their public image. The traits are so familiar as to require listing only: Wilson the moralist and idealist; Harding the exemplar of small-town, "just folks" normalcy; Coolidge the frugal, farm-oriented Puritan; and Hoover the self-made man. If there was any correlation between a people's taste and its Presidents, then the record of this period underscored nostalgia.

Rivalling Hoover in the public mind of the early 1920s as an exponent of self-help and individualism was Edward Bok, the Dutch boy who made good and wrote about it in *The Americanization of Edward Bok* (1920). The book described Bok's immigration from Holland in 1870 at the age of six and his rise from a fifty-cents-a-week window cleaner to editor of the magazine with the largest circulation in the nation, the *Ladies Home Journal.* Bok's autobiography reads as a paean to the American ideal of success. Through luck, pluck, and clean living, he became a confidant and friend of Presidents. Thrift and determination made him rich. Bok played the rags to riches theme to the hilt. "Here was a little Dutch boy," he wrote in his preface, "unceremoniously set down in America . . . yet, it must be confessed, he achieved." His book, Bok promised, would describe "how such a boy, with every disadvantage to overcome, was able . . . to 'make good.' "

In the final chapters of his autobiography, Bok stepped back to comment on the liabilities and advantages of America. He did not slight the former, yet in "What I Owe to America" Bok brushed all debits aside in order to celebrate America's gift of "limitless opportunity: here a man can go as far as his abilities will carry him." For anyone "endowed with honest endeavor, ceaseless industry, and the ability to carry through, . . . the way is wide open to the will to succeed."

The public reception of *The Americanization of Edward Bok* suggests how much Americans in the 1920s wanted to confirm old beliefs. Bok was a hero in the Benjamin Franklin-Horatio Alger mold. His success story demonstrated that passing time and changing conditions had not altered hallowed ideals. His pages suggested no troubling doubts, and, after receiving the Pulitzer Prize for biography in 1921, Bok's book became a best-seller. An inexpensive eighth edition issued in July 1921 enabled it to attain third place on the 1922 lists. But the primary reason for Bok's popularity as hero-author was his ability to tell a nervous generation what it wanted to hear.

It has long puzzled students of the Great Crash of 1929 why even the most informed observers in education and government as well as business did not recognize and heed the prior economic danger signals that in retrospect seem so apparent. Part of the explanation possibly lies in the depth of the general commitment to the ideals of rugged individualism and free enterprise that Hoover and Bok articulated and symbolized. This commitment, in turn, lay in the nervousness of the American people. So much about the twenties was new and disturbing that Americans tended to cling tightly to familiar economic forms. They just could not bear to admit that the old business premises based on individualism and free enterprise might be fraught with peril. With Herbert Hoover leading the way, they chose to go down with the economic ship rather than question and alter its suicidal course.

Respect for the old-time hero was evident in other aspects of postwar thought. The vogue of the Boy Scouts is an example. Although the movement began in 1910, the twenties was the time of its flowering. There were 245,000 Scouts at the beginning of 1917, 942,500 at the end of 1929. In addition, 275,000 adults volunteered their services as leaders. No youth club and few adult organizations matched this record. The Boy Scout Handbook, a manual of ideals and instruction, sold millions of copies. Scouting, apparently, tapped fertile soil in its embodiment of the old-time idea of good citizenship and expertise in the outdoors. The Scout, standing straight in his shorts or knickers and doing the daily good deed that his oath required, was the epitome of the traditional American model of heroic young manhood.

In the late 1920s the Boy Scout *Handbook* featured an unusual drawing. In the foreground was a clean-cut Scout, eyes fixed on adventure. Behind him, signifying the heritage from which he sprang, were the figures of Daniel Boone, Abraham Lincoln, and Theodore Roosevelt, men who were staples in the annals of American heroism. But there was also a new face, that of Charles A. Lindbergh of Minnesota. At the age of just twenty-five Lindbergh rose to the status of an American demigod by virtue of a single feat. On May 20, 1927, he took off in a tiny single-engine airplane from New York City and thirty-three hours later landed in Paris. The nonstop, solo run across the Atlantic catapulted the average American into a paroxysm of pride and joy. Overnight Lindbergh became the greatest hero of the decade. There was but little exaggeration in the contention of one journalist that Lindbergh received "the greatest ovation in history." Certainly his return from Paris to the United States generated a reception extraordinary even for an age that specialized in ballyhoo. The *New York Times* devoted more space to Lindbergh's return than it had to the Armistice ending World War I. A virtual national religion took shape around Lindbergh's person. A 1928 poll of schoolboys in a typical American town on the question of whom they most wanted to be like produced the following results: Gene Tunney, 13 votes; John Pershing, 14; Alfred E. Smith, 16; Thomas A. Edison, 27; Henry Ford, 66; Calvin Coolidge, 110; Charles A. Lindbergh, 363. If the amount of national adulation is meaningful, adults everywhere would likely have responded in similar proportions.

The explanation of Lindbergh's popularity lies less in his feat (pilots had flown across the Atlantic before) and more in the mood of the people at the time it occurred. The typical American in 1927 was nervous. The values by which he ordered his life seemed in jeopardy of being swept away by the force of growth and change and complexity. Lindbergh came as a restorative tonic. He reasserted the image of the confident, quietly courageous, and self-reliant individual. He proved to a generation anxious for proof that Americans were still capable of pioneering. Even in an age of machines the frontier was not dead—a new one had been found in the air.

The reaction to Lindbergh's flight in the national press stressed these ideas. "Lindbergh served as a metaphor," wrote one commentator in *Century*. "We felt that in him we, too, had conquered something and regained lost ground." A writer in *Outlook* made the point

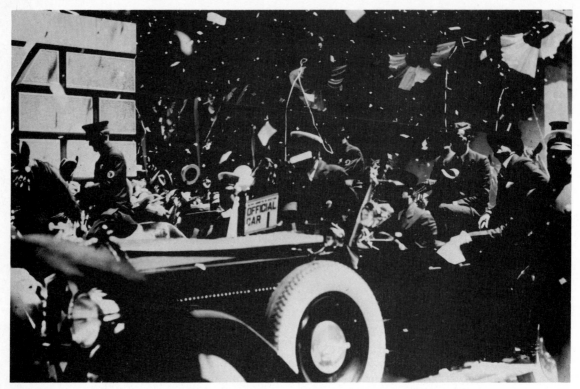

■ ■ *The New York City ticker-tape parade for aviator Charles Lindbergh on June 14, 1927, attracted more than three million wildly enthusiastic spectators.*

more explicitly: "Charles Lindbergh is the heir of all that we like to think is best in America. He is the stuff out of which have been made the pioneers that opened up the wilderness first on the Atlantic coast, and then in our great West." A newspaper cartoon showed a covered wagon leaving for California in 1849 and next to it Lindbergh's plane taking off for Paris in 1927. Colonel Theodore Roosevelt, the son of the President, remarked that Lindbergh "personifies the daring of youth. Daniel Boone, David Crockett, and men of that type played a lone hand and made America. Lindbergh is their lineal descendant." Calvin Coolidge, who personally welcomed Lindbergh home, simply said that he was "a boy representing the best traditions of this country."

For one journalist the most significant part of

the Lindbergh phenomenon was not the flight but the character of the man: "his courage, his modesty, his self-control, his sanity, his thoughtfulness of others, his fine sense of proportion, his loyalty, his unswerving adherence to the course that seemed right." His unassuming manner fit the traditional hero's mold. Many observers of the postflight celebration noted how the hero refused to capitalize financially on his popularity. It was telling evidence as an essayist put it, that the American people "are *not* rotten at the core, but morally sound and sweet and good!" The generalization from the individual to society was easily acceptable because Americans in 1927 desperately wanted to keep the old creed alive. Lindbergh's flight was popularly interpreted as a flight of faith—in the American experience and in the American people.

Looking back over the 1920s F. Scott Fitzgerald remembered in 1931 that "in the spring of 1927, something bright and alien flashed across the sky. A young Minnesotan who seemed to have nothing to do with his generation did a heroic thing, and for a moment people set down their glasses in country clubs and speakeasies and thought of their old best dreams." Also in 1931 Frederick Lewis Allen recalled that Lindbergh had been "a modern Galahad for a generation which had foresworn Galahads." Both Fitzgerald and Allen were right in their assessment of the public reaction to Lindbergh's flight, but wrong about the dreams he engendered being foreign to the 1920s. Fitzgerald notwithstanding, Lindbergh had a great deal to do with his generation. Allen to the contrary, the Lindbergh craze was not a case of Americans returning to ideals they had forsaken; they had never left them.

Popular books as well as heroes revealed the American mind in the 1920s, and the great majority of the best-sellers of the decade were decidedly old-fashioned. Frontier and rural patterns of thought and action dominated the popular novels. Their plots and protagonists operated according to time-honored standards of competition, loyalty, and rugged individualism. Complications were few and usually resolved, in the final pages, with an application of traditional morality. The total effect was a comforting reaffirmation of the old American faith. Such novels, to be sure, made slight contribution to serious American literature. But they were read—by millions! And they both influenced and reflected the mood of Americans who had never even heard of Fitzgerald and Hemingway. Indeed in comparison to best-selling authors, the Fitzgeralds and Hemingways were highly esoteric.

Exact figures are elusive, but it would be difficult to dispute Gene (Geneva) Stratton-Porter's claim to preeminence among popular novelists in the first three decades of the twentieth century. Her vogue began with *Freckles* in 1904 and continued right through the war, into the twenties, and beyond. In 1932 a *Publisher's Weekly*

survey of the best-selling novels of the century revealed Porter in the top four positions with *Freckles, The Girl of the Limberlost* (1909), *The Harvester* (1911), and *Laddie* (1913). Each had sold well over a million copies. With other titles Porter made the "top ten" list in 1918, 1919, 1921, and 1925. Most of her sales were in fifty-cent reprint editions, suggesting that her public consisted of relatively unsophisticated readers.

Gene Stratton-Porter found a publishing bonanza by articulating the values to which a large part of the American reading public subscribed. Chief among them was a belief in the virtue of close association with nature. As a girl Porter ran in the swamps, woods, and fields around Wabash, Indiana, and the characters in her novels do likewise. The experience was represented as inspirational in the highest sense. Nature was not only a source of beauty and contentment but a repository of moral and religious truth. The outdoors provided a constant backdrop in Porter's stories. Indeed the margins of her books were sometimes adorned with pen and ink drawings of birds, animals, and flowers. *The Harvesters* was dedicated to Henry David Thoreau.

Second only to nature in Porter's scale of values was cheerfulness. Her stories expound the benefits of optimism, confidence, courage, and keeping a stiff upper lip. Typically the plots involve the protagonist, frequently a child, in a series of adversities. But looking for the silver lining and heeding the teachings of nature eventually resolve all problems. *Freckles,* for instance, describes a boy who believes himself an orphan, wanders in the Limberlost swamp, and is ultimately found and claimed by his wealthy father. Eleanora of *A Girl of the Limberlost* defies poverty by selling the moths she collected in the swamp. In *Michael O'Halloran* Porter copied the Horatio Alger formula, taking a little newsboy up the success ladder on the wings of determination and pluck.

Porter's novels appealed to the kind of American whose eyes glazed and even dampened when they thought of the good old days when life was simple and generally lived in close proximity to nature. In Porter one basked momentarily in an uncomplicated world where virtue triumphed and right prevailed. Much of Porter's public seemed to consist of people displaced or crushed by modern American civilization. Letters of appreciation poured in to her from sanitariums, rest homes, reform schools, and jails. But in a larger sense the uncertainties and nervousness of the age in general provided a milieu in which her kind of writing could flourish.

William Lyon Phelps once wrote of Gene Stratton-Porter, "she is a public institution, like Yellowstone Park, and I should not think she would care any more than a mountain for adverse criticism." In fact, Porter did care. She habitually replied to her unfavorable reviewers in lengthy letters. In one she responded to a critic who had labelled her writing "molasses fiction." This was really a compliment, rejoined Porter: "molasses is more necessary to the happiness of human and beast than vinegar. . . . I am a molasses person myself. . . . So I shall keep straight on writing of the love and joy of life . . . and when I have used the last drop of my molasses, I shall stop writing." She closed the letter with a hint of conceit: "God gave me a taste for sweets and the sales of the books I write prove that a few other people are similar to me in this."

Harold Bell Wright rivaled Gene Stratton-Porter as a dispenser of wholesomeness, optimism, and the arcadian myth. His *The Winning of Barbara Worth* (1911) had a half million copies in print within a month of its initial publication and maintained sufficient popularity to rank fifth, behind Porter's four books, in the 1932 best-selling novels of the century poll. After *Barbara Worth* Wright produced a novel every other year for two decades. Americans seemed as eager to buy and read his books after the war as before. His first twelve books enjoyed an average sale of nearly 750,000 each.

A sometime minister, Wright sermonized constantly in his novels. Until the final typing no character in any had a name except that of his main trait—Hypocrisy, Greed, Ambition, and so

on. Wright's message was the familiar one: clean living, hard work, and contact with God's great open spaces could save a man from the physical and moral deterioration city life engendered. *When a Man's a Man* of 1916, for example, features a millionaire who goes west to escape the effete, artificial, decadent East. Its setting on an Arizona cattle ranch reflected Wright's own enthusiasm for the Southwest that led him to make his home there. Wright also loved Missouri's Ozark Mountains, and the region figured in a number of his stories. *The Re-Creation of Brian Kent*, third on the best-seller list for 1920, employs an Ozark setting to tell the story of a human wreck who is redeemed by the beauty of nature, the challenge of work, and a woman's love. An elderly schoolmarm, identified only as Auntie Sue, supervises the transformation and extracts the moral.

The stereotyped plots and characters, the wooden dialogue, and the commonplace preaching in Wright's books elicited a barrage of unfavorable criticism. According to one reviewer in 1924, Wright was guilty of perpetuating "the shibboleths and superstitions of our fathers, making old creeds and antique fables sacred in the eyes of all." And so he did. Yet his stories sold millions of copies. A large number of American readers found his message comfortable and meaningful. "Harold," one critic punned, "is always Wright." But for the popular mind of the teens and twenties ethical certainty was highly valued, and traditional mores seemed the most certain. The intellectuals might scoff, but Wright, like Porter, found the goldmine of popular favor.

The western novel, which Owen Wister introduced into American writing in 1902 with *The Virginian*, increased in popularity as the nation moved increasingly further from frontier conditions. The foremost practitioner of the art in the decade after World War I was a one-time dentist from Zanesville, Ohio, named Zane Grey. Blending minor literary talent with a keen sense of the public taste, Grey produced over fifty westerns and provided the basis for dozens of motion pictures, many of which were produced in the early 1920s before the advent of sound tracks. The total sale of all his writings approaches twenty million. From 1917 to 1924 Grey was never *off* the national list of the top ten best-sellers. Twice, 1918 and 1920, he ranked first. He may well have been the most widely read author in the American twenties.

The Zane Grey magic was a blend of violence, heroism, and the frontier. His stories lacked sophistication, but they juxtaposed good and evil in unmistakable terms. Titanic struggles might be waged, but the issues were always clearly defined and the outcome, as Grey fans came to learn, never really in doubt. A simple code of conduct suffused Grey's books. It emphasized courage, self-reliance, fair play, and persistence—the traditional frontier virtues. Those who violated the code always paid the price.

As a mythmaker for the multitudes in the 1920s, Zane Grey became as legendary as his protagonists. Many people believed he spoke for the best parts of the national heritage. John Wanamaker, the department store mogul, addressed him directly: "never lay down your pen, Zane Grey. . . .You are distinctively and genuinely American. You have borrowed none of the decadence of foreign writers. . . . The good you are doing is incalculable." Even the critics treated Grey more tolerantly than they did Porter and Wright. "We turn to him," one commentator wrote, "not for insight into human nature and human problems nor for refinements of art, but simply for crude epic stories, as we might to an old Norse skald, maker of the sagas of the folk."

The concept of escape from the present, so important in the appeal of many of the best-selling popular novels in the twenties, reached a climax in the writing of Edgar Rice Burroughs. A failure for years in business and pulp magazine writing, Burroughs turned to a new theme in 1914 and struck pure gold. *Tarzan of the Apes* has probably sold more copies to date (over five mil-

lion) than any other American book. Over thirty other stories of the English orphan reared in the African jungle by apes followed. As early as 1920 the Tarzan cult was nationwide. Burroughs was syndicated in newspapers; his motion pictures reached millions of people. With his superhuman prowess and his mate, Jane, Tarzan entered public thought and speech to an astonishing degree. For people vaguely repressed by civilization, Tarzan was a potent symbol of freedom, power, and individuality. A new wild man on a new frontier, Tarzan helped sustain traditional American values.

American readers seemed to have an unsatiable appetite for nature novels for the first three decades of the twentieth century. In addition to Porter, Wright, Grey, and Burroughs, a host of others rode the theme to publishing successes that were minor only in comparison. The names of Rex Beach, Peter B Kyne, Emerson Hough, and James Oliver Curwood were quite familiar to readers and moviegoers of the postwar decade even if they are not to most literary historians. Curwood, for instance, published between 1908 and 1926 twenty-six novels that dramatized the theme of courage in the wilderness. The motion pictures made from his books, such as *Back to God's Country* (1919), were intended, so an advertisement ran, for those who "love God's great out-of-doors, the land of frozen forests and everlasting snows where the gaunt wolf stalks its prey, where men loom large and life is big." In 1923 Hough's *The Covered Wagon* became the basis for the most famous western movie of the decade. Stewart Edward White rivalled both Curwood and Hough with books such as *The Blazed Trail, The Silent Places,* and *The Rules of the Game.* And that was it precisely—the game had rules that were at once easily perceived and rooted in the national character. If changing conditions were eroding the old certainties, that was only more reason to grasp them more tightly.

In popular fiction Americans of the 1920s were still inhabitants of the nineteenth century. The sexy novels of flaming youth and the risqué movies satisfied only part of the taste of the twenties. The other, and larger, part thrilled to old-time heroics such as those provided by the man Douglas Durkin sketched in *The Lobstick* *Trail* of 1922: "his blood was clean, his body knit of fibre woven in God's out-of-doors, his mind fashioned under a clear sky in a land of wide horizons."

■■■

STUDY QUESTIONS

1. What caused the nervousness that many Americans experienced in the 1920s?

2. What values were characteristic of America's pioneering past? How did the heroes of the 1920s demonstrate these values?

3. Why were sports so popular during the decade? How did athletic heroes help ease Americans' minds about the national character?

4. How were the popular images of Herbert Hoover and Charles Lindbergh similar? Why were both men considered heroes during the 1920s?

5. What were the characteristics of many popular novels during the 1920s? What type of stories did people enjoy reading about?

6. How were the novels of Gene Stratton-Porter, Harold Bell Wright, Zane Grey, and Edgar Rice Burroughs similar or different?

BIBLIOGRAPHY

The above section comes from Roderick Nash, *The Nervous Generation: American Thought, 1917–1930* (1970), which presents a view of the 1920s vastly different from Frederick Lewis Allen's. A good overview of the role of the hero in American culture is Leo Lowenthal, *Literature, Popular Culture and Society* (1961). The most important athletic heroes of the decade are discussed in Randy Roberts, *Jack Dempsey: The Manassa Mauler* (1979); Robert Creamer, *Babe* (1974); Marshall Smelser, *The Life that Ruth Built* (1975); Paul Gallico, *The Goddess People* (1965); and Frank Deford, *Big Bill Tilden: The Triumphs and the Tragedy* (1975). John W. Ward, "The Meaning of Lindbergh's Flight," *American Quarterly*, 10 (1958), is a classic study of the importance of heroism in the 1920s. On Lindbergh also see Walter S. Ross, *The Last Hero: Charles Lindbergh* (1976).

YOU ARE THE STAR: EVOLUTION OF THE THEATER PALACE, 1908–1929

Lary May

The emergence of a consumer culture was the most important development during the 1920s. Between 1922 and 1929, American industrial output nearly doubled, and the greatest growth took place in industries producing consumer goods—automobiles, household appliances, furniture, and clothing. At the same time, workers' wages rose steadily. To ensure continued growth and prosperity, businessmen and marketing experts encouraged Americans to buy and consume their products. Advertising specialists quickly attempted to associate consumption with the good life in the minds of millions of Americans. Success became associated with what a person owned rather than what he or she had accomplished.

Movie idols became the heroes and Hollywood the capital of this new culture of consumption. As Lary May writes in his study of the development of the motion picture industry, "The vague, mythic term 'Hollywood' connoted a way of life unfolding in the exclusive neighborhoods of Beverly Hills, Santa Monica, and Brentwood. Freed from any nearby reminders of social responsibility . . . the stars could create a new, uplifted life without the inhibitions of the past. Usually homes drew on styles of European, African, or Asian aristocracy, reflecting not only high culture, but the quest for a more exotic life." Perhaps no couple better captured the lure of consumption than Douglas Fairbanks and Mary Pickford. Both at their home Pickfair and on the silver screen, they showed millions of Americans that good healthy consumption was the only way to live.

Few Americans, however, could afford to purchase a Pickfair or live the way dashing Douglas and sweet Mary lived. Nevertheless, most Americans could afford to buy a ticket to see one of their movies. And once in one of the theater palaces, they too were allowed at least momentarily to experience the good life. In the following essay, Lary May discusses the development and meaning of the elaborate theaters of the 1920s.

E *qual opportunity came to mean not merely that each of us had a right to protect his interests with his vote, but that each of us had a right to stalk around in public places and live vicariously the life of the rich.*

CHARLES FERGUSON, "HIGH CLASS"
Harper's Monthly Magazine, 1932

Charles Ferguson's observations concerning the movie theaters spreading over the cities in the late teens and twenties captured a key ingredient of our story. Powerful and innovative as Pickford and Fairbanks were, they alone were not enough to validate the rise of a new economy and morality. Going to a movie meant much more than merely watching the screen. It was a total experience that immersed the fans directly in the life they saw in celluloid. Gradually, theater owners began to realize that they could heighten the immediacy of moviegoing. If entering the theater felt like coming into the star's home, the viewers could become part of that high life they watched in the darkened room. For a brief period during the day or evening, the happy ending was theirs, too. Nowhere was this more obvious than in the cathedrals of the motion pictures, which democratized the styles of elite estates or hotels on an unprecedented scale. A close examination of this phenomenon can help us understand why the masses could so closely identify with the stars. Who went to the movies, and what did they expect from them?

In the early period, theater owners catered to the immigrants' tastes for foreign films, pure entertainment, and shorts portraying their political and economic situation. Yet after 1908, they faced a quandary in attracting a more affluent audience for their recently uplifted product. They saw that movies were spreading. But they also knew that the nickelodeon was merely one

among many amusements appealing to the urban workers. Amid the hurly burly of the streets in 1910 there were 9,000 saloons and just 400 movie houses. An average poorer neighborhood in those days might have twenty nickelodeons which captured the attention of the respectable press and social workers. Still, the same areas might also have nearly a hundred saloons and twenty dance halls. Yet as the movie house moved uptown, it was not just one of many entertainments for the bourgeois. Rather, it was the only legitimized arena where the classes and sexes mingled. But it was left in an ambiguous situation. How could theater owners sanction an amusement that drew audiences precisely because it had been forbidden? Shrewd theater owners realized that if they could remove this unease without losing the allure, they could reap handsome profits.

Theater managers thus did everything possible to raise movies above their disreputable origins. The municipal codes and censorship board played an important role in this process. Like the movies themselves, the theaters benefitted from these reforms. For once the movie house earned a license, a more affluent clientele could enter the arena with some sense of safety. As a result, between 1908 and 1914, as films went from shorts to photoplays, nickelodeons changed from store fronts to more sumptuous buildings. Describing this process of elaboration, Adolph Zukor recalled that the "nickelodeon had to go, theaters replaced shooting galleries, temples replaced theaters, cathedrals replaced temples." Another exhibitor, Marcus Loew, refurbished his Brooklyn store front, and changed its name from the Cozy Corner to the Royal. In Chicago, the future head of Universal Pictures, Carl Laemmle, transformed his chain of nickelodeons into prestigious "White Fronts." Still others, such as A. J. Balaban of Chicago who would soon put together a large chain with Samuel Katz and merge it to Paramount Pictures, made the most of the synthesis of movies and reform. On his marquee he displayed a magnified copy of a letter from Jane Addams:

It is unfortunate that the five cent theaters have become associated in the public mind with the lurid and unworthy. Our experience at Hull House has left no doubt that in time the moving picture will be utilized for all purposes of education. The schools and churches will count film among its most valuable entertainment and equipment.

Balaban's tactics clearly reflected the wisdom of a shrewd businessman, ever ready to change his product for the better market. In New York, Boston, St. Louis, and Chicago, the pattern after 1908 was to open refined theaters in neighborhoods higher up the social order. As movie houses in Boston increased from thirty-one to forty-one in 1914, all the new ones opened in the wealthy suburbs of Roxbury, Dorchester, Cambridge, and Somerville. "For the first time in the history of the town," observed a reporter in the industry's major trade journal, "the selectmen of Brookline, Massachusetts, have decided to grant a license to a photoplay show." In the city's major cultural area of Brighton, three movie houses opened, despite the opposition of Mayor John F. Fitzgerald, grandfather of the future President Kennedy. Another opened across from the Boston Symphony, and the exclusive opera house at Potter Hall converted into a cinema. The same thing was happening all over. In Atlanta, for example, Walter P. Eaton noted in 1914, "You cannot of course draw any hard and fast line which will not be crossed at many points, but in Atlanta, Georgia, for example, you may often see automobiles parked two deep along the curb in front of a motion picture theater, which hardly suggests exclusively proletarian patronage."

Well-heeled motorists spurred theater owners to do everything in their power to keep the wheels pointed toward the movies. In this effort, they developed a whole literature on how to charge higher prices and bring in more wealthy patrons. Among the primary criteria were seating capacity and location. A high-class movie theater had to be located on a well-lit major thoroughfare. In part this was done to make it visible to a wider population. But it was also important to assure patrons of security. Patriotic symbols on the imposing marquees contributed to this respectability. Presumably, a packed house with a "crowded look" indicated that movies were acceptable to everyone, and no longer located in "dirty dives." It was equally crucial to raise the status of the proprietors themselves. One method was to have the well-dressed owner greet patrons at the door. Another was to raise the license fee from $25 for a "common show" to $500, the same as for a legitimate theater. At the same time, seating capacity was increased from a limit of 300 to over 1,000. With large investments at stake, exhibitors did everything to clean up their establishments, for they wanted no "trouble with the police." Finally, operators were cautioned to encourage a "mixed house" by avoiding programs slanted to one nationality, by eliminating ethnic vaudeville acts, and by discarding all songs in foreign languages. By 1916, New York had ten luxury houses, which the trade journals of the industry described as alternatives to the "gay and fatuous forms of degeneracy" among the rich and the "jaded appetites of the unwashed poor."

Theater architects also sought a middle ground between decadence and shabbiness. Between 1908 and 1914, proprietors saw that ladies and gentlemen would come to their establishments if movies houses mirrored the designs fashionable for public buildings at the time. Traditionally, this had required classical forms from Greece and Rome. Democrats equated the balance, clarity, and angularity of these styles with the order so necessary for a self-governing polity. During the Progressive era, the classical designs advocated by the Founding Fathers, combined with their French and Italian derivatives, infused a great architectural revival. Designers for the Chicago World's Fair as well as the City Beautiful movement all contributed to a proliferation of these motifs. When this was applied to the early movie theaters, at times it became a hodgepodge. But the Gothic, Romanesque, and romantic genres were usually framed by the

Doric, Ionic, or Corinthian pillars associated with classicism and reason. While this suggested that movies too were in line with the spirit of reform, it also reflected continuity with historical progress. Upon entering, the patron encountered an atmosphere that made no distinction between public and private values. Like libraries, state houses, and public buildings, the movie house would educate as it entertained.

A major director like Griffith considered these theaters ideal frames for his photoplays. In sober contrast to the ornate feudal styles popular among the very wealthy of New York and other large cities such as San Francisco and Chicago, classical architecture symbolized the moral middle. It also stood out with grandiose pretention against "low-life" structures housing saloons and penny arcades. Both of these high and low cultural styles reflected the values of a feudalistic, European tradition; but Griffith saw that Doric or Ionic styles remained true to "American sentiment and setting." In contrast to Gothic romanticism, classicism fit a public-spirited citizenry, radiating the designs of the early Americans "who drew their spirit from the Greeks and Romans" who "lived their lives with the same severity." Presumably, these theaters would inspire the self-discipline of the founding fathers, stoic men like Washington, Jefferson, Lee, and Patrick Henry. With such places complementing the democratic spirit of Griffith's own work, he explained that "if I had a son I would let him see pictures as he liked, because I believe they would keep his character along the most rigid lines of conduct. No one need fear it will deviate from the Puritan plane."

Classicism also fused the goals of the early film makers to those of the exhibitors. The trade journals in 1910 began calling for better films and more luxurious theaters in which to exhibit them. On the outside of such theaters as The Empress in Owensburg, Kentucky, The Superba in Grand Rapids, Michigan, The Star in Cherry Valley, New York, and The Elite in Carthage, Missouri, Grecian pillars graced the façades, and patriotic symbols and flags adorned the mar-

quees. Inside one might find the Statue of Liberty or American Eagles. Soon each had orchestras, a far cry from the pianos, organs, or even silence that accompanied the nickelodeons. Now operators hired professional musicians; and film makers such as Griffith synchronized their productions with specific pieces. The ride of the Klan in *The Birth of a Nation*, for example, followed the crescendo of Wagner's "The Ride of the Valkyries." Adding to the prestige value of classical music, the better theaters also featured conductors advertised as having studied with European maestros. Patriotic music such as "The Star Spangled Banner," "Yankee Doodle," "Dixie," and "My Country 'Tis of Thee" commonly heralded the openings of new theaters or special films in the period before the War. When these refined orchestras played jazz or ragtime, the honky-tonk quality associated with urban vice evaporated.

Best of all, these refinements were offered on an egalitarian basis. In contrast to the playhouses of the nineteenth century, all peoples mingled at the movies. Even when theaters moved into wealthier neighborhoods, the seating arrangements still were not sharply differentiated by rank. Although loges were slightly more expensive and the balconies still reserved for blacks, even the most expensive seats were not beyond the reach of patrons of modest means. In 1913, when it cost from 40¢ to $1.40 to see stage drama, movie admissions averaged a mere 7¢. There were two prices for cinema tickets, ranging from five to fifteen cents; but people of modest incomes could afford both. While this openness seemed dangerous in the store fronts, owners of refined movie houses encouraged a family crowd, safe even for unchaperoned females. During intermission, the screen often showed a picture of a startled woman being harassed by a strange man, with the caption, "If annoyed, tell the management." In addition, proprietors provided "kindergardens" where childen would be supervised during the picture. All this contributed to a sense of democratic morality. In 1913, one critic commented on the modern film house, which unlike the uptown stage theater had "emancipated the gallery" and created the "great audience" which was "none other than the people without distinction of class."

One of the most successful theater owners of New York City, William Fox, perceived that this required merging low life with high life. Like much of the early audience, Fox was a Jewish immigrant from Eastern Europe. At first he worked as a garment cutter and "sponger" in Manhattan's Lower East Side. Soon this skilled entrepreneur realized that those with a nickel or dime to pay for a show "outnumbered those willing to pay a dollar by a hundred to one." Beginning with nickelodeons, he graduated to store fronts and then luxury houses of classical design. Fox recalled that "the motion picture when it started did not appeal to the native born who had their own forms of recreation . . . its appeal was to foreigners who did not understand our tongue." But when vice crusaders cleaned up the movies, Fox turned New York's notorious Haymarket Saloon—the most famous pub in the vice district—into a white, Grecian-styled movie house. In this symbolic gesture, the up-and-coming theater magnate captured the aura of popular mingling and brought it into a proper atmosphere. As he wrote in 1912,

Movies breathe the spirit in which the country was founded, freedom and equality. In the motion picture theaters there are no separations of classes. Everyone enters the same way. There is no side door thrust upon those who sit in the less expensive seats. There is always something abhorrent in different entrances to theaters . . . in the movies the rich rub elbows with the poor and that's the way it should be. The motion picture is a distinctly American insitution.

A clear testimony to the power of this appeal came in 1913 when *Harper's* magazine asked Olivia Harriet Dunbar to go among the "riotous joy of the multitude" and describe the "lure of the films." While the editors of a prestigious magazine may have questioned the propriety of sending a woman to see the hurly-burly of the movies, they soon discovered that Dunbar actually liked the chaos. Patrons, she observed, flowed in and out of the theaters without paying any attention to formality. Once seated in front of the screen, they seemed to leave their status concerns and social roles behind. Inside the darkened room, the diverse audience was part of one crowd sitting passively "amid the strange turbulence of a nightmare." The half-slumbering viewers were drawn into one "oddly literal dream" after another. In a society noted for energy and order, these theaters seemed to "offer thousands of cases of disproof of all that has been fallaciously said regarding the restless energy of the American." Crowds came and went, films danced on the screen, yet through it all, there was protection for "endangered girlhood" and a refined atmosphere, evoking "emotions in conformity with the orthodox code."

Gradually, theater managers realized that movie patrons wanted more than a perpetuation of civic proprieties; they wanted a release from daily concerns as well. In this, fans appropriately looked to the movies for a new and glamorous facet of urban culture: nightlife. Perhaps the best example of this after 1910 was New York City's Broadway. As the largest thoroughfare of mid-Manhattan, it had long brought together the upper middle-class . . . and the immigrants. . . . In the twentieth century, this common meeting ground was complemented by perhaps one of the most unique developments of the period, the ability of electricity to turn the night into day. Even though gaslight had been available earlier, the brilliance of electricity was magical. Now it was possible for groups to escape the cares of the day on the "Great White Way" at night. Advertisers lit up the evening darkness with huge billboards; and ambitious theater managers capitalized on this electrifying atmosphere by using multicolored bulbs on their marquees. A reporter for *The Atlantic Monthly* described the scene in 1910: "When I walk down Broadway, I want to shout for joy it is so beautiful." Charles Chaplin also appreciated the magnificence of Broadway. Seeing it for the first time as a young immigrant in 1912, he recalled that "it began to light up with myriad colored lights and electric bulbs that sparkled like an electric jewel. And in the warm night, my attitude changed and the meaning of America became clear to me: the tall skyscrapers, the brilliant gay lights, the thrilling display of advertisements stirred me with a sense of hope and adventure."

Realizing this appeal, managers started consciously to identify moviegoing with the atmosphere of nightlife. The dancing marquee lights foreshadowed the medium itself. Seated in a darkened room, the audience participated in an experience that was, in an often quoted phrase, "hypnotic." While a legitimate theater divided the story with a rising and falling curtain, the film continued without break from beginning to end. Instead of actors and actresses performing on an artificial stage, events on film took place in real surroundings. The director "brought the players right into your lap, not the least flicker of emotion was lost." Magnified so many times larger than life, the star seemed to have unusual qualities of emotional power. The viewer entering the theater, consequently, expected to *feel,* as well as see, the star's charisma. As *Reel Life* explained this vicarious thrill, "To have world famous celebrities brought to your very door, to meet people of great renown face to face, to be able to observe their little everyday mannerisms and become really acquainted with them on the motion picture screen, is of absorbing interest to everyone."

After 1914, theater owners were more conscious of infusing their movie houses with these same emotional and personal qualities. This appeared most symbolically in the slow decline of theaters built with classical design, which had been linked to the rational concerns of daytime. As the popularity of film makers such as Griffith gave way to the rebellious quest for newness of Pickford and Fairbanks, owners started to integrate more elaborate foreign motifs into their buildings. Commenting on the decline of classic balanced forms, one theater architect wrote, "It is difficult to reconcile gaiety of architectural expression with the style of ancient Greece." In

other words, no longer could an owner simply imitate the pragmatic, rational look of public buildings. New theaters had to radiate unique exotic qualities capable of standing out in sharp juxtaposition from the surrounding businesses. As one builder explained, "An exterior design in which the curves of graceful arches predominate provides a pleasing contrast to the cold, straightforward lines of the usual service buildings."

One way to heighten the appeal of night time play was to draw on designs of northern Europe, and make the theater a magnificent palace that emulated the hotels, restaurants, and estates of the very rich. Although hotel proprietors of the nineteenth century had utilized this concept to attract settlers to boom towns, or to high-light the splendor of their cities, the quest for magnificence found its greatest model in the innovations pioneered by John Jacob Astor III's son, who built the Waldorf Astoria in New York. This glittering hotel graced the society pages of newspapers in the eighties and nineties, showing urban readers the life of those who had money. Corridors and dining rooms adorned with marble, mahogany, and mirrors gave rich men an opportunity to show off their women laden with fine clothes and jewels. Yet there was no doubt that the wealthy had exclusive entry rights to this prohibitively expensive Renaissance playground. Here and in other French and Italian-styled edifices up and down Fifth Avenue, the industrial titans and their families could "lead an expensive, gregarious life as publicly as possible."

One of the great innovations of theater owners was to bring "big rich" opulence within the reach of millions of urbanites. Precisely at the time when Broadway players were entering the movies, perceptive proprietors were converting luxurious playhouses into cinemas. It was obvious that nothing brought people downtown like a first-run house which emulated the domains of the wealthy uptown. Indeed, the idea was to make aristocratic splendor a modern necessity. The head of New York's largest theater chain, Marcus Loew, articulated this philosophy: "The gorgeous theater is a luxury and it is easy to become accustomed to luxury and hard to give it up once you have tasted it." Given this expanding demand, it was easy to raise prices, for managers knew that the middle-class audience would pay for prestige, as long as it was not prohibitive. "If the patrons don't like it," wrote Carl Laemmle as he raised his entry fees, "tell them that's the way they do it in Europe." In other words, the lavish, expensive environment increased the allure of the movies. It may have been as important as the film itself.

As the movie house drew on extravagant styles, it went even one step further in capturing the appeal of mass culture: it signaled a release from everyday inhibitions, tapping the quest for post-Victorian freedom. In this transformation, motifs became more "barbaric" or "primitive." At first, managers, tried to capture the ambiance of the film by filling the theater with artifacts from the movie's era. Pickford's *Ali Baba and the Forty Thieves,* for example, might be shown in an auditorium laden with Arabian decor. Soon the entire edifice would exude this romance. The exoticism of ancient lands, the Far and Near East, American Indians, India, Latin America, or the "Dark Ages" began inspiring downtown houses in the late teens. Undulating spires, curving pillars, and floating or towering ceilings were a far cry from classical balance and proportion. Another device for accomplishing a similar effect was to duplicate nature inside of the auditorium. In these "atmospherics," explained one designer, the idea was to create the Italian countryside with murals, piazzas, and gardens, complete with artificial shrubbery and domes painted like the sky. In one of the first theaters to employ these devices, the Riviera in Chicago, the interior duplicated the Mediterranean. Here the viewer could feel free from the limits of time and space, similar to the celluloid itself. "With a little architectural hocus-pocus," wrote Lewis Mumford of these theaters, "we transport ourselves to another age, another climate, another historical regime, and best of all to another system of aesthetics.

Everything in the theater palace heightened the break from the "machine-like world." Enter-

ing the lobby, patrons beheld a "world of nations," filled with fine furnishings, tapestries, statues, and rugs from the four corners of the globe. Mirrors covering entire walls let the fans see themselves amid this luxury. Descending the sumptuous staircases in the huge lobby, patrons entered like announced guests at a grand ball. As the stars appeared amid luxury on the screen, the viewers saw their own images framed in elegance in the carefully angled mirrors in the halls. Even one's private moments were graced with the trappings of wealth, for the gilt and tile ladened restrooms were equally lavish. Ladies could adorn themselves under lights that complimented their complexions, so they might resemble their sisters on the screen. Inside the auditorium itself, proprietors utilized a "science" of colored lighting to set the mood: red for Latin passion, pastels for Scandinavian idealism. Fans blowing over ice to "banish the summer heat" further closed out the discomforts of the real world.

Above all, the lavish theater had to be a personalized place where the fan felt unique and important. One of the most successful theater owners, A. J. Balaban, realized how crucial it was to provide a contrast to the anonymity of the city. In 1905 Balaban left his job as a factory laborer and entered the entertainment business. After vice crusades closed his dance hall, where wives and single women often fraternized with foreign males, Balaban opened a movie house approved by the reformers. Soon he became the most successful theater owner in Chicago, and standardized his techniques for the hundreds of first-run cinemas owned by Paramount Pictures in the twenties. First he taught employees how to behave. As extensions of the proprietor, they had to greet patrons at the door. Uniformed ushers served as the palace guard for the democratic nobles. Each young man "picked for educational and home discipline" greeted the customer with a smile and a respectful "Ma'am" or "Sir." He controlled the flow of the crowd, and escorted ladies and gentlemen to their seats. Lights on the side aisles that allowed the ushers to evict disorderly elements contributed to this sense of safety.

Most important, Balaban's ushers had to be young and friendly. This was necessary because, for all its appeal, there was a slightly uncomfortable aura of luxury and status surrounding the theates. In America, this look of aristocratic splendor had been reserved for the industrial titans or mercantile elites, groups disdained by much of the populace. Since the theaters were indeed filled with "fine furnishings" and "fountains fit for mansions and kings," Balaban warned that ushers had to soften the sense of pretension and power that went with this atmosphere. So the youthful ushers were instructed to act without condescension, and to treat all customers as friends as well as ladies and gentlemen, equal to anyone in the outside world. Smiles and cordiality presumably would dissolve any connotations of snobbishness; and the youthfulness promised that moviegoing would be relaxing, free of the power relations and corruptions of the everyday world. The well-stroked patron by this time felt like "somebody," and was now ready for some good, clean fun.

Typical of this ethic were the theaters run by Samuel Lionel Rothafel, the future "Roxy." His establishments clearly showed how the styles of the rich mansions and cabarets were trickling down the social order. Rothafel knew that in an atmosphere of luxury it was necessary to dissolve the upper-class pretension. To stimulate wide participation, the public had to know it was "their theater." At the Regent in 1915, Rothafel first applied the formula he would later take into more elaborate New York theaters like the Capitol and the Roxy. Built near Columbia University, a solidly middle-class area, the Regent was noted for its French Renaissance decor, spread over an elaborate, brightly lit facade. The auditorium included colored lights, a flowing fountain, an elaborate orchestra, and aristocratic furnishings, with "not an ounce of dust." Each patron was made "to feel wanted" by the usher. In his competent hands, the customer was freed from the responsibilities and cares of the day. This formula was duplicated across the country in "Million Dollar" cinemas. As one insightful observer

noted, "They offered a gilded mansion for the weekly invasion of those who lived in stuffy apartments, a gorgeous canopy to spread over a cramped and limited life, a firmament for cliff dwellers, a place where even the most menial can stalk about with the vague feeling for the moment that we have taken hold of romance."

Contributing to the illusion of status was the movie premiere. Long a practice among the elite, the premiere of an opening play provided the opportunity for wealthy and famous people to promenade in public. This idea was brought to the movies almost without alteration starting about 1913. At first trade journals argued that by getting the local leaders to attend a film, they could gain legitimacy for moviegoing itself. Gradually, however, it became more than this. True to their growing conception of themselves as democratic rulers, the Carnegies, the Lodges, Roosevelts, Vanderbilts, and other members of the Four Hundred accepted invitations to opening nights. In 1914, Mrs. Vanderbilt even wrote a letter of commendation to Harry Aitkin of Triangle Company, complimenting him on his fine theater and the patriotism in his films. Aitkin advertised throughout the countryside other big names who had commended his movie, gathering even wider interest. When his productions opened to the public the day following the premiere, fans thronged to partake of what the big rich had sampled, for only fifteen or twenty cents. One shrewd observer recognized how this phenomenon tapped the desire for vicarious status:

Up to the capacities of our tastes and incomes, the rest of us followed in the footsteps of our financial overlords; for whenever we can break from our anonymous cubicles, our standardized offices, our undifferentiated streets, we abandon ourselves to Pure Romance.

By the 1920s, the stars themselves were the notables attending premieres at even more extravagant theaters like the Roxy and Radio City Music Hall in New York. Perhaps the most

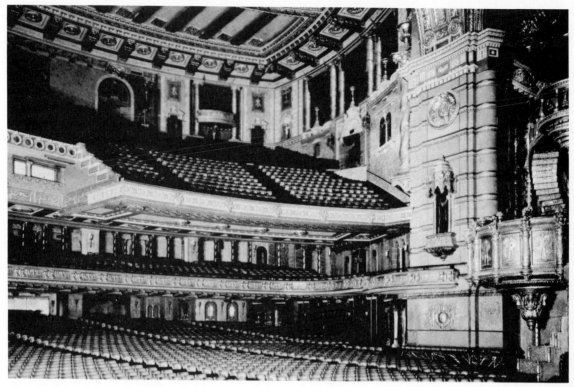

The Roxy Theatre, Manhattan. Opulent surroundings contributed greatly to the whole pleasurable experience of "going to the movies" in the 1920s.

elaborate example of stardom fused to opulence was Sid Grauman's Chinese Theater in Los Angeles. Grauman, the son of an immigrant vaudeville manager, built the Chinese in 1927, modeled on a Mandarin palace from a time when the "world was young." In a grand synthesis, this Jewish entrepreneur borrowed a tradition from European Catholics and placed it in an Oriental setting in the middle of Hollywood: it was Grauman's brainchild to invite celebrities of the industry to place their hands and feet in the wet cement of the theater's patio. Significantly, Pickford and Fairbanks were the first players to be so honored. This served a dual purpose. As the cement dried, leaving an indelible print, it gave the stars a sense of immortality. But it also allowed the patrons to measure their own features against these relics of their saints. After touching the sacred indentations, the viewers entered a mammoth auditorium where they saw these same idols moving before their very eyes. Grauman made certain that everything in the theater provided an "atmosphere in which the patron actually lived with the characters on the screen."

Grauman's Chinese culminated a trend that had penetrated northern urban centers for two decades. Beneath the evolution of the theater palace from 1908 to 1929 lay one key development: from a pariah nickelodeon, the motion picture had become a major urban institution for the middle class. And the sheer number and size of movie houses reflected the overwhelming popularity of the mature movie industry. In New

York City, ninety-seven nickelodeons held licenses in 1900. All observers agreed that they were located either in the cheap business sections or in the poorer amusement centers, and usually frequented by men. Nine years later there were 400, including several "store fronts" which were hastily converted shops showing "flickers" on a screen. Seating capacity was limited to 400. By 1912, movies could show to a 1,000-plus audience, and more luxurious, classically designed theaters began to spread up and down main thoroughfares, catering to men and women of all classes. Over the next fifteen years, the number of cinemas grew to over eight hundred, averaging 1,200 seats each, or one for every six people in the entire metropolis. In other words, while the population of New York doubled between 1910 and 1930, the capacity of movie theaters increased more than eight times. Such growth in less than two decades testifies to the enormous appeal of the movies, and to the advent of a truly new public arena with phenomenal popularity.

Furthermore, this expansion reflected the creation of America's first *mass* amusement—but it was clearly geared toward middle-class aspirations. A number of studies over time verify this pattern. As we have seen, early examinations found that the 1908 patrons were workers; by 1912 25 percent of the audience was clerical and 5 percent was business class of both sexes. Detailed examinations from the twenties and forties show that this expansion continued. Polling the audience, investigators found that high school and college graduates went most often, although they comprised only one fourth of the population in 1920. Likewise, people with higher incomes went more often than workers or farmers; and those under thirty-five comprised the bulk of the audience. Men and women attended in equal numbers; but females were the ones who read the fan magazines, wrote letters to their idols, and knew the film plots by heart. In essence, the core of the new audience was made up of precisely those people who would have not appeared in the neighborhood of a nickelodeon.

It was also no accident that with theaters glorifying mass consumption, moviegoing was unquestionably an urban phenomenon. The theaters were overwhelmingly situated in cities, at a time when half the nation's population lived in rural areas. There were 28,000 theaters in 1928; and over half of them were in the industrial centers of New York, Illinois, Pennsylvania, Ohio, and California. The major cities in these states contained most of the large luxury cinemas. San Francisco, New York, Chicago, and Los Angeles each had from five to eight hundred theaters, averaging over 1,000 seats each, or one for every five to seven people. These movie houses stayed open seven days a week, twelve hours a day, while those in the small towns were only open on weekends. In contrast to a place like New York, whose 800 theaters could contain one sixth of the city's residents, the Southern city of Birmingham, Alabama, had only thirty-one theaters. Although it had a much smaller population, the combined capacity of its movie houses was only one seat for every thirty-two people in the city. All in all, this "mass" media was geared to a Northern and West Coast urban market—precisely where the work week was shortest and the per capita income largest.

The phenomenal popularity of the movies during these years was also unique to the United States. Although other countries had films, the United States was clearly the cinema capital. The audience was between twenty and thirty million weekly; and movies absorbed the largest portion of the average American's recreation budget in the 1920s. During the decade, the number of theaters in the United States grew from 21,000 to 28,000. By comparison, in Germany they went from 2,826 to 5,000; and in France from 1,500 to 3,900. European houses were probably smaller as well. Yet the combined populations of these two countries equalled that of the United States. Moreover, this country had more movie theaters than all of Europe. Part of the explanation lies in economics. America was the most industrialized and wealthy country, particularly after the War had devastated the economies of Europe. Also, American affluence was probably more widespread, making it possible for more people to spend their excess funds at the movies.

Beyond this economic explanation lies a deeper cultural cause. Most western European nations industrialized within a more aristocratic, hierarchical tradition. Consequently, the movies did not become identified with the perpetuation of egalitarianism. Nor were they part of a moral revolution that was eroding Victorian behavioral codes. In twentieth-century America, however, movies and mass culture were key elements in the transition from nineteenth-century values of strict behavior toward greater moral experimentation. As the economy consolidated, the leisure arena preserved a sense of freedom and mobility. Both on the screen and in the theater, moviegoers tasted the life of the rich as it was brought within reach of the masses, breaking down the class divisions of the past. Here was a revitalized frontier of freedom, where Americans might sanction formerly forbidden pleasures through democratized consumption. One theater chain manager noted why the luxury movie house could perpetuate the spirit of the old West in a new age. Using an apt metaphor, he wrote,

Our movie houses have collected the most precious rugs, fixtures and treasures that money can produce. No kings or emperors ever wandered through a more lavish environment. In a sense they are social "safety valves" in that the public can partake of the same environment of the rich and use them to the same extent.

Yet the creation of the lavish theaters suggested that Americans were divided on the meaning of the new life. The "cathedrals" of motion pictures seemed to offer secular salvation; the classless seating and sexual mingling of both sexes in a former lower-class arena suggested a break from formality. After 1914, this break was intensified as classicism gave way to architectural styles that mixed foreign, high and low culture together. Managers heightened the effect of an escape from time and hierarchy of the outside world through the friendly ushers, the nightlife, and the premiere. Here was a place where people could presumably mingle on equal terms with the top people in society. Nevertheless, the ambivalence in this release from restraint required that it be surrounded with all the symbols of high culture which gave status. In order to afford this style of leisure, both sexes would have to pursue success even more diligently. While the "cathedral" of the motion picture glorified consumption and play, it thus kept alive very traditional values. But this experience did not end when the patrons exited. They could see that the message of the movie and its palace was alive and well in the last great component of the motion picture universe: Hollywood.

■ ■ ■

STUDY QUESTIONS

1. How did movie theaters change from the time when they were largely an immigrant entertainment to the period when they were a more middle class entertainment? What was the difference between a nickelodean and a movie palace?

2. What was the significance of the architecture of the movie palace?

3. How did electricity change nightlife?

4. How did movie theaters try to create a haven from the "machine-like world"?

5. Why was Sid Grauman's Chinese Theater so successful?

6. How did the movie palaces encourage and support both the values of consumption and of work?

BIBLIOGRAPHY

The above selection is from Lary May's masterful *Screening Out the Past: The Birth of Mass Culture and the Motion Picture Industry* (1980). The best general history of the motion picture industry in America is Robert Sklar, *Movie Made America: A Social History of American Movies* (1975), which is particularly insightful on the immigrant origins of the industry. Other useful studies include Garth Jowett, *Film, The Democratic Art* (1976); Lewis Jacob, *The Rise of the American Film: A Critical History* (1939); William Everson, *The American Silent Film* (1978); and Leo Rosten, *Hollywood: The Movie Colony, the Movie Makers* (1941). A good inside look at Hollywood during the period is Budd Schulberg, *Moving Pictures: Memories of a Hollywood Prince* (1981).

The emergence and acceptance of consumer values has been traced in a number of fine studies. Among the best are T.J. Jackson Lears, *No Place of Grace: Anti-Modernism and the Transformation of American Culture, 1880–1920* (1981); John F. Kasson, *Amusing the Millions: Coney Island at the Turn of the Century* (1978); Charles E. Funnell, *By the Beautiful Sea: The Rise and High Times of that Great Resort, Atlantic City* (1983); and Lewis A. Erenberg, *Steppin' Out: New York Nightlife and the Transformation of American Culture, 1890–1930* (1981).

ORGANIZED CRIME IN URBAN SOCIETY: CHICAGO IN THE TWENTIETH CENTURY

Mark Haller

In 1919 Congress adopted the Eighteenth Amendment which prohibited "the manufacture, sale, or transportation of intoxicating liquors." Prohibition, however, did not stop Americans from manufacturing, selling, or transporting alcohol; it simply made the actions illegal. During the 1920s and early 1930s, criminals rather than businessmen supplied the public's thirst, and often the distinction between the two occupations grew fuzzy. As "Scarface" Al Capone once noted, "I make my money by supplying a public demand. If I break the law, my customers, who number hundreds of the best people in Chicago, are as guilty as I am. . . . Everybody calls me a racketeer. I call myself a businessman. When I sell liquor it's bootlegging. When my patrons serve it on a silver tray on Lake Shore Drive, it's hospitality."

For many Americans, Capone's point was well taken. As a result, criminals achieved a certain social respect and were able to spread their influence into legitimate business. A 1926 congressional investigation demonstrated that organized crime had made significant inroads into the worlds of labor unions, industry, and city governments. By 1933 when Congress repealed the Nineteenth Amendment, organized crime had become a permanent part of the American scene.

In the following essay, historian Mark H. Haller examines the role of crime in ethnic communities and urban society. Like sports and entertainment, crime served as an avenue out of the ethnic ghettoes and played an important role in the complex urban environment.

Many journalists have written exciting accounts of organized crime in American cities and a handful of scholars have contributed analytical and perceptive studies. Yet neither the excitement in the journalistic accounts nor the analysis in the scholarly studies fully captures the complex and intriguing role of organized criminal activites in American cities during the first third of the twentieth century. The paper that follows, although focusing on Chicago, advances hypotheses that are probably true for other cities as well. The paper examines three major, yet interrelated, aspects of the role of organized crime in the city: first, the social worlds within which the criminals operated and the importance of those worlds in providing social mobility from immigrant ghettos; second, the diverse patterns by which different ethnic groups became involved in organized criminal activities and were influenced by those activities; and third, the broad and pervasive economic impact of organized crime in urban neighborhoods and the resulting influence that organized crime did exert.

Crime and Mobility

During the period of heavy immigrant movement into the cities of the Northeast and Midwest, organized crime provided paths of upward mobility for many young men raised in ethnic slums. The gambling kings, vice lords, bootleggers and racketeers often began their careers in the ghetto neighborhoods; and frequently these neighborhoods continued to be the centers for their entrepreneurial activities. A careful study of the leaders of organized crime in Chicago in the late 1920s found that 31 percent were of Italian background, 29 percent of Irish background, 20 percent Jewish, and 12 percent black; none were native white of native white parents. A recogni-

tion of the ethnic roots of organized crime, however, is only a starting point for understanding its place in American cities.

At a risk of oversimplification, it can be said that for young persons in the ethnic ghettos three paths lay open to them. The vast majority became, to use the Chicago argot, "poor working stiffs." They toiled in the factories, filled menial service and clerical jobs, or opened mom-and-pop stores. Their mobility to better jobs and to homeownership was, at best, incremental. A second, considerably smaller group followed respectable paths to relative success. Some of this group went to college and entered the professions; others rose to management positions in the business or governmental hierarchies of the city.

There existed, however, a third group of interrelated occupations which, although not generally regarded as respectable, were open to uneducated and ambitious ethnic youths. Organized crime was one such occupational world, but there were others.

One was urban machine politics. Many scholars have, of course, recognized the function of politics in providing mobility for some members of ethnic groups. In urban politics, a person's ethnic background was often an advantage rather than a liability. Neighborhood roots could be the basis for a career that might lead from poverty to great local power, considerable wealth, or both.

A second area consisted of those businesses that prospered through political friendships and contacts. Obviously, construction companies that built the city streets and buildings relied upon government contracts. But so also did banks in which government funds were deposited, insurance companies that insured government facilities, as well as garbage contractors, traction companies and utilities that sought city franchises. Because political contacts were important, local ethnic politicians and their friends were often the major backers of such enterprises.

A third avenue of success was through leadership in the city's labor unions. The Irish in Chicago dominated the building trade unions and most of the other craft unions during the first 25 years of this century. But persons of other ethnic origins could also rise to leadership positions, especially in those unions in which their own ethnic group predominated.

Another path of mobility was sports. Boxing, a peculiarly urban sport, rooted in the neighborhood gymnasiums, was the most obvious example of a sport in which Irish champions were succeeded by Jewish, Polish and black champions. Many a fighter, even if he did not reach national prominence, could achieve considerable local fame within his neighborhood or ethnic group. He might then translate this local fame into success by becoming a fight manager, saloon keeper, politician or racketeer.

A fifth area often dominated by immigrants was the entertainment and night life of the city. In Chicago, immigrants—primarily Irish and Germans—ran the city's saloons by the turn of the century. During the 1920s, Greek businessmen operated most of the taxi-dance halls. Restaurants, cabarets and other night spots were similarly operated by persons from various ethnic groups. Night life also provided careers for entertainers, including B-girls, singers, comedians, vaudeville and jazz bands. Jewish comedians of the 1930s and black comedians of our own day are only examples of a larger phenomenon in which entertainment could lead to local and even national recognition.

The organized underworld of the city, then, was not the only area of urban life that provided opportunities for ambitious young men from the ghettos. Rather, it was one of several such areas. Part of the pervasive impact of organized crime resulted from the fact that the various paths were interrelated, binding together the worlds of crime, politics, labor leadership, politically related businessmen, sports figures and the night life of the city. What was the nature of the interrelationships?

To begin with, organized crime often exerted important influences upon the other social worlds. For aspiring politicians, especially during the early years after an ethnic group's arrival

in a city, organized crime was often the most important source of money and manpower. (By the turn of the century, an operator of a single policy wheel in Chicago could contribute not only thousands of dollars but also more than a hundred numbers writers to work the neighborhoods on election day.) On occasion, too, criminals supplied strongarm men to act as poll watchers, they organized repeat voters; and they provided other illegal but necessary campaign services. Like others engaged in ethnic politics, members of the organized underworld often acted from motives of friendship and common ethnic loyalties. But because of the very nature of their activities, criminal entrepreneurs required and therefore sought political protection. It would be difficult to exaggerate the importance of organized crime in the management of politics in many of the wards of the city.

Furthermore, it should not be thought that the politics of large cities like Chicago was peculiarly influenced by organized crime. In a large and heterogeneous city, there were always wards within which the underworld exercised little influence and which could therefore elect politicians who would work for honest government and law enforcement. But in the ethnic and blue-collar industrial cities west or southwest of Chicago, the influence of organized crime sometimes operated without serious opposition. In Cicero, west of Chicago along major commuting lines, gambling ran wide open before the 1920s; and after 1923 Capone's bootlegging organization safely had its headquarters there. In other towns, like Stickney and Burnham, prostitution and other forms of entertainment often operated with greater openness than in Chicago. This symbiotic relationship, in which surrounding blue-collar communities provided protected vice and entertainment for the larger city, was not limited to Chicago. Covington, Kentucky, had a similar relationship to Cincinnati, while East St. Louis serviced St. Louis.

The organized underworld was also deeply involved in other areas of immigrant mobility. Organized criminals worked closely with racketeering labor leaders and thus became involved in shakedowns, strike settlements and decisions concerning union leadership. They were participants in the night life, owned many of the night spots in the entertainment districts, and hired and promoted many of the entertainers. (The comedian Joe E. Lewis started his career in Chicago's South Side vice district as an associate and employee of the underworld; his case was not atypical.) Members of the underworld were also sports fans and gamblers and therefore became managers of prize fighters, patrons at the race tracks and loyal fans at ball games. An observer who knew many of Chicago's pimps in the 1920s reported:

The pimp is first, last and always a fight fan. He would be disgraced if he didn't go to every fight in town. . . .

They hang around gymnasiums and talk fight. Many of them are baseball fans, and they usually get up just about in time to go to the game. They know all the players and their information about the game is colossal. Football is a little too highbrow for them, and they would be disgraced if they played tennis, but of late the high grade pimps have taken to golf, and some of them belong to swell golf clubs.

However, criminals were not merely sports fans; some ran gambling syndicates and had professional interests in encouraging sports or predicting the outcome of sports events. Horse racing was a sport conducted primarily for the betting involved. By the turn of the century, leading gamblers and bookmakers invested in and controlled most of the race tracks near Chicago and in the rest of the nation. A number of successful gamblers had stables of horses and thus mixed business with pleasure while becoming leading figures in horse race circles. At a less important level, Capone's organization in the late 1920s owned highly profitable dog tracks in Chicago's suburbs.

The fact that the world of crime exerted powerful influences upon urban politics, business, labor unions, sports and entertainment does not adequately describe the interrelations of these worlds. For many ambitious men, the worlds were tied together because in their own lifetimes they moved easily from one area to another or else held positions in two or more simultaneously. In some ways, for instance, organized crime and entertainment were barely distinguishable worlds. Those areas of the city set aside for prostitution and gambling were the major entertainment districts of the city. Many cabarets and other night spots provided gambling in backrooms or in rooms on upper floors. Many were places where prostitutes solicited customers or where customers could find information concerning local houses of prostitution. During the 1920s, places of entertainment often served liquor and thus were retail outlets for bootleggers. In the world of entertainment, the distinction between legitimate and illegitimate was often blurred beyond recognition.

Take, as another example, the career of William Skidmore. At age fourteen, Billie sold racing programs at a race track near Chicago. By the time he was twenty-one, in the 1890s, he owned a saloon and cigar store, and soon had joined with others to operate the major policy wheels in Chicago and the leading handbook syndicate on the West Side. With his growing wealth and influence, he had by 1903 also become ward committeeman in the thirteenth ward and was soon a leading political broker in the city. In 1912 he was Sergeant-at-Arms for the Democratic National Convention and, afterwards, aided Josephus Daniels in running the Democratic National Committee. Despite his success as gambler and politician, his saloon, until well into the 1920s, was a hangout for pickpockets and con men; and "Skid" provided bail and political protection for his criminal friends. In the twenties Skidmore branched into the junk business and made a fortune selling junk obtained through contracts with the county government. Not until the early 1940s did he finally go to prison, the victim of a federal charge of income tax evasion. In his life, it would be impossible to unravel the diverse careers to determine whether he was saloon keeper, gambler, politician or businessman.

The various social worlds were united not

simply by the influence of organized crime and by interlocking careers; the worlds also shared a common social life. At local saloons, those of merely local importance met and drank together. At other restaurants or bars, figures of wider importance had meeting places. Until his death in 1920, Big Jim Colossimo's restaurant in the South Side vice district brought together the successful from many worlds; the saloon of Michael (Hinky Dink) Kenna, first ward Alderman, provided a meeting place in the central business district. Political banquets, too, provided opportunities for criminals, police, sports figures and others to gather in honor of a common political friend. Weddings and funerals were occasions when friends met to mark the important passages through life. At the funeral of Colossimo—politician, vice lord and restauranteur—his pallbearers included a gambler, two keepers of vice resorts, and a bailbondsman. Honorary pallbearers were five judges (including the chief judge of the criminal courts), two congressmen, nine resort keepers or gamblers, several aldermen and three singers from the Chicago Opera. (His good friend, Enrico Caruso, was unable to be present.) Such ceremonial events symbolized the overlapping of the many worlds of which a man like Colossimo was a part.

Thus far we have stressed the social structure that linked the criminal to the wider parts of the city within which he operated. That social world was held together by a system of values and beliefs widely shared by those who participated in crime, politics, sports and the night life of the city. Of central importance was the cynical—but not necessarily unrealistic—view that society operated through a process of deals, friendships and mutual favors. Hence the man to be admired was the smart operator and dealer who handled himself well in such a world. Because there was seen to be little difference between a legal and an illegal business, there was a generally tolerant attitude that no one should interfere with the other guy's racket so long as it did not interfere with one's own. This general outlook was, of course, widely shared, in whole or in part, by other groups within American society so that

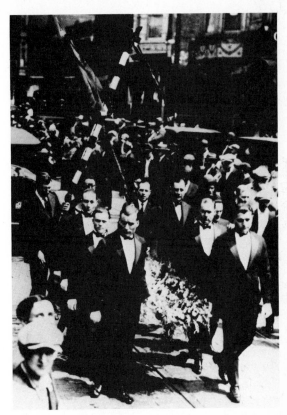

■ ■ *The lavishly bedecked casket and banners in the funeral cortege of a not-very-famous Chicago gangster of the 1920s. Bootlegging and racketeering in life gave way to ritual and pageantry in death.*

there was no clear boundary between the social world of the smart operators and the wider society.

In a social system held together by friendships and favors, the attitude toward law and legal institutions was complex. A basic attitude was a belief that criminal justice institutions were just another racket—a not unrealistic assessment considering the degree to which police, courts and prosecutor were in fact used by political factions and favored criminal groups. A second basic attitude was a belief that, if anyone cooperated with the law against someone with whom he was associated or to whom he owed favors, he was a stoolpigeon whose behavior was beneath contempt. This does not mean that criminal justice institutions were not used by members of organized crime. On a day-to-day basis, members of the underworld were tied to police, prosecutors and politicians through payments and mutual favors. Criminal groups often used the police and courts to harass rival gangs or to prevent the development of competition. But conflicts between rival groups were also resolved by threats or violence. Rival gambling syndicates bombed each others' places of business, rival union leaders engaged in bombing and slugging, and rival bootlegging gangs after 1923 turned to assassinations that left hundreds dead in the streets of Chicago. The world of the rackets was a tough one in which a man was expected to take his knocks and stand up for himself. Friendship and loyalty were valued; but so also were toughness and ingenuity.

Gangsters, politicians, sports figures and entertainers prided themselves for being smart guys who recognized how the world operated. They felt disdain mixed with pity for the "poor working stiffs" who, ignorant of how the smart guys operated, toiled away at their menial jobs. But if they disdained the life of the working stiff, they also disdained the pretensions of those "respectable" groups who looked askance at the world within which they operated. Skeptical that anyone acted in accordance with abstract beliefs or universalistic principles, the operators believed that respectable persons were hypocrites. For instance, when Frank J. Loesch, the distinguished and elderly lawyer who headed the Chicago Crime Commission, attacked three criminal court judges for alleged political favoritism, one politician declared to his friends:

Why pick on these three judges when every judge in the criminal court is doing the very same thing, and always have. Who is Frank Loesch that he should holler? He has done the same thing in his day. . . . He has asked for plenty of favors and has always gotten them. Now that he is getting older and is all set and doesn't have to ask any more favors, he is out to holler about every one else. . . . There are a lot of these reformers who

are regular racketeers, but it won't last a few years and it will die out.

In short, the world view of the operators allowed them to see their world as being little different from the world of the respectable persons who looked down upon them. The whole world was a racket.

Ethnic Specialization

Some have suggested that each ethnic group, in its turn, took to crime as part of the early adjustment to urban life. While there is some truth to such a generalization, the generalization obscures more than it illuminates the ethnic experiences and the structure of crime. In important respects, each ethnic group was characterized by different patterns of adjustment; and the patterns of involvement in organized crime often reflected the particular broader patterns of each ethnic group. Some ethnic groups—Germans and Scandinavians, for instance—appear not to have made significant contributions to the development of organized crime. Among the ethnic groups that did contribute, there was specialization within crime that reflected broader aspects of ethnic life.

In Chicago by the turn of the century, for example, the Irish predominated in two areas of organized crime. One area was labor racketeering, which derived from the importance of the Irish as leaders of organized labor in general.

The second area of Irish predominance was the operation of major gambling syndicates. Irish importance in gambling was related to a more general career pattern. The first step was often ownership of a saloon, from which the owner might move into both politics and gambling. Many Irish saloon keepers ran handbooks or encouraged other forms of gambling in rooms located behind or over the saloon. Those Irishmen who used their saloon as a basis for electoral politics continued the gambling activities in their saloons and had ties to larger gambling syndicates. Other saloon keepers, while sometimes taking important but backstage political positions such as ward committeeman, developed the gambling syndicates. Handbooks required up-to-the-minute information from race tracks across the country. By establishing poolrooms from which information was distributed to individual handbooks, a single individual could control and share in the profits of dozens or even hundreds of handbooks.

The Irish also predominated in other areas of gambling. At the turn of the century they were the major group in the syndicates that operated the policy games, each with hundreds of policy writers scattered in the slum neighborhoods to collect the nickels and dimes of the poor who dreamed of a lucky hit. They also outfitted many of the gambling houses in the Loop which offered roulette, faro, poker, blackjack, craps and other games of chance. Furthermore, many top police officers were Irish and rose through the ranks by attaching themselves to the various political factions of the city. Hence a complex system of Irish politicans, gamblers and police shared in the profits of gambling, protected gambling interests and built careers in the police department or city politics. Historians have long recognized the importance of the Irish in urban politics. In Chicago, at any rate, politics was only part of a larger Irish politics-gambling complex.

The Irish politics-gambling complex remained intact until about World War I. By the 1920s, however, the developing black ghetto allowed black politicians and policy operators to build independent gambling and political organizations linked to the Republicans in the 1920s and the Democratic city machine in the 1930s. By the 1920s, in addition, Jewish gamblers became increasingly important, both in the control of gambling in Jewish neighborhoods and in operations elsewhere. Finally, by the mid-1920s, Italian bootleggers under Capone took over gambling in suburban Cicero and invested in Chicago gambling operations. Gambling had become a complex mixture of Irish, Negro, Jewish and Italian entrepreneurship.

Although the Irish by the twentieth century played little direct role in managing prostitution, Italians by World War I had moved into important positions in the vice districts, especially in the notorious Levee district on the South Side. (Political protection, of course, often had to be arranged through Irish political leaders.) Just as the Irish blocked Italians in politics, so also they blocked Italians in gambling, which was both more respectable and more profitable than prostitution. Hence the importance of prohibition in the 1920s lay not in initiating organized crime (gambling continued both before and after prohibition to be the major enterprise of organized crime); rather, prohibition provided Italians with an opportunity to break into a major field of organized crime that was not already monopolized by the Irish.

This generalization, to some extent, oversimplifies what was in fact a complex process. At first, prohibition opened up business opportunities for large numbers of individuals and groups, and the situation was chaotic. By 1924, however, shifting coalitions had emerged. Some bootlegging gangs were Irish, including one set of O'Donnell brothers on the far West Side and another set on the South Side. Southwest of the stockyards, there was an important organization, both Polish and Irish, coordinated by "Pollack" Joe Saltis. And on the Near North Side a major group—founded by burglars and hold-up men—was led by Irishmen . . . and Jews. . . . There were, finally, the various Italian gangs, including the Gennas, the Aiellos, and, of course, the Capone organization.

The major Italian bootlegging gang, that associated with the name of Al Capone, built upon roots already established in the South Side vice district. There John Torrio managed houses of prostitution for Big Jim Colossimo. With Colossimo's assassination in 1920, Torrio and his assistant, Capone, moved rapidly to establish a bootlegging syndicate in the Loop and in the suburbs south and west of the city. Many of their associates were persons whom they had known during humbler days in the South Side vice district and who now rose to wealth with them. Nor was their organization entirely Italian. Very early, they worked closely with Irishmen like Frankie Lake and Terry Druggan in the brewing of beer, while Jake Guzik, a Jew and former South Side pimp, became the chief business manager for the syndicate. In the bloody bootlegging wars of the 1920s, the members of the Capone organization gradually emerged as the most effective organizers and most deadly fighters. The success of the organization brought wealth and power to many ambitious Italians and provided them with the means in the late 1920s and early 1030s to move into gambling, racketeering and entertainment, as well as into a broad range of legitimate enterprises. Bootlegging allowed Italians, through enterpreneurial skills and by assassination of rivals, to gain a central position in the organized underworld of the city.

Although Jewish immigrants in such cities as Cleveland and Philadelphia were major figures in bootlegging and thus showed patterns similar to Italians in Chicago, Jews in Chicago were somewhat peripheral figures. By World War I, Chicago Jews, like Italians, made important inroads into vice, especially in vice districts on the West Side. In the 1920s, with the dispersal of prostitution, several Jewish vice syndicates operated on the South and West Sides. Jews were also rapidly invading the world of gambling. Although Jews took part in vice, gambling and bootlegging, they made a special contribution to the organized underworld by providing professional or expert services. Even before World War I, Jews were becoming a majority of the bailbondsmen in the city. By the 1920s, if not before, Jews constituted over half the fences who disposed of stolen goods. (This was, of course, closely related to Jewish predominance as junk dealers and their importance in retail selling.) Jews were also heavily overrepresented among defense attorneys in the criminal courts. It is unnecessary to emphasize that the entrepreneurial and professional services of Jews reflected broader patterns of adaptation to American urban life.

Even within relatively minor underworld positions, specialization by ethnicity was important. A study of three hundred Chicago pimps in the early 1920s, for instance, found that 109

(more than one-third) were black, 60 were Italian, 47 Jewish and 26 Greek. The large proportion of blacks suggests that the high prestige of the pimp among some elements of the lower-class black community is not a recent development but has a relatively long tradition in the urban slum. There has, in fact, long been a close relationship of vice activities and Negro life in the cities. In all probability, the vice districts constituted the most integrated aspect of Chicago society. Black pimps and madams occasionally had white girls working for them, just as white pimps and madams sometimes had black girls working for them. In addition, blacks held many of the jobs in the vice districts, ranging from maids to entertainers. The location of major areas of vice and entertainment around the periphery and along the main business streets of the South Side black neighborhood gave such activities a pervasive influence within the neighborhood.

Black achievements in ragtime and jazz had their roots, at least in part, in the vice and entertainment districts of the cities. Much of the early history of jazz lies among the talented musicians—black and white—who performed in the famous resorts in the Storyville district of New Orleans in the 1890s and early 1900s. With the dissolution of Storyville as a segregated vice district, many talented black musicians carried their styles to Chicago's South Side, to Harlem, and to the cabarets and dance halls of other major cities. In the 1920s, with black performers like King Oliver and Louis Armstrong and white performers like Bix Beiderbecke, Chicago was an important environment for development of jazz styles. Just as Harlem became a center for entertainment and jazz for New Yorkers during prohibition, so the black and tan cabarets and speakeasies of Chicago's South Side became a place where blacks and whites drank, danced and listened to jazz music—to the shock of many respectable citizens. Thus, in ways that were both destructive and productive, the black experience in the city was linked to the opportunities that lay in the vice resorts, cabarets and dance halls of the teeming slums. In the operation of entertainment facilities and policy rackets, black entrepreneurs found their major outlet and black politicians found their chief support.

Until there has been more study of comparative ethnic patterns, only tentative hypotheses are possible to explain why various ethnic groups followed differing patterns. Because many persons involved in organized crime initiated their careers with customers from their own neighborhood or ethnic group, the degree to which a particular ethnic group sought a particular illegal service would influence opportunities for criminal activities. If members of an ethnic group did not gamble, for instance, then ambitious members of that ethnic group could not build gambling syndicates based upon local roots. The general attitude toward law and law enforcement, too, would affect opportunities for careers in illegal ventures. Those groups that became most heavily involved in organized crime migrated from regions in which they had developed deep suspicions of government authority—whether the Irish fleeing British rule in Ireland, Jews escaping from Eastern Europe, Italians migrating from southern Italy or Sicily, or blacks leaving the American South. Within a community suspicious of courts and government officials, a person in trouble with the law could retain roots and even respect in the community. Within a community more oriented toward upholding legal authority, on the other hand, those engaged in illegal activities risked ostracism and loss of community roots.

In other ways, too, ethnic life sytles evolved differently. Among both Germans and Irish, for instance, friendly drinking was part of the pattern of relaxation. Although the Irish and Germans by 1900 were the major managers of Chicago's saloons, the meaning of the saloon was quite different for the two groups. German saloons and beer gardens were sometimes for family entertainment and generally excluded gambling or prostitution; Irish saloons, part of an exclusively male social life, often featured prostitution or gambling and fit more easily into the world of entertainment associated with organized crime. Finally, it appears that south Ital-

ians had the highest homicide rate in Europe. There was, in all probability, a relationship between the cultural factors that sanctioned violence and private revenge in Europe and the factors that sanctioned the violence with which Italian bootleggers worked their way into a central position in Chicago's organized crime.

There were, at any rate, many ways that the immigrant background and the urban environment interacted to influence the ethnic experience with organized crime. For some ethnic groups, involvement in organized crime was not an important part of the adjustment to American urban life. For other groups, involvement in the organized underworld both reflected and influenced their relatively unique patterns of acculturation.

Economic Impact

The economic role of organized crime was an additional factor underlying the impact of organized crime upon ethnic communities and urban society. Organized crime was important because of the relatively great wealth of the most successful criminals, because of the large numbers of persons directly employed by organized crime, and because of the still larger numbers who supplemented their income through various part-time activities. And all of this does not count the multitude of customers who bought the goods and services offered by the bootleggers, gambling operators and vice lords of the city.

During the first thirty or forty years after an immigrant group's arrival, successful leaders in organized crime might constitute a disproportionate percentage of the most wealthy members of the community. (In the 1930s at least one-half of the blacks in Chicago worth more than $100,000 were policy kings; Italian bootleggers in the 1920s may have represented an even larger proportion of the very wealthy among immigrants from southern Italy. The wealth of the successful criminals was accompanied by extensive political and other contacts that gave them considerable leverage both within and outside the ethnic community. They had financial resources to engage in extensive charitable activ- ities, and often did so lavishly. Projects for improvement of ethnic communities often needed their support and contacts in order to succeed. Criminals often invested in or managed legitimate business enterprises in their commu- nities. Hence, despite ambiguous or even antag- onistic relations that they had with "respect- able" members of their ethnic communities, suc- cessful leaders in organized crime were men who had to be reckoned with in the ethnic communi- ty and who often represented the community to the outside world.

In organized crime, as in other economic activities, the very successful were but a minori- ty. To understand the economic impact of crime, it is necessary to study the many persons at the middle and lower levels of organization. In cities like Chicago the number of persons directly employed in the activities of organized crime was considerable. A modest estimate of the number of fulltime prostitutes in Chicago about 1910 would be 15,000—not counting madams, pimps, procurers and others in managerial posi- tions. Or take the policy racket. In the early 1930s an average policy wheel in the black ghet- to employed 300 writers; some employed as many as 600; and there were perhaps 6,000 pol- icy writers in the ghetto. The policy wheels, in this period of heavy unemployment, may have been the major single source of employment in the black ghetto, a source of employment that did not need to lay off workers or reduce wages merely because the rest of the economy faced a major depression. Finally, during the 1920s, bootlegging in its various aspects was a major economic activity employing thousands in man- ufacture, transportation and retailing activities.

Yet persons directly employed constituted only a small proportion of those whose income derived from organized crime. Many persons supplemented their income through occasional or parttime services. While some prostitutes walked the streets to advertise their wares, oth- ers relied upon intermediaries who would direct customers in return for a finder's fee. During cer-

tain periods, payments to taxi drivers were suffi- ciently lucrative so that some taxi drivers would pick up only those passengers seeking a house of prostitution. Bellboys, especially in the second- class hotels, found the function of negotiating between guests and prostitutes a profitable part of their service. (Many of the worst hotels, of course, functioned partly or wholly as places of assignation.) Bartenders, newsboys and waiters were among the many helpful persons who pro- vided information concerning places and prices.

Various phases of bootlegging during the 1920s were even more important as income sup- plements. In the production end, many slum families prepared wine or became "alky cook- ers" for the bootlegging gangs—so much so that after the mid-1920s, explosions of stills and the resulting fires were a major hazard in Chicago's slum neighborhoods. As one observer report- ed:

During prohibition times many respectable Sicilian men were employed as "alky cookers" for Capone's, the Aiello's or for personal use. Many of these people sold wine during prohibition and their children delivered it on foot or by streetcar without the least fear that they might be arrested. . . . During the years of 1927 to 1930 more wine was made than during any other years and even the "poorest people" were able to make ten or fifteen barrels each year—others making sixty, seventy, or more barrels.

Other persons, including policemen, moonlight- ed as truck drivers who delivered booze to the many retail outlets of the city. Finally, numerous persons supplemented their income by retailing booze, including bellboys, janitors in apartment buildings and shoe shine boys.

The many persons who mediated between the underworld and the law were another group that supplemented its income through under- world contacts. Large numbers of policemen, as well as bailiffs, judges and political fixers, received bribes or political contributions in return for illegal cooperation with the underworld. Defense attorneys, tax accountants and bailbondsmen, in return for salaries or fees, provided expert services that were generally legal.

For many of the small businessmen of the city, retailing the goods or services of the underworld could supplement business income significantly. Saloons, as already mentioned, often provided gambling and prostitution as an additional service to customers. Large numbers of small businesses were outlets for handbooks, policy, baseball pools, slot machines and other forms of gambling. A substantial proportion of the cigar stores, for example, were primarily fronts for gambling; barber shops, pool halls, newsstands, and small hotels frequently sold policy or would take bets on the horses. Drug stores often served as outlets for cocaine and, during the 1920s, sometimes sold liquor.

The organized underworld also influenced business activity through racketeering. A substantial minority of the city's labor unions were racketeer-controlled; those that were not often used the assistance of racketeer unions or of strongarm gangs during strikes. The leaders of organized crime, as a result, exercised control or influence in the world of organized labor. Not so well known was the extensive racketeering that characterized small business organizations. The small businesses of the city were generally marginal and intensely competitive. To avoid cutthroat competition, businessmen often formed associations to make and enforce regulations illegally limiting competition. The Master Barbers Association, for example, set minimum prices, forbad a shop to be open after 7:30 P.M., and ruled that no shop could be established within two blocks of another shop. Many other types of small businesses formed similar associations: dairies, auto parts dealers, garage owners, candy jobbers, butcher stores, fish wholesalers and retailers, cleaners and dyers, and junk dealers. Many of the associations were controlled, or even organized, by racketeers who levied dues upon association members and controlled the treasuries; they then used a system of fines and violence to insure that all businessmen in the

trade joined the association and abided by the regulations. In return for control of the association's treasury, in short, racketeers performed illegal services for the assocation and thereby regulated much of the small business activity of the city.

Discussion of the economic influence of organized crime would be incomplete without mentioning the largest group that was tied economically to the underworld, namely, the many customers for the illegal goods and services. Like other retailers in the city, some leaders of organized crime located their outlets near the center of the city or along major transportation lines and serviced customers from the entire region; others were essentially neighborhood businessmen with a local clientele. In either case, those providing illegal goods and services usually attempted to cultivate customer loyalty so that the same customers would return on an ongoing basis and advertise among their friends. Organized crime existed because of wide customer demand, and a large proportion of the adult population of the city was linked to organized crime on a regular basis for purchase of goods and services.

Heroism and Ambiguity

Because of the diverse ways that successful criminal entrepreneurs influenced the city and ethnic communities, many of them became heroes—especially within their own communities. There were a variety of reasons for the admiration that they received. Their numerous philanthropies, both large and small, won them reputations as regular guys who would help a person in need. Moreover, they were often seen as persons who fought for their ethnic communities. They aided politicians from their communities to win elections in the rough and often violent politics of the slums and thereby advanced their ethnic group toward political recognition. Sometimes they were seen as fighters for labor unions and thus as friends of labor. And, on occasion, they fought directly for their ethnic group. There was, for instance, the case of the three Miller brothers from Chicago's West Side Jewish ghetto. In typical ghetto pattern, one became a boxer, one a gangster and one a policeman. The boxer and gangster were heroes among Jews on the West Side, where for many years Jewish peddlers and junk dealers had been subjected to racial slurs and violent attacks by young hoodlums from other ethnic groups. "What I have done from the time I was a boy," Davy Miller told a reporter,

was to fight for my people here in the Ghetto against Irish, Poles or any other nationality. It was sidewalk fighting at first. I could lick any five boys or men in a sidewalk free-for-all.

When the Miller brothers and their gang protected the Jews of the West Side, the attacks against them abated.

Particularly for youngsters growing up in the ghettos, the gangsters were often heroes whose exploits were admired and copied. Davy Miller modestly recognized this when he said:

Maybe I am a hero to the young folks among my people, but it's not because I'm a gangster. It's because I've always been ready to help all or any of them in a pinch.

An Italian student at the University of Chicago in the early 1930s remembered his earlier life in the Italian ghetto:

For 26 years I lived in West Side "Little Italy," the community that has produced more underworld limelights than any other area in Chicago. . . .

I remember these men in large cars, with boys and girls of the neighborhood standing on the running board. I saw them come into the neighborhood in splendor as heroes. Many times they showered handfuls of silver to youngsters who waited to get a glance at them—the new heroes— because they had just made headlines in the newspapers. Since then I have seen many of my playmates shoot their way to the top of gangdom and seen others taken for a ride.

Nevertheless, despite the importance of gangsters and the world within which they moved, their relations to ethnic groups and the city were always ambiguous. Because many of their activities were illegal, they often faced the threat of arrest and, contrary to common belief, frequently found themselves behind bars. Furthermore, for those members of the ethnic community who pursued respectable paths to success, gangsters gave the ethnic group a bad name and remained a continuing source of embarrassment. St. Clair Drake and Horace R. Cayton, in their book on the Chicago black ghetto, describe the highly ambiguous and often antagonistic relations of the respectable black middle class and the policy kings. In his book on Italians in Chicago, Humbert S. Nelli explains that in the 1920s the Italian language press refused to print the name of Al Capone and covered the St. Valentine's Day massacre without suggesting its connection with bootlegging wars.

The respectable middle classes, however, were not the only ones unhappy about the activities or notoriety of gangsters. Organized crime sometimes contributed to the violence and fear of violence that pervaded many of the ghetto neighborhoods. Often local residents feared to turn to the police and lived with a stoical acceptance that gangs of toughs controlled elections, extorted money from local businesses and generally lived outside the reach of the law. Some immigrant parents, too, resented the numerous saloons, the open prostitution and the many gambling dens—all of which created a morally dangerous environment in which to raise children. Especially immigrant women, who watched their husbands squander the meager family income on liquor or gambling, resented the activities of organized crime. Within a number of neighborhoods, local churches and local leaders undertook sporadic campaigns for better law enforcement.

Organized crime, then, was an important part of the complex social structure of ethnic communities and urban society in the early twentieth century. For certain ethnic groups, organized crime both influenced and reflected the special patterns by which the groups adjusted to life in urban America. Through organized crime, many members of those ethnic groups could achieve mobility out of the ethnic ghettos and into the social world of crime, politics, ethnic business, sports, and entertainment. Those who were successful in organized crime possessed the wealth and contacts to exercise broad influence within the ethnic communities and the city. The economic activities of the underworld provided jobs or supplemental income for tens of thousands. Despite the importance of organized crime, however, individual gangsters often found success to be ambiguous. They were not always able to achieve secure positions or to translate their positions into respectability.

■■■

STUDY QUESTIONS

1. What was the primary occupational paths out of the ghetto for uneducated but ambitious ethnic youths? How were the paths interrelated?

2. How did organized crime exert influence upon other social worlds? What in particular was the relationship between organized crime and urban politics?

3. What social values did criminals share with the leaders in politics, sports, labor unions, entertainment, and business? What was the attitude of the men in these professions toward law and legal institutions?

4. What does Haller mean by "ethnic specialization" in crime? What factors account for the criminal specialization of the different ethnic groups?

5. What was the economic impact of organized crime on the ethnic and urban environment?

6. Why did a number of criminals become ethnic heroes? What role did the "criminal heroes" play in their ethnic neighborhoods?

BIBLIOGRAPHY

Because of the secretive nature of organized crime, it has proven an illusive subject for scholars. Nevertheless historians and sociologists have produced several valuable studies. Andrew Sinclair, *Prohibition: The Era of Excess* (1962), examines the impact of the Eighteenth Amendment on the rise of organized crime. Humbert S. Nelli, *The Italians in Chicago, 1880–1930: A Study in Ethnic Mobility* (1970), and *The Business of Crime* (1976) deal admirably with the subject of ethnic crime. John A. Gardiner, *The Politics of Corruption: Organized Crime in the American City* (1970), is also valuable. William F. Whyte, *Street Corner Society: The Social Structure of an Italian Slum* (1955), is a classic sociological study of an ethnic urban environment. Finally, Daniel Bell, *The End of Ideology* (1961), considers crime as a means of social and economic mobility.

Part Five

DEPRESSION
AND WAR

Despite all the talk about prosperity and progress in the 1920s, there were disturbing signs that the economy was not as healthy as people assumed. Throughout the decade agricultural prices steadily declined as production rose, in what many called a "poverty of abundance." In face of high protective tariffs, foreign trade gradually declined and the production of durable, domestic goods peaked in 1927. When the bubble burst with the crash of the stock market in October 1929, most Americans were shocked. The shock soon turned to despair as banks failed in record numbers, small businesses closed their doors, and unemployment reached unheard-of levels. How could it have been? For three centuries the world viewed America as the land of opportunity. Suddenly, people were losing their jobs, homes, and life savings. The American dream had become a nightmare.

Bewildered with their plight, most Americans were desperate for answers. Socialists and communists blamed capitalism, arguing that, just as Karl Marx had predicted, the system was collapsing under the weight of its own corruption and exploitation. The technocrats claimed that industrialization had run its course and that a new social order, based on science and technology, would soon emerge out of the rubble of the depression. Businessmen blamed politicians for the trouble. Farmers saw bogeymen in bankers and commodities speculators. Some Americans even blamed Jews for the collapse. Abandoning laissez-faire economics, Hoover modestly tried to reorganize the federal government to fight the depression, but his efforts failed. In the next presidential election Americans put Franklin D. Roosevelt into the White House.

Roosevelt was an unlikely hero for an impoverished nation. Born to old wealth and raised in splendor, he had little understanding of economics and no empathy

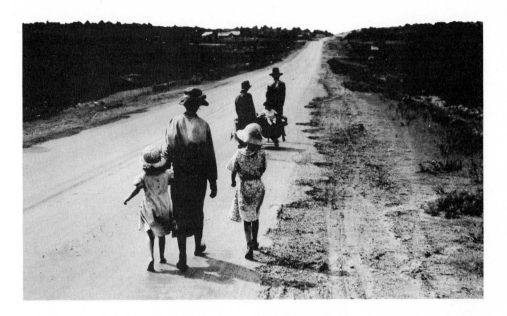

for poverty. But he did have keen political instincts and few philosophical inhibitions. In a whirlwind of activity, the New Deal greatly increased relief spending, attacked specific problems in the money markets, and tried, usually in a haphazard way, to stimulate an industrial recovery. Although it took World War II to finally lift the country out of the depression, Franklin D. Roosevelt nevertheless became one of the most beloved presidents in American history, popular enough to win reelection in 1936, 1940, and 1944. People remembered him for the spark in his eye, his smiling face and cocked head, and his uncompromising exuberance. To men working on government projects, it was Roosevelt who took them away from the soup lines. To farm wives living in poverty, it was Roosevelt who brought the electric transmission lines, the subsidy check, and the refinanced mortgage. To mass production workers, it was Roosevelt who sanctioned their labor unions and brought minimum wages. And to old people, it was Roosevelt who provided for their futures with Social Security.

But just as Roosevelt was easing fears about the economic future, political developments in Europe were bringing new tensions to a weary nation. Adolf Hitler's designs on Austria, Czechoslovakia, and Poland in 1938 and 1939 convinced many that another war was imminent and that the problems of the depression, as bad as they were, would only be child's play compared to a new global conflagration. Hitler's conquest of France and the Low Countries in 1940, the assault on Great Britain, and the invasion of the Soviet Union in 1941 only confirmed those fears. For a brief time, the United States was caught between its historic need for isolation and its responsibilities as a global leader. On December 7, 1941, Japan resolved America's uncertain position.

F.D.R.'S
EXTRA BURDEN

Bernard Asbell

When President Franklin D. Roosevelt collapsed and died of a stroke on April 12, 1945, the nation went into a state of depression unknown since the death of Abraham Lincoln. Like Lincoln, Roosevelt had become inseparably linked with a series of national crises—in his case the Great Depression and World War II. And like Lincoln, Roosevelt was viewed as a savior, a man who had redeemed his people, first from starvation and then from the spector of fascist oppression. Put simply, FDR enjoyed the elusive charisma so prized by politicians. Blessed with enormous self-confidence and an ingratiating personality, he inspired tremendous loyalty among most Americans. They loved him and put him in the White House on four separate occasions—1932, 1936, 1940, and 1944. But like all charismatic leaders, Roosevelt also generated tremendous hostility in some circles, particularly in corporate boardrooms and the parlors of the well-to-do. They viewed him as a "traitor to his class," a politician so seduced by power that he posed a threat to property and the social order.

Franklin D. Roosevelt was a complicated man, a beloved acquaintance of thousands but an intimate of very few. Born rich and raised in pampered splendor, he nevertheless led a virtual revolution in public policy, giving ethnic minorities, labor unions, and poor people their first taste of influence at the federal level. Although Roosevelt inspired a legion of intellectuals to invest their energies in public service, he was not an innovative thinker himself. He preferred the give and take of politics, and the inherent excitement of its risks, to the intricate nuts and bolts of social and economic policy. His public persona was overwhelming, but there was also a private side to his life that the American people understood only superficially. During the summer of 1921, little more than a decade before he became president, Roosevelt contracted polio, or infantile paralysis, a disease that crippled him for the rest of his life. In "F.D.R's Extra Burden," Bernard Asbell describes that paralysis and how Roosevelt, the press, and the nation handled it.

Every campaigner, especially for leadership of a large and complex state or for national office, is a cripple.

His legs are bound against running faster than his constituents are able to keep in step. His hands are tied by the limited powers of the office he seeks; he had better not promise what he knows he cannot deliver. His tongue is gagged against pronouncements that may make new friends if those pronouncements will also make new enemies. His balance is threatened by the pulls and tugs of conflicting demands for justice—shall money go for this urgent need or that one?—shall this group's freedom be expanded at the expense of that one's?

Immobilized by these paralyzing constraints, the candidate has to make himself appear able-bodied, attractive, confident, and powerful. At least more so than his opponent.

Being crippled—not in metaphor, but in reality—is perhaps good schooling for politics.

To this day, more than a quarter century after his death, people keep wondering aloud and speculating, "If Roosevelt had not been a cripple, would he have been the same kind of President?" Of course not. "If a different kind, how?" Impossible to say. "If he had not been a cripple, would he have become President at all?" Again, imponderable.

Did F.D.R.'s private battle teach him to identify with those who suffer? Unquestionably. Moreover it taught him the uses of patience (never a strong suit with crusaders who relied upon him, upon whom he relied, yet who continually harassed him). It heightened his sense of time and timing. "It made him realize"—an observation of Egbert Curtis, a Warm Springs companion—"that he was not infallible, that everything wasn't always going to go his way." More than anything, it forced him to study the uses of handicap, paradoxically giving him a leg up in a profession of able-bodied crippled men.

Let's not carry theory and speculation too far. Instead, let's try to observe firsthand, insofar as the written word permits, the connections between suffering and Roosevelt's acquired capacity for patience, for tolerance and respect of the wills and ambitions of others, for turning handicap into power.

We begin with his own words. A sufferer identifies with sufferers; and "Doctor" Roosevelt of Warm Springs also identified with other doctors. In F.D.R.'s early days at Warm Springs a South Carolina physician wrote to Roosevelt for a personal case report that might help him treat any polio patients who came his way. Roosevelt's reply is the only detailed personal account of what he had recently endured. The letter, dictated to Missy LeHand, his private secretary, during their first stay at Warm Springs, says in part:

. . . I am very glad to tell you what I can in regard to my case and as I have talked it over with a great many doctors can, I think, give you a history of the case which would be equal to theirs.

First symptoms of the illness appeared in August, 1921. . . . By the end of the third day practically all muscles from the chest down were involved. Above the chest the only symptom was a weakening of the two large thumb muscles making it impossible to write. There was no special pain along the spine and no rigidity of the neck.

For the following two weeks I had to be catheterized and there was slight, though not severe, difficulty in controlling the bowels. The fever lasted for only 6 or 7 days, but all the muscles from the hips down were extremely sensitive to the touch and I had to have the knees supported by pillows. This condition of extreme discomfort lasted about 3 weeks . . . [but] disappeared gradually over a period of six months, the last remaining point being the calf muscles.

As to treatment—the mistake was made for the first 10 days of giving my feet and lower legs rather heavy massage. This was stopped by Dr.

"F.D.R.'s Extra Burden" by Bernard Asbell, from *American Heritage* (June, 1973). Reprinted by permission of Curtis Brown, Ltd. Copyright © 1973 by Bernard Asbell.

Lovett, of Boston, who was, without doubt, the greatest specialist on infantile paralysis. In January, 1922, 5 months after the attack, he found that the muscles behind the knees had contracted and that there was a tendency to footdrop in the right foot. These were corrected by the use of plaster casts during two weeks. In February, 1922, braces were fitted on each leg from the hips to the shoes, and I was able to stand up and learned gradually to walk with crutches. At the same time gentle exercises were begun, first every other day, then daily, exercising each muscle 10 times and seeking to avoid any undue strain by giving each muscle the correct movement with gravity. These exercises I did on a board placed on the bed.

The recovery of muscle paralysis began at this time, though for many months it seemed to make little progress. In the summer of 1922 I began swimming and found that this exercise seemed better adapted than any other because all weight was removed from the legs and I was able to move the legs in the water far better than I had expected. . . .

I still wear braces, of course, because the quadriceps are not yet strong enough to bear my weight. One year ago I was able to stand in fresh water without braces when the water was up to my chin. Six months ago I could stand in water up to the top of my shoulders and today can stand in water just level with my arm pits. This is a very simple method for me of determining how fast the quadriceps are coming back. Aside from these muscles the waist muscles on the right side are still weak and the outside muscles on the right leg have strengthened so much more than the inside muscles that they pull my right foot forward. I continue corrective exercises for all the muscles.

To sum up I would give you the following ''Don'ts'':

Don't use heavy massage but use light massage rubbing always towards the heart.

Don't let the patient over-exercise any muscle or get tired.

Don't let the patient feel cold, especially the legs, feet or any other part affected. Progress stops entirely when the legs or feet are cold.

Don't let the patient get too fat.

The following treatment is so far the best, judging from my own experience and that of hundreds of other cases which I have studied:

1. Gentle exercise especially for the muscles which seem to be worst affected.

2. Gentle skin rubbing—not muscle kneading—bearing in mind that good circulation is a prime requisite.

3. Swimming in warm water—lots of it.

4. Sunlight—all the patient can get, especially direct sunlight on the affected parts. It would be ideal to lie in the sun all day with nothing on. This is difficult to accomplish but the nearest approach to it is a bathing suit.

5. Belief on the patient's part that the muscles are coming back and will eventually regain recovery of the affected parts. There are cases known in Norway where adults have taken the disease and not been able to walk until after a lapse of 10 or even 12 years.

I hope that your patient has not got a very severe case. They all differ, of course, in the degree in which the parts are affected. If braces are necessary there is a man in New York . . . who makes remarkable light braces of duraluminum. My first braces of steel weighed 7 lbs. apiece—my new ones weigh only 4 lbs. apiece. Remember that braces are only for the convenience of the patient in getting around—a leg in a brace does not have a chance for muscle development. This muscle development must come through exercise when the brace is not on—such as swimming, etc.

At Hyde Park, before discovering Warm Springs, this powerful man, to the shock of his children and friends, practiced dragging himself crablike across the floor, explaining that the one fear he ever knew was that of being caught in a fire. Then, showing off his inordinately strong shoulders and arms, he filled the house with laughter, wrestling his boys on the floor two at a time. His mother ordered an electric tricycle from Europe, but F.D.R. used it only once. He didn't want his muscles *worked;* he wanted to work them himself.

John Gunther describes Roosevelt's determination to get from floor to floor unaided: "Day after day he would haul his dead body weight up the stairs by the power of his hands and arms, step by step, slowly, doggedly; the sweat would pour off his face, and he would tremble with exhaustion. Moreover he insisted on doing this with members of the family or friends watching him, and he would talk all the time as he inched himself up little by little, talk, talk, and make people talk back. It was a kind of enormous spiritual catharsis—as if he had to do it, to prove his independence, and had to have the feat witnessed, to prove that it was nothing."

At Warm Springs in 1924 he concentrated on the day he would be able to walk unaided with braces. Braces, which he once said he "hated and mistrusted," which he could not put on or take off by himself, made him like a man on stilts. Unable to flex his toes, he had no balance. In 1928, after seven years of immobility and more than four years of daring and persevering, one day, finally, triumphantly, he hobbled most of the way across the living-room floor of his cottage—with braces, but without human help. The achievement was exhausting—and was never to be accomplished again. Years later, according to Grace Tully, "Missy's eyes filled up when on occasions she reminisced about those days." Roosevelt liked to maintain the belief that if he had had another year before the demand that he run for governor, he'd have mastered walking with a single brace.

In the summer of 1928 at Warm Springs, shortly after Roosevelt agreed to address the Democratic National Convention at Houston, son Elliott, eighteen, was visiting. One evening Roosevelt was lost in concentrated thought when suddenly he burst out:

"With my hand on a man's arm, *and one cane*—I'm sure. Let's try it!"

A fellow polio victim, Turnley Walker, Roosevelt's dinner guest, described what then happened and was repeated over and over:

First Roosevelt would get over to the wall and balance there with his cane. It was an ordinary cane but he held it in a special way, with his

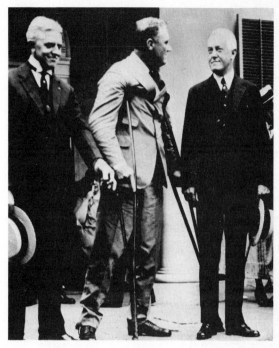

A 1924 photo of FDR taken three years after he was stricken with polio, shows him standing with crutches and leg braces. In later years, as governor of New York and president of the United States, he was rarely photographed in a full-length view.

index finger extended down along the rod from the handle. This finger acted as a rigid cleat . . . so that the strength of the massive arm and shoulder rammed straight along the cane to its tip against the floor.

"Now, Elliott, you get on the left, my weak side." Elliott watchfully took his place and [Helena] Mahoney [a physiotherapist] came forward to show him how to hold his right arm against his middle at the proper angle and lock it there with a clenching of his biceps.

"Remember that a polio needs more than a fingertip of guidance—he needs an iron bar," *said Mahoney, "Make a habit of holding that arm there. Never forget the job it's got to do."*

"Let's go," said Roosevelt, and he reached out to find the proper grip. Elliott had never felt his father's hand touching him that way. He had been grabbed and hugged, and even tossed and caught

*with wild energy when he was younger. But now
the fingers sought their grip with a kind of ruthless
desperation. . . . The pressure became stronger
than he had expected as his father pressed down to
hitch one braced leg forward for the first step.
"You must go right with him," said Mahoney
sternly. "Watch his feet. Match your strides with
his." Elliott stared down as the rigid feet swung
out slowly, and through the pressing hand he
could feel the slow, clenching effort of his father's
powerful body.*

*"Don't look at me, Son. Keep your head up,
smiling, watching the eyes of people. Keep them
from noticing what we're doing."*

*The cane went out, the good leg swung, the
pressure came, the weak leg hitched up into its arc
and then fell stiffly into the proper place against
the floor. Elliott carefully coordinated his own legs,
and they moved across the room.*

*Roosevelt set his hips against the far wall and
told Elliott to rest his arm. "We'll do beautifully,"
he said.*

*They went across the room and back again. It
was becoming somewhat easier.*

*"As soon as you feel confident, Son, look up
and around at people, the way you would do if I
weren't crippled."*

*"But don't forget," Mahoney warned, "if he
loses his balance, he'll crash down like a tree."*

"Don't scare us," said Roosevelt.

*. . . The cane, the swing, the pressure, the
swing. Elliott found that he could look up now
and then as they advanced. He caught his father's
eyes, the broad smile which was held with a very
slight rigidity. . . . Only then did he notice that
his father was perspiring heavily.*

Yet except when a public show required such
extraordinary exertion, Roosevelt was as helpless as a baby. When no strangers were around
to see, he let himself be carried by practiced
attendants. When F.D.R. became governor, his
cousin Nicholas Roosevelt spent a weekend at
Hyde Park and later recalled: "His mother and I
stood on the veranda watching his son Elliott

and Gus Gennerich, the state trooper who acted
as his personal bodyguard, carry him down the
steps and place him in the car. As they turned
and left him, he lost his balance (his powerful
torso was much heavier than his crippled legs),
and he fell over on the car seat. I doubt if one
man in a thousand as disabled and dependent on
others would have refrained from some sort of
reproach, however mild, to those whose care-
lessness had thus left him in the lurch. But
Franklin merely lay on his back, waved his
strong arms in the air and laughed. At once they
came back and helped him to his seat behind the
wheel, and he called me to join him."

Louis Howe, F.D.R's indispensable factotum,
set an iron rule—one that F.D.R. was not inclined to resist—that he never be carried in public.

Frances Perkins remembered the gubernatori-
al campaign.

*I saw him speak in a small hall in New York
City's Yorkville district. The auditorium was
crowded. . . . The only possible way for any
candidate to enter the stage without being crushed
by the throng was by the fire escape. I realized
with sudden horror that the only way he could get
over that fire escape was in the arms of strong
men. That was how he arrived.*

*Those of us who saw this incident, with our
hands on our throats to hold down our emotion,
realized that this man had accepted the ultimate
humility which comes from being helped
physically. . . . He got up on his braces, adjusted
them, straightened himself, smoothed his hair,
linked his arm in his son Jim's, and walked out
on the platform as if this were nothing
unusual. . . . I began to see what the great
teachers of religion meant when they said that
humility is the greatest of virtues, and that if you
can't learn it, God will teach it to you by
humiliation.*

Was humility—or humiliation—Roosevelt's
great teacher? Many have speculated. Harold

Ickes, after a day in a campaign car with press secretary Steve Early:

"[Early] recalled the campaign trips that he had made with Roosevelt when the latter was a candidate for Vice President in 1920. He said that if it hadn't been for the President's affliction, he never would have been President of the United States. In those earlier years, as Steve put it, the President was just a playboy. . . . He couldn't be made to prepare his speeches in advance, preferring to play cards instead. During his long illness, according to Steve, the President began to read deeply and study public questions."

Perkins: ". . . He had become conscious of other people, of weak people, of human frailty. I remember thinking that he would never be so hard and harsh in judgment on stupid people— even on wrongdoers. . . . I remember watching him [as governor] in Utica. . . . Certainly some of the Democratic rank-and-file were pretty tiresome, with a lot of things to say that were of no consequence. However, he sat and nodded and smiled and said, 'That's fine,' when they reported some slight progress. I remembered, in contrast, how he had walked away from bores a few years earlier when he was in the State Senate.

"Now he could not walk away when he was bored. He listened, and out of it learned . . . that 'everybody wants to have the sense of belonging, of being on the inside,' that 'no one wants to be left out,' as he put it years later in a Columbus, Ohio, speech. . . ."

A considerably more speculative observation by Noel F. Busch, childhood neighbor of the Oyster Bay Roosevelts who grew up to be a *Time* correspondent and avid F.D.R.-watcher: "Loss of the use of one's legs has several effects on the human psyche. One is that, when deprived of the power to move around, the mind demands a substitute or compensation for this power, such as the ability to command other people to move around. That is why almost all invalids tend to be peevish and demanding. However. . . Roosevelt sublimated and refined the pardonable peevishness of the normal invalid into an adminis-

trative urge which would have had profound consequences for him even if he had never become President."

Biographer Emil Ludwig: "The privilege of remaining seated, which everyone concedes him because of his affliction, starts him off with an advantage in his intercourse with others, in the same way as the smallness of Napoleon's stature compelled everyone standing before him to bend his back a little. Certainly giants like Bismarck or Lincoln had an advantage when they appeared before men, but the same effect can be produced by the opposite, by a weakness, and as Roosevelt looks up at everyone standing in front of him, he has accustomed himself to an upward and therefore very energetic gesture of the chin which counteracts the danger of his conciliatory smile."

While never mentioning his paralysis in public (until his last speech to Congress in 1945) and seldom privately, F.D.R. could come down fiercely on those he felt mentioned it unfairly. Huey Long's tapping a straw hat on the useless Presidential knee he could take as bad manners—the other fellow's problem, not his. But when Fulton Oursler brought him a manuscript of a profile of F.D.R. by Jay Franklin to be published in *Liberty*—the editor courteously seeking F.D.R.'s reaction—Oursler saw "a red flush rise on his neck like the temperature in a thermometer." Assuming that Roosevelt was angered over some political needling, he learned otherwise:

"Mr. Oursler, there is only one statement in this article that I want corrected. The author says in this line here that I have 'never entirely recovered from infantile paralysis.' *Never recovered what?* I have never recovered the complete use of my knees. Will you *fix* that?"

His reticence to mention it—and the released heat that accompanied exceptions—were shared by Mrs. Roosevelt. At an Akron, Ohio, lecture she was asked: "Do you think your husband's illness has affected his mentality?" Betraying no emotion as she read the written question aloud, she paused for an extra cooling moment and replied: 'I am glad that question was asked. The answer is Yes. Anyone who has gone through great suffering is bound to have a greater sympathy and understanding of the problems of mankind." The audience rose in an ovation.

He was frequently torn between keeping his silence and protesting his case. On April 6, 1938, he wrote to an "old friend"—Elliott's description—mentioning his affliction. The important thing is not what he wrote but his decision not to mail it. Instead, he marked it "Written for the Record" and filed it away. It said in part:

. . . I do not mind telling you, in complete 100% confidence, that in 1923, when I first went to Florida . . . my old running mate, Jim Cox, came to see me on my house-boat in Miami. At that time I was, of course, walking with great difficulty— braces and crutches. Jim's eyes filled with tears when he saw me, and I gathered from his conversation that he was dead certain that I had had a stroke and that another one would soon completely remove me. At that time, of course, my general health was extremely good. . . .

Jim Cox from that day on always shook his head when my name was mentioned and said in sorrow that in effect I was a hopeless invalid and could never resume any active participation in business or political affairs.

As late as 1931—I think it was—when I was coming back from the Governors' Conference in Indiana, I stopped off at Dayton to see Jim Cox. He had had a very serious operation, followed by a thrombosis in his leg, and was very definitely invalided. His whole attitude during the two hours I spent with him alone was the same—that it was marvelous that I could stand the strain of the Governorship, but that in all probability I would be dead in a few months. He spent the greater part of the time asking me solicitously how I was, though he was a much sicker man than I was.

He made a fine come-back and is furious today if anybody ever refers to the thrombosis he had in his leg—but I still think he expects me to pop off at any moment.

While deciding not to mail that letter, at other times he could be as open as a billboard. Son Jimmy recalls that on one of Madame Chiang Kai-shek's visits to the White House the grande dame thoughtlessly told the President not to stand up as she rose to leave the room. He gently replied, "My dear child, I couldn't stand up if I had to."

In a wheelchair or an automobile, getting F.D.R. into or out of an overcoat was an awkward exercise. With a stage sense of costume, F.D.R. took to a velvet-collared, braid-looped regulation Navy cape that, along with his cigarette holder, became a personal mark. Again, disadvantage was the fabric from which, with flair and style, he fashioned advantage.

Out of deference to his office as well as personal affection, newsmen virtually never mentioned the President's disability. So effective was their conspiracy, even upon themselves, that, as John Gunther recalled, "hard-boiled newspaper men who knew that he could not walk as well as they knew their own names could never quite get over being startled when F.D.R. was suddenly brought into a room. The shock was greater when he wheeled himself and, of course, was greatest when he was carried; he seemed, for one thing, very small. . . . During the 1930s when I lived in Europe I repeatedly met men in important positions of state who had no idea that the President was disabled."

The people of the United States—his constituents, those from whom he drew strength and, more importantly, those who drew strength from him—knew, yet didn't know. They, too, waiting at tiny railroad depots, straining to see through the autumn sunshine the commanding figure of their President, froze at the sight of the painfully slow-motion, brace-supported step-pause-step across what seemed a torturous mile of observation platform from the train's rear door to the microphone.

It was an unexpected, unforgettable drama of frailty and strength.

STUDY QUESTIONS

1. Did Roosevelt's illness give him the capacity to identify with the suffering of others? How much? Why?

2. Describe the physical course of Roosevelt's disease? How physically restricted was he in his activities?

3. What would you say about his mental attitude? What does it reveal about his personality?

4. How did the press handle the illness? Why were they so respectful of Roosevelt's privacy? Would today's press be equally respectful? Why or why not?

5. Why was Roosevelt so secretive of his illness? What were the possible political ramifications of the public understanding the extent of his handicap?

BIBLIOGRAPHY

The best survey of the era of Franklin D. Roosevelt is William E. Leuchtenburg, *Franklin D. Roosevelt and the New Deal, 1932–1940* (1963). For a critical approach to the Roosevelt administration, see Paul Conkin, *The New Deal* (1967). Arthur M. Schlesinger, Jr.'s pro-Roosevelt trilogy still makes for outstanding reading. See *The Crisis of the Old Order* (1957), *The Coming of the New Deal* (1959), and *The Politics of Upheaval* (1960). An excellent political biography of Roosevelt is James Macgregor Burns, *Roosevelt: The Lion and the Fox* (1956). Also see Burns's *Roosevelt: The Soldier of Freedom* (1970) for a discussion of World War II. Joseph Lasch, *Eleanor and Franklin* (1971) describes the relationship between the president and his wife. For descriptions of opposition to Roosevelt and the New Deal, see George Wolfskill, *Revolt of the Conservatives* (1962); Donald McCoy, *Angry Voices* (1958); and Alan Brinkley, *Voices of Protest: Huey Long, Father Coughlin, and the Great Depression* (1982).

THE SAD IRONS

Robert A. Caro

For millions of older Americans, the Great Depression remains a vivid memory, a haunting reminder of the time when the promise of prosperity failed. For their descendents, the Great Depression is a chapter or two in a textbook, marked by pictures of gaunt faces and skinny Texas panhandle farmers leaning into the fierce winds of the Dust Bowl. Most descriptions of the Great Depression and New Deal revolve around images of what was lost and what was regained, of how the nation underwent the glittering but superficial prosperity of the 1920s, the poverty of the 1930s, and the boom years of World War II, and how public policymakers struggled to gain control of vast economic forces.

But there is another side of the New Deal. While economic recovery was the primary objective of the Roosevelt administration, the New Deal also introduced some sections of the country to modern technology. In the nineteenth century the Industrial Revolution began its transformation of American life, bringing people together in large cities, organizing life into bureaucracies and interest groups, and relieving drudgery through technology. By 1920s, the nation had become intoxicated with the marvels of the light bulb, the internal combustion engine, and the electric motor, all of which revolutionized the way people lived. But millions of people were still unable to take advantage of the new gadgets. Instead, they lived as their ancestors had, tied to the soil in backbreaking, relentless labor. In "The Sad Irons" Robert Caro describes the "Hill Country" of Central Texas before the Rural Electrification Administration brought farm families into the modern age. The extension of electric transmission lines into the remote corners of the Hill Country transformed their lives, and for the next fifty years they remembered the New Deal as their savior.

Obtaining the financing and the authorization for the four dams being built along the Lower Colorado had been difficult. Now Lyndon Johnson undertook a task more difficult still. By ensuring completion of the dams, he had ensured the creation of electric power, which would be generated by the fall of water through dam penstocks. Now he was going to try to get the power to the people. He was going to try to bring electricity to the Hill Country.

Electricity had, of course, been an integral part of life in urban and much of small-town America for a generation and more, lighting its streets, powering the machinery of its factories, running its streetcars and trolleys, its elevated trains and subways, moving elevators and escalators in its stores, and cooling the stores with electric fans. Devices such as electric irons and toasters (which were in widespread use by 1900), refrigerators (which were widely sold beginning in 1912), and vacuum cleaners, dishwashers, hot plates, waffle irons, electric stoves and automatic washing machines for clothes had freed women from much of the drudgery of housework. In the evenings, thanks to electricity, there were the movies, and by 1922, forests of radio antennae had sprouted on tenement roofs. By 1937, when Lyndon Johnson went to Congress, electricity was so integral a part of life that it was hard to remember what life had been like without it.

It was not a part of life in the Hill Country. In Lyndon Johnson's congressional district, the sole source of power had been Texas Power & Light, a subsidiary of the New York-based utility holding giant, Electric Bond & Share. TP&L had, in 1927, agreed to "electrify" a handful of Hill Country towns (Johnson City was one), but not with power from its central generating station at Marble Falls; according to TP&L, which put the cost of building electric lines at $3,000 per mile,

From *The Years of Lyndon Johnson: The Path to Power* by Robert A. Caro. Copyright © 1982 by Robert A. Caro. Reprinted by permission of Alfred A. Knopf, Inc.

the limited use such small communities would make of electric power would never justify the investment required to build lines across the wide spaces of the Edwards Plateau. The TP&L "power plant" in each of these towns was, therefore, no more than a single thirty-horsepower diesel engine; it generated only enough voltage for ten-watt bulbs, which were constantly dimming and flickering—and which could not be used at all if an electric appliance (even an electric iron) was also in use. Since the "power plant" operated only between "dark to midnight," a refrigerator was useless. To most of the residents in these towns, such problems were academic: so high were TP&L's rates that few families hooked up to its lines. And in any case, the diesel engine was constantly breaking down under the strain placed on it. On the rare occasions on which a movie was shown, there was as much suspense in the audience over whether the electricity would hold out to the end of the film as there was in the film itself. Recalls Lucille O'Donnell of Burnet: "I'd be watching *The Perils of Pauline* and I'd just be about to see whether or not the train was going to run over her and the lights would go out." And the residents of these towns were the only inhabitants of the Hill Country with any electricity at all. TP&L refused even to consider building lines to the area's tens of thousands of individual farms and ranches.

As a result, although the electric milking machine had been invented almost two decades before, the Hill Country farmer had to milk his cows by hand—arising at three-thirty or four o'clock in the morning to do so, because milking was a time-consuming chore (more than two hours for twenty cows) and it had to be finished by daylight: every hour of daylight was needed for work in the fields. Milking was done by the dim light of kerosene lanterns; although Sears, Roebuck was boasting in 1937 that a new, deluxe kerosene lamp provided as much illumination as a forty-watt electric bulb, the lamps in use in the Hill Country furnished—at most—twenty-five watts of light. Or it was done in the dark. And there was a constant danger of fire with kerosene lamps, and even a spark could burn down a hay-filled barn, and destroy a farmer's last chance of holding on to his place, so many farmers were afraid to use a lantern in the barn. "Winter mornings," recalls one, "it would be so dark . . . you'd think you were in a box with the lid shut." Because without electricity there could be no refrigerator, the milk was kept on ice. The ice was expensive and farmers had to lug it from town at enormous cost in time. Though they kept it underground—covered with sawdust—it still, as farmer Chester Franklin of Wimberley puts it, "melted away so quick." And often even the ice didn't help. Farmers would have to take the milk out of their pit and place it by the roadside to be picked up by the trucks from Austin dairies, but often—on those unpaved Hill Country roads on which flat tires were a constant occurrence—the trucks would be late, and the milk would sit outside in the Hill Country heat. Even if it was not actually spoiled, the dairy would refuse to accept it if its temperature was above fifty degrees Fahrenheit—and when the truck driver pulled his thermometer out of the milk, a farmer, seeing the red line above fifty, would know that his hours of work in the barn in the dark had been for nothing.

Because there was no electricity, moreover, a Hill Country farmer could not use an electric pump. He was forced not only to milk but to water his cows by hand, a chore that, in dry weather, meant hauling up endless buckets from a deep well. Because he could not use an electric auger, he had to feed his livestock by hand, pitchforking heavy loads of hay up into the loft of his barn and then stomping on it to soften it enough so the cows could eat it. He had to prepare the feed by hand: because he could not use an electric grinder, he would get the corn kernels for his mules and horses by sticking ears of corn—hundreds of ears of corn—one by one into a corn sheller and cranking it for hours. Because he could not use electric motors, he had to unload cotton seed by hand, and then shovel it into the barn by hand; to saw wood by hand,

by swinging an axe or riding one end of a ripsaw. Because there was never enough daylight for all the jobs that had to be done, the farmer usually finished after sunset, ending the day as he had begun it, stumbling around the barn milking the cows in the dark, as farmers had done centuries before.

But the hardness of the farmer's life paled beside the hardness of his wife's.

Without electricity, even boiling water was work.

Anything which required the use of water was work. Windmills (which could, acting like a pump, bring water out of a well into a storage tank) were very rare in the Hill Country; their cost—almost $400 in 1937—was out of the reach of most families in that cash-poor region, and the few that had been built proved of little use in a region where winds were always uncertain and, during a drought, non-existent, for days, or weeks, on end. And without electricity to work a pump, there was only one way to obtain water: by hand.

The source of water could be either a stream or a well. If the source was a stream, water had to be carried from it to the house, and since, in a country subject to constant flooding, houses were built well away from the streams, it had to be carried a long way. If the source was a well, it had to be lifted to the surface—a bucket at a time. It had to be lifted quite a long way: while the average depth of a well was about fifty feet in the valleys of the Hill Country, in the hills it was a hundred feet or more.

And so much water was needed! A federal study of nearly half a million farm families even then being conducted would show that, on the average, a person living on a farm used 40 gallons of water every day. Since the average farm family was five persons, the family used 200 gallons, or four-fifths of a ton, of water each day—73,000 gallons, or almost 300 tons, in a year. The study showed that, on the average, the well was located 253 feet from the house—and that to pump by hand and carry to the house 73,000 gallons of water a year would require someone

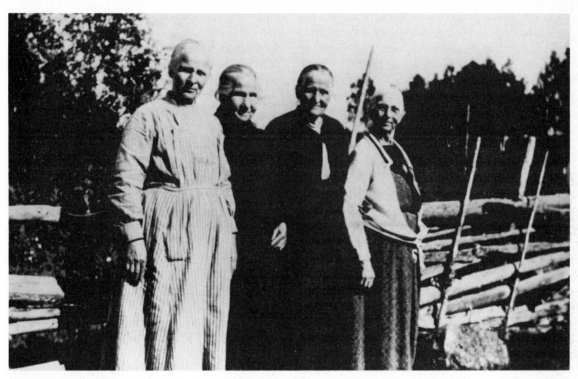

■ ■ *Members of the Peterson family in Travis County, Texas. These farm women of the Hill Country had to haul wood and water for washing and cooking day in and day out until the end of the 1930s.*

to put in during that year 63 eight-hour days, and walk 1,750 miles.

A farmer would do as much of this pumping and hauling as possible himself, and try to have his sons do as much of the rest as possible (it was Lyndon Johnson's adamant refusal to help his mother with the pumping and hauling that touched off the most bitter of the flareups with his father during his youth). As soon as a Hill Country youth got big enough to carry the water buckets (which held about four gallons, or thirty-two pounds, of water apiece), he was assigned the job of filling his mother's wash pots before he left for school or the field. Curtis Cox still recalls today that from the age of nine or ten, he would, every morning throughout the rest of his boyhood, make about seven trips between his house and the well, which were about 300 feet apart, on each of these trips carrying two

large buckets, or more than sixty pounds, of water. "I felt tired," he says. "It was a lot of water." But the water the children carried would be used up long before noon, and the children would be away—at school or in the fields—and most of the hauling of water was, therefore, done by women. "I would," recalls Curtis' mother, Mary Cox, "have to get it, too—more than once a day, more than twice; oh, I don't know how many times. I needed water to wash my floors, water to wash my clothes, water to cook. . . . It was hard work. I was always packing [carrying] water." Carrying it—after she had wrestled off the heavy wooden lid which kept the rats and squirrels out of the well; after she had cranked the bucket up to the surface (and cranking—lifting thirty pounds fifty feet or more—was very hard for most women even with a pulley; most would pull the rope hand over hand, as if they were climbing it, to get their body weight into the effort; they couldn't do it with their arms alone). Some Hill Country women make wry jokes about getting water. Says Mrs. Brian Smith of Blanco: "Yes, we had running water. I always said we had running water because I grabbed those two buckets up and ran the two hundred yards to the house with them." But the joking fades away as the memories sharpen. An interviewer from the city is struck by the fact that Hill Country women of the older generation are noticeably stooped, much more so than city women of the same age. Without his asking for an explanation, it is given to him. More than once, and more than twice, a stooped and bent Hill Country farm wife says, "You see how round-shouldered I am? Well, that's from hauling the water." And, she will often add, "I was round-shouldered like this well before my time, when I was still a young woman. My back got bent from hauling the water, and it got bent when I was still young."

The Hill Country farm wife had to haul water, and she had to haul wood.

Because there was no electricity, Hill Country stoves were wood stoves. The spread of the cedar brakes had given the area a plentiful supply of wood, but cedar seared bone-dry by the Hill Country sun burned so fast that the stoves seemed to devour it. A farmer would try to keep a supply of wood in the house, or, if he had sons old enough, would assign the task to them. (Lyndon Johnson's refusal to chop wood for his mother was another source of the tension between him and Sam). They would cut down the trees, and chop them into four-foot lengths that could be stacked in cords. When wood was needed in the house, they would cut it into shorter lengths and split the pieces so they could fit into the stoves. But as with the water, these chores often fell to the women.

The necessity of hauling the wood was not, however, the principal reason so many farm wives hated their wood stoves. In part, they hated these stoves because they were so hard to "start up." The damper that opened into the fire-box created only a small draft even on a breezy day, and on a windless day, there was no draft—because there was no electricity, of course, there was no fan to move the air in the kitchen—and a fire would flicker out time after time. "With an electric stove, you just turn on a switch and you have heat," says Lucille O'Donnell, but with a wood stove, a woman might have to stuff kindling and wood into the firebox over and over again. And even after the fire was lit, the stove "didn't heat up in a minute, you know," Lucille O'Donnell says—it might in fact take an hour. In part, farm wives hated wood stoves because they were so dirty, because the smoke from the wood blackened walls and ceilings, and ashes were always escaping through the grating, and the ash box had to be emptied twice a day—a dirty job and dirtier if, while the ashes were being carried outside, a gust of wind scattered them around inside the house. They hated the stoves because they could not be left unattended. Without devices to regulate the heat and keep the temperature steady, when the stove was being used for baking or some other cooking in which an even temperature was important, a woman would have to keep a constant watch on the fire, thrusting logs—or corncobs, which ignited quickly—into the firebox every time the heat slackened.

Most of all, they hated them because they were so hot.

When the big iron stove was lit, logs blazing in its firebox, flames licking at the gratings that held the pots, the whole huge mass of metal so hot that it was almost glowing, the air in the kitchen shimmered with the heat pouring out of it. In the Winter the heat was welcome, and in Spring and Fall it was bearable, but in the Hill Country, Summer would often last five months. Some time in June the temperature might climb to near ninety degrees, and would stay there, day after day, week after week, through the end of September. Day after day, week after week, the sky would be mostly empty, without a cloud as a shield from the blazing sun that beat down on the Hill Country, and on the sheet-iron or corrugated tin roofs of the box-like kitchens in the little dog-run homes that dotted its hills and valleys. No matter how hot the day, the stove had to be lit much of the time, because it had to be lit not only for meals but for baking; Hill Country wives, unable to afford store-bought bread, baked their own, an all-day task. (As Mrs. O'Donnell points out, "We didn't have refrigerators, you know, and without refrigerators, you just about have to start every meal from scratch.") In the Hill Country, moreover, Summer was harvest time, when a farm wife would have to cook not just for her family but for a harvesting crew—twenty or thirty men, who, working from sun to sun, expected three meals a day.

Harvest time, and canning time.

In the Hill Country, canning was required for a family's very survival. Too poor to by food, most Hill Country families lived through the Winter largely on the vegetables and fruit picked in the Summer and preserved in jars.

Since—because there was no electricity—there were no refrigerators in the Hill Country, vegetables or fruit had to be canned the very day they came ripe. And, from June through September, something was coming ripe almost every day, it seemed; on a single peach tree, the fruit on different branches would come ripe on different days. In a single orchard, the peaches might be reaching ripeness over a span as long as two weeks; "You'd be in the kitchen with the peaches for two weeks," Hill Country wives recall. And after the peaches, the strawberries would begin coming ripe, and then the gooseberries, and then the blueberries. The tomatoes would become ripe before the okra, the okra before the zucchini, the zucchini before the corn. So the canning would go on with only brief intervals—all Summer.

Canning required constant attendance on the stove. Since boiling water was essential, the fire in the stove had to be kept roaring hot, so logs had to be continually put into the firebox. At least twice during a day's canning, moreover—probably three or four times—a woman would

have to empty the ash container, which meant wrestling the heavy, unwieldy device out from under the firebox. And when the housewife wasn't bending down to the flames, she was standing over them. In canning fruit, for example, first sugar was dropped into the huge iron canning pot, and watched carefully and stirred constantly, so that it would not become lumpy, until it was completely dissolved. Then the fruit—perhaps peaches, which would have been peeled earlier—was put in the pot, and boiled until it turned into a soft and mushy jam that would be packed into jars (which would have been boiling—to sterilize them—in another pot) and sealed with wax. Boiling the peaches would take more than an hour, and during that time they had to be stirred constantly so that they would not stick to the pot. And when one load of peaches was finished, another load would be put in, and another. Canning was an all-day job. So when a woman was canning, she would have to spend all day in a little room with a tin or sheet-iron roof on which a blazing sun was beating down without mercy, standing in front of the iron stove and the wood fire within it. And every time the heat in that stove died down even a bit, she would have to make it hotter again.

"You'd have to can in the Summer when it was hot," says Kitty Clyde Ross Leonard, who had been Johnson's first girlfriend. "You'd have to cook for hours. Oh, that was a terrible thing. You wore as little as you could. I wore loose clothing so that it wouldn't stick to me. But the perspiration would just pour down my face. I remember the perspiration pouring down my mother's face, and when I grew up and had my own family, it poured down mine. That stove was so hot. But you had to stir, especially when you were making jelly. So you had to stand over that stove." Says Bernice Snodgrass of Wimberley: "You got so hot that you couldn't stay in the house. You ran out and sat under the trees. I couldn't stand it to stay in the house. Terrible. Really terrible. But you couldn't stay out of the house long. You had to stir. You had to watch the fire. So you had to go back into the house."

And there was no respite. If a bunch of peaches came ripe a certain day, that was the day they had to be canned—no matter how the housewife might feel that day. Because in the fierce Hill Country heat, fruit and vegetables spoiled very quickly. And once the canning process was begun, it could not stop. "If you peeled six dozen peaches, and then, later that day, you felt sick, you couldn't stop," says Gay Harris. "Because you can't can something if it's rotten. The job has to be done the same day, no matter what." Sick or not, in the Hill Country, when it was time to can, a woman canned, standing hour after hour, trapped between a blazing sun and a blazing wood fire. "We had no choice, you see," Mrs. Harris says.

Every week, every week all year long—every week without fail—there was washday.

The wash was done outside. A huge vat of boiling water would be suspended over a larger, roaring fire and near it three large "Number Three" zinc washtubs and a dishpan would be placed on a bench.

The clothes would be scrubbed in the first of the zinc tubs, scrubbed on a washboard by a woman bending over the tub. The soap, since she couldn't afford store-bought soap, was soap she made from lye, soap that was not very effective, and the water was hard. Getting farm dirt out of clothes required hard scrubbing.

Then the farm wife would wring out each piece of clothing to remove from it as much as possible of the dirty water, and put it in the big vat of boiling water. Since the scrubbing would not have removed all of the dirt, she would try to get the rest out by "punching" the clothes in the vat—standing over the boiling water and using a wooden paddle or, more often, a broomstick, to stir the clothes and swish them through the water and press them against the bottom or sides, moving the broom handle up and down and around as hard as she could for ten or fifteen minutes in a human imitation of the agitator of an automatic—electric—washing machine.

The next step was to transfer the clothes from the boiling water to the second of the three zinc washtubs: the "rinse tub." The clothes were lifted out of the big vat on the end of the broomstick, and held up on the end of the stick for a few minutes while the dirty water dripped out.

When the clothes were in the rinse tub, the woman bent over the tub and rinsed them, by swishing each individual item through the water. Then she wrung out the clothes, to get as much of the dirty water out as possible, and placed the clothes in the third tub, which contained bluing, and swished them around in *it*— this time to get the bluing all through the garment and make it white—and then repeated the same movements in the dishpan which was filled with starch.

At this point, one load of wash would be done. A week's wash took at least four loads: one of sheets, one of shirts and other white clothing, one of colored clothes and one of dish towels. But for the typical, large, Hill Country farm family, two loads of each of these categories would be required, so the procedure would have to be repeated eight times.

For each load, moreover, the water in each of the three washtubs would have to be changed. A washtub held about eight gallons. Since the water had to be warm, the woman would fill each tub half with boiling water from the big pot and half with cold water. She did the filling with a bucket which held three or four gallons— twenty-five or thirty pounds. For the first load or two of wash, the water would have been provided by her husband or her sons. But after this water had been used up, part of washday was walking—over and over—that long walk to the spring or well, hauling up the water, hand over laborious hand, and carrying those heavy buckets back. Another part of washday was also a physical effort: the "punching" of the clothes in the big vat. "You had to do it as hard as you could—swish those clothes around and around and around. They never seemed to get clean. And those clothes were heavy in the water, and it was hot outside, and you'd be standing over that boiling water and that big fire—you felt like you were being roasted alive." Lifting the clothes out of the vat was an effort, too. A dripping mass of soggy clothes was heavy, and it felt heavier when it had to be lifted out of that vat and held up for minutes at a time so that the dirty water could drip out, and then swung over to the rinsing tub. Soon, if her children weren't around to hear her, a woman would be grunting with the effort. Even the wringing was, after a few hours, an effort. "I mean, wringing clothes might not seem hard," Mrs. Harris says. "But you have to wring every piece so many times—you wring it after you take it out of the scrub tub, and you wring it after you take it out of the rinse tub, and after you take it out of the bluing. Your arms got tired." And her hands—from scrubbing with lye soap and wringing—were raw and swollen. Of course, there was also the bending—hours of bending—over the rub boards. "By the time you got done washing, your back was broke," Ava Cox says. "I'll tell you—of the things of my life that I will never forget, I will never forget how much my back hurt on washdays." Hauling the water, scrubbing, punching, rinsing: a Hill Country farm wife did this for hours on end—while a city wife did it by pressing the button on her electric washing machine.

Washday was Monday. Tuesday was for ironing.

Says Mary Cox, in words echoed by all elderly Hill Country farm wives: "Washing was hard work, but ironing was the worst. Nothing could be as hard as ironing."

The Department of Agriculture finds that "Young women today are not aware of the origin of the word 'iron,' as they press clothes with light-weight appliances of aluminum or hollow stainless steel." In the Hill Country, in the 1930s an iron was *iron*—a six- or seven-pound wedge of iron. The irons used in the Hill Country had to be heated on the wood stove, and they would retain their heat for only a few minutes—a man's shirt generally required two irons; a farm wife would own three or four of them, so that several could be heating while one was working.

An iron with a wooden handle cost two dollars more than one without the handle, so Hill Country wives did their weekly loads of ironing—huge loads because, as Mary Cox puts it, "in those days you were expected to starch and iron almost everything"—with irons without handles. They would either transfer a separate wooden handle from one iron to another, or they would protect their hands with a thick potholder.

Since burning wood generates soot, the irons became dirty as they sat heating on the stove. Or, if any moisture was left on an iron from the sprinkled clothes on which it had just been used, even the thinnest smoke from the stove created a muddy film on the bottom. The irons had to be cleaned frequently, therefore, by scrubbing them with a rag that had been dipped in salt, and if the soot was too thick, they had to be sanded and scraped. And no matter how carefully you checked the bottom of the irons, and sanded and scraped them, there would often remain some little spot of soot—as you would discover when you rubbed it over a clean white shirt or dress. Then you had to wash that item of clothing over again.

Nevertheless, the irons would burn a woman's hand. The wooden handle or the potholder would slip, and she would have searing metal against her flesh; by noon, she might have blister atop blister—on hands that had to handle the rag that had been dipped in salt. Ironing always took a full day—often it went on into Tuesday evening—and a full day of lifting and carrying six- or seven-pound loads was hard on even these hardy Hill Country women. "It would hurt so bad between the shoulders," Elsie Beck remembers. But again the worst aspect of ironing was the heat. On ironing day, a fire would have to be blazing in the wood stove all day, filling the kitchen, hour after hour, with heat and smoke. Ironing had to be done not only in the Winter but in the Summer—when the temperature outside the kitchen might be ninety or ninety-five or one hundred, and inside the kitchen would be considerably higher, and because there was no electricity, there was no fan to so much as stir the air. In a speech in Congress some years later, Representative John E. Rankin described the "drudgery" a typical farm wife endured, "burning up in a hot kitchen and bowing down over the washtub or boiling the clothes over a flaming fire in the summer heat." He himself remembered, he said, "seeing his mother lean over that hot iron hour after hour until it seemed she was tired enough to drop." Rankin was from Mississippi, but his description would have been familiar to the mothers of the Edwards Plateau. The women of the Hill Country never called the instruments they used every Tuesday "irons," they called them "sad irons."

Washing, ironing—those were chores that were performed every week. Then, of course, there were special occasions—harvest time and threshing time, when a woman had to cook not just for her family but for a crew of twenty or thirty men; the shearing, when, because there was no electricity and her husband had to work the shears, she had to crank the shearing machine, pedaling as if she were pumping a bicycle up a steep hill, pedaling, with only brief pauses, hour after hour; "He was always yelling 'Faster, faster,' Mrs. Walter Yett of Blanco recalls. "I could hardly get up the next morning, I was so tired after that." Washing, ironing, cooking, canning, shearing, helping with the plowing and the picking and the sowing, and, every day, carrying the water and the wood, and because there was no electricity, having to do everything by hand by the same methods that had been employed by her mother and grandmother and great-great-great-grandmother before her—"They wear these farm women out pretty fast," wrote one observer. In the Hill Country, as many outside observers noted, the one almost universal characteristic of the women was that they were worn out before their time, that they were old beyond their years, old at forty, old at thirty-five, bent and stooped and tired.

A Hill Country farm wife had to do her chores even if she was ill—no matter how ill. Because

Hill Country women were too poor to afford proper medical care, they often suffered perineal tears in childbirth. During the 1930s, the federal government sent physicians to examine a sampling of Hill Country women. The doctors found that, out of 275 women, 158 had perineal tears. Many of them, the team of gynecologists reported, were third-degree tears, "tears so bad that it is difficult to see how they stand on their feet." But they *were* standing on their feet, and doing all the chores that Hill Country wives had always done—hauling the water, hauling the wood, canning, washing, ironing, helping with the shearing, the plowing and the picking.

Because there was no electricity.

The lack of electricity meant that the days of the people of the Hill Country were filled with drudgery; at night they were denied the entertainment—movies, radio—that would have made the drudgery more bearable. The radio could, moreover, have ended the area's isolation. The feeling of the Hill Country youngsters of the 1920s—Lyndon Johnson's generation— that "we were completely cut off out here," that "we were back in the woods, compared to the rest of the world," that "everything had already happened before we found out about it," was the feeling of the 1930s generation as well. Because there was no electricity, the only radios in the Hill Country were the occasional crystal sets with earphones and poor reception. Amos 'n' Andy, Lum 'n' Abner, Ma Perkins—theirs were voices familiar to most of America; it was a rare inhabitant of the Edwards Plateau who had not heard them even once. "What we missed most was the fireside chats," says Mary Cox. "I mean, we loved Franklin D. Roosevelt in this country, and we kept reading about these wonderful fireside chats. But we never got to hear them."

Even reading was hard.

Evening was often the only time in which Hill Country farm couples could read ("There was no other time," says Lucille O'Donnell. "There was never a minute to read during the day, it seemed"), but the only light for reading came from kerosene lamps. In movies about the Old West, these lamps appear so homy that it is difficult for a city dweller to appreciate how much—and why—some farm dwellers disliked them so passionately.

Lighting the kerosene lamp was a frustrating job. "You had to adjust the wick just right," says Curtis Cox of Bryan. "If you turned it too high, it would flame up and start to smoke. The chimney—that's the glass part—would get all black, and your eyes would start to smart." Keeping it lit was even more frustrating. It burned straight across for only a moment, and then would either flare up or die down to an inadequate level. Even when the wick was trimmed just right, a kerosene lamp provided only limited illumination. The approximately twenty-five watts of light provided by most such lamps was adequate for children doing their homework—although surveys would later find that the educational level of rural children improved markedly immediately upon the introduction of electricity—but their parents, whose eyes were not so strong, had more difficulty. Mary Cox says that she couldn't read with their lamp for more than a short period: "I always loved to read," she recalls. "But I couldn't enjoy it on the farm. It was hard on the eyes, a strain on the eyes. I had to force myself to read at night." Lucille O'Donnell came to Burnet from Virginia, where she had liked to read in bed; she couldn't do that on her farm, she says, because she couldn't afford the kerosene. When she did read at night, she could't read in bed. Her husband, Tom, "would be asleep," she recalls, "and I would put the lamp beside him on the bed, and sit on that little stool and read in the most awkward position." Pointing to deep vertical lines between her eyebrows, more than one Hill Country farm wife says: "So many of us have these lines from squinting to read."

The circle of light cast by a kerosene lamp was small, and there were seldom enough lamps in the home of an impoverished farm family. If a family had so many children that they completely surrounded the one good lamp while studying, their mother could not do her sewing until they were finished. And outside the small circles of light, the rooms of a farmhouse were dark. "The house looked scary," says Mary Cox. "If I was alone at night, it was awfully lonely." And, of course, there were no lamps in the outhouse. Many a Hill Country farm wife echoes the words of Betty MacDonald: "I had a horrible choice of either sitting in the dark and not knowing what was crawling on me or bringing a lantern and attracting moths, mosquitoes, nighthawks and bats."

No radio; no movies; limited reading—little diversion between the hard day just past and the hard day just ahead. "Living was just drudgery then," says Carroll Smith of Blanco. "Living— just *living*—was a problem. No lights. No plumbing. Nothing. Just living on the edge of starvation. That was farm life for us. God, city people think there was something fine about it. If they only knew . . ."

So many conveniences taken for granted in American cities were unknown on the Edwards Plateau: not just vacuum cleaners and washing machines but, for example, bathrooms, since, as a practical matter, indoor plumbing is unfeasible without running water, which requires an electric pump. In the Summer, bathing could be done in the creek (when the creek wasn't dry); in the Winter, it entailed lugging in water and heating it on the stove (which entailed lugging in wood) before pouring it into a Number Three washtub. Because bathing was so hard, "you bathed about once a week," Bernice Snodgrass says. Children went barefoot, so "we'd make them wash their feet [at the pump outside] you know. We [adults] would wash our face and hands and ears in washpans but we didn't take a bath but once a week." There were few toilets, and most Hill Country outhouses were the most primitive sort. Many had no pit dug under them. "It would just drop on the ground," Guthrie Taylor recalls. "No, it wouldn't be cleared away"; every so often the flimsy little shelter would just be moved to another spot. Since toilet paper was too expensive, pages from a Sears,

Roebuck catalogue, or corncobs, were used. And some families did not have outhouses. When the Snodgrasses moved to Mount Gaynor from Austin, Bernice Snodgrass says, "We were the only people in the neighborhood that had one. You know what everybody else did? They went out behind the barn, or behind a tree, or something." Frederick Law Olmsted had found the same situation—houses at which there was "no other water-closet than the back of a bush or the broad prairies"—on his journey through the Hill Country in 1857. He had been shocked then, because the America he knew had advanced beyond such primitive conditions. Now it was 1937; four more generations had been living in the Hill Country—with no significant advance in the conditions of their life. Many of the people of Lyndon Johnson's congressional district were still living in the same type of dwelling in which the area's people had been living in 1857: in rude "dog-run" shelters one board thick, through which the wind howled in the winter. They were still squatting behind a bush to defecate. Because of their poverty, they were still utterly bereft not only of tractors and feed grinders, but of modern medical assistance—and were farming by methods centuries out of date.

Although they understood that, as Louise Casparis says, "we were behind the rest of the world," natives of the Hill Country did not realize how *far* behind the rest of the world.

How could they be expected to realize? Without many books to read—or, in general, newspapers, either, except for those pathetic four-page local weeklies; without radio to listen to, with only an occasional movie to watch—how was news of advances in the rest of the world to reach them? Since many of them never saw that world for themselves—an astonishing high proportion of Hill Country residents would never visit even Austin or San Antonio—the Hill Country's awareness of the outside world was dim. The life of Hill Country natives was, more-

over, the same life that their mothers and fathers—and grandmothers and grandfathers—had lived; how were they to know, except in general, vague, terms, that there was another kind of life? When they heard about the wonders of electricity, they thought electricity was the electricity they saw in Johnson City, the dim, flickering lights hardly better than lamplight; the wonders they imagined were the electric iron and the radio, little more; "I remember when someone started telling me about these washing machines," recalls Ava Cox. "A machine that *washed?* I couldn't picture that *at all!*" Even the concept of the toilet was difficult for them to accept completely; when Errol Snodgrass, newly arrived in Mount Gaynor, began not only to build an outhouse but to dig a pit underneath it, a neighbor asked him: "What do you want that pit for?" And when he explained, Bernice Snodgrass recalls, the reaction of the neighborhood was, " 'They're so highfalutin that they have to have a toilet.' They thought an outhouse with a pit under it—they thought that that was what people meant when they spoke about a toilet!" Natives of the Hill Country couldn't understand why families that had moved away from the Hill Country never returned. It is not, therefore, by lifelong residents of the Hill Country that the contrast between life there and in the outside world is most clearly enunciated, but by newcomers: from families which, due to economic necessity, moved to the Hill Country in the 1930s.

The Depression had cost Brian and Mary Sue Smith their home and their once-profitable automobile-repair shop in Portland, Texas, a town near Corpus Christi. In 1937, they moved with their three children to the Hill Country—to a fifty-three-acre farm near Blanco—because "that was the only place where land was cheap enough so we could buy a farm."

Portland had electricity—had had it for years. "You never even thought about electricity," Mrs. Smith says. "I just accepted it. I mean, if I thought about it, I suppose I would have thought, 'Doesn't *everyone* have electricity?' "

Now she found out that not everyone did.

The Smiths had brought their radio, a big black Atwater Kent with an amplifying horn on top, to their new home, but it could not be played. "You know, it was very lonely on that farm," Mrs. Smith says. "The quiet was nice sometimes. But sometimes it was so quiet it hurt you." They had brought their washing machine, but that could not work, either. Mrs. Smith loved to read, but "The light was hard on your eyes. My eyes just weren't good enough to read at night." In Portland, she had crocheted at night, but she found the light was too dim for her to do that at night. And, of course, there was no time to do it during the day; what time wasn't consumed by her household chores was taken up husking, shelling and grinding corn by hand for feed for the 150 hens whose eggs she was selling; by cranking the sheep-shearing machine. Soon after she arrived on the farm, her husband became very ill, and for more than a year she had to care for the livestock too, and to plow behind a pair of mules—although she had never plowed before. "Up before daylight. Build the fire in the wood range. Put on the biscuits. Go out and milk the cows. Breakfast. Work was all there was. It was a bare existence."

Getting the water, from a well some 200 yards from the house, was the chore that bothered her most. "The children had had running water in Portland, of course, and they acted like they still had it," she says. When she started meeting other Hill Country women, she noticed that many of them were round-shouldered, and they told her it was from carrying heavy buckets of water. She didn't want to be round-shouldered. But there seemed no solution. "Carry and carry. Back and forth. Sometimes I would get awfully discouraged. When I first moved there [to the Hill Country], I felt like a pioneer lady, like one of the women who had come here in covered wagons. I said, if they could do it, I could, too. But it was very hard. After you spent all morning lugging those big buckets back and forth, you felt more like an ox or a mule than a human being. Portland was just a little town. It was no great metropolis. But moving from Portland into the Hill Country was like moving from the twentieth century back into the Middle Ages."

■■■

STUDY QUESTIONS

1. Why had electric transmission lines never been built in large areas of the Hill Country?

2. Why was the lot of these women so difficult before the arrival of electricity?

3. Why was water such a critical item to Hill Country women? Describe the efforts required to get water into the typical home in this area.

4. Why did Hill Country women hate their stoves?

5. How did these women iron clothes? Why did they hate the chore of ironing?

6. When electricity arrived at a Hill Country farm, what changes did it bring in the way people lived?

BIBLIOGRAPHY

For the best description of the Hill Country, see Robert A. Caro, *The Years of Lyndon Johnson. The Path to Power* (1982). Also see John Graves, *Hard Scrabble* (1974) and *Texas Heartland: A Hill Country Year* (1975). The best descriptions of southern agriculture during the New Deal years are Richard S. Kirdendall, *Social Scientists and Farm Politics in the Age of Roosevelt* (1966) and David Conrad, *The Forgotten Farmers* (1965). The latter deals with those who did not benefit from the Agricultural Adjustment Administration. On the problem of poverty in the South, see Paul Mertz, *The New Deal and Southern Rural Poverty* (1978). The best discussion of the Rural Electrification Administration is D. Clayton Brown, *Electricity for Rural America: The Fight for REA* (1980).

"UNCONTROLLED DESIRES": THE RESPONSE TO THE SEXUAL PSYCHOPATH, 1920–1960

Estelle B. Freedman

The contemporary American preoccupation with crime is nothing new. In the nineteenth century, bank and train robberies gave rise to a hero worship of sorts, with criminals like Jesse James and Billy the Kid enjoying a degree of notoriety that rivaled the fame of lawmen like Wyatt Earp and Wild Bill Hickock. During the 1920s, Prohibition spawned the new industry of organized crime, and Americans were both fascinated and appalled by the violent excesses of people like Al Capone and Dion O'Bannion. When the Great Depression ended Prohibition, and as people tried to forget their poverty, the focus of American popular culture shifted to a new set of criminals—to outlaws like Bonnie and Clyde, John Dillinger, Ma Barker, and Pretty Boy Floyd—and to the "G-Men," like J. Edgar Hoover, who were out to get them. After World War II, the country's attention turned to the search for Communist spies and Mafia hit men. People followed with fascination the fates of Alger Hiss and Lucky Luciano.

Many of the criminals who captured the American imagination managed to achieve almost a folk-hero status. The public resented their crimes but often applauded their audacity and admired their power. One group of criminals, however, inspired only loathing from the American public—the psychopathic sexual offenders: rapists, voyeurs, exhibitionists, and child molesters. Victorian values had made sex a controversial and difficult issue in American society, and the association of violent criminality with sexuality especially outraged the country. Today that attitude remains. The crimes committed during the 1960s, 1970s, and 1980s by serial murderers, rapists, and child molesters such as John Wayne Gacy, Richard Speck, Henry Lee Lucas, and Theodore Bundy were unimaginable to most Americans and inspired the revival of capital punishment in many states. In " 'Uncontrolled Desires': The Response to the Sexual Psychopath, 1920–1960," Estelle B. Freedman looks at how Americans of that era tried to come to terms with sexual offenders and how that response influenced prevailing attitudes about gender, sexuality, and mental illness.

In the 1931 German film *M*, Peter Lorre portrayed a former mental patient who stalked innocent school girls, lured them with candy and balloons, and then, offscreen, murdered them in order to satiate his abnormal erotic desires. Two years later, when the film opened in the United States, the *New York Times* criticized director Fritz Lang for wasting his talents on a crime "too hideous to contemplate." Despite the reviewer's distaste for the public discussion of sexual crimes, the American media soon began to cater to a growing popular interest in stories of violent, sexual murders committed by men like "M." In 1937 the *New York Times* itself created a new index category, "Sex Crimes," to encompass the 143 articles it published on the subject that year. Cleveland, Detroit, and Los Angeles newspapers also ran stories about sexual criminals, while national magazines published articles by legal and psychiatric authorities who debated whether a "sex-crime wave" had hit America.

The sex crime panic soon extended beyond the media and into the realm of politics and law. Between 1935 and 1965, city, state, and federal officials established commissions to investigate sexual crime, passed statutes to transfer authority over sex offenders from courts to psychiatrists, and funded specialized institutions for the treatment of sex offenders. As a result, in most states, a man accused of rape, sodomy, child molestation, indecent exposure, or corrupting the morals of a minor—if diagnosed as a "sexual psychopath"—could receive an indeterminate sentence to a psychiatric, rather than a penal, institution. The laws defined the sexual psychopath as someone whose "utter lack of power to control his sexual impulses" made him "likely to attack . . . the objects of his uncontrolled and uncontrollable desires."

A close look at the sex crime panics that began in the mid-1930s, declined during World

War II, and revived in the postwar decade reveals that those episodes were not necessarily related to any increase in the actual incidence of violent, sexually related crimes. Although arrest rates for sexual offenses in general rose throughout the period, the vast majority of arrests were for minor offenses, rather than for the violent acts portrayed in the media. Moreover, when arrest rates accelerated sharply during World War II, the popular discourse on sex crimes quieted, and no new psychopath laws were enacted. The historical evidence also prohibits a conspiratorial interpretation in which power-hungry psychiatrists manipulated the public and politicians to create a sex crime panic and psychiatric solutions to it. Most psychiatrists remained skeptical about psychopath laws. Rather, the media, law enforcement agencies, and private citizens' groups took the lead in demanding state action to prevent sex crimes. In the process, they not only augmented the authority of psychiatrists, but also provoked a redefinition of normal sexual behavior.

The new image of aggressive male sexual deviance that emerged from the psychiatric and political response to sex crimes provided a focus for a complex redefinition of sexual boundaries in modern America. For one thing, public outrage over rare, serious sexual crimes facilitated the establishment of legal and psychiatric mechanisms that were then used to regulate much less serious, but socially disturbing, behaviors. The response to the sexual psychopath, however, was not merely expansion of social control over sexuality by psychiatry and the state. Rather, by stigmatizing extreme acts of violence, the discourse on the psychopath ultimately helped legitimize nonviolent, but nonprocreative, sexual acts, within marriage or outside it. At the same time, psychiatric and political attention to the psychopath heightened public awareness of sexuality in general, and of sexual abnormality in particular, between 1935 and 1960.

Thus the response to the sexual psychopath must be understood in the context of the history

Freedman, Estelle B., " 'Uncontrolled Desires': The Response to the Sexual Psychopath, 1920–1960," *Journal of American History* (June 1987), 83–106.

of sexuality, for it evidenced a significant departure from the nineteenth-century emphasis on maintaining female purity and a movement toward a modern concern about controlling male violence. In the nineteenth century, the ideal of female purity had served symbolically to control male lust and to channel sexual impulses into marital, reproductive relationships. In practice, of course, individuals deviated from the ideal, and periodic sexual reform movements—such as moral reform, social purity, and anti-prostitution—attempted to uphold female purity and restore the deviant to the fold. Antebellum sexual reformers typically employed moral suasion and social sanctions, but by the early twentieth century, reformers had increasingly turned to the state to enforce their vision of moral order. During the Progressive Era, for example, city and state governments investigated white slavery, Congress passed the Mann Act to prohibit the interstate transportation of women for immoral purposes, and during World War I the United States Army mobilized against prostitution, incarcerating suspected prostitutes found in the vicinity of military training camps.

By the 1920s the Victorian ideal of innate female purity had disintegrated. Stimulated by Freudian ideas, a critique of "civilized morality" infiltrated American culture. Meanwhile, working-class youth, blacks, immigrants, and white bohemians had created visible urban alternatives to the old sexual order. They engaged in a sexually explicit night life, used birth control, or accepted sexuality outside marriage. Even for the middle classes, a recognition of female sexual desire and of the legitimacy of its satisfaction—preferably in marriage but not necessarily for procreation—came to dominate sexual advice literature by the 1920s. As birth control, companionate marriage, and female sexual desire became more acceptable, female purity lost its symbolic power to regulate sexual behavior. Not surprisingly, by the 1930s calls to wipe out prostitution could no longer mobilize a social movement. Reformers now had to base

their arguments more on "social hygiene"—the prevention of venereal disease—rather than on the defense of female virtue.

If the Victorian ideal divided women into the pure and the impure, modern ideas about sexuality blurred boundaries in ways that made all women more vulnerable to the risks once experienced primarily by prostitutes. "If woman in fact should be a sexual creature," Victorian scholar Carol Christ has asked, "what kind of beast should man himself become?" One response to her query was heralded in England during the 1880s by the crimes of Jack the Ripper, whose sexual murders of prostitutes, Judith R. Walkowitz has argued, created a powerful cultural myth associating sex with "violence, male dominance and female passivity." In twentieth-century America, the image of the sexual psychopath further specified both the "kind of beast" man might become and the kind of victims he now sought. The sexual psychopath represented man unbounded by the controls of female purity, a violent threat not only to women, but to children as well. But violence against women and children was not the underlying concern of the sex crime panics. Rather, the concept of the sexual psychopath provided a boundary within which Americans renegotiated the definitions of sexual normality. Ultimately, the response to the sexual psychopath helped legitimize less violent, but previously taboo, sexual acts while it stigmatized unmanly, rather than unwomanly, behavior as the most serious threat to sexual order.

To understand how and why this controversial psychiatric diagnosis attracted so much public attention and found its way into American criminal law requires three levels of analysis: of psychiatric ideas, of political mobilization, and of sexual boundaries. Taken together, they reveal a complex relationship between psychiatry, social change, and sexuality. Psychiatrists, journalists, and politicians all helped create the sexual psychopath, but a public concerned with changing gender relationships seized upon the threat of "uncontrolled desires" to help redefine sexual normality and deviance in modern America.

When it first appeared in Europe in the late nineteenth century, the diagnosis of psychopathy did not refer exclusively either to sexual abnormality or to men. Akin to the concept of moral insanity, it was applied to habitual criminals who had normal mentality but exhibited abnormal social behavior. The German psychiatrist Emil Kraepelin used the term psychopathic personality in his influential 1904 textbook to refer primarily to criminals with unstable personalities, vagabonds, liars, or beggars, although he also listed prostitutes and homosexuals. In 1905, Adolf Meyer introduced the concept of the psychopath into the United States, where sexual crime remained synonymous with female immorality. William Healy's pathbreaking study, *The Individual Delinquent* (1915), mentioned female hypersexuality and described psychopaths as egocentric, selfish, irritable, antisocial, nervous, and weak willed, but Healy refused to discuss male sexual abnormality and recommended that most readers "should leave the unpleasant subject alone." Until the 1920s American psychiatrists who diagnosed mental patients as psychopaths typically applied the term to either unemployed men or "hypersexual" women.

The transformation of the psychopath into a violent, male, sexual criminal occurred gradually as a result of three convergent trends. First, as courts and prisons became important arenas into which American psychiatry expanded beyond its earlier base in state mental hospitals, the recently established specialization of forensic psychiatry sought new explanations for criminal behavior. Second, the social stresses of the depression drew attention to the problems of male deviance. Third, the social scientific study of sexuality became respectable, and the influence of psychoanalytic theories on American psychiatry during the 1930s provided an intellectual base for a sexual theory of crime.

American criminologists began to use the psychopathic diagnosis during the 1920s partly because of weaknesses in the dominant theory that low mentality ("mental defect" or "feeblemindedness"), if not the cause of crime, was highly correlated with it. During the Progressive Era, several states had established separate institutions for the indeterminate commitment of mentally defective prisoners. In practice, however, many of the suspected "defective delinquents" turned out to have normal IQs. With the influx of psychiatrists into courts and prisons after 1915, criminologists increasingly turned to psychiatric diagnoses, such as "constitutional psychopath," to help explain these troublesome prisoners. In 1921, the Massachusetts legislature enacted the Briggs Law, which required psychiatric evaluation of recidivist felons and those convicted of capital offenses. Many of those prisoners who could not be diagnosed as insane or mentally defective were eventually labeled "psychopathic." Such redefinitions expanded the category of insanity and helped create a new deviant population, the psychopaths. In 1918, for example, psychiatrist Bernard Glueck diagnosed almost 20 percent of the inmates at New York's Sing Sing prison as "constitutional inferior, or psychopathic" and recommended a new state institution to house psychopathic and defective delinquents. Between 1919 and 1926, the percentage of inmates classified as psychopaths at one men's reformatory in New York rose from 11.6 to 50.8, while diagnoses of mental defect declined sharply.

Despite increased use of the psychopathic diagnosis, male sexual crimes rarely received the attention of psychiatrists and criminologists during the 1920s. When sexuality and psychopathy were linked at that time, women, not men, remained the likely subjects. Indeed, the first specialized institution for psychopathic criminals, a hospital operated at the Bedford Hills Reformatory for Women between 1916 and 1918, had been established because of John D. Rockefeller, Jr.'s interest in eliminating prostitution. Glueck's Sing Sing study did note an absence of sexual morality among psychopathic male inmates, 10 percent of whom had committed sexual crimes. However, his characterization of the psychopath emphasized recidivism, drug and alcohol use, and unstable work patterns, rather than abnormal sexual impulse. Even when sexual crimes against children first became the focus of governmental reports in the 1920s, the psychopath was not associated with such offenses. Nevertheless, the malleable diagnostic category of psychopath had become more widely applied and would soon take on new meanings.

The sexualization of the male psychopath occurred during the 1930s, when American criminologists became increasingly interested in sexual abnormality and male sexual crime. The disruption of traditional family life during the depression, when record numbers of men lost their status as breadwinners, triggered concerns about masculinity. Psychologist Joseph Pleck has argued that during the 1930s psychologists elaborated on sex differences and investigated sexual deviance in order to shore up the psychological basis of masculinity at a time when social and economic support for the traditional male role seemed to be eroding. In the process, the male sexual deviant became the subject of special attention, particularly if he was inadequately masculine (the effeminate homosexual) or hypermasculine (the sexual psychopath). Both categories of deviant males were thought to attack children, thus simultaneously threatening sexual innocence, gender roles, and the social order. The psychopath neatly fit these concerns. From the origin of the concept, the psychopath had been perceived as a drifter, an unemployed man who lived beyond the boundaries of familial and social controls. Unemployed men and vagabonds populated the depression-era landscape, signaling actual family dissolution and symbolizing potential social and political disruption. Like the compulsive child murderer "M," the psychopath could represent the threat of anarchy, of the individual unbound by either social rules or individual conscience.

The apparent "sexualization" of the drifter reflected, in part, a merging of economic and psychological identities in modern America.

In this social context, Americans embarked on the serious study of human sexuality, measuring normality and defining deviance. During the twenties and thirties, classic texts by European sexologists, such as Richard von Krafft-Ebing, Havelock Ellis, and Magnus Hirschfeld, became more widely available. A growing number of American researchers, including Katharine Bement Davis and Robert Latou Dickinson, conducted survey and case studies of sexual practices. Within criminology, older biological theories combined with the recent identification of sex hormones to stimulate studies of the mentality of homosexuals, the impact of castration on rapists, and the levels of endocrines in senile sex offenders. New funding sources supported the investigation of sexuality. In 1931, the Rockefeller Foundation helped establish the National Research Council Committee for Research on Problems of Sex, which later supported the work of Alfred Kinsey. The Committee for the Study of Sex Variants, founded in 1935 and chaired by Eugen Kahn (an authority on the psychopath), sponsored a pioneering, two-volume study of homosexuality by psychiatrist George Henry.

A second intellectual current helps account for psychiatric interest in sex criminals, in general, and the sexual component of psychopathic personality, in particular. In the 1920s, Freudian concepts of psychosexual development had begun to filter through the fields of psychiatry and criminology, a process that accelerated after the immigration of European analysts to this country. In the early 1930s, a few discussions of the psychopath—such as Kahn's important text, translated into English in 1931—referred to infantile sexuality and to arrested sexual development. In the same year, psychiatrist Franz Alexander elaborated on the contribution to criminality of the Oedipal complex and of anal and oral eroticism. A 1937 article in the *Psychoanalytic Review* indicated the new direction in psychiatric interpretations when it characterized the psychopath as "the phallic man," fixated at an infantile stage of boundless bisexual energy. By the late 1930s, most discussions of the psychopath included at least a section on sexual types, such as "overt homosexuals, exhibitionists, sadists, masochists, and voyeurs." Some authors explicitly linked such deviants to the commission of sexual crimes.

The most prolific advocate of the psychosexual interpretation of psychopathic behavior was Benjamin Karpman, chief psychotherapist at St. Elizabeth's Hospital in Washington, D.C. In voluminous case studies of criminals, Karpman attributed most habitual criminality to arrested sexual development and identified psychopaths by their incapacity to repress or to sublimate their overly active sexual impulses. The typical sexual psychopath was, he believed, "all instinct and impulse." Karpman once claimed, for example, that the psychopath was "always on the go for sexual satisfaction . . . like a cancer patient who is always hungry no matter how much he is fed." Later investigators would attribute sexual psychopathy to underdeveloped, rather than overdeveloped, libido, but Karpman held firmly to his belief that sexual psychopaths always had insatiable and uncontrollable desires. Although his views were extreme among psychiatrists, Karpman's vision of the psychopath as emotionally primitive and sexually ravenous resonated with popular stereotypes that harked back to the theory of the born criminal. Thus, an older, hereditarian tradition merged with new psychiatric concepts to produce a crude model of the psychopath as oversexed, uninhibited, and compulsive. It was this image that found its way into the popular press and ultimately into the law.

The incorporation of the sexual psychopath into American criminal law began in the late 1930s in the wake of the first of two waves of popular concern about violent sexual crimes. Three constituencies—the media, citizens' groups, and law enforcement agencies—created the sex crime panic and demanded that politicians offer solutions to the problems of rape and sexual murder of children. Politicians, in turn, seized upon the sexual psychopath as the villain in the sex crime drama and called on psychiatrists as the heroes who might rid society of the danger they posed.

Each of the two major sex crime panics—roughly from 1937 to 1940 and from 1949 to 1955—originated when, after a series of brutal and apparently sexually motivated child murders, major urban newspapers expanded and, in some cases, sensationalized their coverage of child molestation and rape. Between 1937 and 1940, and again during the postwar decade, the *New York Times*, previously silent on the subject, averaged over forty articles per year on sex crimes. In 1937, magazines ranging from *Science* and the *Christian Century* to the *Nation* and the *New Masses* reported on the sex crime panic. After World War II news and family magazines, including *Time, Newsweek,* and *Parents' Magazine,* carried articles titled "Queer People," "Sex Psychopaths," and "What Shall We Do About Sex Offenders?" In its 1950 series on "Terror in Our Cities," *Collier's* magazine summarized the newspaper headlines in St. Louis ("The City that *DOES* Something About Sex Crime") in a representative composite.

KINDERGARTEN GIRL ACCOSTED BY MAN—CLERK ACCUSED OF MOLESTING 2 GIRLS IN MOVIE—MAN ACCUSED BY 8-YEAR-OLD BOY OF MOLESTING HIM IN THEATRE—6-YEAR-OLD GIRL AT ASHLAND SCHOOL MOLESTED—LABORER ARRESTED FOR RAPE OF 10-YEAR-OLD GIRL—FINED FOR MOLESTING 2 BOYS, AGED 8 AND 10—ARRESTED ON SUSPICION OF MOLESTING 4-YEAR-OLD GIRL—YOUTH WHO MOLESTED BOY 4, IS FINED $500—9 CHARGES AGAINST MOLESTER OF GIRLS.

Despite the lack of evidence that the incidence of rape, child murder, or minor sex offenses had increased, public awareness of individual acts of sexual brutality led to demands

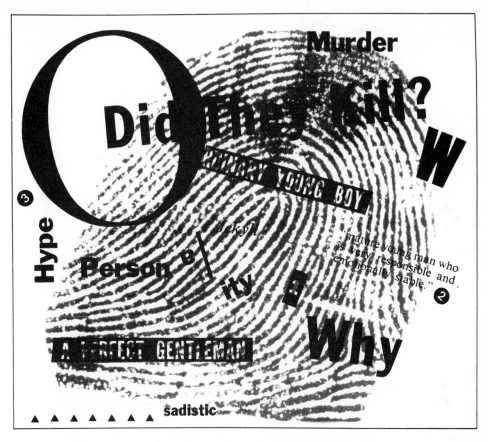

that the state crack down on sex crimes. In 1937, after two child murders had occurred in New York City, residents of Ridgewood, Queens, held a protest meeting and demanded that police be given more power to "take suspicious characters in hand before they commit the crimes." In Chicago, after the rape-murder of two nurses, a police squad was formed to "round up attackers." When a Philadelphia man confessed to attacks on both male and female children, that city's mayor recommended sterilization of sex offenders. In New Jersey, when six men were indicted for assaulting girls, the New Jersey Parents and Teachers Congress urged denial of parole to those convicted of sex crimes. In 1937 a mob in Inglewood, California, threatened lynching while the police sought the murderers of three local girls. In 1950, a Connecticut mob attempted to lynch a suspected sex criminal,

while the national American Legion called for life sentences without parole for sex offenders.

Federal Bureau of Investigation director J. Edgar Hoover played an important role in fueling the national hysteria and channeling it into support for stronger law enforcement. In 1937 Hoover called for a "War on the Sex Criminal" and charged that "the sex fiend, most loathsome of all the vast army of crime, has become a sinister threat to the safety of American childhood and womanhood." In a popular magazine article published in 1947, Hoover claimed that "the most rapidly increasing type of crime is that perpetrated by degenerate sex offenders." Implying that this threat to social order required total mobilization, Hoover continued: "Should wild beasts break out of circus cages, a whole city would be mobilized instantly. But depraved human beings, more savage than beasts, are permitted to rove America almost at will."

In response to the sex crime panic, police roundups of "perverts" became common, especially in the wake of highly publicized assaults on children. The targets of crackdowns were often minor offenders, such as male homosexuals. A rare glimpse of the reaction of "perverts" to such roundups appeared in a letter written in 1946 by one homosexual male to another after a brutal child murder in Chicago: "I suppose you read about the kidnapping and killing of the little girl in Chicago—I noticed tonight that they 'thought'(in their damn self-righteous way) that perhaps a pervert had done it and they rounded up all the females [male homosexuals]—they blame us for everything and incidentally it is more and more in the limelight everyday—why they don't round us all up and kill us I don't know." In this case and in others, police justified increased surveillance of all deviant sexual behavior, whether violent or not, by the need to protect women and children from sexual violence.

While some politicians supported the call for law and order, others turned to psychiatrists for solutions to the sex crime problem. In the 1930s, the New York State legislature called on institutional psychiatrists to explain how to prevent sex crimes. Mayor Fiorello LaGuardia appointed psychiatrists, lawyers, and criminologists to a Mayor's Committee for the Study of Sex Offenses. In a move that foreshadowed the national political response to sex crimes, LaGuardia also instituted an emergency program that transferred accused and convicted sex criminals from city penitentiaries to Bellevue Hospital for medical observation.

Some psychiatrists expressed discomfort about the sex crime panic. Karl Bowman, then director of the psychiatric division at Bellevue, observed that most of the men transferred there were minor offenders who did not belong in a mental hospital. At a 1938 symposium on "The Challenge of Sex Offenders" sponsored by the National Committee on Mental Hygiene, psychi-

atrists argued that no sudden increase in sex crime had occurred and cautioned against new legislation that would establish either castration or prolonged imprisonment for sex offenders. Bowman and other panelists called for more frank, rational discussions of sexuality and claimed that sexual repression caused sex offenses. Other psychiatrists, such as Ira Wile, wrote articles opposing prolonged imprisonment or castration for sex offenders. They recommended instead hospital care, psychiatric exams, and research on sex crimes.

Despite psychiatric ambivalence about proposed legislation that would incorporate the psychopathic diagnosis into the law, and despite strong criticism of such statutes within the legal profession, five states—Michigan, Illinois, Minnesota, Ohio, and California—passed "sex psychopath" laws between 1935 and 1939. That not simply psychiatric leadership, but the public mobilization to combat the alleged sex crime wave explains their passage is evident in the case of Ohio. In 1934, psychiatrists in that state's mental hospitals had failed to get the legislature to fund separate treatment for psychopathic criminals. In 1938, however, after the *Cleveland Plain Dealer* ran in a series of articles on sex offenders, civic groups created sufficient pressure to achieve quick passage of the Ascherman Act, which permitted the indefinite commitment of psychopaths to the state mental hospital.

Although the psychopath laws were avowedly enacted to protect women and children, they were the product of men's political efforts, not women's. Several women's clubs publicly favored stronger criminal penalties for sex crimes, and male politicians frequently called on representatives of conservative women's organizations to testify in favor of psychopath legislation. However, in contrast to earlier movements for moral reform and social purity, in which organizations such as the Woman's Christian Temperance Union had played a major part, the campaign for sexual psychopath laws had little female, and no feminist, leadership.

The hiatus in the sex crime panic during the early 1940s further suggests that its central concern was men, not women. The legitimization of male aggression during World War II and the shift of national attention toward external enemies combined to reduce the focus on violent sexual crimes. Although arrest rates remained high during the war, both newspaper and magazine coverage of sex crimes tapered off markedly, and only one state—Vermont—enacted a psychopath law. The wartime entry of men into the military and of women into jobs formerly held by men restored the "hypersexual" woman to the foreground. Social workers and government agencies condemned the phenomenon of "victory girls," young women who willingly had sex with soldiers and sailors, and antiprostitution campaigns revived briefly in the name of protecting soldiers from venereal disease.

The postwar years, however, provided a climate conducive to the reemergence of the male sexual psychopath as a target of social concern. The war had greatly increased the authority of psychiatrists, who had been drafted to screen recruits and to diagnose military offenders. Postwar psychiatric and social welfare literature stressed the adjustment problems of returning servicemen, some of whom, it was feared, might "snap" into psychopathic states. In addition, demobilization and reconversion to a peacetime economy stimulated concerted efforts to reestablish traditional family life. Returning male veterans needed jobs that had been held by women, who were now encouraged to marry, bear children, and purchase domestic products. Moreover, the onset of the Cold War, with its emphasis on cultural conformity, intensified efforts to control deviant behavior. Nonconformity—whether political, social, or sexual—became associated with threats to national security. And, amid the pressures for social and sexual stability, Alfred Kinsey published his study of male sexual behavior, igniting unprecedented public debate about normal and abnormal sexuality.

During the postwar decade, the sex crime panic gathered renewed momentum, peaking in the mid-1950s. As if to signal—or to enforce—the return of prewar gender relations, sex crimes once again became a subject of media attention and political action. Although arrests for rape and other sex offenses fell after the war, legislatures revised earlier sexual psychopath laws, and between 1947 and 1955, twenty-one additional states and the District of Columbia enacted new psychopath laws. In the early 1950s, arrest rates returned to prewar levels, but only after the second phase of the sex crime panic had begun.

The sexual psychopath laws enacted during the two periods of panic operated alongside older penal codes that punished crimes such as rape and murder with incarceration in state penitentiaries or execution. Most sex offenders continued to be processed under the older codes. During the early 1950s, for example, California superior courts sentenced only 35 percent of convicted sex offenders to mental institutions as psychopaths; 54 percent went to prisons and 11 percent to the youth authority. Prior to 1953 annual commitments of psychopaths averaged thirty-seven in each state with a special law. Revised laws and new facilities in the 1950s increased commitments in several states; Michigan and Maryland, for example, each averaged one hundred per year. Few of those committed, however, were the homicidal sex maniacs on whom the sex crime panic had originally focused. They tended to be white men, often professionals or skilled workers, who were overrepresented among those convicted of sexual relations with children and minor sexual offenses. Black men, who continued to be overrepresented among those convicted of rape, were more likely to be imprisoned or executed than to be treated in mental institutions. In short, white men who committed sexual crimes had to be mentally ill; black men who committed sexual crimes were believed to be guilty of willful violence.

The sexual psychopath laws did not necessarily name specific criminal acts, nor did they differentiate between violent and nonviolent, or consensual and nonconsensual, behaviors. Rather, they targeted a kind of personality, or an identity, that could be discovered only by trained psychiatrists. Whether convicted of exhibitionism, sodomy, child molestation, or rape, sexual psychopaths could be transferred to state mental hospitals or psychiatric wards of prisons for an indefinite period, until the institutional psychiatrists declared them cured. The laws rested on the premise that even minor offenders (such as exhibitionists), if psychopaths, posed the threat of potential sexual violence. Indefinite institutionalization of sex offenders would protect society from the threat of violent sexual crimes, and psychiatric care would be more humane than castration, life imprisonment, or execution.

In addition to passing laws, elected officials in ten states appointed special commissions to investigate the nature of sexual offenders, the problem of sex crimes, or the legislative means to prevent them. The documents published by such commissions varied in depth and tone from superficial accounts of popular attitudes to serious discussions of the psychiatric, legal, and ethical issues raised by sex-offender legislation. In general, the state reports echoed themes raised by the earlier New York mayor's committee. They found little evidence of increases in local sex crime rates, bemoaned the vagueness of the classification "sexual psychopath," called for scientific study of these mysterious offenders, and recommended new or revised psychopath laws that would, unlike many of the earlier statutes, require conviction of a crime before institutionalization. The preventive measures suggested by state commissions took two forms: specialized psychiatric institutions for men convicted of sex crimes and preventive measures, such as psychiatric screening of potential psychopaths through schools or behavior clinics and sex education to promote healthy family life.

Whatever ambivalence psychiatrists may have had about incorporating the psychopathic diagnosis into law, the postwar response to sexual crimes helped to solidify psychiatric authority within the criminal justice system in two important ways. Following state commission recommendations for more research, a half dozen states provided funding for psychiatric studies of sex offenders. In California, for example, the sex crime panic enabled Karl Bowman, director of the Langley Porter Psychiatric Clinic of the University of California, to obtain funds from the state legislature for programs on sexual deviates, although his previous requests for state funding had been denied. The New Jersey Sex Offender Acts of 1949 and 1950 established a Diagnostic Center for the study of juvenile and adult offenders, and New York State's Sex Delinquency Research Project funded studies of sex offenders at Sing Sing prison.

The second means by which the state expanded both its own and psychiatrists' authority was the establishment of specialized institutions to treat sexual offenders. Under the initial sexual psychopath statutes, men committed for sexual offenses served their indeterminate sentences either on mental wards of prisons or on criminal wards of mental hospitals, such as Howard Hall at St. Elizabeth's Hospital. In 1949, the Ohio legislature appropriated over one million dollars to build a specialized facility for mentally defective and psychopathic criminals at the Lima State Hospital. Maryland legislators authorized the maximum security Patuxent Institution, which opened in 1951, for the psychiatric treatment of habitual offenders, mental defectives, and sexual criminals. In 1954, California transferred the men who had been sentenced as psychopaths from state mental hospitals to the newly completed, ten-million-dollar Atascadero State Hospital. Once institutionalized, the psychopath received treatments according with the therapeutic trends of the era: Metrazol, insulin shock or electro-shock; hormonal injections; sterilization; group therapy; and, in some cases, frontal lobotomy. According to the clinical literature, none of these proved effective in reducing "uncontrolled desires."

The sexual psychopath laws, always controversial among psychiatrists and lawyers, came under renewed criticism in the 1950s and 1960s. In 1949 the Committee on Forensic Psychiatry of the liberal Group for the Advancement of Psychiatry issued a report that argued that the concept of the psychopath was too vague and controversial to be written into law. The following year, in the New Jersey state report on sex offenders, sociologist Paul Tappan attempted to refute the myth of escalation from minor to violent sex crimes, noting that sex offenders had the lowest recidivism rates of all criminals. Legal scholars stepped up their critique of the sexual psychopath laws, and during the 1960s, a "due process revolution" in mental health inspired constitutional challenges to sexual psychopath laws on the grounds that they denied both due process and equal protection to accused sex offenders. By 1968, when Michigan repealed the first of the original state psychopath laws and abolished the legal category of "criminal sexual psychopath," an experiment in psychiatric criminology seemed to have come full circle.

As they debated the treatment of the sexual psychopath, psychiatrists and politicians spoke to deeper social concerns about the meaning of sexuality. At a time when the standards of sexual behavior for both women and men were changing rapidly, the psychopath became a malleable symbol for popular fears about the consequences of new sexual values. A close reading of the popular, legal, and psychiatric literature related to the sex crime panics and the psychopath laws reveals at least three ways in which the concept of the sexual psychopath served to create or to clarify boundaries between normal and abnormal behavior. First, the discussion of the sexual psychopath influenced the redefinition of rape as not only a male psychological aberration, but also an act in which both women and children contributed to their own victimization. Second, it drew a strict boundary between heterosexual and homosexual males, labeling the latter as violent child molesters. Finally, the creation of the psychopath as an extreme deviant figure helped Americans adjust to a sexual system in which nonprocreative acts were no longer considered abnormal.

Unlike the Progressive-Era antiprostitution crusade, the sex crime panic of the thirties, forties, and fifties virtually ignored women as perpetrators, while redirecting concern about victims to include not only women, but especially children of both sexes. Child molestation, like rape, clearly predated the sex crime panics, but for the first time the sexual victimization of children became a subject of popular concern. The gradual acceptance of female sexual desire helped focus attention on children, for if women now actively sought sexual fulfillment, they were less accessible as symbolic victims, while childhood innocence remained a powerful image. In the film M, for example, a real-life rapist of women was transformed into a child murderer, as if rape alone were not enough to horrify the modern audience. At the same time, Freudian ideas about childhood sexuality and Oedipal desire raised the specter of children's participation in sexual acts. Finally, just as the continued entry of women into the paid labor force evoked fears about unattended children becoming juvenile delinquents, it may have also heightened fears of children's susceptibility to the sexual advances of strangers.

A close investigation of the psychopath literature suggests that women—and to some extent children as well—were paying a high price for the modern recognition of their sexual desire and the removal of female purity as a restraint on male sexuality. Female victims were often portrayed as willing participants in the acts of which men were accused. For example, the New York mayor's committee on sex offenses explained that "In most sex crimes, the fact that a particular girl is a victim of a sex assault is no accident. Generally, there is to be found something in the personality, the environmental background, or the family situation of the victim . . . which predisposes her to participation in sex delinquency." The theme that victims were in some way delinquent themselves recurred during the 1950s in the work of relatively liberal critics of the laws, such as Bowman and Bernice Engle, of the influential California Sex Deviate Research Project, and Morris Ploscowe, a lawyer and judge who championed liberalization of laws regulating sexuality. These critics reiterated doubts that a woman could be raped without some predisposition. The legal reforms that they recommended to improve the treatment of the psychopath included corroboration of rape charges by witnesses, investigation of victims' past sexual activity, and proof of "complete sexual penetration"—in short, the very legal mechanisms that feminists would seek to dismantle a decade later. Moreover, in a major study of child sexual abuse and incest, conducted at California's Langley Porter Clinic, the authors described the majority of the victims (80 percent of whom were female) as "seductive," "flirtatious," and sexually precocious. They labeled those for whom abuse persisted over time as "participating victims." Thus, in a movement allegedly based upon the urgent need to protect women and children, the victims were ultimately as stigmatized as the perpetrators. As in the case of the Southern rape complex, in which black men lived in fear of accusation and white women lived in fear of assault, the threat of the sexual psychopath served to regulate sexual behavior not only for "deviant" men, but also for women.

The image of the rapist in the psychopath literature further attests to the marginal influence of women's interests on the response to the sexual psychopath. The laws rested on the premise that most rapists were "sick" men, suggesting that rape was an isolated act committed by crazed strangers. In fact, recent scholarship has shown that sexual assault is a common experience for women, its perpetrators as likely to be family members or acquaintances as strangers. Even more interesting is a shift in the psychiatric and legal interpretations that occurred by the 1950s. Critics of the psychopath laws increasingly suggested that, in the words of one state report, "aggression is a normal com-

ponent of the sexual impulse in all males." By this logic, as long as he did not mutilate or murder his victim, the rapist might be considered almost normal and certainly more "natural" than men who committed less violent, and even consensual, sexual acts such as sodomy and pedophilia. Accordingly, men diagnosed as psychopaths were more likely to be accused of pedophilia and homosexuality than of rape or murder.

The response to the sexual psychopath was not, then, a movement to protect female purity; its central concern was male sexuality and the fear that without the guardianship of women, either men's most beastlike, violent sexual desires might run amok, or men might turn their sexual energies away from women entirely. Adult women were now suitable objects for "normal" male sexual desire, even normal male aggression, but the discourse on the psychopath mapped out two new forbidden boundaries for men: sex with children or with other men. The literature frequently played on fears of child molestation, and a significant minority of psychopaths were charged with male homosexual acts, either with children or adults. This fact, and the frequent overlap in use of the terms *sex criminal, pervert, psychopath,* and *homosexual,* raises the question of whether *psychopath* served in part as a code for *homosexual* at a time of heightened public consciousness of homosexuality.

Social historians have recently identified the 1940s as a critical period in the formation of a public homosexual world in the United States. Although homosexual subcultures had begun to form in American cities as early as the 1890s, it was not until the 1930s that literature and the theatre drew national attention to the existence of homosexuals in this country. The war years provided new opportunities for young men and women to discover homosexuality as they left their families and hometowns to enter the military or defense industries. During the 1940s both homosexual men and lesbians created visible social institutions, including bars, social clubs, and political organizations. By 1950 the early homophile rights movement, the forerunner of gay liberation, was articulating a positive view of homosexuals as a cultural minority group. However, society as a whole remained strongly homophobic. As Barbara Ehrenreich has argued, during the 1950s, "Fear of homosexuality kept heterosexual men in line as husbands and breadwinners." Despite efforts to remove the stigma from homosexuality, the American Psychiatric Association categorized it as a mental disease until 1973. Moreover, in the 1950s the federal government launched a campaign to remove homosexuals from government jobs.

The psychopath literature did reinforce the fear of male homosexuality. At times it appeared that a major motive of the psychopath laws was to prevent the contagion of homosexuality from spreading from adults to youths. Such contagion might corrupt the entire community and might ultimately result in violent death. For example, a 1948 article in the *American Journal of Psychiatry* argued that when adults indulged in homosexual acts with minors, "The minors in turn corrupted other minors until the whole community was involved." As evidence the authors cited "the recent killing of a 7-year-old boy by a 13-year-old because he [the younger child] would not perform the act of fellatio." Furthermore, the beliefs that homosexuals actively recruited among youth and that seduction in youth or childhood was the "commonest single environmental factor" explaining homosexuality were both used to support psychopath legislation. Dr. J. Paul de River, a crude popularizer of theories of sexual psychopathy, stated the case for vigilance in his book *The Sexual Criminal*:

All too often we lose sight of the fact that the homosexual is an inveterate seducer of the young of both sexes, and that he presents a social problem because he is not content with being degenerate himself; he must have degenerate companions and is ever seeking for younger victims.

Thus, homosexuality was increasingly linked to violence and, especially, to the allegedly coercive recruitment of minors for illicit sexual activity.

The panic over the sexual psychopath, however, did not merely shore up traditional sanctions against male homosexuality by associating it with violence. Rather, even the seemingly repressive aspects of the campaign promoted a new, more open, public discourse on nonmarital, nonprocreative sexuality. The literature on the sexual psychopath helped break down older taboos simply by discussing sexual deviance. At the same time, the literature encouraged a reevaluation of heterosexual behavior during a time of rapid flux in sexual standards. At a basic level, the psychopath literature helped disseminate information about sexual practices that had previously been outside the bounds of proper discourse. Now, in the name of preventing children from either becoming or succumbing to sexual psychopaths, professionals began to argue that sex education should not ignore such practices as oral and anal sex. The state commissions on sex crimes took an especially active part in this educational campaign, holding extensive public hearings and conducting attitudinal surveys on sexual abnormality. For example, the Michigan Governor's Study Commission distributed "A Citizens' Handbook of Sexual Abnormalities and the Mental Hygiene Approach to Their Prevention." An Oregon social hygiene council published a fourteen-page "Introduction to the Problem of the Sex Deviate." The city of Long Beach, California, distributed a cartoon-illustrated booklet for children as its "answer to sex fiends." Like the antimasturbation literature of the nineteenth century, the sexual perversion literature of the postwar era was, no doubt, as educative as it was preventive.

In commenting on the widespread concern about psychopaths, many writers pointed to the influence of Kinsey's study of male sexuality, published in 1948, which revealed the extensive practice of nonprocreative sexual acts, within and outside marriage. An editor of the *American*

Journal of Psychiatry even argued that Kinsey's evidence of a "gap between cultural mores and private behavior" might have set off a "reaction formation against anxiety and guilt" that led, in turn, to the scapegoating of extreme sexual offenders. Liberal critics of the psychopath laws also referred to Kinsey's study, citing his results to argue that sexual variations were now so common among "normal" couples that they should be excluded from the psychopath laws. For example, Bowman and Engle attempted to differentiate between the dangerous acts of the psychopath and the newly acceptable practices of masturbation, premarital petting, and "unnatural acts" (i.e., oral and anal sex) performed in private between consulting adults. Thus, they assured the public that "serious" perversions did require psychiatric treatment but that healthy sexuality might include nonprocreative heterosexual acts. In this way, the discourse on the psychopath helped redefine the boundaries of normal sexuality and may well have contributed to the sexual liberalism of the 1960s.

From the 1930s through the 1950s, the sexual psychopath provided the focus for public discussions of sexual normality and abnormality, while the state played an increasingly important role in defining sexual deviance and in prescribing psychiatric treatment. The debates on the psychopath statutes did more than expand the legal authority of psychiatry. The critics of the laws ultimately helped to legitimize nonprocreative heterosexual acts; the media and national commissions helped educate the public about both "natural" and "perverse" sexual behaviors. At the same time, the psychopath literature tended to stigmatize female and child victims of sexual assault and to draw a firm sexual boundary proscribing all homosexual activity and linking it with extreme violence, especially against youths.

It is difficult to assign any simple meaning to the response to the sexual psychopath. Like "M," or like his later American counterpart in Alfred Hitchcock's film, *Psycho*, the image of the sexual psychopath revealed a deep discomfort with the potential violence of male sexuality unconstrained by female purity—of "uncontrolled desires." The response to the sexual psychopath also confirms that, as in the case of lynching, the fear of sexual violence can provide an extremely powerful tool for mobilizing political support against nonconforming individuals. The ultimate historical legacy of the response to the sexual psychopath, however, was to expand the public discourse on sexuality, to focus attention on male violence, and to heighten the importance of sexuality as a component of modern identity. In so doing, the sexual psychopath helped to redefine the boundaries of acceptable sexual behavior in modern America.

■ ■ ■

STUDY QUESTIONS

1. In what ways did Freudian ideas influence popular and psychiatric views of criminality in the 1920s?

2. How did the Great Depression of the 1930s affect prevailing attitudes toward sexual psychopathy?

3. What were the Victorian ideals of female and male sexuality? How did those ideals change during the 1920s?

4. Why were there sex crime panics late in the 1930s and early in the 1950s? What role did the media play in magnifying public fears?

5. Why did concern with psychosexual crime decline during World War II?

6. How did the issue of psychopathic sexual crimes influence the development of psychiatry between 1920 and 1960?

7. During the years between 1920 and 1960, how did American attitudes about legitimate and illegitimate sexual activities change? What role did sexual psychopathy play in those changes?

BIBLIOGRAPHY

David J. Pivar's *Purity Crusade: Sexual Morality and Social Control, 1868–1900* (1973) looks at the rise of Victorian attitudes in the United States, while Paul Robinson's *The Modernization of Sex* (1976) looks at the decline of Victorian values. The impact of Sigmund Freud on American culture is explained in Nathan G. Hale, Jr., *Freud and the Americans: The Beginning of Psychoanalysis in the United States, 1876–1917* (1971); Gerald Grob, *Mental Illness and American Society, 1815–1940* (1983); and Albert Deutsch, *The Mentally Ill in America* (1949). On changing attitudes toward women, see William Chafe, *The American Woman: Her Changing Social, Economic, and Political Roles, 1920–1970* (1972). Attitudes toward sexual minorities are described in John D'Emilio, *Sexual Politics, Sexual Communities: The Making of a Homosexual Minority in the United States, 1940–1970* (1983), and Ronald Bayer, *Homosexuality and American Psychiatry: The Politics of Diagnosis* (1981).

WAR OF
THE WORLDS

William Manchester

It's a truism today that the mass media influences the lives of Americans. Society is constantly barraged with questions and criticisms about such issues as the quality of children's programming, the political bias of newscasters, the ethics of television advertising, the domination of political campaigns by the media, and the decline of literacy and the written word. More than any other technological innovation, the development first of radio and then of television has transformed American life, changing the way people live and relate to one another. The first radio station in the United States began broadcasting out of Pittsburgh in 1920. Three years later there were more than 500 stations doing the same thing, and by 1929 more than 12 million families listened to the radio at home every night. The communications revolution that radio stimulated contributed to the creation of a mass, national culture.

The influence of the radio, however, did not immediately dawn on people. In 1927 the National Broadcasting Company became the first national network, and by 1933 President Franklin D. Roosevelt was effectively using the radio for his famous "fireside chats." But it was not until 1938, when Orson Welles broadcast his famous "War of the Worlds" program, that Americans realized the potential of radio to shape public attitudes. With Adolf Hitler making his designs on Czechoslovakia well known, Americans were worried that another global conflict was in the making. Battered by the frustration of the Great Depression and nervous about the safety of the world, millions of people panicked when Orson Welles described over national radio an invasion of the East Coast by Martians. In the following essay, historian William Manchester describes the broadcast and the controversy it inspired.

The journalistic hoax has a long, picaresque, and not entirely dishonorable history. Edgar Allan Poe became famous on the strength of his "Unparalleled Adventure of One Hans Pfall"; H. L. Mencken's spurious account of how the first bathtub was invented became a national joke and found its way into some encyclopedias. The most successful of all, Richard Adams Locke's Moon Hoax of 1835, told wide-eyed readers of the *New York Sun* that one "Sir John Herschel," using "an immense telescope based on an entirely new principle," had identified bat-man inhabitants of the moon. Poe, Mencken, and Locke were quickly forgiven, for newspapers, being what Marshall McLuhan calls a "cool medium," are not likely to incite a riot. The mass media are "hot," and radio has never been hotter than the night before Halloween in 1938.

The recipient of that heat was then the most versatile and successful young man on Broadway. Actor-director, producer, at the age of twenty Orson Welles had been radio's "Lamont Cranston" *(The Shadow)*. He had dressed Julius Caesar in a business suit, put on a Negro *Macbeth* with Haiti as the background—and made money with both. When his WPA production of *The Cradle Will Rock* was ordered canceled on opening night by Washington—on political grounds—Welles defied the government. He and his theatrical company led the customers through the streets to an empty theater. The play became an enormous success, and CBS invited the prodigy of show business to broadcast a one-hour drama from the network's Studio One each Sunday evening at 8 P.M. There were no sponsors; the program was what was called "sustaining." CBS wasn't making much of a gesture. It couldn't sell the time, because its NBC competitor, the Chase and Sanborn Hour, was the most popular program of the week. Don Ameche was the master of ceremonies there, Dorothy Lamour

From *The Glory and the Dream: A Narrative History of America, 1932–1972* by William Manchester. Copyright © 1973, 1974 by William Manchester. Reprinted by permission of Little, Brown and Company.

the singer, and high comedy was provided by ventriloquist Edgar Bergen and his redheaded dummy Charlie McCarthy. Carved by a Chicago bartender for $35, and based on a Bergen sketch of a Chicago newsboy, Charlie had been No. 1 for eighteen months. His witty, insolent personality dominated Sunday prime time.

When it came to a choice between great theater and listening to Bergen talk to himself, most Americans preferred Bergen. Both the Crosley and Hooper radio censuses conducted the week before that Halloween gave the Chase and Sanborn Hour 34.7 percent of the total possible audience and Welles's Mercury Theater 3.6 percent. (There was a hidden factor here, withheld from advertisers because it would damage their morale; we shall encounter it presently. Still, the figures doubtless held up on an average Sunday.) Of the 32 million families then living in the United States, about 27.5 million owned radios. Thus when CBS played the opening strains of the Tchaikovsky Piano Concerto in B Flat Minor—the Mercury's opening theme each week—Welles could assume that about a million people were tuned to him. On October 30 that figure would grow.

Roosevelt had sent a personal message to Hitler on September 26 asking him to stop issuing ultimatums and proposing instead a conference of "nations directly interested in the present controversy" as an alternative to the battlefield. He suggested it be held immediately in some "neutral spot in Europe." It never came off—other conferences were being arranged—but on that same day Orson Welles had an inspiration. Why not dramatize H. G. Wells's *War of the Worlds?* His agent thought the idea silly, and Howard Koch, his writer believed it was impossible. The young producer insisted. Being a strong personality, he won, and Koch went off to translate Wells into Welles. On Tuesday, October 25, five days before the show, he phoned John Houseman, the Mercury's editor. He was throwing in the towel, he said; science fantasy couldn't be turned into radio drama. The Mercury's secretary agreed. "You can't do it!" she cried. "Those old Martians are just a lot of nonsense! We're going to make fools of ourselves! Absolute fools!" Houseman thought of substituting *Lorna Doone,* but Orson wouldn't discuss it, so writing the Wells script became a team effort. By Thursday they had a show—a dull show, everyone agreed.

Then someone—later no one remembered who—made a suggestion. Wouldn't it be a good idea to make the whole thing a simulated news broadcast? As realistic as possible? Even a voice like Roosevelt's? It was all possible, including the voice; Kenneth Delmar, whom Fred Allen would later make famous as Senator Claghorn, could summon commanding tones. The actor who would play Carl Phillips, the first network "announcer," dug into the CBS record library and listened, over and over, to the semihysterical radio commentator's descripton of the *Hindenburg* exploding at Lakehurst. Welles himself would appear as a Princeton scientist. They were to open with a weather report, dance music, and then the special bulletins. The cast thought Welles dragged this part much too long. He shook his head; that, he explained, was what gave it authenticity.

It certainly did. The public had become accustomed to sudden interruptions during the Czech crisis; each had provided a significant development later confirmed in the newpapers. Radio, indeed, had become the accepted vehicle for important announcements. And there were other circumstances which would increase authenticity. Since the 1936 election, *Fortune* had found, people had more faith in commentators than in newspapers. Indeed, for many the line between reality (news) and fantasy (drama) had become hopelessly blurred. In one of the more penetrating postmortems of the performance, *Variety* doubted that "any explanation would have prevented some people taking the whole thing in deadly earnest," because "evidence of the seriousness with which many listeners take radio dramas is the concerned letters numerous dialers write in about the characters and happenings in the daily serial shows."

It was, furthermore, an era in which people still respected authority, and Kenneth Delmar would be identified as "the Secretary of the Interior." For audiences in New York and New Jersey, real streets were to be named: the Pulaski Skyway, South Street, route 23. Added to all these, a Princeton University study later found, were intellectual and emotional immaturity, Depression insecurity ("Things have happened so thick and fast since my grandfather's day that we can't hope to know what might happen now," one respondent said afterward) and, outweighing everything else, the "recent war scare in Europe."

Welles seems to have had some apprehension. The script opened and closed with explanations that this was only a play, and four CBS station breaks were to interrupt the actors and say the same thing. All that was fine, given their assumption that listeners would join them at eight o'clock and stay till the end. But the assumption was unsound. Here the rating surveys' little secret assumed tremendous significance. Their discovery, which would have discouraged sponsors, was that when a commercial or an unpopular entertainer came on, people reached over and twisted their radio dials. Everyone enjoyed Edgar Bergen and Charlie McCarthy, but they were only part of a variety show.

The Mercury's relatively small but faithful audience heard the Tchaikovsky theme, the introduction, an authentic weather report, and "We now take you to the Meridian Room in the Hotel Park Plaza in downtown New York, where you will be entertained by the music of Ramón Raquello and his orchestra." Periodic bulletins traced the progress of Carl Phillips and Professor Pierson to the New Jersey town of Grovers Mill. There were sirens and crowd noises in the background. At that moment, 8:12 P.M., Charlie McCarthy finished his first skit and a soothing voice began to recommend the rich flavor of Chase and Sanborn coffee.

Nearly six million people spun dials to CBS. This is what they heard:

ANNOUNCER: . . . I'll move the microphone nearer. Here, (Pause) Now we're not more than
twenty-five feet away. Can you hear it now?
Oh, Professor Pierson!

PIERSON: Yes, Mr. Phillips?

ANNOUNCER: Can you tell us the meaning of that
scraping noise inside the thing?

PIERSON: Possibly the unequal cooling of its surface.

ANNOUNCER: Do you still think it's a meteor, Professor?

PIERSON: I don't know what to think. The metal
casing is definitely extraterrestrial . . . not
found on this earth. Friction with the earth's
atmosphere usually tears holes in a meteorite.
The thing is smooth and, as you can see, of cylindrical shape.

PHILLIPS: Just a minute! Something's happening!
Ladies and gentlemen, this is terrific. The end
of the thing is beginning to flake off! The top is
beginning to rotate like a screw! The thing must
be metal!

Excited crowd voices were heard; then back to
the microphone.

ANNOUNCER: Ladies and gentlemen, this is the
most terrifying thing I have ever witnessed! . . .
Wait a minute! Someone's crawling out of the
hollow top. Someone or . . . something. I can
see peering out of that black hole two luminous
discs . . . are they eyes? It might be a face. It
might be . . .

(Shout of awe from the crowd)

ANNOUNCER (sobbing and retching): Good heav-
ens, something's wriggling out of the shadow
like a gray snake. Now it's another one, and
another! They look like tentacles to me. There, I
can see the thing's body. It's large as a bear
and it glistens like wet leather. But that face. It
. . . it's indescribable. I can hardly force myself
to keep looking at it. The eyes are black and
gleam like a serpent. The mouth is V-shaped
with saliva dripping from its rimless lips that
seem to quiver and pulsate. . . .

The announcer temporarily loses control.
Silence. A few bars of "Clair de Lune." A second
announcer, cool and professional, says, "We are
bringing you an eyewitness account of what's
happening on the Wilmuth farm, Grovers Mill,
New Jersey." A few more bars of Debussy, then
the cool announcer again: "We now return you
to Carl Phillips at Grovers Mill." Policemen, it
develops, are advancing on the thing, but the
Martians turn a sheet of flame upon them.
Screams are heard, and unearthly shrieks. A
barn blows up; then the mike goes dead. In
comes the second announcer, saying quietly,
"Ladies and gentlemen, due to circumstances
beyond our control, we are unable to continue
the broadcast from Grovers Mill. Evidently
there's some difficulty with our field transmission. However, we will return you to that point
at the earliest opportunity." Now the action
escalates. The state police have been burned to
cinders. "Brigadier General Montgomery Smith,
commander of the State Militia in Trenton,"
makes an official statement, in behalf of the governor of New Jersy, placing the counties of Mer-
cer and Middlesex, as far west as Princeton and
east to Jamesburg (all real places), under martial
law. New spaceships are landing, and Pierson,
who has made a miraculous escape, says the
invaders are armed with something which "for
want of a better term, I shall refer to . . . as a
heat-ray."

Now the second announcer is upset:

ANNOUNCER: Ladies and gentlemen, I have a
grave announcement to make. Incredible as it
may seem, both the observations of science and
the evidence of our eyes lead to the inescapable
conclusion that those strange beings who landed
in the Jersey farmlands tonight are the vanguard of an invading army from the planet
Mars.

In shocked tones he reveals that Martians
have annihilated the New Jersey National
Guard. Marital law is declared throughout New
Jersey and eastern Pennsylvania. The President
has declared a national emergency. The Secre-

tary of the Interior, sounding like FDR and even using his phrases, begs the country to do its duty and pray God for help. The Army Air Corps is wiped out. An operator comes on jerkily:

OPERATOR: *This is Newark, New Jersey. . . . This is Newark, New Jersey! . . . Warning! Poisonous black smoke pouring in from Jersey marshes. Reaches South Street. Gas masks useless. Urge population to move into open spaces . . . automobiles use routes 7, 23, 24. . . . Avoid congested areas. Smoke now spreading over Raymond Boulevard. . . .*

In the last sequence before the middle break, Ray Collins, the only surviving announcer, is standing on a New York rooftop. Bells are ringing in the background warning New Yorkers that it's time to evacuate the city; the Martians are coming. "Hutchinson River Parkway is still kept open for motor traffic. Avoid bridges to Long Island . . . hopelessly jammed." Voices in the background are singing a hymn; you can just hear them as Collins, his voice choking, reads a bulletin announcing that "Martian cylinders are falling all over the country. One outside Buffalo, one in Chicago, St. Louis. . . ."

Toward the end of Collins's speech (8:32 P.M.) Davidson Taylor, a CBS program supervisor, was asked to leave the Studio One control panel; an urgent phone call awaited him. He left and returned, his face a white knot. Already 60 per cent of local stations had broken into the broadcast to reassure listeners that all this was make-believe, and New York policemen were surrounding the CBS Building. None of the performers or technicians would be allowed to leave after the show; some urgent questions needed answering. When Taylor came back to the control booth, Collins was describing the Martians, tall as skyscrapers, astride the Pulaski Skyway, preparing to wade through the Hudson River. It was seconds before the break, so Taylor decided to let Collins end, which he did in a voice ravaged by gas:

COLLINS: *. . . Now they're lifting their metal hands. This is the end now. Smoke comes out*

. . . black smoke, drifting over the city. People in the streets see it now. They're running toward the East River . . . thousands of them, dropping like rats. Now the smoke's spreading faster. It's reached Times Square. People are trying to run away from it, but it's no use. They're falling like flies. Now the smoke's crossing Sixth Avenue . . . Fifth Avenue . . . 100 yards away . . . it's 50 feet . . .

OPERATOR FOUR: *2X2L calling CQ . . . 2X2L calling CQ . . . 2X2L calling CQ . . . New York. Isn't there anyone on the air? Isn't there anyone . . . 2X2L . . .*

Now came the break; now a regular CBS announcer told them that they were listening to a CBS presentation of Orson Welles and his Mercury Theater. The second half of the program followed. It was sensitively written, with no hysterics, but that didn't matter any more. Before the break hundreds of thousands of screaming Americans had taken to the streets, governors were begging their constituents to believe that martial law had *not* been declared, and the churches were jammed with weeping families asking for absolution of their sins before the Martians came to *their* town. Altogether, the Princeton study discovered, approximately 1,700,000 believed the program to be a news broadcast, and about 1,200,000 were sufficiently distressed to do something about it. "For a few horrible hours," the study concluded, "people from Maine to California thought that hideous monsters armed with death rays were destroying all armed resistance sent against them; that there was simply no escape from disaster; that the end of the world was near."

In every state, telephone operators were overwhelmed. Local stations reported a 500 percent increase in incoming calls. In New York CBS and police switchboards were jammed. Riverside Drive became impassable; it was packed with mobs of sobbing people. Conditions were worse in northern New Jersey, where the first Things had been "discovered." Weeping families clung to one another, terrified men ran blindly across

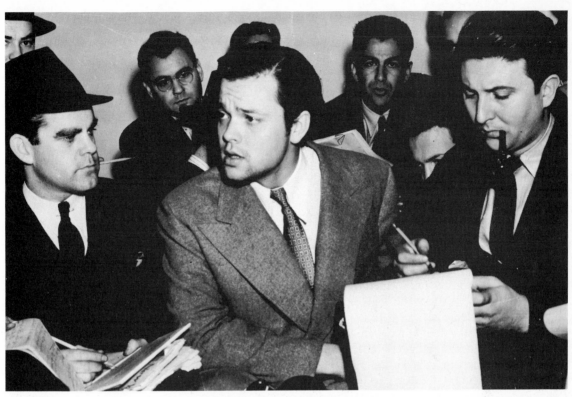

■ ■ *Orson Welles, besieged by reporters the day after the 1938 broadcast of the ''War of the Worlds.'' Welles expressed amazement and regret that his dramatization had created panic among millions of radio listeners.*

fields, and drivers raced about in all directions, all hoping to escape asphyxiation and flaming death. Train terminals and bus stations were filled with wild-eyed people demanding tickets to anywhere; one New York woman phoning the Dixie Bus Terminal for information gasped, "Hurry, please, the world is coming to an end and I have a lot to do."

When Dorothy Thompson wrote, "Nothing about the broadcast was in the least credible," there was a tendency among those who had not heard the program to dismiss the stricken mobs as ignorant. It was untrue. Miss Thompson to the contrary, *War of the Worlds* was a magnificent technical achievement; even today a transcription of it is chilling. And while there was some correlation between fear, education, and eco-

nomic status—the most vulnerable were listeners who had not completed grammar school and had been on relief for more than three years—the well-to-do could not be let off so easily. Princeton found that 28 percent of the college graduates who were tuned to the program, and 35 percent of those with high incomes, believed they were hearing straight news. On a southern university campus, sorority girls wept in each other's arms and took turns telephoning their parents for a last goodbye, and an Ivy League senior, driving back from a Vassar check-in, was convinced when he flipped on the car radio that "Princeton was wiped out and gas was spreading over New Jersey and fire."

In Studio One, Welles signed off jovially: "Goodbye everybody, and remember, please, for the next day or two the terrible lesson you learned tonight . . . and if your doorbell rings and nobody's there, that was no Martian! It's Halloween." The red light went out; the Mercury Theater was off the air. But it was Studio One's doorbell that was ringing, and somebody was out there—not Martians but New York's finest, determined to teach Orson Welles a lesson he would never forget. Before opening the door, Welles and Houseman answered a shrill telephone in the control room. As Houseman later remembered it, the call came from "the mayor of some Midwestern city, one of the big ones. He is screaming for Welles. Choking with fury, he reports mobs in the streets of his city, women and children huddled in the churches, violence and looting. If, as he now learns, the whole thing is nothing but a crummy joke—then he, personally, is coming up to New York to punch the author of it on the nose!"

They hung up, the door burst open, the studio was suddenly crowded with dark blue uniforms, and what Houseman called "the nightmare" began—interrogations hinting darkly at countless suicides, traffic deaths, and a "fatal stampede in a Jersey hall." At the moment the police could think of no law that had been broken, so the two men were released to a more terrible fate: the press. It seemed to Houseman that the press was being vindictive because radio had eclipsed newspaper coverage of the Czech crisis. Reporters countered that the broadcast was a big story, which it certainly was. Next morning scare headlines read:

RADIO WAR TERRORIZES U.S.

PANIC GRIPS NATION
AS RADIO ANNOUNCES
"MARS ATTACKS WORLD"

TIDAL WAVE OF TERRORISM
SWEEPS NATION

PHONE CALLS SWAMP POLICE
AT BROADCAST OF FANTASY

"The show came off," Houseman said wryly. There was no doubt about that. For two days it drove Hitler off front pages, while CBS put to rest the fears of those still distressed by following its hourly time signal ("9 P.M. B-u-l-o-v-a, Bulova Watch Time") with an explanation that "the entire story and all of its incidents were fictitious." The Federal Communications Commission issued a statement describing the program as "regrettable" and proposing a new radio code. For a while there was talk of criminal action, but it died away. By then Orson Welles had rocketed to national fame, and his Mercury Theater, no longer CBS's poor relation, had acquired a lavish sponsor in Campbell Soups. Eventually Welles was invited to a White House function. The President took him off to one side and said, "You know, Orson, you and I are the two best actors in America." He seemed serious, but Welles wasn't sure how to take it, so he merely bowed.

■ ■ ■

STUDY QUESTIONS

1. How would you describe the personality of Orson Welles? Did he sense at the outset the kind of controversy he was about to trigger?

2. How significant was the Czech crisis as a background to the reaction to the broadcast?

3. What does the incident indicate about public gullibility and the capacity of people to distinguish between truth and fiction?

4. In your opinion, was the broadcast unethical and dangerous? Would television networks risk such a broadcast today? Why or why not?

5. Manchester also argues that a struggle was going on in the United States between the broadcast and print media. Why? How important was that struggle? In your opinion, which medium has prevailed in the United States.

BIBLIOGRAPHY

For discussions of the role of advertising in the 1920s, see Stuart Ewen, *Captains of Consciousness* (1976). The influence of films on American culture is ably portrayed in Robert Sklar, *Movie-Made America* (1975) and Larry May, *Screening Out the Past* (1980). Paul Carter's *Another Part of the Twenties* (1977) is an excellent description of popular social attitudes during the infancy of the radio industry. Although there is not much literature on the history of radio, see Erik Barnouw, *A Tower of Babel: A History of Broadcasting in the United States* (1966) and Francis Chase, *Sound and Fury: An Informal History of Broadcasting* (1942).

HITLER'S LEGIONS IN AMERICA

Arnold Krammer

After a decade of poverty, unemployment, and economic uncertainty, the United States was transformed by the Nazi invasion of France in June 1940. Considered at the time to be one of the premier military powers on earth, France succumbed in less than a month to the German assault, and suddenly the United States was lifted out of its isolationist malaise. The country also left behind the Great Depression. In Franklin D. Roosevelt's words, "Dr. New Deal" gave way to "Dr. Win the War." Employment and government spending increased enormously because of military production. After the Japanese attack on Pearl Harbor in December 1941, the country entered a period of massive mobilization. Men marched off to war and women marched off to the factories. Unprecedented populations shifts occurred as people moved to where they could work or be close to loved ones.

One great challenge had given way to another. World War II had a moral clarity about it which sanctioned sacrifice. Arrayed against the United States were the forces of evil, symbolized in Adolf Hitler's outstretched hand, Benito Mussolini's arrogant demeanor, or Hideki Tojo's tight smile. World War II seemed a global struggle between good and evil, and Americans spent a great deal of time between 1941 and 1945 convincing themselves of their own virtue as well as the of malignancy of fascism and its supporters. But amidst that great ideological crusade, some Americans had the opportunity to confront the enemy firsthand. By the end of World War II, there were more than 400,000 German prisoners-of-war in American camps. Their presence in small towns and cities across the country gave Americans a different image of the Axis "supermen." In "Hitler's Legions in America," historian Arnold Krammer describes those German POWs in the United States.

I n the early morning in a small town, people might have been eating breakfast, businesses opening their doors for their first customers, and traffic coming to life. In the distance, people might have heard crisp, guttural commands being shouted in German, and they might have shaded their eyes against the bright morning sun to stare at the columns of young men—blond, deeply-tanned, and healthy—as they marched through town to harvest the crops in the surrounding fields. A rural town in Nazi Germany? People across the United States who remember World War II know better. This scene could have taken place in Trinidad, Colorado; Algona, Idaho; Dermott, Arkansas; West Ashley, South Carolina; Evelyn, Michigan; or in any of several hundred other cities and towns across the country.

The scene would have been enacted by Americans by the second year of war, 1943, when the population was adjusting to the scarcity of certain products and to the daily influx of war news. People were exhorted to produce at extraordinary levels; farmers were moving to the city for higher-paying jobs in war industries; the scarcity of tires, gasoline, and batteries was patriotically endured; OPA ration books were the housewives' bibles; and "Mairzy Doats" was at the top of the charts. Young boys avidly followed the course of the war by shifting pins on their bedroom wall maps. People were amused to find that "Kilroy" (whoever he was) had gotten there ahead of them, and every advertisement reminded readers to "Buy War Bonds." The war touched everyone by then. But for most civilians the first contact with the enemy came when large numbers of German prisoners of war appeared in their communities.

When the United States entered the war, the question of enemy prisoners was among the last

"Hitler's Legions in America," by Arnold Kramer from *American History Illustrated* (June, 1983). Copyright © 1983 by Historical Times, Inc. Reproduced through the courtesy of Historical Times, Inc., publisher of *American History Illustrated*.

consideration of a country recovering from a Japanese attack in the Pacific and feverishly preparing for a war in Europe. We had never held large numbers of foreign POWs in our history and were unprepared for the problems of managing them. But prepared or not, we suddenly found ourselves receiving captured German soldiers. More than 150,000 men arrived after the North African campaign in the spring of 1943, and between May and October of that year, an average of 20,000 POWs arrived each month. The Normandy invasion the following June sent the numbers soaring to 30,000 prisoners a month, and by the end of the year, they poured in at the rate of 60,000 a month. By the end of the war, the United States held more than 400,000 enemy captives in 511 camps across the country.

Some of the problems dealing with the POWs were minor, others nearly fatal to the program. No initial attempt was made, for example, to segregate hardened Nazis (many of whom were among the early prisoners from the elite Afrika Korps) from the anti-Nazis, which made later control and re-education of the POWs extremely difficult. German-speaking interpreters among the American guards were scarce since qualified linguists were immediately transferred to intelligence units overseas. This not only prevented the authorities from monitoring the political activities of their prisoners, but it made it easy for the POWs to playfully take advantage of the guards, or interchange identities and ranks when the opportunities arose.

In Washington, government agencies jealously competed for jurisdiction over the POW program. The Justice Department demanded responsibility for the prisoners' security, the War Department for control of the camps, the State Department for control over their eventual repatriation, and the War Production Board for issues involving their labor. Meanwhile, prisoners were already arriving from the battlefields of North Africa and Sicily, and the War Department, together with the Army Corps of Engineers, began scouring the country for camp sites.

Every available country fairground, municipal auditorium, and abandoned CCC camp was held in readiness, and military bases were ordered to prepare a section of the installation for arriving POWs. Construction began on hundreds of POW camps, designed for between 2,000 and 4,000 men and built to standard specifications. The major considerations in site selection were that the area have plenty of available land and that the camp be as far as possible from any critical war industries. As a result, two-thirds of all camps in the United States were located in the south and southwest. The camps had to be located two to three miles from towns and railroad lines—close enough to transport prisoners and provide work projects, but far enough from populated areas to minimize escapes and acts of sabotage. Each camp was made up of two to four compounds of about five hundred men each, and these compounds were surrounded by a heavy wire fence, as was the entire camp. The barracks were designed for utility, not comfort: a concrete slab floor, a structure covered with tarpaper or corrugated tin, rows of cots and footlockers, and a potbellied stove in the center aisle. Stark as they were, many Americans felt that the camps were too good for the prisoners and referred to their local camp as the "Fritz Ritz."

Local communities seldom had more than ten or twelve weeks to adjust to the prospect of hosting a POW camp. Most received word during late autumn of 1942, and while speculation ran high regarding the nationality of the prospective prisoners—relocated Nisei Japanese, German, or Italian military captives—both townspeople and farmers were generally optimistic about the economic and labor potential. The camps were quickly completed by the Corps of Engineers, and the communities settled back to await their new "neighbors."

"When the day arrived for the first trainload of prisoners to reach Hearne," recalled Norman L. McCarver, a local Texas chronicler, "the roadways leading from the outskirts of town to the main entrance of the camp were lined with curious citizens waiting to get a good look at the German prisoners. They were still wearing the clothes they had on when captured several weeks previous. Bloodstains were still visible on those who had been wounded during the fighting in North Africa." In West Ashley, South Carolina, townspeople lined up along Main Street to stare at the 3,250 men in desert-khaki uniforms who disembarked from the train. "Holy Cow!" exclaimed septuagenarian resident Val Horn in recalling that November afternoon. "The line of prisoners stretched the whole distance from town, along Highway 61, all the way out to camp. Remember, we were a town of only 6,000 people!" The community of Rockford, Illinois, hosted 3,865 Germans at the nearby army training installation at Camp Grant; at Camp Como, Mississippi, more than 7,000 German prisoners were isolated on a section of the army base out of the way of the more than 60,000 G.I.s who passed through that training camp; at Camp Indianola, Nebraska, some 4,800 Germans spent the war years in relative comfort; and Somerset, Maryland, nearly tripled its population with the arrival of 3,760 Afrika Korps veterans. Even such tiny towns as Jerome, Arkansas; Ashwood, Virginia; Ysleta, Texas; and Worland, Wyoming, found themselves caught up in the POW program when small work camps of 100-300 prisoners sprang up nearby.

While every community contained some people who were disturbed at having Germans in their midst while their sons and husbands were overseas fighting Nazism, their animosity softened as the war progressed to victory and as the "humanness" of the prisoners became evident. Eventually, most people realized the logic of the POW program and the potential advantage of the prisoners to labor-starved farmers.

The prisoners themselves were relieved and somewhat astonished at the conditions and treatment which greeted them. Unlike the more security-conscious British, the American War Department allowed incoming prisoners to retain most of their personal belongings. At their first meal they saw foods that most had not tasted in years: beef, tomatoes, green vegetables, milk, even ice cream. To their delight they found that cigarettes and, in some camps, even beer and wine were available at the camp PX, purchasable with the canteen coupons that the government paid to them for daily work. "We thought we were in heaven," recalled a former POW. "Food which was not even found in our Mothers' kitchens at home! White bread, and real coffee! We were dumbstruck!" Such treatment caused some grumbling among Americans who resented the quality and quantity of food being fed to the POWs.

The government, however, realized that the better we treated the enemy prisoners in our custody, the better our own soldiers—some 90,000—in enemy hands might be treated. The logic worked. While Russian prisoners in Germany drank melted snow and ate rodents, and French prisoners were humiliated and kept on short rations, American POWs, while certainly not comfortable, received adequate, if not decent, treatment. Unfortunately the War Department never disclosed these motives to an anxious public living with red meat stamps and counting up ration points.

The German prisoners began settling into a daily routine. Following the Geneva Convention of 1929 as the only guideline, the POW camps were separated into different compounds for officers and enlisted men. High-ranking German officers were provided with individual rooms and the use of their enlisted valets. Like American officers in German camps, they were not required to work, seldom volunteered, and received a standard monthly salary: lieutenants received $20.00 a month; captains received $30.00; and majors and higher received $40.00. Enlisted men lived less luxuriously in barracks and were paid 10¢ per day in canteen coupons, plus an additional 80¢ in coupons for every day of mandatory labor. "That may not sound like much today," recalled a former German prisoner, "but that 80¢ would buy us 8 beers or 8 packs of cigarettes!"

The prisoners themselves maintained camp discipline. Long lines of Germans moved to and from their work without resistance or disorganization, led only by several noncommissioned German officers. German enlisted men snapped to attention whenever one of their officers strolled by, and there is no case on record of a German enlisted POW refusing to obey an order from his officer. Washington was greatly relieved that the combat-hardened veterans continued their iron discipline throughout the war, since they required fewer guards and allowed more G.I.s to be shipped overseas. Townspeople were also pleased and gratefully relaxed their vigilance as their earlier fears of mass escapes faded away.

In their spare time, the POWs had a variety of programs in which they could participate. They preferred sports as the most popular pastime, and both officers and enlisted men organized soccer games on the camp parade grounds at every opportunity. Families out for a Sunday afternoon drive often stopped beside their local POW camp to join the cheering crowds of POWs and guards watching young Germans aggressively kicking a soccer ball across a makeshift field. Some prisoners took up weightlifting, others participated in handball, and still others, curious about the customs of their hosts, learned to play baseball. Those prisoners who preferred intellectual to physical exercise had more than enough to occupy their time. Each camp contained men who had been carpenters, mechanics, linguists, or professors of history before the war, and they jumped at the opportunity to conduct classes in their specialties. Regular courses were taught in everything from physics and chemistry to American government, English, and journalism. Some camps even offered piano lessons and such courses as the history of Amer-

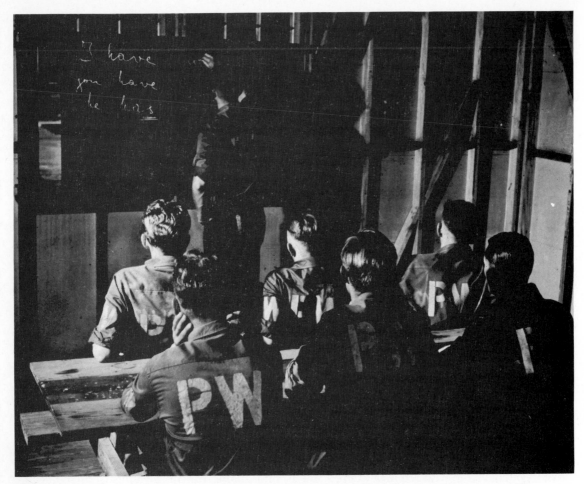

■ ■ *Education played a key role in every compound, with English classes usually the most popular courses. At Camp Blanding, Florida, the prisoners' senior officer served as the instructor in English classes held daily.*

ican comic strips. These mini-universities required examinations, encouraged discussion, and issued final grades and even graduation certificates.

For those prisoners who showed an interest in subjects unavailable inside their camps, the War Department arranged for them to enroll in extension courses through local sponsoring universities. While there is no way of knowing how many POWs became dedicated fans of the Wisconsin Badgers, Texas Longhorns, or the Missouri Tigers, many prisoners of war did return to Germany with substantially improved educations.

As the war progressed through 1944, the War Department arranged for these POW students to receive university credit through the German Ministry of Education, and some of the men eventually graduated from German universities after finishing part of their undergraduate work at POW camps in the United States. Many have become successful German businessmen and professionals following their return. Today, Willibald Bergmann is a manufacturer in Nurem-berg; Dan Kwart von Arnim is the director of a medical clinic; Carl Amery became a well-known writer, as did Hans Werner Richter; Wer-ner Baecker is the New York representative for a German television network; and Heinrich Mat-thias is a high official in the Import-Export Department of Germany's second largest finan-cial institution, the Dresdener Bank. Alfred Klein went back into the military when the *Bundes-wehr* was authorized in 1956, and today he is a lieutenant colonel in the German air force and head of the Air Warfare Department at the Ger-man air force academy at Fürstenfeldbrück. Scratch many an influential German, and you may find an ex-POW who learned his basic English in Pennsylvania, Virginia, Oklahoma, or Tennessee. The two most important German officials in the United States today—Baron Rüdiger von Wechmar, president of the General Assembly of the United Nations, and Brigadier General Hans A. Link, German military repre-sentative to the United States and Canada—fin-ished their service in the Afrika Korps in Camps Carson and Trinidad, Colorado.

Prisoners with additional spare time or who did not care to study or play soccer pursued per-sonal hobbies or made handicrafts. Officers, in particular, were fond of gardening, while other prisoners built furniture, painted murals on the walls of camp theaters, mess halls, and clinics, or sculpted statues to be placed outside of the pris-oners' canteen buildings. One enterprising pris-oner at Camp Ruston, Louisiana, made a clock from some tin cans and used two soda bottles for weights, and it kept perfect time. At Camp Hearne, Texas, a group of Germans painstaking-ly constructed a waist-high replica of an old Ger-man castle complete with detailed turrets and moats. A curious visitor can still examine a medieval *schloss* rising just above the weeds in a corner of the empty landscape of the long-aban-doned Texas camp site.

Too much leisure time is the deadly enemy of any prisoner, and prison memoirs are replete with stories of devices to keep prisoners occu-pied. Without sufficient work the military pris-oner in particular, feeling abandoned by his country and despised by his captors, could become increasingly frustrated, hostile, and, in response to his training as a soldier, aggressive against his captors. The best solution was daily and tiring work. Fortunately, the government desperately needed agricultural labor, and the needs of the prisoners coincided with the needs of the government. Following a long period of bureaucratic debate involving the War Depart-ment, Department of Labor, Provost Marshal General's Office, union representatives, and lob-byists from a number of industries and agricul-tural pressure groups, the government ham-mered out a series of directives in the fall of 1943 outlining the use of POW labor in accordance with the restrictions laid out in the Geneva Con-vention.

The forced labor of enemy personnel had been a time-honored practice, and while the Geneva Convention did not prevent their employment, it did restrict their use. The prison-ers had to be physically able, and the work nei-ther dangerous nor unhealthy. Most important, no work projects could be directly related to the war effort or instrumental in the defeat of the prisoners' homeland. Consequently, the men could work in two areas: at military installa-tions, and as labor contracted out to private busi-nesses, farms, and small industries.

Within weeks of the labor directive, thou-sands of prisoners were assigned to various mil-itary bases to replace American personnel as administrative clerks, bakers, carpenters, electri-cians, garbage collectors, sign painters, and in many other capacities. Returning American sol-diers were startled and often angered to find themselves being processed by indifferent clerks wearing Wehrmacht uniforms with the letters "PW" stenciled across the back. Wounded G.I.s recovering at Halloran General Hospital in New York or Glennan Hospital in Oklahoma were no less outraged to be helped by German-speaking orderlies whose Afrika Korps uniforms were visible beneath their open white smocks. Security was understandably heavy during the first few months because army officials feared the damage that POWs might accomplish when allowed to work inside active military bases and hospitals.

Despite the lack of incidents and the apparent ease with which the prisoners accepted their tasks, the army issued an official *Handbook for Work Supervisors of Prisoner of War Labor* which instructed American guards to "be aloof, for the German only respects firm leadership. . . . Allow them to rest only when necessary. DRIVE!" The American General Wilhelm D. Styer put it more succinctly. When his aide questioned some aspect of prisoner labor, General Styer grunted, "We must overcome the psychology that you cannot do this or that. I want to see these prisoners work like ants!"

And work they did. Within a year of the beginning of the war, the domestic labor market was already feeling the pinch, especially in the agricultural sector since so many able-bodied young men were being drafted into the armed forces. By mid-1942 even the government admitted that the situation was alarming. The practical decision was to provide POWs to the labor-starved market on a contract basis.

This bureaucratic rat race eventually untangled itself, and by mid-1944 the requirements for POW labor became so informal that in many cases a telephone call or personal visit to the county agent's office would be sufficient to obtain a truckload of POWs. Soon even the most skeptical farmers were waiting in line to get their share of these efficient and inexpensive workers. Hardly any eligible industry failed to use at least a few truckloads of prisoners during the war, and the POWs saw "action" in jobs that ranged from logging, food processing, flood control, and quarrying to their ironic but far from unenjoyable assignment as Kosher meat packers in Farmington, New Jersey. Their greatest contribution, however, was in agriculture.

In Louisiana, prisoners worked in the rice, cotton, and sugar cane fields, harvesting more than 246,000 acres of cane in 1944 alone. In Missouri, they dug potatoes, shocked oats, and harvested wheat. They picked tomatoes in Indiana, potatoes and sugar beets in Nebraska, wheat and seed crops in Kansas, and peanuts in Georgia.

They were young, farmers recalled, about twenty years old on the average and very eager to learn. The prisoners worked a steady ten-hour day, broken only by a lunch of bologna sandwiches supplied by the farmers and eaten out in the fields. They were guarded by a minimum number of armed G.I.s from the camp, and due to the low incidence of escapes, supervision was negligible. "I remember a number of occasions when we were being trucked out of Camp Rucker, Alabama," said former POW Alfred Klein, "and the guard would ask me to hold his rifle until he had climbed in or out of the truck. Almost as an after-thought, he would ask me to hand it up to him a few minutes later."

There were some difficulties, to be sure. Many prisoners were inexperienced in farm work and, as a result, did not produce as much as "free" labor. Another problem voiced by American farmers concerned the fact that they would train one group of POW laborers only to be assigned a different group the following day. Finally, there was the language barrier, and the resulting difficulties were more often humorous than not. One day in the spring of 1944, an American sergeant was marching a large group of prisoner-laborers the several miles from a farm to the prisoner compound at Camp Reynolds, Pennsylvania, when he found himself groping in his vocabulary for the German equivalent of "Halt!" (which happens to be "Halt!"). He threw up his arm to stop them, and the entire platoon of prisoners came to attention, shot their arms upward, and chorused, "Heil Hitler!"

The stories and anecdotes about the prisoners are as varied and numerous as the men and tasks involved, and without a doubt, readers of these pages who used POW labor or lived near a camp will smile as they recall an amusing incident.

Despite the extensive work, education, and recreation programs, prisoners escaped, approximately 100 per month or slightly more than three per day. Working on agricultural sites under the minimal supervision, some prisoners walked away from their work parties to find female company. Others wanted to shop in local stores, or mingle with people, or only wanted to be alone. Indeed, prisoner escapes were as varied as imagination and circumstances allowed. They dug tunnels under the wire fences, jumped from barracks roofs, hung under laundry trucks, and posed as American guards. Whatever the method of escape, the prisoners were almost always rounded up within hours of their disappearance.

Sheriff Harold Ellsworth of Lewiston, Illinois, near Camp Ellis, described his feelings about the escapees. "They made us feel kind of sorry for them, these German escapees," recalled the sheriff. "We would find them there in the streets, without a word of English, in Bloomington, in Peoria, in Galesburg; or else in the woods, completely lost like strayed sheep. Yes, I tell you, it was rather pitiful. Besides, local people weren't afraid of them. When they met up with one, they called us; we came, put a hand on their shoulder, and gently brought them back to camp."

Unlike American prisoners in Germany who had the help of the French underground and could escape to Switzerland, German prisoners in the United States found little sympathy among Americans. Even if they did, there was no place for them to go. Such logic, however, did not stop 2,222 men from trying.

In Wyoming, two German escapees succeeded in getting almost three miles from their camp and were already celebrating their new-found freedom when they ran headlong into a detachment of American troops on maneuvers. They were returned to Camp Douglas at gun point and presented to the startled camp author-

ities who were not yet aware of their escape. On another occasion, a German was captured outside of Lisbon, New Hampshire, when he accepted an automobile ride from the local police chief. On another occasion, an escapee made it from Camp Grant, Illinois, to Chicago in time to celebrate New Year's Eve 1945 in a tavern. When the party moved to a private home for sandwiches, Paul Stachowiak went along too. Everybody thought he was the guest of somebody else, but when he began to boast that he had just escaped from the POW camp in nearby Rockford, one of the more sober partygoers called the police. Another prisoner was captured by a Pennsylvania railroad detective in Oil City, Pennsylvania, when he failed to understand that his ticket did not entitle him to remain in the parlor car. Five others were captured in a hen house outside of Indianola, Nebraska, by several country boys armed with shotguns. Still another escapee was captured near Camp Como, Mississippi, as he sat down in the back of a southern bus directly beneath the sign that read: "Colored Only."

A few prisoners had greater success. Georg Gaertner was a former draftsman who escaped from his POW compound at Deming Army Air Corps Base, New Mexico, on September 21, 1945. The last statement he made to his comrades before his escape was that he had no intention of returning home to the devastation of postwar Germany, and he apparently made good on his promise. Gaertner simply melted into the mainstream of American life. Despite an intensive search by the FBI and his photo appearing in post offices across the country, he has never been located. In 1963, on the authority of the U.S. Attorney General, the FBI ended its search for Georg Gaertner, and at the moment of this writing, the now sixty-two-year-old German is the only former POW who remains at large.

As the war drew to a close, the question of repatriation became an immediate and thorny problem, and the United States was torn between two opposing points of view. One segment of public opinion warned that to send the German prisoners home so soon would be detrimental to our labor situation and dangerous to the Allied occupation effort to prevent the rise of Neo-Nazism. The other side argued that with the war over, the country no longer had any legal right to hold or work the POWs. The latter position prevailed. Repatriation finally began in November 1945, and the POWs were returned to Germany at the rate of 50,000 a month. The final boatload of 1,500 German prisoners sailed from Camp Shanks, New Jersey, on July 22, 1946, "waving an indifferent farewell." The commander of Camp Shanks, Colonel Harry W. Maas, echoed the feelings of the country at large, sighing "Thank God, that's over!" With the exception of 188 German prisoners still in hospitals, psychiatric wards, military prisons, or on the run in the United States, it was indeed over.

People living in communities that once hosted large numbers of German prisoners have forgotten the experience as nearby camps gradually disappeared. One by one, they were shut down during the postwar months and the facilities sold at auction. But if the townspeople have forgotten about those days, the prisoners have not.

Announcements appear periodically in German newspapers and military journals reminding former POWs from particular camps about an upcoming reunion or social function. More than 300 former prisoners from Camp Mexia, Texas, gathered for such a reunion in Heidelberg in June 1978. They crammed their signatures on several 6"×8" photo postcards and mailed them to favorite guards and townspeople. Some even return with their families to their old camp sites to stroll through the "old neighborhood," noting changes, taking photographs, and reminiscing with welcoming friends, farmers, and even community dignitaries.

During one of these visits, a former POW named Wilhelm Sauerbrei best summarized the experience of the prisoners. Driving from Houston to Hearne, Texas, in a car full of reporters and friends, the former Afrika Korps corporal regaled the occupants with stories and recollections about his camp days.

"You must have had it pretty easy," a Houston reporter commented.

"I'll tell you, pal," Sauerbrei said confidently, "if there is ever another war, get on the side that America isn't, then get captured by the Americans—you'll have it made!"

■ ■ ■

STUDY QUESTIONS

1. What problems did the United States have in administering the POW program?

2. How did the government decide where to build the prisons? How did American communities react to the POWs? Did their reactions change over time? Why or why not?

3. In general, what kind of treatment was extended to the POWs? How did the Germans feel about their care? Why?

4. What was the day-to-day routine in the camps? Why did the camps require relatively little security?

5. What kind of work did the POWs do? How did they respond to the work?

6. Why did relatively few German POWs try to escape? How successful were they? Why?

BIBLIOGRAPHY

An excellent study of the impact of World War II on American society is John Morton Blum, *V Was for Victory* (1976). Also see Richard Polenberg, *War and Society* (1972). Philip Knightley treats the affect of World War II on American journalism and culture in *The First Casualty* (1975), as does Alan Winkler in *The Politics of Propaganda* (1978). An excellent study of Franklin D. Roosevelt as a wartime leader is James MacGregor Burns, *Roosevelt: The Soldier of Freedom* (1970). The impact of World War II on the American economy is treated in Donald Nelson, *Arsenal of Democracy* (1946) and Bruce Catton, *The War Lords of Washington* (1946).

Part Six

AMERICA IN THE AGE OF ANXIETY: 1945–1960

The fallout of Hiroshima lasted many years. The most immediate result of the atomic bombs which America dropped on Japan on August 6 and August 9, 1945, was the end of World War II. V-J Day was celebrated with an emotional outpouring of relief. Most Americans believed that the United States had saved the world from the totalitarian threat of the Axis Powers. They also assumed that America would now return to its traditional foreign policy posture of isolationism. Such was not the case. World War II had made the United States the most powerful country in the world. Retreat into isolationism was impossible. During the next few years, America accepted the responsibilities that went with being a world power and replaced Great Britain as the globe's policeman.

Almost as soon as the war was over, the Soviet Union emerged as America's leading rival. Joseph Stalin, Russia's leader, was by nature suspicious, and the complexities and uncertainties of Soviet politics made him even more so. He resented America and Great Britain for delaying the second front against Germany during World War II. He was also upset that the United States refused to share its nuclear secrets with the Soviet Union. Fears, anxieties, and ambitions degenerated into a new type of power conflict. Called the Cold War, the object was to control, either through economic or military means, as much of the world as possible.

America originated the policy of "containment" as a strategy for the Cold War. The policy was essentially defensive in nature, and it forced America to react to Soviet movements. Although the policy scored several notable successes—particularly in Turkey, Greece, and Western Europe—it had a number of real weaknesses.

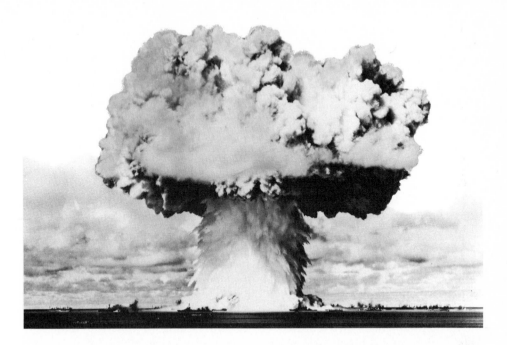

Most important, it committed American troops to prevent the expansion of Communism. In Korea and later in Vietnam, Americans came to understand the limitations and constraints of the containment doctrine.

The Cold War and the fear of a nuclear confrontation shaped domestic politics as well as foreign affairs. If Americans distrusted Stalin's motives, they also questioned the actions of their own leaders. They asked pointed and complex questions, yet sought simple answers. Why had Stalin gained so much territory at Yalta? How was Russia able to develop its own atomic weapons so rapidly? Who lost China? Politicians such as Senator Joseph McCarthy of Wisconsin and Congressman Richard Nixon of California provided easy answers. They said that Communist sympathizers in the American government had worked to insure the success of the Soviet Union. The publicity lavished on the trials of Alger Hiss and Julius and Ethel Rosenberg, and the activities of McCarthy and the House Un-American Activities Committee increased the public's distrust of its own officials.

In the following section the essays deal with the fallout of Hiroshima and the Cold War. Although they examine very different subjects—television scandals, Korean War POWs, science fiction movies, and investigations of sexual behavior—they contain a unifying theme. They all discuss Americans' attitudes toward themselves. The underlying assumption was that something deep and troubling was wrong, that the American character had changed for the worse. The search for exactly what was wrong took many different turns and helped illuminate the psychological, cultural, and social landscape of the 1950s.

THE SCIENTIST AS SEX CRUSADER: ALFRED C. KINSEY AND AMERICAN CULTURE

Regina Markell Morantz

During the late 1940s and early 1950s a series of unsettling events shocked Americans and disturbed their sense of postwar complacency and optimism. Communism—its spread and increased dangerousness—inspired much of the fear. In late 1949 the National leader Chiang Kai-shek and his followers fled mainland China for sanctuary on Formosa. In Chiang's place came Communist Mao Tse-tung. Although Mao's victory was predictable and the result of internal Chinese forces, Americans tended to view the "fall of China" as a victory for Soviet foreign policy. Other shocks came rapidly. In September 1949 President Truman announced that the Russians had detonated a nuclear device, thus ending the American monopoly of the bomb. And throughout the period, the trials of Alger Hiss raised questions about the loyalty of American government officials.

No less sensational and disturbing was the publication of Alfred Kinsey's *Sexual Behavior in the Human Male* (1948), which quickly sold over 275,000 copies. For many Americans, Kinsey's "message" was as insidious as those of Marx and Lenin. He told Americans about themselves, about their sexual practices, fears, and desires. And what Kinsey said was not what most Americans wanted to believe. In the following essay historian Regina Markell Morantz discusses the reception, influence, and implications of Kinsey's scientific pioneering work. She demonstrates the limits of Kinsey's scientific objectivity and the nature of his liberalism. More importantly, however, Morantz uses the findings of Kinsey and more recent sex researchers to explore the changing character and behavior of millions of Americans. As she suggests, sex has become less a liberating, revolutionary force than simply another aspect of America's consumer economy.

In January 1948, Robert Latou Dickinson, noted gynecologist and sex researcher, dashed off a note to his friend and colleague Alfred Charles Kinsey. Dickinson's copy of the newly published *Sexual Behavior in the Human Male*, which he had awaited "with one of the keenest anticipations of a lifetime," had arrived. "I have my copy at last of SBHM!" he informed Kinsey. "Glory to God!" In a lively correspondence throughout the 1940s the two men shared enthusiasm for Kinsey's studies in human sexuality, their mutual respect enhanced by appreciation of the social significance of this work. Given the chance to see Kinsey's labors in print, Dickinson's excitement grew: "Dear ACE:" he wrote Kinsey in February, "In sex education, and marriage counsel [*sic*] and v.d. and prostitution attacks . . . we would, in America, hereafter, speak of the Pre-Kinsey and the Post-Kinsey eras."

The press, the public, and expert opinion subsequently confirmed Dickinson's assessment. Writers dubbed *Sexual Behavior in the Human Male* "the most talked about book of the twentieth century." Others ranked it with *Das Kapital, The Origin of Species,* and *Wealth of Nations.* Indeed, the reception accorded Kinsey's work was unprecedented. Although Kinsey's publishers authorized an inadequate first printing of 5,000 copies, less than two months after publication *Sexual Behavior in the Human Male* had sold 200,000 copies and stood in second place on the non-fiction best-seller list. George Gallup reported that one out of every five Americans had either read or heard about the book, while five out of six of those interviewed judged its publication "a good thing." Multiple reviews appeared in literary periodicals. Medical and lay organizations held symposia to assess its impact.

Overnight "Kinsey" became a household word, his name forever embedded in popular culture.

Response to the Kinsey report testified more than anything else to the revolution in sexual mores that its text, charts, and statistical tables so laboriously documented. No one would now dispute that a generation of Americans who had come of age in the first decades of the twentieth century had begun to lift the mantle of fear and shame from their sexual activities. Since 1913 American newspapers had been hailing what one headline writer called "sex o'clock in America." Even the scientific study of sex had gotten underway years before Kinsey: The Male Report cites 19 prior investigations of human sexuality. But journalists who wrote about America's sex obsession before World War I rarely elaborated on what factors underlay the new freedom in manners, while post-war professionals who had begun to analyze its components increasingly avoided sharing their findings with a popular audience. What made Kinsey different—indeed, what made him unique—was his confidence that Americans were ready for a confrontation with their own sexuality. In dispassionate prose he laid bare the facts.

Most of his contemporaries understood Kinsey's research to be a monumental achievement of twentieth-century science. He managed where others had failed to discuss sexual matters before a public still ignorant and uncomfortable with the subject. His own liberalism was grounded in the conviction that nothing human should be alien to the realm of science.

Of course Kinsey's detractors were vindictive. Some disputed his findings, questioning his evidence and doubting his methods; others condemned him for publicizing his facts. But though Kinsey may have underestimated the reaction of those ill-equipped to handle his candor, his faith in the American people was not misplaced. Accepting the legitimacy of his research with respect they afforded all science, they rapidly made his work part of the conventional wisdom. After summarizing the origins of sex research in America, this essay will attempt to analyze this

"The Scientist as Sex Crusader: Alfred C. Kinsey and American Culture" by Regina Markell Morantz, from *American Quarterly XXIX* (Winter, 1977). Published by the American Studies Association. Copyright © 1977. Reprinted by permission of American Quarterly and the author.

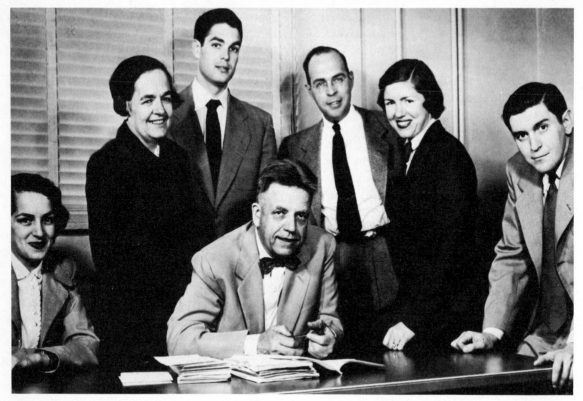

■ ■ *Dr. Alfred C. Kinsey, shown here with his family, pioneered sex research in two studies (1948 and 1953) that brought sex out of the bedroom and into America's parlor.*

process of acceptance. It will focus on Kinsey the man, the content of his reports and the critical response they evoked, and the larger cultural meaning of Kinsey's work.

Victorian aversion to the investigation of sexual matters relegated sex to the backroom almost as effectively in 1900 as in the previous century. Scientists and physicians either shared their society's view of what was proper, or else kept quiet about it. Research into the socially taboo took courage; chastisement was often swift and forceful. When the distinguished Chicago physician, Denslow Lewis, proposed in 1899 to speak to the American Medical Association on the "Gynecologic Consideration of the Sexual Act," he was denounced by Howard A. Kelly of Johns Hopkins. "The discussion of the subject," Kelly

asserted, "is attended with filth and we besmirch ourselves by discussing it in public." Characteristically, the Association refused to publish Lewis' paper.

Nineteenth-century moralism gradually succumbed in the first decades of the twentieth century to the combined attack of purity advocates (including feminists, clergymen, and social reformers), idealistic physicians inspired by bacteriological discoveries facilitating the control of venereal disease, and the diverse but insistent proponents of the Freudian revolution. Social and economic factors also underlay the emergence of new sexual attitudes. As early as 1907 Simon Patten predicted the gradual economic shift away from austerity and production to a concern with consumption. An interest in leisure and luxury fostered pleasure and personal fulfillment as positive goods, and undermined Victorian prescriptions of thrift, self-denial, and personal control. Urbanization eroded community and religious controls on behavior. In addition, the increasingly visible women joining the labor force were freed from some of the constraints of home and family.

Though sex was discussed in the Progressive era, sex research remained controversial. Not until 1921 did scientists and social reformers organize a two-day conference under the auspices of the National Research Council to examine the status of American sex research. Acknowledging the importance of such investigation, conference members decried the "enshrouding of sex relations in a fog of mystery, reticence and shame." Sensing the national faith in science, participants argued that scientists were best qualified to study sex because "their standing in the community would prevent fears that their findings would be put to propaganda purposes." The meetings resulted in the formation of a Committee for Research on Problems in Sex chaired by Yale psychologist Robert Yerkes and connected with the National Research Council. Funded largely by the Rockefeller Foundation, and working closely with the Bureau of Social Hygiene, another Foundation project, the Committee directed most sex studies in the next two decades. Alfred Kinsey turned to this committee for financial support in 1939. Aid for his project opened the door to a new and controversial era in sex research.

While the Committee for the Study of Problems in Sex quietly encouraged research on sexuality in the 1920s and 1930s, Kinsey built his career as a leading expert on the gall wasp. Twenty-six years old in 1920, Kinsey came to Indiana University as an assistant professor of zoology. For the next two decades he taught courses in entymology, general biology, and insect taxonomy, and by the mid-thirties he had published two specialized books, numerous articles, and an innovative high school biology text.

Few facts are available to explain Kinsey's subsequent interest in sex. His own sexual history, like those of the people he interviewed, will presumably remain locked forever in the confidential files at the Institute for Sex Research. Though he spoke little of his past, it is clear that his parents were strict and puritanical. The product of a deeply religious home, Kinsey suffered as a youngster because of his proficiency in the natural sciences and his fascination with Darwinian evolution. When Kinsey rebelled, science offered him a set of values which emotionally rivalled his juvenile commitment to religion. His sympathetic attitude toward the sexual dilemmas of the young may have grown out of memories of his own pain, frustration, and ignorance; science granted him the tools to make his sympathy more objective. But cloaked in the unbiased empiricism of the dispassionate scientist lay the emotional preferences of a moral crusader.

Kinsey's involvement with sex research began quietly in 1938 when he was chosen as the faculty coordinator of a newly established marriage course. The course consisted of interdisciplinary guest lecturers, with Kinsey lecturing on biology. His class notes reveal sophistication with published works on sex. Indeed, in a letter to Robert Latou Dickinson written in 1941, he admitted: "It was your own work which turned my attention to the purposes of research in this field some ten or twelve years ago although circumstances were not propitious for starting the work until three years ago." In a talk delivered in 1935 to a faculty discussion club he had proved himself familiar with previous sex studies by G. V. Hamilton and Katherine B. Davis. The lectures displayed his concern with both the influence of social institutions on sexual behavior and the "sexual conflicts of youth." Significantly, he reflected that such conflicts arose because of the "long frustration of the normal sexual activities."

Kinsey emphasized the central importance of sexual adjustment to stable unions. "I know of no evidence," he stated flatly, "that this biological basis can be completely sidestepped and still lead to a successful home." He accused modern education "through its system of mores, laws, and ethics," of conditioning attitudes toward sex which were "wrong in the sense that they interfere with the successful consummation of the marriage . . . [and] develop the sexual maladjustments that appear most often after marriage. Our ignorance of copulatory techniques," he continued, "which is the direct outcome of the impressions that are imprinted on the young, our ignorance of satisfactory contraceptive devices above all, produce attitudes which make our concepts of sex wrong." By delaying sexual activity until marriage, he argued, young people only made the achievement of successful marriage more problematic. Responses repressed for ten or twelve years after an individual is first capable of sexual activity could hardly be changed by a marriage ceremony. Distorted attitudes formed in adolescence required years of adjustment after marriage. "Why offer a marriage course?" Kinsey asked his listeners. "Society," he answered, "has been responsible for interfering with what would have been normal biological development. . . . It behooves us to make amends to society by taking you as you approach the time of marriage and giving you the results of scholarly thinking on these several problems." Repeatedly, Kinsey the scientist would side with biology when it conflicted with accepted social mores.

In the summer of 1938 Kinsey began taking the sex histories of his students and within a year had scheduled interviews outside the university to vary his sampling. Aware of their potential significance, he termed these histories "a scientific goldmine" and wondered to a colleague if they would not account "for the largest volume of research I will yet publish." Under mounting pressure from conservative elements of the community, Kinsey terminated his connection with the marriage course in 1940. Soon afterward he received his first grant from the Committee for Research in Problems of Sex. Abandoning his interest in the gall wasp, he prepared to devote himself solely to the study of human sexual behavior.

The current permissiveness surrounding sex research should not obscure the fact that thirty years ago Kinsey's findings disturbed, shocked, and threatened not just ordinary men and women but professionals as well. A good deal of the hostile criticism directed at Kinsey's work had little to do with its scientific value. Princeton University president Harold Dodds likened the Male volume to "the work of small boys writing dirty words on fences." The Chicago *Tribune* termed Kinsey a "menace to society." The Reverend Henry Van Dusen, president of Union Theological Seminary and a member of the Rockefeller Foundation, called for a "spontaneous ethical revulsion from the premises of the study," and chided the Foundation for its sponsorship. Kinsey's work, he lamented, revealed "a prevailing degradation of American morality approximating the worst decadence of the Roman era." Harvard sociologist Carle C. Zimmerman labelled the Male volume an "attack on the Western family," and accused Kinsey of irresponsibility in making it public. Millicent McIntosh, indomitable president of Barnard College and mother of five, worried in 1954 that Kinsey's books had already contributed "to the difficulties encountered by young people in establishing a good relationship between the sexes."

Hysteria reached Congress when New York Representative Louis B. Heller called upon the Postmaster General to bar the Female Report from the mails until it could be investigated, charging Kinsey with "hurling the insult of the century against our mothers, wives, daughters and sisters." Soon rumors spread that the Special House Committee founded during the McCarthy era to inquire into the use of funds by tax-exempt foundations would ask Kinsey to testify regarding financial aid from the Rockefeller Foundation. Others accused Kinsey of aiding communism. Shortly thereafter the Rockefeller Foundation informed Kinsey that his grant would not be renewed.

Much of the criticism of Kinsey's work, however, was not hysterical. Most commentators admired his research and welcomed its publication. Yet serious critics also offered objections. The debate centered on two issues: the possibility of conducting a scientific investigation that was value-free (and whether Kinsey had done so); and the extent to which a behavioristic approach could solve fundamental questions of human existence.

Kinsey never admitted publicly that scientists based their investigations on cultural assumptions. He remained deaf to the charge that his work reflected his own biases. Yet his objectivity was itself polemical: his research subverted the status quo specifically because it examined individual deviance dispassionately. Many critics were repelled by the idea of studying sexual nonconformity objectively. By definition norms are not always rational. Kinsey's non-judgmental approach aligned him with the twentieth-century rebels against Victorian repression. Though many critics shared the Progressive faith that the truth would make men free, they resisted applying this conviction to sex research. In this instance the truth was dangerous and might help destroy the American value system. Reinhold Niebuhr passionately argued this point of view when he declared that Kinsey's assumptions represented "a therapy which implies a disease in our culture as grievous or more grievous than the sickness it pretends to cure."

Soon after the publication of the Male volume, Lionel Trilling wrote of Kinsey and his coauthors that "nothing comes more easily to their pens than the criticism of the subjectivity of earlier writers on sex, yet their own subjectivity is sometimes extreme." A retrospective reading of both volumes reveals why Kinsey was an easy mark for Trilling's pen. In neither book did he disguise either his admiration for the sexually active or his suspicion of the sexually repressed. His statistical interpretations fell invariably on the side of sexual liberalism. In a chapter on the onset of male puberty, for example, he recorded his approval of men who began their sexual activities early. On scant evidence he asserted

that early-adolescent males were often "the more alert, energetic, vivacious, spontaneous, physically active, socially extrovert, and/or aggressive individuals in the population," while late-maturing males tended to be "slow, quiet, mild in manner, without force, reserved, timid, taciturn, introvert, and/or socially inept." He revealed his own biases most clearly when he linked the aggressive, success-oriented personality type—an American paragon—to vigorous sexuality.

Equally controversial were Kinsey's interpretations of the data concerning the relationship between premarital intercourse and marital adjustment. Although he admitted that premarital petting contributed "definitely to the effectiveness of the sexual relations after marriage," he nevertheless remained contemptuous of the hypocrisy involved in adolescent petting behavior. "It is amazing," he wrote,

to observe the mixtures of scientifically supported logic, and utter illogic, which shapes the petting behavior of most of these youths. That some of them are in some psychic conflict over their activities is evidenced by the curious rationalizations which they use to satisfy their consciences. They are particularly concerned with the avoidance of genital union. The fact that petting involves erotic contacts which are as effective as genital union, and that it may even involve contacts which have been more taboo than genital union, including some that have been considered perversions, does not disturb the youth so much as actual intercourse would. By petting, they preserve their virginities, even though they may achieve orgasm while doing so.

Coupled with his disdain for this hypocrisy was his finding of a "marked, positive correlation between experience in orgasm obtained from premarital coitus [for women], and the capacity to reach orgasm after marriage." Over half the female sample who had experienced premarital coital orgasm had reached sexual climax in nearly all of their coitus during the first year of marriage. Only 29 percent of women without such premarital experience were able to achieve regular orgasm during the first year.

Kinsey dismissed selective factors as accounting for the correlation, and emphasized that almost half of those women sampled who had premarital intercourse had it exclusively with their fiancés. This figure led some critics to question whether such behavior could properly be termed "premarital coitus" at all. Kinsey found that the overall number of women achieving orgasm *at least occasionally* within the first year of marriage was as high as 75 percent. Indeed, the percentage rose steadily according to the number of years married. What Kinsey's statistics seemed to indicate was that reaching orgasm for women was a *learned* skill that took time to develop. Kinsey's data, critics argued, could or could not be interpreted to justify premarital intercourse.

Kinsey nevertheless used his findings to suggest that traditional mores regarding premarital intercourse were outmoded. In an impassioned paragraph, he made his sympathies clear. His carefully selected phrases, typical of numerous passages in the books, bristled with an aggressive undertone barely couched in the language of scientific neutrality: "The attempt," he wrote

to ignore and suppress the physiologic needs of the sexually most capable of the population, has led to more complications than most persons are willing to recognize. This is why so many of our American youth, both females and males, depend upon masturbation instead of coitus as a premarital outlet. Restraints on premarital heterosexual contacts appear to be primary factors in the development of homosexual activities among both females and males. . . .

The considerable development of petting, which many foreigners consider one of the unique aspects of the sexual pattern in this country, is similarly an outgrowth of this restraint on premarital coitus.

The law specifies the right of the married adult to have regular intercourse, but it makes no

provision whatsoever for the approximately 40 per cent of the population which is sexually mature but unmarried. Many youths and older unmarried females and males are seriously disturbed because the only sources of sexual outlet are either legally or socially disapproved.

Such statements challenged the 1950s social and sexual standards. Most marriage manuals still preached the virtues of premarital chastity, while only a few professionals had given serious thought to the problems of sexual adjustment for the unmarried.

Kinsey's detractors feared that his premises implied an animalistic philosophy of sex devoid of emotional and social content. They accused him of a crude behaviorism that failed to place sexual activity within the larger context of human values. Thoughtful reviewers, many of them psychiatrists and psychologists, chided him for his recurrent neglect of the psycho-dynamics of sex. Denying that as a biologist Kinsey was equipped to examine complex psycho-social questions, analysts decried his measure of sex activity in terms of outlet and orgasm. By reducing sex to the mechanistic Kinsey ignored motivation. Should orgasm in and of itself, they asked, be the goal of human sexual behavior? Where was the place of love in Kinsey's universe? Speaking of sex solely in terms of outlet negated its relationship to the creative, integrative, and inspirational aspects of human life. Sexuality, though important, remained only one dimension of the human personality. "It was Freud's idea," wrote Karl Menninger, "that sexuality in the broad sense, the life instinct, was represented not nearly so much by orgasm as by human love, and that the goal of all sexual behavior was better integration, better inter-human concern, and thereby less mutual destructiveness."

The psychoanalytic case against Kinsey extended beyond his failure to consider the emotional content of the sex act. Kinsey avoided placing sexuality within a developmental framework. Except for confirming infantile sexuality, he refused to see any substantiation for other central tenets of psychoanalytic theory. His animus toward psychoanalysts remained clear. He denied that "normal" psychosexual development preceded from narcissism through homosexual to heterosexual activities. In a final affront to Freudian theory, he questioned the significance to women of such concepts as penis envy, castration fear, defense against incestuous wishes, and fixation at the clitoral stage. "The psycho-sexual pattern in the human animal," he wrote, "originates in indiscriminate sexual responses which as a product of conditioning and social pressures, become increasingly restricted in the directions of traditional interpretations of what is normal or abnormal in sexual behavior. . . . It is simply a picture of physiologic response and psychologic conditioning in terms that are known to the biologist and psychologist." Psychoanalysts found this approach simplistic. "Frigidity," argued Marie Robinson, "is in the vast majority of cases, essentially a psychological problem. No amount of mechanical manipulation can make a difference. Anybody who tells you differently," she cautioned her patients, "is . . . wrong." "Kinsey's credo," wrote Edmund Bergler and William S. Kroger, "amounts to naiveté of the first order. . . . It overlooks the complex mechanisms of inner-unconscious-conscious. . . . Sex, though biologically present in every human being, goes through complicated (not simple) transformations before maturity is reached."

While psychoanalysts worried over Kinsey's behaviorism, theologians accused him of materialism. Kinsey's animal analogy represented a conscious tool in his revolt against Victorian sexual attitudes which for a century had exalted ecstasy of the spirit and devalued the pleasures of the flesh. In contrast, Kinsey embraced man's mammalian heritage. Admiring Freud for reasserting the primacy of physical drives, Kinsey believed that man's pretensions to uniqueness had accounted for untold sexual unhappiness. As a biologist he took for granted that, in the long run, physiological factors were more effec-

tive than man-made regulations in determining patterns of human behavior. Reinhold Niebuhr read him correctly when he charged Kinsey with referring consistently to analogies between man and the sex practices of infrahuman species "without once calling attention to uniquely human characteristics of man's sexual life."

This alleged materialism led Kinsey to the controversial assumption that the prevalence of certain types of behavior indicated both their mammalian origins and their biological normality. The frequency of types of behavior socially labelled "deviant" testified to the persistence of biologic over cultural determinants. Such a view demanded a reevaluation of homosexuality. Regarding the "normality" of such behavior Kinsey wrote:

In view of the data which we now have on the incidence and frequency of the homosexual, in particular on its coexistence with the heterosexual in the lives of a considerable portion of the male population, it is difficult to maintain the view that psychosexual reactions between individuals of the same sex are rare and therefore abnormal or unnatural, or that they constitute within themselves evidence of neuroses or even psychoses.

Theologians and other humanists united in their revulsion against this view of sex. Man, they reminded their readers, was not just a little above the apes, but a little below the angels. The difference between human beings and animals lay in the capacity of men to control their instincts, to use language, and to develop creativity, imagination, and culture. In the end, critics maintained, sex was a social activity, culturally and psychologically influenced.

Many of Kinsey's difficulties with the humanists may have arisen from his narrow philosophy of science. He often argued that as a scientist he reserved the right to limit his investigation in any way he saw fit. Though he never denied the significance of the social and psychologic components of human behavior, he insisted that science was "by its method limited to the consideration of material phenomena. The accumulation of scientific data depends upon the reduction of such material to quantifiable units which can be measured." He implied that any other order of facts or values than his could be explored only by non-scientific or ultra-scientific means. He accused psychiatrists studying Freudian stages in psycho-sexual development of investigating "mystic impulses." Theologians, and those "concerned with the moral values of sexual behavior" he considered to be antagonistic to science altogether.

Kinsey's refusal to answer the criticism of the humanists also revealed his shortcomings as a sexual theorist. Kinsey's work is peculiarly joyless. "If someone," wrote Karl Stern in *Commonweal*, "attempted to set the stage for a dehumanized, de-personalized society, for the great beehive—he would start out with things like the Kinsey Report." Ironically, the Victorians themselves had been accused of joylessness, though for different reasons. Kinsey, it seemed to some, represented a new kind of puritan. "There is in all this," Stern remarked with considerable irony, "a subtle, hidden despising of nature."

In the present period of sexual permissiveness, the arguments of the humanists loom more salient than they did thirty years ago. A general theory of sexuality cannot remain grounded in only one academic discipline, but must seek to integrate the methods and findings of many. Undoubtedly Kinsey would have renounced the role of sexual theorist. He died too soon for us to speculate on whether subsequent research would have led him beyond a crude empiricism. Yet in stubbornly labelling even thoughtful critics as Victorian moralists in disguise, perhaps Kinsey had a point. His findings may not have helped to cure the sexually neurotic, but, given the prevailing atmosphere surrounding the public discussion of sex, his behavioristic approach may have liberated sexually active men and women still haunted with Victorian prudery. *Look* magazine recognized this therapeutic effect: "What they [the authors] have learned and will learn may have a tremendous effect on the future social history of mankind. For they are presenting facts. They are revealing not what *should be*, but what *is*. For the first time data on human sex behavior is entirely separated from questions of philosophy, moral values, and social customs."

The fact that Kinsey himself had been raised under the canons of sexual puritanism probably made him sensitive to the problems of ordinary men and women. Certainly his democratic tendencies convinced him that for most people questions concerning the ultimate significance of sexuality were not only unimportant, they were irrelevant. The first task was to unshackle a generation from its repressive past. Relieving guilt and reassuring readers that everyone had similar sexual impulses, Kinsey's books contributed to a changing sexual climate in which ordinary people lived and worked. They probably had the same emancipating effect on the unpsychoanalyzed masses that Freud's work achieved for generations of intellectuals.

Not long after the publication of the Female volume, Kinsey's health began to deteriorate. For over a decade he had maintained a schedule which left him little free time. The emotional criticism that accompanied the release of his second book hurt him deeply. Cessation of foundation backing left the future of his research in the balance; for three years he struggled to reestablish the Institute for Sex Research on a solid financial footing. In 1956, at the age of 64, he died of a heart attack.

In the years between the publication of the Male Report and his premature death, Kinsey grew petrified of yellow journalism and the danger of misinterpretation. The importance of his scientific approach in achieving acceptance for his work cannot be overstressed. Indeed, his insistence on the legitimacy of his research and his scientific credentials eventually made him a heroic figure, even in the eyes of his enemies. Nowhere was this fact more poignantly demonstrated than in the following obituary published in the *Catholic Record*, one of his most severe critics:

The death of Dr. Kinsey, famous Indiana University zoologist, and compiler of the controversial studies on human sex life, removes a truly dedicated scholar from the Bloomington campus. Few could disagree more strongly than we with Dr. Kinsey's views or deplore more deeply the evil influence such views could have on individuals and society. Yet one cannot deny that Dr. Kinsey's unremitting efforts, his patient, endless search, his disregard for criticism and ridicule, and his disinterest in financial gain should merit him high marks as a devoted scholar. While we have hurled our share of brick-bats at some of Dr. Kinsey's ideas when he was living, and still hold these ideas to be poisonously wrong, we must admit that we would welcome on our side many more scholars with something of Kinsey's devotion to knowledge and learning.

Kinsey hoped that his work would be widely publicized and that its effect would be educational, not trivializing. Contemporary observers credited him with achieving his goal. Donald B. Hileman's study of magazine coverage of the Female volume in 1953 found that Kinsey had already forced a reorientation of attitudes toward sexual matters among journalists. *Time* magazine agreed. Kinsey's biggest impact, they argued, was "conversational." Despite the increase in talk about sex after World War I, printed and public discussion remained taboo. "No single event," they concluded, "did more for open discussion of sex than the Kinsey Report, which got such matters as homosexuality, masturbation, coitus and orgasm into most papers and family magazines.

Though some critics feared that the reports would have an immediate adverse effect on public behavior, there is little evidence that such fears were justified. On the other hand, studies undertaken soon after publication suggested that Kinsey's work did liberalize attitudes, especially among the young. His findings publicized not only the sexual diversity but also the gap between ideals and reality in America. Such information about the prevalence of certain "questionable" practices tended to alter attitudes in the direction of tolerance. In this sense Kinsey's books probably were a catalyst. With consummate skill he dispelled ignorance about changes in sexual mores which had already taken place, *sub rosa*, since World War I. In presenting Americans with a *fait accompli*, his work demanded more realistic, more humane sex mores. He forced a public debate over the meaning of sex in modern life as no other author had except Freud.

Marriage counselors and sex therapists hailed the reports' role in alleviating guilt and promoting understanding between the sexes. For over a generation liberal therapists had struggled with their own ignorance and the greater ignorance of their patients. Lack of sexual harmony was deemed the most frequent cause of family disruptions. Dr. Lena Levine, director of the Margaret Sanger Research Bureau, recalled the early period of marriage counseling "with no nostalgia whatever."

We had no authorities to turn to, no reference books to give the women. We listened to the same story over and over again, and we counseled patients as best we could on technique. The worst job was to get the message across to the husbands, who were usually at fault, chiefly because they hadn't the slightest idea how a woman was put together and what she needed in the way of stimulation.

Kinsey paved the way for modern approaches to sex therapy. Masters and Johnson built on the groundwork laid by their more controversial predecessor.

Ironically, Kinsey's friends as well as his enemies responded only to the obvious Kinsey: the broad-minded, democratic rebel, the sexual libertarian. While he was surely all of these things, there was another side to this complex and subtle man, more easily understood only in historical retrospect. In many ways Kinsey remained bound to his Victorian past. Despite his studied neutrality concerning the various forms of sexual outlet, his acceptance of homosexuality, and his tolerance of extramarital sexuality, Kinsey was not a social revolutionary. His revolt against his society's outmoded sexual mores did not lead him to question other aspects of the value structure. Like most of his contemporaries, he had an attachment to happy, stable marriages, and he expected his research to ease the majority of Americans into a permanent monogamy so satisfying that social stability would be guaranteed. His data suggesting that sexual liberation had *not* destroyed cherished social institutions should have reassured his detractors, had they been composed enough to pay careful attention. It was no accident that Kinsey admired other personality traits of sexually precocious youths— their aggressive energy, their drive and spontaneity. Here he is most candid and also most reactionary: sexual abandon is coupled with the time-honored assumptions of enterprising capitalistic society.

Kinsey's faith in this social order is evident in his lecture notes for the 1938 marriage course, and in his special relationship with the American Association of Marriage Counselors. For many years an associate member, Kinsey was made an affiliate in 1952. Many critics erroneously interpret the failure to treat reproductive issues in the two reports as evidence of Kinsey's lack of interest. Yet approximately ten percent of Kinsey's standard interview was devoted to this subject and his silence on these matters reflects anything but indifference. He withheld his statistics on pregnancy, contraception, and abortion because the AAMC had convinced him to devote an entire book to these questions. Thus Masters and Johnson have only followed in the direction that Kinsey led. Like him they emerge as resolute foes of guilt and shame; like him they do not champion the cause of premarital chastity. But their ideal sexual order, like Kinsey's, leads to a retreat into privatism. They link greater sexual permissiveness with happier marriages, and they conceive of sexual life in terms of "enduring, heterosexual relationships of substantial affection.

Thus the cultural and intellectual revolution

that Kinsey touched off was archetypically American: its purpose was to keep basic institutions the same, especially at a time when, in the aftermath of world war, they might have been fundamentally altered.

In the thirty years since Kinsey published his volumes, his data have become a rich potential source for measuring social change. Unfortunately, historians have yet to mine his findings with any persistence. Used primarily to verify the "sexual revolution" in the first decades of this century, Kinsey's work has been virtually ignored by students interested in broader social and cultural issues. Few commentators, for example, have explored the implications of Kinsey's discovery that men from different classes exhibit divergent sexual behavior. The report maintained that lower-and working-class males had a decidedly higher incidence of premarital intercourse than college-educated men, tended to frown on extended foreplay in intercourse as "unnatural," were less likely to make love in the nude, masturbated less frequently, and viewed sex more as an uncontrollable impulse, less as a question of right and wrong. Middle-class and college-educated youths were moralistic; they tended to be virgins at marriage, although they petted and masturbated more often. The upwardly or downwardly mobile male, moreover, tended to form such attitudinal and behavioral patterns *long before he moved into his destined class.*

Kinsey's findings raise questions about the relationship of sex behavior, character structure, social mobility, and class, some of which might be read back into the past. Indeed, his data suggest a connection between twentieth-century middle-class behavior patterns and the emergence of the "modern" temperament, a primary attribute of which seems to be, at least for the nineteenth century, the ability to defer present gratification for future rewards. Historians of the nineteenth century have been struggling to link Victorian sexual repression to the emergence of a personality type comfortable with industrial capitalism. Thrift in semen, they argue, mirrored the injunction to be frugal materially. The ability to control passion and the denigration of personal pleasure as a goal created men and women who fit the demands of the take-off period of industrialization, when production, economy, and austerity took precedence over consumption. Marx eloquently characterized this stage in capitalistic growth:

Political economy, the science of wealth, is therefore, at the same time, the science of renunciation, of privation and of saving. . . . The science of a marvelous industry is at the same time the science of asceticism. . . . The less you eat, drink, buy books, go to the theater or to balls, or to the public house, and the less you think, love, theorize, sing, paint, fence, etc. the more you will be able to save. . . .

Historians have based their theories about nineteenth-century sexuality on evidence drawn from the prescriptive literature—advice books, political and social writings, medical treatises. Surely Kinsey's statistics give us some hard evidence that the repressive Victorian sexual theory was somehow linked to the behavior patterns of an upwardly mobile middle class.

Yet when we examine Kinsey's data more closely we must qualify Marx's contention that deferred gratification was always a prerequisite for capitalistic growth. By the 1920s, at least, it seems clear that middle-class youths were no longer deferring *gratification;* they were merely delaying *copulation.* The upwardly mobile petted and masturbated frequently despite guilt. Kinsey's figures for *total* sexual outlet (achieving orgasm by any means) showed only minor class differences. Presumably, the mature industrial economy no longer requires the full repression of sexual desires, it merely demands that those desires be gratified in particular ways. Thus, middle-class youths, in order to contribute to the system, deferred not necessarily sexual pleasure, but intercourse, marriage, children, and family obligations. Lower-class men, on the other hand, postponed neither early copulation, nor

marriage, nor large families, all of which probably helped to insure their docility, if not contentedness, in the factory.

Recent sex surveys report that the behavioral gap between men of different classes has substantially narrowed since Kinsey. Probably because of the widespread dissemination of effective contraceptive devices, premarital intercourse has increased among college-educated males, while sex behavior among the lower classes has differentiated to include nudity, extended foreplay, and increasing oral-genital contacts. Indeed, it appears that in an economy characterized by abundance and oriented toward the production of luxury items and consumer goods, sexual pleasure has become a means of recreation for all classes. Character structure and child rearing practices have shifted accordingly, away from an emphasis on autonomous self-control and toward the rational acceptance of pleasure, personal fulfillment, and happiness. Education, mass media, and the increase in leisure time among all social strata have tended to homogenize popular culture and narrow behavioral differences between social groups.

These developments suggest that we have entered a third phase of capitalistic growth. As yet we have proved incapable of dealing with problems of overproduction. The goal of the system remains consumption, and sexual liberation is encouraged primarily through advertising, as a means of orienting people toward new *things,* new ideas, new forms of luxury and pleasure. The encouragement of hedonism in all spheres seems essential for the affluent society. Thus sexual freedom has not been tied to social revolution. Championing privatism and the concern with individual adjustment, the new permissiveness has focused on self-fulfillment, not social change. Social historians interested in generational shifts in personality structure would do well to explore the implications of these changes in sexual behavior.

Kinsey's findings also indicate that knowledge of female sexuality has gradually become more sophisticated. If a sexual revolution has occurred, its base has been changes in female attitudes and behavior. While male trends shifted only minimally between generational cohorts in Kinsey's sample, women moved steadily toward the male standard. The evidence of the Female Report that women born after 1900 were more likely to reach orgasm in marriage, and that educated middle-class women achieved greater sexual satisfaction than their lower-class sisters deserves special attention. It would seem that sexual liberation, fostered by greater educational opportunities, presupposes and encourages the development of individuality and autonomy among women.

On the other hand, students of lower-class sexual patterns have found that among the less educated "both husbands and wives feel that sexual gratification for the wife is much less important than for the husband." Lower-class lovemaking tends to be less "technically versatile," lacking in the extended foreplay intended to facilitate the wife's satisfaction. Lower-class women, perhaps as a consequence, view sex primarily as a duty. Yet although they enjoy sex less they rarely refuse intercourse. Sociologist Lee Rainwater links these sexual patterns to a patriarchal family structure, a radical separation between male and female spheres, and a lack of meaningful communication between sexual partners, all characteristic of lower-class groups. Recent work on nineteenth-century sex roles has pictured a similar family structure exhibiting the same well-defined differentiation between male and female culture. One is tempted to use Kinsey's statistics to posit the prevalence among the middle class in the last century of contemporary lower-class patterns of lovemaking, oriented toward male satisfaction. For an age which barely accepted the legitimacy of female pleasure and still linked intercourse with reproduction, such a thesis appears plausible and is borne out by Kinsey's data revealing a gradual increase in female orgasm in the twentieth century.

The evolution of consciousness over the last century has altered expectations concerning what is sexually natural and possible. Human needs diversify with changing social and cultural conditions, and things become desirable merely because they are suddenly possible. Kinsey's data offer us an insight into this transformation in the meaning of marriage and sexual relations. His findings suggest that this century has witnessed a merging of spiritual love and passion in a novel way. His evidence indicates that middle-class lovemaking techniques are a recent dimension of the popular imagination. The emergence of almost universal petting in the 1920s and 1930s represents a new psycho-sexual intimacy. The increasing sexual responsiveness of middle-class women may be a function of this.

It has become fashionable to mourn the passing of the old sexual order in which the omnipresence of guilt, anxiety, and dread over the violation of taboos guaranteed at least that life would be interesting. "If . . . nothing is grave," a recent commentator has written, "satire cannot bite and tragedy gives way to the social illness of maladjustment. For many, human life under such conditions would lose its music." Such an attitude offers further proof of the distance we have travelled from the sexual culture of Kinsey's generation. Privy to the tragic ways in which people's sexual lives were blighted by society, Kinsey welcomed a new order while he helped to bring it about. We are the richer for Kinsey's conviction that human beings should get more joy out of all sexual activity.

Yet Kinsey was no revolutionary. Though he wished that the world would be a better place because of his books, his vision required no fundamental social or economic changes. He understood neither the revolutionary nor the disintegrative potentialities inherent in sexual liberation. In the end, Kinsey's hedonism has become a conservative force, and he himself the unwitting agent of an increasingly callous and wasteful society.

STUDY QUESTIONS

1. What factors explain the remarkable popular success of *Sexual Behavior in the Human Male*?

2. What characterized the study of sexual behavior before Kinsey? How did Kinsey's study change people's beliefs and attitudes?

3. What does Regina Morantz mean when she describes Kinsey as "the scientist as sex crusader"? Did the passionate or dispassionate side of Kinsey's personality influence his life?

4. How did the American people react to the publication of *Sexual Behavior in the Human Male*? What were the major issues raised by the debate over Kinsey's book?

5. How were Kinsey's research and results culturally biased? How was his sexual liberalism demonstrated in his work? How did he challenge the 1950s social and sexual standards? What place did love play in Kinsey's study of sexual relations?

6. How did Kinsey's work set the stage for a dehumanized, depersonalized society? What long-range effects did Kinsey's writing have on society? Was Kinsey a social revolutionary? Why or why not?

7. What links are there between sexual activity and economic and class behavior?

BIBLIOGRAPHY

Sexual Behavior in the Human Male (1948) and *Sexual Behavior in the Human Female* (1953) are the classic sexual studies by Alfred C. Kinsey. Gay Talese, *Thy Neighbor's Wife* (1980), is a popular and useful examination of changing sexual behavior in America. Reay Tannahill, *Sex in History* (1980), discusses changing sexual behavior and attitudes in world history. A number of useful articles deal with the subject of American and English sexual attitudes. Among the best are John Burham, "The Progressive Era Revolution in American Attitudes Toward Sex," *Journal of American History*, 59 (1973); Charles Rosenberg, "Sexuality, Class, and Role," *American Quarterly*, 25 (1973); and Peter Cominos, "Late Victorian Sexual Respectability and the Social System," *International Review of Social History*, 8 (1963). Two other innovative books are Steven Marcus, *The Other Victorians: A Study of Sexuality and Pornography in Mid-Nineteenth Century England* (1974), and John S. Haller and Robin M. Haller, *The Physician and Sexuality in Victorian America* (1974).

AMERICAN PRISONERS OF WAR IN KOREA: A SECOND LOOK AT THE 'SOMETHING NEW IN HISTORY' THEME

H. H. Wubben

Contrary to what most people had anticipated, the end of World War II did not bring a feeling of security to the United States. The war was barely over when the Soviet Union replaced the Germans and Japanese as mortal enemies of the Americans. The Soviet threat seemed particularly ominous because of the Marxist prediction of revolutionary upheavals in capitalist countries. In the late 1940s, United States foreign policy revolved around the idea of "containment," an economic and military commitment to keep Russian influence behind the "Iron Curtain." The Truman Doctrine of 1946, the Marshall Plan of 1947–48, the North Atlantic Treaty Organization, and the Berlin Airlift of 1948–49 were all directed at stopping Soviet expansion in Western Europe. In order to secure Congressional funding of that foreign policy, the Truman administration talked unceasingly of the international communist conspiracy, and in the process created a tense, suspicious political atmosphere inside the United States. Many Americans became convinced there was a subversive, internal Communist plot to overthrow the United States government.

The American fear of the Soviet Union and Communism intensified in 1950 with the outbreak of the Korean War. North Korean troops poured across the 38th parallel into South Korea, and the United States implemented the containment policy by sending hundreds of thousands of troops into the peninsula. When the armistice was reached three years later, the United States had had its first taste of undeclared war—a "police action." And when the prisoners of war began filtering home with their horror stories of deprivation, torture, and "brainwashing," Communism became even more sinister to the American people. The experiences of the POWs also gave rise to serious doubts about the "American character." In the following selection, historian H. H. Wubben discusses the significance of the POW problem in the context of the Cold War.

Americans have long been intrigued by speculations about their national character. In particular they have been receptive to assessments which credit them with immunity against certain human frailties, an immunity not possessed by most other peoples. Out of the Korean War came a controversy which impinged annoyingly upon such assessments and which provided grist for the mill of those who now preferred to believe that in recent decades the character had deteriorated.

Throughout the conflict reports coming out of North Korea indicated that the communists were subjecting American prisoners of war to a re-education process popularly described as "brainwashing." Prisoner returnees during Operation Little Switch in May and Operation Big Switch in August and September 1953 corroborated some of these reports. But it also became clear that such re-education was largely ineffective. Nevertheless, 21 prisoners chose not to return home. A few who did return admitted that they were "progressives," that is, men partially converted by the Chinese re-education program. Some who did not confess to such leanings faced accusations from other prisoners that they had taken the "progressive" line.

In addition it became apparent that a number of men had engaged in collaborative or criminal behavior detrimental to the welfare of their fellows. Consequently, the armed services made special efforts to find out what had happened. Psychiatrists and psychologists interviewed the newly-freed prisoners during the repatriation process and on the journey home. Intelligence officers also interviewed them, compiling dossiers on each man. Information acquired by these specialists eventually provided the data upon which subsequent formal studies of the

"American Prisoners of War in Korea: A Second Look at the 'Something New in History' Theme" by H. H. Wubben, from *American Quarterly, XXII* (Spring, 1970). Published by the American Studies Association. Reprinted by permission of American Quarterly and the author.

prisoners and their behavior in captivity were based.

In 1955 came the official government view of the POW behavior issue, the report of the Secretary of Defense's Advisory Committee on Prisoners of War. But the committee's judgment was hardly definitive. On the one hand, the group declared, "the record [of the prisoners] seems fine indeed . . . they cannot be found wanting." On the other it concluded, "The Korean story must never be permitted to happen again." Then in 1956 the Army issued a training pamphlet on the subject of POW behavior. It was even more ambiguous. Readers learned that the Chinese "lenient policy" designed to lessen resistance "resulted in little or no active resistance to the enemy's indoctrination." Later, however, they read that the "large majority . . . resisted the enemy in the highest tradition of the service and of our country."

Findings of the major formal studies, financed by or undertaken by the armed services in most cases, are much more satisfying to the scholar who desires more consistency in both raw material and analysis. These include research projects done for the Department of the Army, the Surgeon General's Office, the Air Force and the Walter Reed Army Institute of Research. Also engaged in examination of POW experiences was the Society for the Investigation of Human Ecology. The studies never achieved wide circulation although the research scientists who engaged in them reported their substance in professional journals. Eventually one scholarly book-length treatment appeared, Albert Biderman's *March to Calumny*. Biderman, a sociologist who was active in several of these projects, demolished in a convincing manner those interpretations which accused the prisoners of being singularly deficient in the attributes expected of American servicemen unfortunate enough to become prisoners of war.

The work of such specialists, however, has had little impact compared with that of those whose reports convey a largely, if not exclusively, negative version of the prisoners' actions during captivity. That version, in general, declares that American prisoners of war in Chinese and North Korean hands were morally weak and uncommitted to traditional American ideals. Consequently, some, though not a majority, were infected to a degree with the virus of communism. Furthermore, they were undisciplined. They were unwilling to aid each other in their travail. And they succumbed too easily under limited duress or no duress at all to the pressures of their captors to engage in collaborative behavior, including informing on each other. Their death rate, 38%, was the highest in history, and most deaths resulted from "give-up-itis" and lack of concern for one another among the prisoners themselves, not from communist mistreatment. Also, no prisoners successfully escaped from communist prison camps, a "first" in U.S. military experience. Other nationality groups, particularly the Turks, successfully resisted communist blandishments, and only the Marines among the Americans consistently adhered to patterns of honorable conduct. Finally, the POWs in Korea were the first Americans in captivity to so act, a "fact" which calls for a reassessment of mid-century American values and the culture which spawned them.

Among those who accepted this as history, in part or in whole, were President Dwight Eisenhower, FBI Director J. Edgar Hoover and Senator Strom Thurmond of South Carolina. Political scientist Anthony Bouscaren saw the "record" as evidence that American education had flunked a significant test. Another critic of education, Augustin Rudd, viewed the prisoner performance as evidence that the chickens of progressive education had come home to roost. The editors of *Scouting* magazine in 1965 cited it in urging continued efforts to implant the ideals of the Boy Scout Code among youth in that organization. And as late as 1968, California educator and political figure Max Rafferty employed it in some of his campaign literature during his senatorial race.

These individuals, however, have not been so influential as two others in promoting this "his-

tory." They are the late Eugene Kinkead, a freelance writer, and Lt. Col. William E. Mayer, one of the psychiatrists who participated in the interviewing of the repatriates. Kinkead's major contribution was a book entitled *In Every War But One* which sold around fifteen thousand copies. Col. Mayer's contributions, mainly public addresses, have won even wider circulation than Kinkead's, thanks to the tape recorder and the mimeograph. Both men have modified from time to time their indictment of the prisoners, if not of recent trends in American society. Mayer, for instance, toward the end of one of his speeches said, "Finally, the great majority of men didn't become communists, didn't suffer any kind of moral breakdown, no matter what the communists did to them." But by then the negative point had been so strongly stressed that few listeners were aware of his significant caveat.

That they were not aware resulted from a number of circumstances. Many conservative Americans were disgruntled at the absence of a decisive American victory in the war. They blamed communist subversion at home for the result. This subversion in turn they blamed on "socialistic" influences originating in the 1930s which, they charged, had weakened the capacity and will of home, church and school to develop good character among the nation's youth. Thus, the prisoners served as evidence to verify their beliefs. Many liberals accepted the prisoners as examples of societal sickness also, although they rejected the communist subversion theme. They claimed that American materialism lay at the root of the problem. Both groups professed to view the prisoners with pity rather than scorn, as men who through no fault of their own were simply unfortunate products of a society on the verge of decay. Both were impressed by Mayer's credentials and the literate, entertaining manner in which he employed tendentious illustrations to document a general picture of moral and morale breakdown resulting from defective precaptivity nurture. Given these general dispositions on the part of many Mayer listeners, it is no wonder that they let his muted but significant qualifier slip by. They weren't interested in it. Finally many Americans, including academicians who would ordinarily have demanded more intellectual rigor in their own disciplines, simply took Mayer's and Kinkead's revelations at face value because they seemed to meet the test of reasonableness.

Historians have long known a great deal about the behavior of Americans in prisoner camps prior to the Korean War, particularly about prison behavior in World War II camps. As Peter Karsten wrote in the spring of 1965 issue of *Military Affairs*, the motivation and conduct of American servicemen, in or out of prison camps, have been a source of concern from the American Revolution to the Present. George Washington had numerous unkind words for defectors, mutineers and those of his forces who lacked "public spirit." The activities of the reluctant warriors of the War of 1812, the defectors and the short-term volunteers who departed the service when their time was up—if not sooner—wherever they were during the Mexican and Civil Wars, are a matter of record. "Give-up-itis," called "around the bends," was not unknown at Andersonville and Belle Isle. Draft dodgers and deserters numbered over 170,000 in World War I. By the early 1940s, "around the bends" had several new names, the most common being "Bamboo disease" and "fence complex."

Even in a "popular" war, World War II, the Army worried about the lack of dedication among its troops. Indoctrination programs were overhauled and beefed up with negligible success. A Social Science Research Council team which analyzed data collected by the Army during the war, concluded that the average soldier "gave little concern to the conflicting values underlying the military struggle . . . . [and] Although he showed a strong but tacit patriotism, this usually did not lead him in his thinking to subordinate his personal interests to the furtherance of ideal aims and values."

As to moral and morale breakdown under sever conditions, two military physicians report-

ed that in Japanese POW camps "moral integrity could be pretty well judged by inverse ratio to one's state of nutrition." And, they added, "Although some of these prisoners sublimated their cravings by giving aid to their fellows, there was, in general, a lowering of moral standards. Food was often obtained by devious means at the expense of other prisoners." Though a buddy system did function to some extent, particularly among small cliques who shared both companionship and food, there were few group activities, and most men tended to be taciturn and seclusive. Being unable to defy their captors and survive, they expressed considerable verbal resentment toward each other. In particular they disparaged their own officers and their behavior. Another physician, who was a prisoner himself in the Philippines and Japan, write that most POWs, whether sick or well, suffered periods of apathy or depression which, if not countered forcefully, would lead to death. "Giving up" occurred earliest and easiest among younger men as in Korea. In a sentence strikingly reminiscent of the Kinkead-Mayer critique, except that he omitted the "something new in history" theme, the physician wrote, "Failures in adjustment were most apparent in the 18-to-23-year-old group who had little or no previous experience and much overprotection. These men demonstrated marked inability to fight physical diseases and the initial shock of depression of captivity."

Dr. Harold Wolff, a consultant to the Advisory Committee, reported that in World War II German prison camps where the pressures were much less severe than in Japanese and Korean camps, about 10% of the Americans "offered remarkably little resistance, if not outright collaboration." Wolff also noted that the escape record of Americans in World War II was not exceptional. Less than a dozen prisoners of the Japanese out of twenty-five to thirty thousand men escaped from permanent camps, all in the Philippines. Less than one hundred out of ninety-four thousand Americans captured by the Nazis successfully escaped from camps, of which less than half returned to Allied control.

Autobiographical accounts of former World War II prisoners also tell much which shows that the Korean POW behavior was not unique. Edward Dobran, an airman held by the Germans, reported that a G.I. mess hall crew at his camp took care of itself well but skimped on the rest of the men's rations. Nor could those who apportioned food in the squads be trusted to do their job honestly more than a few days at a time. Dobran concluded, "In a place such as this, every man is strictly for himself. This sort of living and hardships showed what a human being is really made of. If you didn't look out for yourself here, nobody else did.

Physician Alfred Weinstein's book-length recital of prison-camp life in the Philippines and Japan tells about a Marine officer's extensive collaboration with the Japanese and about the stealing of medicine by the same officer and some enlisted men medics at Cabanatuan. Some POW mechanics and truck drivers, put to work by the Japanese, lived high, using their positions to smuggle from Manila desperately needed food and medicine which they then sold for outrageous prices to the rest of the prisoners who were in dire need of both. Nor was Weinstein complimentary about behavior in an officers' ward at a prisoner hospital at Cabanatuan. These officer-patients demanded so many special privileges, food and medicine because of their rank that the senior American officer had to break up the group by distributing the men throughout the other wards. Also not complimentary about the self-seeking of a few officers incarcerated in Japan is Hugh Myers in a recently published memoir. Myers has described how four veteran Navy chiefs from the garrison at Guam assumed control over prison life at one stage in his POW experience when it became apparent that the officers were too concerned about their privileges, too inexperienced, or both, to do the job fairly or well.

Nevertheless, in all the accounts discussed above which were written by men who had been POWs there is no tendency to denigrate American civilization because of the failings of a greater or lesser number of men in prison camps. Nor is it assumed by them that men under conditions of stress will uniformly conduct themselves in exemplary fashion. Weinstein, for instance, wrote, "Hard living, disease, and starvation made heroes out of few men. More frequently does it make animals out of men who, in the normal course of living would go through life with a clean slate."

Two aspects of the Korean POW story, then, should be of particular interest to the historian. First, there is the fact that a poorly understood historical experience is interpreted in such a way that it makes a thoroughly inaccurate comparison between Americans past and Americans present. Second, there is the acceptance by the general public of this "nonhistory" as history, largely without the aid of historians. Critical to the development of these two aspects is the misuse of the data derived from the prisoner's experiences. This data, largely collected at the time of their repatriation, was not originally intended to provide raw material for behavioral or historical studies per se. It was, rather, gathered with the intention of providing information for possible court martial action against men accused of collaboration or criminal activity while in captivity, to identify men who merited commendation and decoration, and to identify repatriates who needed psychiatric care.

Consequently, the generally accepted percentage classification of POWs by behavior, 5% resistor, 15% participator (or collaborator), and 80% middlemen, needs to be viewed more as suggestive than as absolutely definitive. Biderman, for instance, reports that placement of a POW in the collaborator category required only that he be "accused of committing isolated but serious acts of collaboration" which could be corroborated. Placement in this category remained firm, moreover, even if the prisoner were otherwise regarded as having been a hardcase resistor throughout his captivity, as some of them were.

With regard to the evidence that the POWs

were peculiarly weak in moral fibre, uncommitted to American ideals and ignorant of the institutions and history of their country, a change in perspective is revealing. If one accepts the idea that it takes moral fibre to resist, actively *and* passively, ideological conversion attempts by a captor who is very concerned about "correct thoughts" and who has overwhelming power which he uses as it suits his purpose, then one must grant that most prisoners had it to some meaningful degree. The Chinese regarded passive resistance to indoctrination, including "going through the motions," as "insincere" and "stupid," if not actually reactionary behavior, as many of the scholars of POW behavior have noted. They made strenuous efforts to overcome such "insincerity" and "stupidity." But in May of 1952 they abandoned compulsory indoctrination, keeping classes only for the relatively small number of progressives. Their extensive efforts had resulted in disappointing returns among their stubborn captives.

Many prisoners did supply evidence that there was often a lack of discipline in their ranks. Autobiographies, both American and British, speak of a dog-eat-dog system prevailing during several of the "death marches" and in the temporary holding camps during the harsh winter of 1950–51. They also tell of prisoners in need being refused assistance by other prisoners. In these respects, however, they differ little from World War II POW memoirs which described the same kind of reaction to stress during those periods in which captivity conditions were the worst. Conversely, those who give testimony to such animalistic behavior also testify to behavior of a different order. Morris Wills, one of the original 21 who refused repatriation, only to return over a decade later, has written: "You really can't worry about the other fellow; you are at the line of existence yourself. If you go under that, you die. You would help each other if you could. Most would try; I wouldn't say all."

"Reactionary" Lloyd Pate wrote a similar, if more positive, vein. "After the first shock of our capture wore off, the G.I.'s with me on those Korean mountain roads began to act like soldiers this country could be proud of." He told of prisoners helping each other to keep up the pace when dropping out meant death; and he credited two such good Samaritans with saving his life. Captive British journalist Philip Deane in one poignant passage revealed the context within which many prisoners faced life or death under brutal march conditions. In it he inadvertently answers many who charge that the prisoners "shamefully" abandoned their weaker fellows en route. A young American lieutenant, faced with a bitter choice, allowed five men to drop out, in effect "abandoning" them, contrary to the orders of the North Korean march commander. He could not, he told the North Korean, order them carried because "That meant condemning the carriers to death from exhaustion." For this decision, the lieutenant's captors executed him on the spot.

The same kinds of sources, supplemented again by the studies of research scientists and journalists, reveal that the physical duress to which prisoners allegedly succumbed so easily, presumably leading widespread collaboration, ranged all the way from calculated manipulation of necessities of life to murder. One former prisoner labeled a reactionary by his captors told the author of many instances of physical brutality practiced by the Chinese. Among those brutalized were Chinese-appointed squad leaders who couldn't or wouldn't promote group compliance with the indoctrination program. Some, he maintained, were murdered. Others were subjected to severe beatings and then denied medical treatment for the injuries inflicted; death sometimes resulted. Some bad treatment, he declared, resulted from caprice, citing a case of one man in his squad, a "middleman" who underwent several nighttime beatings over a period of one month for no apparent reason. Nevertheless, those who disparage prisoner behavior tend to take at face value the Chinese contention that they did not commit atrocities or torture their captives. An official U.S. Army report issued in June 1953, however, declared that after Chinese entrance into the war they were "fully as active as the North Koreans" in commission of war crimes.

So far as the POW death rate, 38%, is concerned, this figure is speculative. It does not include atrocity deaths, which numbered over a thousand. Nor does it include well over two thousand missing in action. The Chinese kept no dependable records, and throughout much of the first year of the war the prisoners were in no position to do so themselves. Whatever the true death rate, critics of the prisoners and of the alleged "softness" of American society see it as "too high." By implication they blame most of the deaths on prisoner negligence, or worse, on loss of will to live. Five prisoner physicians, however, reported otherwise shortly after the war. They wrote:

The erroneous impression has been created that prisoners of war who were in good physical health gave up and died; this is not true. Every prisoner of war in Korea who died had suffered from malnutrition, exposure to cold, and continued harassment by the Communists. Contributing causes to the majority of deaths were prolonged cases of respiratory infection and diarrhea. Under such conditions, it is amazing not that there was a high death rate, but that there was a reasonably good rate of survival.

Another example of misuse of data to demonstrate weakness on the part of the POWs and their nurture is the "no escape" theme. While it is true that no American successfully escaped from permanent prison camps in the Yalu River region, several hundred did escape before permanent camps were established, some after several months of captivity. From these camps, furthermore, at least 46 verifiable escape attempts involving nearly 4% of the POWs have been authenticated. Nevertheless, both Mayer and Kinkead have insisted that failure to escape from permanent camps is significant. Mayer, in one speech, praised American prisoners in the Philippines for attempting and completing escapes despite the Japanese practice of putting prisoners

in blood-brother groups of ten. If one escaped the rest were to be shot. But, according to Weinstein, the POWs took the Japanese at their word and established MP patrols to halt just such escape attempts.

The assumption of Turkish superiority in POW camps also rests on a misreading of evidence. Turkish prisoners were, in the first place, a select group of volunteers. Furthermore, half of them were captured after the worst period of captivity was over, the winter of 1950–51. Well over 80% of the American POWs were not so fortunate. Turkish prisoners, unlike the Americans, were not split up. Officers and enlisted men remained together most of the time, an aid to maintenance of discipline. Nor were the Turks the objects of intense re-education efforts as the Americans were. Yet, one Turk served on a peace committee. One refused to accept repatriation until he had a late change of heart. And some communist propaganda materials show Turkish involvement in communist-sponsored POW programs. In 1962, Brigadier General S. L. A. Marshall (ret.), military historian and author of *The River and the Gauntlet* and *Pork Chop Hill*, bluntly told a Senate subcommittee that the Turks were overrated. Said Marshall, "The story about the Turks being perfect prisoners is a continuation of the fable that they were perfect soldiers in the line which was not true at all."

The assumption of Marine superiority to soldiers in prisoner-camp behavior also rests upon misreading of evidence. Marines may have retained more esprit de corps as prisoners, but they, like the Turks, were more of an elite unit. However, at Kangyye in 1951, some Marines made speeches, signed peace petitions (often with illegible signatures and wrong or misspelled names), and wrote articles for a "peace camp" paper called *The New Life*. Told by the Chinese that rewards for being a "good student" could include early release, some made up stories of hungry childhood and living on relief. Others said they joined the Corps in order to get decent food and clothing. Two described the criteria for a satisfactory article: "All you had to do was string stuff together in fairly coherent sentences such words as 'warmongers' . . . 'Wall Street big shots' . . . 'capitalistic bloodsuckers' and you had it made." Eighteen Marines and one soldier who convinced the Chinese of their "sincerity" eventually were selected for early repatriation. Taken close to the front, they crossed up their captors by escaping ahead of schedule.

The experience of the eighteen Marines is discussed in a University of Maryland history master's thesis on Marine POWs in Korea by Lt. Col. Angus MacDonald. MacDonald notes with disapproval that the Marines gave far more information to their captors than name, rank and serial number. But he correctly views these as gambits designed to secure release from captivity. The Army, however, seems to have taken a less pragmatic, and, consequently, more humorless view of similar efforts by its enlisted men. MacDonald, on the other hand, does not deal adequately with the joint investigations of all services which, when concluded, revealed that only 11% of the Army repatriates compared with 26% of the Marine repatriates warranted further investigation on possible misconduct charges. Instead he quotes with approval an address by Col. Mayer which praised Marine performance, and by implication, criticized that of Army POWs. Eventually both services made the further investigations suggested, the Army possibly applying a broader set of standards to define misconduct, since it initially cleared only 58% of the 11% thought to warrant further investigation. The Marines cleared 94%. Finally, only fourteen cases came up for trial, all Army cases, out of which eleven convictions resulted.

In view of the commonly accepted belief that the Marines performed better than soldiers as POWs, it is interesting to note the comment by retired Air Corps Major General Delmar T. Spivey in a John A. Lejeune Forum on prisoner behavior. In this Marine-sponsored forum, Spivey, who while imprisoned in Germany during World War II was senior officer in the Center Compound of Stalag III, made the unrebutted statement that:

Even with all these things ["survival courses, physical conditioning programs, instruction in our American heritage, information about the enemy, courses and exercises designed to instill pride and self-respect and belief in one's service and country, and the assurance that our country will stand by an individual, both in combat and as a prisoner"] . . . we cannot assume that every fighting man will be completely prepared for his responsibilities as a prisoner. History is not on our side, and neither is human nature when we consider the past conduct of prisoners of war.

The conclusions of professional and semi-professional scholars and writers about American POW behavior are mixed. Stanley Elkins in his search for suggestive experience to support his description of the effects of a closed system on slave psychological development turned to the POWs. Unfortunately he exaggerated some of the findings of his source, Edgar Schein, one scholar involved in the POW studies. Elkins wrote of "profound changes in behavior and values" being "effected without physical torture or extreme deprivation" and of "large numbers" of American informers and men who cooperated in the indoctrination program. But Schein said only that mandatory discussion and mutual criticism sessions which followed communist indoctrination lectures probably created "considerable doubt concerning ideological position in some of the men." They were, as a whole, he declared, "not very effective." Nor did he give any estimates of the numbers of informers or cooperators relative to the total POW population.

Betty Friedan has seen the average Korean prisoner as an "apathetic, dependent, infantile, purposeless being . . . a new American man . . . reminiscent of the familiar 'feminine' personality." Edgar Friedenberg described the POW as a new model of being, but an international one, not just American. He wrote, "this sort of young man is a character in existentialist novels and post-World War II Italian films." Miss Friedan, however, discovered parallels closer to home. She found them in the youth of the 1950s, in their "new passivity," bored and passionless, demonstrated variously in: the annual spring-time collegiate riots at Fort Lauderdale; a teen-age call girl service in a Long Island suburb; ado-lescent grave defiling in Bergen County, New Jersey; drug-taking parties in Westchester Coun-ty, New York, and Connecticut; and the "help-less, apathetic state" of the female student body at Sarah Lawrence College.

It is doubtful whether the typical Korean POW would recognize himself in all this. His schooling averaged somewhat less than nine years. His social class was hardly comfortable middle. And his withdrawal from activity was certainly in part a shrewd way of fending off the ubiquitous Chinese indoctrinators.

Among historians, Walter Hermes, author of the second volume of a projected five-volume official history of the war, took note of the Kin-kead book. But he accepted Biderman's view, calling it a "convincing rebuttal" of Kinkead's thesis. Robert Leckie, however, relied heavily on Kinkead and called the POW record "sorry . . . the worst in American history." Apathy, he declared, was responsible for the failure of any men to escape. But in the same paragraph he asserted that the Caucasian appearance of the Americans was the "more likely reason for this failure." T. R. Fehrenbach, too, has generally taken a dim view of the prisoners' behavior. "Chemistry and culture," the Doolittle Board's democratization reforms and American educa-tion, among other culprits, were at fault, he wrote. His analysis of sources, like Leckie's, was less than rigorous.

Harry Middleton, while acknowledging that the percentage of collaborators was small, also looked askance at the prisoners' record. His book, though published later (1965) than Feh-renbach's narrative, displayed less acquaintance with or close reading of the available literature on the subject. An English scholar, David Rees, in *Korea: the Limited War*, after devoting a lengthy chapter to the subject, leaned to the point of view that POW behavior was not unusual considering the fallible nature of man and considering the unique nature of the prison-ers' experiences. S. L. A. Marshall, a consultant to the Advisory Committee, is a defender of the prisoners. And Russell Weigley in his *History of the United States Army* also concluded that the Korean POWs were not a discredit to the nation.

In 1962, 21 scholars familiar with the POW behavior materials signed a paper entitled "Statement: to Set Straight the Korean POW Episode." This paper, drawn up by two of the signers, Edgar Schein and Raymond Bauer, who had worked extensively on the subject, directly refuted the popular version of the POW story expounded by Kinkead and Mayer. The "State-ment" included these challenging assertions:

The behavior of the Korean prisoners did not compare unfavorably with that of their countrymen or with the behavior of people of other nations who have faced similar trials in the past.

Instances of moral weakness, collaboration with the enemy, and failure to take care of fellow soldiers in Korea did not occur more frequently than in other wars where comparable conditions of physical and psychological hardship were present. Indeed, such instances appear to have been less prevalent than historical experience would lead us to expect. . . .

It is our opinion that any serious analysis of American society, its strengths and weaknesses, should rest on historically correct data. It is unfortunate that the Korean POW episode has been distorted to make the case for one view of American society. We hope that this Statement will be the first step toward setting the historical facts of this episode straight.

Historically correct data, however, were insufficient for many Americans in the 1950s and 1960s. They seemed to feel that any com-munist success at eliciting collaborative behavior or inducing ideological doubt among any Amer-ican soldiers, no matter how small the number, signified a general American failure. Such failure to them was not to be taken lightly. It might reflect, after all, the existence of a more danger-ous cancer in the American character than even they had suspected.

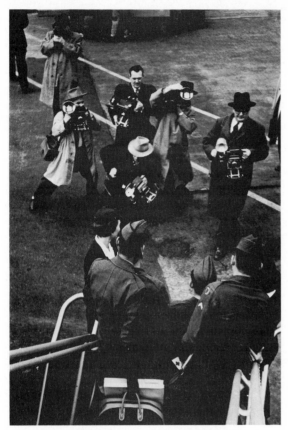

American GIs returning from North Korean prison camps after the end of the Korean War. Contrary to popular opinion, which was gripped by fear of Communist subversion, Korean War POWs did not conduct themselves much differently than did POWs of earlier wars.

the West's battle against communism, had these efforts taken place over the length of time and under circumstances comparable to those endured by the Korean POWs, there might be a rough basis for comparison. But those American POWs weren't so subjected. Dobran did report some anti-Semitism among his POW group upon which the Germans might have capitalized. But one can speculate a little in the other direction that the American reaction to this divisive ploy might have been similar to that in one group of Negro POWs in Korea among whom the Chinese tried to foment ideological change by hammering upon the existence of racial discrimination in the United States. Wrote Lloyd Pate, "A few colored guys got up and said it was our business what we did in the United States and for the Chinks to mind their own damn business."

Second, never before had the American public been so gullible as to believe that such a chimera as the enemy's self-proclaimed "lenient policy" was, in fact, lenient. During the first year of the war in particular the Chinese and North Koreans, often in systematic fashion, fostered brutalizing captivity conditions which were in significant part responsible for prisoner behavior which did not measure up to "ideal" standards.

And, finally, for the first time the public seemed to assume that such selfish undisciplined behavior as existed among the POWs was something new in American military experience and that it was a direct consequence of a characterological deterioration in the nation itself.

Whether or not such a deterioration has been taking place in American society, from the advent of the New Deal and the impact of progressive education as the critics strongly imply, is not under contention here. What is being contended, rather, is that if one really believes this and wants evidence to prove it, one will have to find examples other than among those Americans who died and those who survived in the prison camps of North Korea, 1950–53.

What is really "new in history," then, about the whole Korean POW episode?

First, never before Korea were American POWs confronted by a captor who worked hard to change their ideological persuasion. This point is worth a brief examination. Had American POWs of the Germans, for instance, been subjected to ideological thought reform efforts designed to inculcate virulent racist attitudes or to inculcate the idea that Germany was fighting

STUDY QUESTIONS

1. What is the meaning of "brainwashing" and "reeducation?"

2. By the mid-1950s, what was the prevailing opinion about the behavior of America POWs in Korea? Why did that issue seem to be so important to the American public? How did Americans explain the behavior and "failure" of the POWs?

3. Compare the behavior of American POWs in German prisons during World War II with the Americans in Japanese or Korean prisoner-of-war camps. Was there much difference? Why or why not?

4. Does POW behavior reveal anything about American civilization? Why or why not?

5. Did large numbers of POWs die because of a "loss of the will to live"? Why or why not? Was the behavior of U.S. Marines any different from other groups of POWS? Why or why not?

6. Summarize Wubben's feelings about the behavior of American POWs during the Korean War.

BIBLIOGRAPHY

For a general discussion of the Korean War, see Joseph C. Goulden, *Korea: The Untold Story of the War* (1982). Also see Bruce Cummings, *The Origins of the Korean War* (1980). Ronald Caridi's *The Korean War and American Politics* (1969), analyzes the domestic impact of the conflict. The internal tension inspired by the Cold War is discussed in Edward Shils, *The Torment of Secrecy* (1956); David Caute, *The Great Fear* (1978); and Alan Harper, *The Politics of Loyalty* (1969). The most critical account of American POW behavior during the Korean War is Eugene Kincaid, *In Every War But One* (1959). For a devastating critique of Kincaid's book, see Albert D. Biderman, *March to Calumny: The Story of American POWs in the Korean War* (1963). Also see Louis J. West, "Psychiatry, 'Brainwashing,' and the American Character," *American Journal of Psychiatry* CXX (1964).

INTELLECT ON TELEVISION: THE QUIZ SHOW SCANDALS OF THE 1950S

Richard S. Tedlow

In 1854, Henry David Thoreau wrote, "We are in great haste to construct a magnetic telegraph from Maine to Texas; but Maine and Texas, it may be, have nothing important to communicate." More than one hundred years later, Thoreau's observation, greatly expanded, is still valid. Possessing the technological means of communication is no guarantee of meaningful communication. Nowhere is this situation more evident than in the commercial television industry. In the following essay, Richard S. Tedlow examines the problems inherent in commercial broadcasting, especially as they relate to the television quiz scandals of the late 1950s. The picture he presents is not a flattering one; the object of commercial television is quite simply to sell products, not to educate or uplift its audience. The result is an industry dominated by monetary values and generally oblivious to all ethical or moral consideration. In the specific case of quiz shows, television has produced an additional side effect: it has cheapened the meaning of education and intelligence. As Tedlow cogently observed, "If any crime had been committed in the quiz show episode, it was surely the broad conspiracy to portray as genuine intellectual activity the sprouting of trivia." In today's America where books of lists and trivia make the best sellers list, Tedlow's discussion of the quiz shows has a haunting familiarity.

On the 7th of June, 1955, *The $64,000 Question* made its debut on the CBS television network. No programming idea could have been more thoroughly foreshadowed by previous shows. Since the mid-1930s radio had been exploiting the American passion for facts with contests and games. For years, small amounts of cash or manufacturer-donated merchandise had been given away through various formats. What was new about *Question* was the size of the purse. The giveaway had taken a "quantum jump"; losers received a Cadillac as a consolation prize.

Question's format was simple. The producers selected a contestant who chose a subject about which he or she answered increasingly difficult questions which were assigned monetary values ranging from $64 to $64,000. The contestants could quit without attempting the succeeding plateau, but if he chose to continue and missed, he forfeited his winnings and was left with only his Cadillac.

By a few deft touches, the producers heightened the aura of authenticity and tension. The questions used were deposited in a vault of the Manufacturers Trust Company and brought to the studio by a bank officer flanked by two armed guards. As the stakes increased, the contestant entered a glass-enclosed "isolation booth" on stage to the accompaniment of "ominous music which hinted at imminent disaster" in order to prevent coaching from the audience. Since the contestant returned week after week rather than answering all the questions on one broadcast, the audience was given time to contemplate whether he would keep his winnings or go on to the next plateau and also a chance to worry about how difficult the next question might be.

The program became an immediate hit. In September, an estimated 55 million people, over twice as many as had seen the Checkers speech, viewing 84.8% of the television sets in operation at the time, saw Richard S. McCutchen, a 28-year-old marine captain whose category was gourmet foods, become the first grand prize winner.

Most early contestants were seemingly average folks who harbored a hidden expertise in a subject far removed from their workaday lives. Thus McCutchen was asked about *haute cuisine* rather than amphibious assault. This separation was no accident. Its purpose was not only to increase the novelty of the show by providing something odd to the point of being freakish but also to integrate the viewer more intimately into the video melodrama. Everyone who had ever accumulated a store of disconnected, useless information could fantasize about transforming it into a pot of gold.

In a few months, *Question* had created a large new "consumption community," Daniel Boorstin's label for the nonideological, democratic, vague, and rapidly shifting groupings which have characterized twentieth-century American society. Suddenly, a third of the country had a common bond about which total strangers could converse. Paradoxically, in order to belong to this community, the individual had to isolate himself physically from others. Families stayed at home to watch the show, rather than celebrating it in the company of a large crowd. Movie theaters reported a precipitous decline in business, and stores and streets were empty when it came on the air.

Everyone whose life was touched by the show seemed to prosper. In addition to their prize money, some contestants received alluring offers to do public relations work for large companies or to star in movies. *Question's* creator, an independent program packager named Louis Cowan, became president of CBS-TV, an indication of how pleased the network executives were to present so successful a show. Even the banker who brought the sealed questions from the vault

"Intellect on Television: The Quiz Show Scandals of the 1950s" by Richard S. Tedlow, from *American Quarterly* (Fall, 1979) Volume XXVIII No. 4. Published by the American Studies Association. Copyright © 1976. Reprinted by permission of American Quarterly and the author.

found himself promoted to a vice presidency. But the greatest beneficiary was the sponsor.

In March of 1955, the show was purchased by Revlon, which soon began reaping the rewards of well-constructed advertising on a popular television program. Several products quintupled their sales, and advertising for one had to be discontinued because it sold out nationally. George F. Abrams, the company's vice president in charge of advertising, gloated that *Question* ". . . is doing a most fantastic sales job. It certainly is the most amazing sales success in the history of the cosmetics industry. There isn't a single Revlon item that hasn't benefitted. . . ." Net sales for 1955 increased 54% over the previous year, and in 1956 they soared another 66%. When Revlon shares were first offered on the New York Stock Exchange at the end of 1955, the issue's success was "so great it was almost embarrassing."

Question's greatest liability was its own success; it spawned imitators around the world. In the United States, a spate of programs featuring endless variations of gift-giving for answering questions further retarded "TV's already enfeebled yearning to leaven commercialism with culture." Most of these have mercifully been consigned to oblivion, but one rivaled *The $64,000 Question* in the impact it made upon the nation.

The *21* program was developed by another firm of independent program packagers, Barry and Enright, Inc. The format was different, especially in having two contestants compete against each other and no limit on their winnings, but the basic idea was the same. Questions were given point values, and the points were worth money. Once again, the "wiles of a riverboat gambler" were combined with the memory of sundry bits of information which was passed off as intellectual acumen, with the result a spectacularly profitable property.

Barry and Enright leased the show to Pharmaceuticals, Inc., now known as the J. B. Williams Company, and it first appeared on NBC on October 12, 1956. Pharmaceuticals, whose most well-known product was Geritol, soon had good

reason to be pleased with its quiz show. *21* did not attain quite the ratings of *Question*, but it competed successfully against *I Love Lucy*, one of the most popular programs in television history, and attracted much notice. Although its advertising director was reluctant to give complete credit to the program for the increased sales of Geritol, it could hardly have hurt. Sales in 1957 bettered the previous year's mark by one-third.

Unlike *Question*, *21* did not shun the highly educated, and one of its contestants became a symbol to the nation of the profitability of intellectual achievement. Charles Van Doren provided evidence that an intellectual could be handsome, that he could get rich, and that he could be a superstar. Like a football player, the intellectual athlete could win fame and wealth. Van Doren's family could lay genuine claim to membership in an American aristocracy of letters. Descended from seventeenth-century Dutch immigrants, Van Doren's uncle Carl was a literary critic whose 1939 biography of Benjamin Franklin won a Pulitzer Prize. His father Mark won the Prize for poetry the following year, and he was equally famous for his accomplishments in the classroom as a professor of English at Columbia. The wives of the Van Doren brothers were also literary, rounding out a remarkably cultivated quartet. Van Doren's family divided its time between a country estate in Connecticut and a Greenwich Village townhouse where guests over the years included Sinclair Lewis, Mortimer Adler, Joseph Wood Krutch, and Morris Ernst. The family was the symbol of intellectual vitality.

Van Doren established himself on the program by defeating the swarthy, seemingly impoverished previous champion Herbert Stempel on December 5, 1956, after having played three tie matches with Stempel on November 28. It was smooth sailing for the weeks that followed.

On the TV screen [Eric Goldman has written] he appeared lanky, pleasant, smooth in dress and manner but never slick, confident but with an engaging way of understating himself. The long, hard questions would come at him and his eyes would roll up, squeeze shut, his forehead furrow and perspire, his teeth gnaw at his lower lip. Breathing heavily, he seemed to coax information out of some corner of his mind by talking to himself in a kind of stream-of-consciousness. Like a good American, he fought hard, taking advantage of every rule. . . . Like a good American, he won without crowing. And, like a good American, he kept on winning, drowning corporation lawyers or ex-college presidents with equal ease on questions ranging from naming the four islands of the Balearic Islands to explaining the process of photosynthesis to naming the three baseball players who each amassed more than 3,500 hits. Charles Van Doran was "the new All-American boy," the magazines declared, and to millions he was that indeed. . . .

Van Doran's victories on the quiz show brought him greater rewards than had accrued to any of his predecessors. He received thousands of letters from parents and teachers around the world, thanking him for popularizing the life of the mind. Little services such as dry cleaning, which he had had to pay for when supporting himself on his $4,400 yearly salary as an English instructor at Columbia, were now donated *gratis* by star-struck shopkeepers. Several colleges expressed an interest in hiring him away from Columbia, and he found himself referred to in print as "Doctor" despite not yet having earned his Ph.D. And then, of course, there was the money. Van Doren won $129,000 during his 14 weeks on *21*. Soon after he left, he was awarded a $50,000 contract to appear on the *Today* show, where for five minutes each morning he would speak of science, literature, history. "I think I may be the only person," he once remarked, "who ever read 17th century poetry on a network television program—a far cry from the usual diet of mayhem, murder, and rape."

Rumors of improper practices surfaced soon after the quiz shows made their debut. By the

end of 1956, articles were appearing in the trade and general circulation press discussing the "controls" exercised by the producers to keep popular contestants alive and eliminate the unpopular. "Are the quiz shows rigged?" asked *Time* magazine in the spring of 1957, a year in which the networks were investing a small fortune in them. The answer: producers could not "afford to risk collusion with contestants," and yet, because of pretesting, they were able to ask questions which they knew the contestants would or would not know. They could thus manipulate the outcome "far more effectively than most viewers suspect." The report noted, however, that Van Doren "feels certain that no questions were being formfitted to his phenomenal mind."

A number of contestants had been disappointed at their treatment on the shows. The most important of these, and the John Dean of this piece, was the man Van Doran first defeated, Herbert Stempel.

Stempel's motives were very mixed. One was money. He had quickly squandered his winnings and had failed in an attempt to blackmail more out of producer Dan Enright. A more important reason was his bruised ego. Stempel had been forced to portray himself as a poor boy from Brooklyn, when in fact he had married into a well-to-do family and was from Queens. Enright insisted that he wear ratty suits and a cheap wristwatch to project this imagine and that he address the emcee, Jack Barry, deferentially as Mr. Barry while other contestants called him Jack. He had an I.Q. of 170 and was infuriated by having to "miss" answers he knew "damn well." And he was beside himself at the unearned praise accorded to Van Doren. Here was ". . . a guy that had a fancy name, Ivy League education, parents all his life, and I had the opposite. . . ." He would hear passing strangers remark that he was the man who had lost to this child of light, and he could not stand it. But it was more than greed or envy that prompted Stempel to turn state's evidence. Even before he was ordered to "take a dive" and before he had ever heard of Charles Van Doren, he was telling friends that the show was fixed. Stempel knew all the real answers about the quiz shows, and he was bursting to show the nation how smart he was.

In 1957, Stempel tried to interest two New York newspapers in the truth, but both papers refused to print what would have been one of the biggest scoops of the decade because they feared libel action. It is a commentary on the state of investigative journalism at the time that not until August, 1958, after the discovery that a giveaway show called *Dotto* was fixed, was Stempel able to make his charges in public. At this time also, New York County District Attorney Frank Hogan began an investigation, and the inexorable process of revelation had been set in motion. For almost a year, the grand jury interviewed about 150 witnesses. The producers tried to arrange a cover-up by persuading the show's alumni to perjure themselves. Many of the most well known did just that. It was one thing to fix a quiz show, however, and quite another to fix a grand jury probe. Realizing that the day of reckoning was at last approaching, the producers hurried back to change their testimony. This they did without informing the contestants, leaving them, to put it mildly, out on a limb.

For reasons which remain unclear, the judge sealed the grand jury's presentment, but the Subcommittee on Legislative Oversight (over the FCC) of the House Interstate and Foreign Commerce Committee determined to get to the bottom of the matter. Its public hearings, held in Washington in October and November of 1959, attracted worldwide attention.

On October 6, a bitter Herbert Stempel exposed the whole sordid story of *21*. He had originally applied to take part in what he thought was an honest game but was approached by Enright who talked him into becoming an actor rather than a riverboat gambler. Every detail of his performances was prearranged: his wardrobe, his diffidence, his hesitations, and his answers. He was instructed on the proper way to mop his brow for maximum

effect, and he was guaranteed to sweat because the air conditioning in the isolation booth was purposely kept off. From his testimony, it became clear that Van Doren was implicated as well. On the following two days, other contestants, producer Enright, and his assistant Albert Freedman testified to the fix. No one contradicted Stempel.

In the months preceding the hearings Van Doren had consistently and ever more vehemently proclaimed that no matter what others had done, his appearances on *21* had been strictly legitimate. When Stempel's charges were first published in the papers, Van Doren was "... horror struck. . . . I couldn't understand why Stempel should want to proclaim his own involvement." A representative of D.A. Hogan interviewed him toward the end of the year, and he denied everything. He retained a lawyer, to whom he lied about his involvement, and then proceeded to perjure himself before the New York County Grand Jury in January, 1959. He was assured by Enright and Freedman that they too would cover up.

Van Doren's day of reckoning came on November 2, 1959, before the subcommittee. Herb Stempel hurried down from New York City to get a seat from which he could clearly see his former adversary. Pale and jittery, Van Doren walked into the crowded hearing room and delivered himself of one of the most pathetic confessions in the history of American public speech.

He wished that he could erase the past three years but realizing the past may be immutable resolved to learn from it. When he had first contacted Barry and Enright, he had assumed that their programs were honest. Before his appearance on *21*, Albert Freedman summoned him to his apartment and, taking him into the bedroom, explained that Stempel had to be defeated in order to make the show more popular. Van Doren asked to go on the air honestly, but Freedman said he had no chance to defeat the brilliant Stempel. "He also told me that the show was merely entertainment and that giving help to quiz contests was a common practice and merely a part of show business.'' Besides, said Freedman, Van Doren had an opportunity to help increase respect for intellectual life and education. ''I will not,'' said Van Doren, ''bore this committee by describing the intense moral struggle that went on inside me.'' The result of that struggle was history. Freedman coached him on how to answer questions to increase suspense and several times gave him a script to memorize. When Van Doren missed the questions which were slated for the evening, Freedman ''. . . would allow me to look them up myself. A foolish sort of pride made me want to look up the answers when I could, and to learn as much about the subject as possible.''

As time went on the show ballooned beyond my wildest expectations. . . . [F]rom an unknown college instructor I became a celebrity. I received thousands of letters and dozens of requests to make speeches, appear in movies, and so forth—in short, all the trappings of modern publicity. To a certain extent this went to my head.

He realized, however, that he was misrepresenting education and was becoming more nervous about the show. He urged the producers to let him quit, but it was only after they could arrange a sufficiently dramatic situation that he was defeated.

Van Doren's brief testimony was the climax of the subcommittee's investigation as it was of this scandal as a whole. Nevertheless, the hearings continued, including an investigation of *The $64,000 Question. Question* was also fixed, and although the details differed from the *21* case, the deception was no less pervasive.

It is no exaggeration to say that the American public was transfixed by the revelation of quiz show fraud. A Gallup Poll found the highest level of public awareness of the event in the history of such surveys. Questioned about the shows at successive news conferences, President Eisenhower said he shared ''the American general reaction of almost bewilderment'' and compared the manipulations to the Black Sox scandal of 1919. The quiz show episode affords an opportunity to discuss feelings toward Van Doren, the hero unmasked, and also the general arguments which swirled around television at decade's turn.

For Van Doren, humiliation came in the wake of confession. Just as institutions had been happy to associate themselves with quiz show geniuses, they hurried to dissociate themselves when the geniuses turned out to be hustlers. NBC fired Van Doren, while Columbia ''accepted his resignation.'' The actions of these two institutions were scrutinized along with those of Van Doren in the period following his confession.

From the first, both NBC and CBS had maintained the highly implausible stand that they were fooled about the shows along with the public. They unquestionably could have uncovered the rigging had they really wanted to, and in the end they were left holding the bag. They had lost millions of dollars and, what was worse, had suffered what at the time loomed as a potentially mortal blow to a very pleasant way of making a lot of money. The popular uproar threatened to force government to restrict the broadcasting prerogatives of management. In this state of affairs, Van Doren had to go. CBS took the next step eliminating quiz shows altogether, from which NBC refrained.

Few were surprised by NBC's stand. The network was, after all, a business, and Van Doren had become a liability. Columbia's treatment of him aroused different issues. Some students had no patience with him, but hundreds rallied to his defense with petitions and demonstrations. They pointed out that his teaching was excellent and that having made public relations capital out of his victories, Columbia would be craven to desert him now. The Columbia College dean, however, maintained, ''The issue is the moral one of the honesty and integrity of teaching.''

The dean found Van Doren's deceptions contrary to the principles a teacher should have and should try to instill in his students.

The academic community holds in especial contempt, as *Love Story* author Eric Segal was to discover, those "willing to play the fool" for limitless publicity. In defense of Columbia's action, political scientist Hans J. Morgenthau published two essays purporting to show that Van Doren had actually violated "the moral law" as handed down from Moses, Plato, Buddha, and other worthies. Apparently no such law would have been violated had Van Doren's participation in what thinking people very well knew was a cheap stunt been unrigged. If any crime had been committed in the quiz show episode, it was surely the broad conspiracy to portray as genuine intellectual activity the spouting of trivia. But while the shows were on and winning high ratings, there was neither from Morgenthau nor Columbia a peep of protest.

The most devastating but also perhaps the fairest indictment of Van Doren's role was penned by a Columbia colleague, Lawrence S. Hall, who demonstrated that Van Doren's confession had been as thoroughly fraudulent as his conduct on *21*. He had not confessed because of a letter from a fan of his on the *Today* show as he had claimed but only because of a congressional subpoena. "To the very end he never did perform the ethical free act of making up his mind. . . . Van Doren did not *decide* to tell the truth; what he did was adapt himself to the finally inescapable necessity of telling it." Worst of all, asserted Hall, was his "concealing under [the] piously reflexive formulas" of his silken prose "the most maudlin and promiscuous ethical whoredom the soap opera public has yet witnessed."

Unlike Hall the average American seemed rather sympathetic. A Sindlinger poll asked respondents to rate those most blameworthy for the fixes. Asked to assess the responsibility of network, sponsor, producer, and Van Doren, only 18.6% blamed Van Doren the most while 38.9% blamed him the least. A substantial number even favored a continuation of the shows rigged or not. Many man-in-the-street interviewees said they would have done no differently, and most newspaper editorials treated him extraordinarily gently.

Investigators discovered not a single contestant on *21*, and only one on *The $64,000 Question*, who refused to accept money once they learned the shows were fixed. Most were quite "blithe" about it. Pollsters at the end of the 1950s were finding the belief widespread that the individual did not feel it was his place to condemn. Moral relativism, it seemed, rather than adherence to Professor Morgenthau's moral absolutism, was the rule. So many people lived polite lies that though it may have been titillating to discover them, they were hardly worth preaching about.

Other factors, in addition to this general willingness to partake in a fraud such as the quiz shows, help explain why the outrage was muted and transient. First, as Boorstin has pointed out, television unites many people in a community, but their union is tenuous and easily forgotten. Secondly, although many were taken in by the seeming reality of the shows, they had believed and been disabused so many times in the past that the shock soon wore off. For underneath the belief in the shows there probably lingered skepticism. Robert Merton observed in 1946 that cynicism about public statements from any source, political or commerical, was pervasive. Television was a new medium which some may have thought was simply too big to play by the rules of the oldtime newspaper patent medicine advertiser. The quiz shows taught them that it was not, and some critics asserted that it was the naked selfishness of commercial radio and television, more than the machinations of particular producers or contestants, that was truly to blame. The quiz shows excited to a new pitch of intensity long-running arguments about commercial broadcasting and the public interest.

The growth of commercial broadcasting cannot be explored here at length, but suffice it to say that it was opposed every step of the way by intellectuals, educators, and journalists who deplored what they saw as the perversion of a medium of great potential for the sake of the desire of private business to push products. As early as the 1920s, when radio was first coming into its own, articulate voices spoke up against its use for advertising. Bruce Bliven thought such "outrageous rubbish" should be banned from the air, and at least one congressman considered introducing legislation to that end. Herbert Hoover, whose Commerce Department supervised the granting of broadcast licenses, felt that radio would die if it allowed itself to be "drowned in advertising chatter," but he favored self-regulation rather than government action. The Radio Act of 1927 demanded that licensees operated their stations not solely for profit but with due regard for the "public interest, convenience, and necessity."

As charted by broadcasting's foremost historian, Erik Barnouw, the ascendancy of commercial programming was established in a fit of absence of mind. "If such a system [as exists today] had been outlined in 1927 or 1934, when our basic broadcasting laws were written," he concluded, "it certainly would have been rejected." Critics believed that the quiz shows and the radio "payola" scandals that followed that broadcasting was too important to be left in the hands of those whose primary, if not sole, motive was to turn a profit for the stockholders.

Television executives insisted that the scandals were the exception in a generally well run industry, but critics thought they were the tip of the iceberg. In themselves, the scandals were relatively unimportant, held the *New Republic*. "A real investigation would center on the simple question: why is television so bad, so monstrous?" It was the thirst for profit which forced the industry to a state of thralldom to the ratings. It was profit which mandated such dreadful children's programming. Advertising agencies and their clients, with profit always uppermost in mind, forced absurd restrictions on what could

be broadcast. When commentators complained about the astounding amount of violence on the tube, defenders warned of the danger of censorship. Critics replied that the most stultifying censorship was already being exercised in behalf of the manufacturers of the pointless nostrums of an overindulgent society. In its quest for ratings, television seemed consistently to avoid satisfying the intelligent minority.

The industry had now been caught red-handed, Walter Lippmann wrote, in ". . . an enormous conspiracy to deceive the public in order to sell profitable advertising to the sponsors." The situation which had made this shameful occurrence possible could not be allowed to survive intact. Television had "to live up to a higher, but less profitable, standard." What America needed was prime time TV produced "not because it yields private profits but because it moves toward truth and excellence." What was needed, said Lippmann, was public service television.

Industry spokesmen had traditionally defended themselves as true democrats. The president of CBS, Frank Stanton, soon after *The $64,000 Question* was first aired, declared, "A program in which a large part of the audience is interested is by that very fact . . . in the public interest." By such a standard, the quiz shows can be seen not as "cynical malpractices . . . in one corner of television," as Robert Sarnoff tried to represent them, but rather as the perfect expression of the industry.

Sarnoff recognized the charges being hurled at TV in 1959 and 1960 as the "long-familiar [ones] of mediocrity, imbalance, violence, and overcommercialism." These charges had been unjustified in the past and were unjustified in 1960, but because ". . . those who press them are now armed with the cudgels represented by the quiz-show deceptions" they could not be sloughed off. Sarnoff's response was to promise careful scrutiny of such programs in the future and vigorous self-regulation. As a special bonus to the viewing public in a gesture to wipe the slate clean, he offered to donate time for a series of debates between the major Presidential candi-

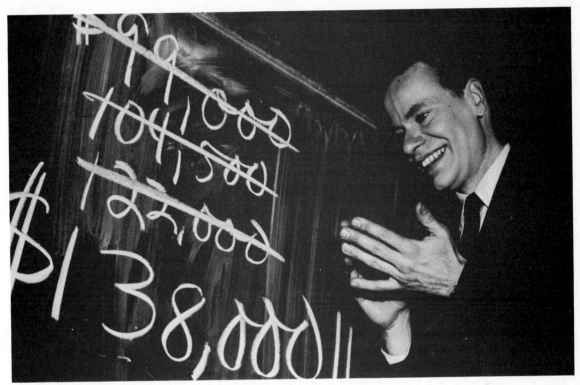

■ ■ *Charles Van Doren, winner of $129,000 in a rigged TV quiz show, pleaded guilty to perjury in his testimony to the New York County Grand Jury and received a suspended sentence in 1962.*

dates of 1960, which eventually resulted in the televised confrontations between Kennedy and Nixon.

Sarnoff's offer was enthusiastically welcomed by such politicians as Steward Udall, who had been working for a suspension of equal time regulations in order to permit broadcast debates between Democratic and Republican Presidential nominees in the upcoming election. Paradoxically, the four "Great Debates" which ensued showed unmistakably the influence of the supposedly discredited quiz programs. The similarity in formats was obvious, As in *21*, two adversaries faced each other and tried to give point-scoring answers to questions fired at them under the glare of klieg lights. The debates bore as little relationship to the real work of the presidency as the quiz shows did to intellectuality. Boorstin has remarked on how successful they

were ". . . in reducing great national issues to trivial dimensions. With appropriate vulgarity, they might have been called the $400,000 Question (Prize: a $100,000-a-year job for four years)." No President would act on any question put to him by the reporters without sustained and sober consultation with trusted advisors. But the American people, conditioned by five years of isolation booth virtuosity, expected the "right" answer to be delivered pithily and with little hesitation. They did not want to be told that some questions did not have simple answers— or any answers at all.

The technological advances which led to radio and television grew out of the tinkerings of amateur experimenters. These two new forms of mass communication, with unprecedented drama and immediacy, developed independently of the desire to say anything. In 1854, Henry David

Thoreau wrote, "We are in great haste to construct a magnetic telegraph from Maine to Texas; but Maine and Texas, it may be, have nothing important to communicate." This observation has been yet more relevant during the last half century. Except for the military, which was always seeking more direct means for locating ships at sea and soldiers on the battlefield, no one knew what to broadcast and telecast. The federal government, dominated by the ideology of free enterprise, declined to fill this void. To be sure, regulations did prohibit certain messages over the air, but there has never been a national statement on the positive purposes of the new media which the industry was obliged to take seriously.

Businessmen soon discovered that broadcasting was a powerful instrument for increasing sales. Those advertisers who had financed the print media, including manufacturers of patent medicines, cosmetics, and cigarettes, quickly adopted the same role with radio and television. Left to their own devices, they sought programs which would constitute a congenial frame for their selling message. They soon hit upon the idea, among others, of parlor games, of which the quiz shows were direct descendants.

Such programs had been popular since the thirties, but in the 1950s, clever producers learned how to make them even more so. They combined large sums of money with the American fondness for facts, dressed up as intellectuality, and the result was *The $64,000 Question* and *21*. When these programs were exposed as frauds, a jaded public, inured to mendacity, was quick to forgive.

Critics have often complained, as they did with vigor after the scandals, that television—"a medium of such great potential"—was being so ill-used. But no one seems to have a clear vision of what that potential is. The lack of direction which characterized the early years of American broadcasting has never been overcome. Commentators such as Lippmann have won their public broadcasting system, but commercial television has not upgraded its fare in order to compete. If anything, public TV may act as a lightning rod deflecting complaints about the commercial industry by providing an outlet for those demanding alternative viewing.

For its part, the industry has usually ignored what enlightened guidance has been available in favor of traditional forms of entertainment guaranteed not to distract the viewer from the advertisements. Thus, recently, quiz and game shows have made a comeback. There has even been talk of resurrecting *The $64,000 Question*, despite the risk of reviving along with it memories of past chicanery. Such programming represents a distressing devotion to Philistinism and a failure of imagination, the solution for which is not in sight.

■ ■ ■

STUDY QUESTIONS

1. What is implied by the concept of a "consumption community"? How is this sort of a community different from any other community?

2. Compare how Charles Van Doren and Herbert Stempel were presented on the television quiz show *21*. Why was Stempel told to appear poor and deferential on the show? Is there a political statement in the images of both men?

3. How did most Americans respond to the disclosure that *21* and other quiz shows were rigged?

4. What does Tedlow mean by the concept of "moral relativism"? Is morality ever absolute?

5. What issues are involved in the debate between advocates of commercial broadcasting and proponents of public service broadcasting?

6. How were the Nixon-Kennedy television debates in 1960 similar to or different from the format of the television quiz show *21*? What does this say about the importance of television in a political campaign?

BIBLIOGRAPHY

The television industry has received far less historical attention than the film industry. This is perplexing, considering that television "touches" more people—American as well as non-American—than the movies. The fact that some movie directors have consciously cultivated reputations as "artists" undoubtedly has something to do with academic interest in their product that is not apparent with television. There are, however, several very good books on television. Among the best are Erik Barnauw, *The Golden Web* (1968), and *The Image Empire: A History of Broadcasting in the United States* (1970); Raymond Williams, *Television: Technology and Cultural Form* (1975); and Robert Sklare, *Prime-Time America: Life on and Behind the Television Screen* (1980). Also of interest are two books by Daniel Boorstin, *The Americans: The Democratic Experience* (1974), and *The Image: A Guide to Pseudo-Events in America* (1961).

The Van Doren case is dealt with in Kent Anderson, *Television Fraud* (1978), and Eric Goldman, *The Crucial Decade and After: America, 1945–1960* (1960). Douglas Miller and Marian Novak discuss social and cultural developments in the 1950s in *The Fifties: The Way We Really Were* (1977).

THE AGE OF CONSPIRACY AND CONFORMITY: INVASION OF THE BODY SNATCHERS

Stuart Samuels

During the late 1940s and early 1950s several investigations by the House Un-American Activities Committee (HUAC) focused on the subversive nature of Hollywood films. Walt Disney told HUAC that screenwriters had tried to make Mickey Mouse follow the Communist Party line, and Committee members criticized such openly pro-Soviet films as Warner Brothers' *Mission to Moscow* (1943) and MGM's *Song of Russia* (1943). Given the anticommunist mood of the period, it was clear that heads would have to roll. And roll they did. In 1947 a group of filmmakers, the Hollywood Ten, challenged HUAC's authority to pry into their personal and political beliefs. As a result, the members of the Hollywood Ten found themselves on a blacklist and for more than a decade the heads of the major studios refused to hire them. In 1951 HUAC resumed their investigation of Hollywood. Many producers, screenwriters, actors, and directors were called before the Committee. About one-third cooperated with HUAC. The two-thirds that refused to cooperate were black-listed.

This disruption of the Hollywood community spilled over into the films made during the period. Most studios, eager to publicize their anticommunist credentials, turned out violently anticommunist films. The result was such movies as *My Son John* (1952) and *I Was a Communist for the FBI* (1951). Other films reflected the political and cultural mood of the country in a less overt manner. In the following essay, Stuart Samuels demonstrates that *Invasion of the Body Snatchers* (1956) is far more than a class "B" science-fiction film. Rather, it is a film that exemplifies the fear and anxieties of the 1950s.

In what way can a seemingly absurd science fiction/horror film, *Invasion of the Body Snatchers*, give us insight into the history and culture of America in the mid-1950s? How is a film about people being taken over by giant seed pods "reflective" of this critical period in our history?

Films relate to ideological positions in two ways. First, they *reflect*, embody, reveal, mirror, symbolize existing ideologies by reproducing (consciously or unconsciously) the myths, ideas, concepts, beliefs, images of an historical period in both the film content and film form (technique). Secondly, films *produce* their own ideology, their own unique expression of reality. Films can do this by reinforcing a specific ideology or undercutting it.

All films are therefore ideological and political insomuch as they are determined by the ideology which produces them. Fictional characters are only prototypes of social roles and social attitudes; every film speaks to some norm. Some behaviors are deemed appropriate, others not. Some acts are condemned, others applauded. Certain characters are depicted as heroic, others as cowardly. Film is one of the products, one of the languages, through which the world communicates itself to itself. Films embody beliefs, not by a mystic communion with the national soul, but because they contain the values, fears, myths, assumptions, point of view of the culture in which they are produced.

While films relate to ideology, they also relate to specific historical and social events, most obviously when the content of a film deals directly with a subject that is identifiable in its own period. In the 1950s, for example, such films as *I Was a Communist for the FBI* (1951) and *My Son John* (1952) spoke to a society increasingly concerned with the nature of the internal communist threat. Similarly, in the previous

decade such films as *The Best Years of Our Lives* (1946) attempted to analyze some of the problems and confusions of the immediate post-World War II period and *The Snake Pit* (1948) addressed a society trying to deal with the tremendous increase in the hospital treatment of the mentally ill. As far back as Griffith's *Intolerance* (1916), which relayed a pacifist message to a nation struggling to stay out of war, films have reflected society's attempts to come to grips with contemporary problems.

Film "reflects" an agreed-upon perception of social reality, acceptable and appropriate to the society in question. Thus, in the 1950s when a conspiracy theory of politics was a widely accepted way of explaining behavior (being duped), action (being subversive), and effect (conspiracy), one would expect the films of the period to "reflect" this preoccupation with conspiracy. But *Invasion of the Body Snatchers* is not *about* McCarthyism. It is about giant seed pods taking over people's bodies. Indirectly, however, it is a *statement about* the collective paranoia and the issue of conformity widely discussed in the period.

The idea for the film came from Walter Wanger, the producer, who had read Jack Finney's novel of the same name in serial form in *Collier's Magazines* in 1955. Wanger suggested the project to his friend Don Siegel, who in turn assigned Daniel Manwaring to produce a screenplay from Finney's book.

The story of the film is contained within a "framing" device—a seemingly insane man, Miles Bennell (Kevin McCarthy), telling a bizarre story to a doctor and a policeman. In flashback we see Bennell's tale—of giant seed pods taking over the minds and bodies of the people of Santa Mira, a small town in California, where Bennell was the local doctor. Returning home after a medical convention, Miles finds the pretty little town and its peaceful inhabitants in the grip of a "mass hysteria." People seem obsessed by the conviction that relatives and friends are not really themselves, that they have been changed. Despite the outward calm of San-

"The Age of Conspiracy and Conformity: Invasion of the Body Snatchers" from *American History/American Film: Interpreting the Hollywood Image* by Stuart Samuels. Copyright © 1979 by Frederick Ungar Publishing Co., Inc. Reprinted by permission.

ta Mira, there is a creeping contagion of fear and paranoia, of wives not knowing their husbands, children fleeing from their parents.

Miles's friend Becky (Dana Wyntner) struggles against this delusion, tends to dismiss it as improbable, but nevertheless finds her own Uncle Ira slightly changed: "There's no emotion in him. None. Just the pretense of it." The improbable becomes real when Miles's friend Jack calls him to report something fantastic: a semihuman body, without features, has been found on Jack's billiard table. From this point on events move rapidly. The unformed body is clearly growing into an exact duplicate of Jack, and in the greenhouse Miles stumbles upon giant seed pods, each containing a half-formed body. In Becky's basement Miles finds still another embryonic shape—this time a model of Becky herself. Now Miles believes the fantastic stories, and determines to escape and warn the world of this danger.

But escape is not simple. The town of Santa Mira has nearly been taken over by the pods, who while the inhabitants sleep form themselves into precise replicas of human beings—even-tempered, peaceful, but soulless automatons. Miles is terrified and drags Becky from her bedroom, to flee in his auto. But the town has now mobilized against them; the pod-people cannot allow the story to be told, and the "people" of Santa Mira organize to catch Miles and Becky. In a desperate escape attempt, they flee over the mountains, pursued by those who had once been friends and neighbors.

The horror mounts when, in a tunnel, Becky succumbs to the pods. She falls asleep and soon her mind and body are taken over, cell by cell. In a moment of utmost panic, Miles looks into her eyes and realizes the awful truth. Continuing on alone, he comes to a highway where he makes wild attempts to flag down motorists who are terrified by his insane behavior. Eventually, he is picked up by the police, who naturally consider him mad, and taken to a hospital for medical examination. The doctors agree that he is psychotic, but then fate intervenes. An intern reports an accident to a truck from Santa Mira, and in a casual aside, he tells how the driver of the wreck had to be dug out from under a pile of strange giant seed pods. The truth dawns on the police inspector, who orders the roads to Santa Mira closed, and in the final shot tells his assistant to "call the FBI."

The political, social, and intellectual atmosphere of the era that created *Invasion* must be understood in light of several preoccupations: the "Red Menace," which crystallized around the activities of Senator Joseph McCarthy and the somewhat less spectacular blacklisting of figures in the communications and entertainment industry, who were seen as a nefarious, subversive element undermining the entire fabric of American society; learning to cope with the consequences of a modern, urban, technologically bureaucratized society; and the pervasive fear of atomic annihilation. All these factors undermined the traditional American myth of individual action. The experience of the Depression, the rise and threat of totalitarianism, the loss of American insularity, the growth of technocracy all in one form or another challenged the integrity of the individual. It is therefore not surprising to note that film genres like science fiction or horror films proliferated in the 1950s. The central themes of these films show a preoccupation with depersonalization and dehumanization. Moreover, as Susan Sontag has suggested, it is by no means coincidental that at a time when the moviegoing public had over ten years been living under the constant threat of instant atomic annihilation films of the 1950s should be concerned with the confrontation of death. As Sontag expressed it: "We live[d] under continued threat of two equally fearful, but seemingly opposed destinies: unremitting banality and inconceivable terror." On the surface there existed a complacency that disguised a deep fear of violence, but conformity silenced the cries of pain and feelings of fear.

In response to the threats of social banality and universal annihilation, three concepts dominated the decade: (1) conformity, (2) paranoia,

(3) alienation. Each concept had its keywords. *Conformity:* "silent generation," "status seekers," "lonely crowds," "organization men," "end of ideology," "hidden persuaders." *Paranoia:* "red decade," "dupes," "front organization," "blacklisting," "un-Americanism," "fifth column," "fellow travelers," "pinkos." *Alienation:* "outsiders," "beats," "loners," "inner-directed men," "rebels." For the most part, the decade celebrated a suburbanized, bureaucratized, complacent, secure, conformist, consensus society in opposition to an alienated, disturbed, chaotic, insecure, individualistic, rebel society. Each of those three concepts dominating the 1950s finds obvious expression in *Invasion of the Body Snatchers.* First—conformity.

During the 1950s a concern for respectability, a need for security and compliance with the system became necessary prerequisites for participation in the reward structure of an increasingly affluent society. Conformism had replaced individuality as the principal ingredient for success. This standard extended to all aspects of life. Tract-built, identical, tidy little boxlike ranch houses on uniform fifty-foot plots bulldozed to complete flatness were the rage. Conformity dictated city planning in the form of Levittowns, the same way it silenced political dissidents in Congress. Creativity meant do-it-yourself painting-by-numbers. One created great artistic masterpieces by following directions.

The concern with conformity grew out of a need to escape from confusion, fear, worry, tension, and a growing sense of insecurity. It was accentuated by a sense of rootlessness and increased mobility. Consensus mentality offered a refuge in an anxious and confusing world. It represented an attempt to shift the burden of individual responsibility for one's fate to an impersonal monolithic whole. Excessive conformity, as in the 1950s, was a salve to smooth over obvious conflict and turmoil. A country that emerged from war victorious around the globe feared internal subversion at home; a society powered by a new technology and a new structure (corporate bureaucracy) feared a loss of personal identity. In the White House was a person whose great appeal was that he represented a politics of consensus, classlessness, and conformism—Eisenhower.

By the time *Invasion* was released (May, 1956) the intensity of the drive for consensus politics had diminished—the Korean War had ended, McCarthy had been censored, Stalin was dead, the spirit of Geneva had thawed the Cold War, the imminent threat of atomic annihilation had subsided, witch hunting had lost its appeal, and the threat of internal subversion had lessened. But the context of fear was still active. The political reality might not seem as frightening, but the mind-set of the period was always ready at any moment to raise its repressive head. To many people, the fact that the enemy appeared less threatening only meant that he was better at concealing his subversion and that the eternal vigilance of good Americans had to be even more effective.

David Riesman's *The Lonely Crowd* (1955) spoke of a society obsessed by conformity. His now-famous formulation about inner-directed and other-directed men, focuses on the same conflicts outlined by Siegel in *Invasion.* Miles Bennell is "inner directed"—a self-reliant individualist who has internalized adult authority, and judged himself and others by these internalized self-disciplined standards of behavior. The "pods" are "other-directed" beings whose behavior is completely conditioned by the example of their peers. While inner-directed individuals like Miles felt concern and guilt about violating their inner ideals—in fact, were driven by them—the other-directed pods had no inner ideals to violate. Their morality came from the compulsion to be in harmony with the crowd. Their guilt developed in direct proportion to how far they deviated from group consensus. The other-directed pods were uncritical conformists. It was no coincidence that the most popular adult drug of the 1950s was not alcohol or aspirin, pot or cocaine—but Miltown and Thorazine—tranquilizers.

The second basic concept in 1950s America,

the natural corollary to the drive toward confor- mity, was the notion of conspiracy. Conformity is based on the idea that there is a clear-cut divi- sion between *them* and *us*. In periods of overt conflict, like wars or economic crises, the divi- sion between the good and the bad is obvious. But in periods of confusion, the identification of enemies becomes more problematic. Covert expressions of subversion are more common than overt challenges; the enemy attacks— whether real or imagined—through subversion and conspiracy rather than war. In the 1950s subversion seemed to be everywhere. Appear- ances were deceptive; to many, nothing was what it appeared to be. Schools named after American heroes like Jefferson, Lincoln, Walt Whitman, Henry George were rumored to be fronts for communists, calls for free speech were seen as pleas for communism, and racial unrest as being formented by party activists. To many, taking the Fifth Amendment in order not to incriminate oneself was just another way of dis- guising one's political treason.

Threats to social order in the 1950s were not so much associated with personal violence as with an indefinable, insidious, fiendishly cold undermining of the normal. Conspiracy theories feed off the idea of the normal being deceptive. In *Invasion*, the pods, the alien invaders, take on the appearance of normal people. It becomes physically impossible to tell the difference between the aliens and the normals. In *Invasion* all forms of normalcy are inverted. Friends are not friends, "Uncle Ira" is not Uncle Ira, the police do not protect, sleep is not revivifying, telephones are no longer a way of calling for help but a device to tell the pod-people where the remaining non-pod-people are. Even the name of the town is paradoxical. Mira in Spanish means "to look," but the people of San- ta Mira refuse to look; they stare blankly into the unknown. A patina of normalcy hides a deep- seated violence. A man holds a giant seed pod and calmly asks his wife, "Shall I put this in with the baby?" "Yes," she replies, "then there'll be no more crying." In another scene, what appears

to be a quiet Sunday morning gathering in the town square turns out to be a collection point where fleets of trucks filled with pods quietly dis- pense these "vegetables" to people who carry them to their cars and buses, ready to spread the invasion to neighboring towns. It is during a typ- ical home barbeque among friends that Miles finds the pods in his greenhouse.

At the end of the film, when all avenues of help seemed closed, Miles and Becky, hiding in an abandoned cave, hear sweet, loving music— a Brahms lullaby. Miles decides that such beauty and feeling could not possibly be the singing of unemotional pods. He scrambles off to find out where this music is coming from—only to dis- cover that its source is a radio in a large truck being loaded by robotlike people with seed pods destined for far-off towns. The familiar is fraught with danger. It is no wonder that Miles comes to the edge of madness, no wonder that he treats people with a paranoid suspicion. Paranoia becomes the logical alternative to podlike con- formism.

Finally, conformism and conspiracy signaled a new age of personal alienation. From the very beginning of our history, one of the most persis- tent myths about American society has been the myth of natural harmony. The idea is derived from the notion made popular by Adam Smith and John Locke that there is a *natural* and har- monious relationship between the desires of individuals and the demands of social necessity, that individuals who act out of self-interest will automatically move the society as a whole in the direction of natural perfection. At the heart of this notion was the belief that nothing in the sys- tem prevented people from achieving their own individual goals, and that the traditional barriers of class, religion, and geography were absent in the American experience. The concept of natural harmony is further based on the belief of abun- dance. Individual failure had to be due to per- sonal shortcomings because a society of abun- dance offered opportunity to anyone capable of grasping it—conflict was not built into the sys- tem. People were basically good. Solutions were always within grasp. Control was inevitable. Progess was assured.

This underlying belief in natural harmony was one of the casualties of the post-1945 world. In the 1930s American films had portrayed people ordering their environment. "The people," the Mr. Smiths, the Mr. Deeds, the Shirley Temples, and the Andy Hardys saw to it that control and harmony were restored. Individual "good acts" reinforced "social good" in the desire to control life. In the 1940s the theme of conquest, control, and restoration of the natural was the underlining statement of war films. Commitments to courage, self-sacrifice, and heroism were shown instead of Senate filibusters, talks with Judge Hardy, or faith in "the people." Depictions of failure, helplessness, and feelings of inadequacy were introduced as muted themes in the postwar films. Although we had won the war, conquered the Depression, and tamed nature by splitting the atom, things seemed out of control in the 1950s as conflict emerged between the desire for personal autonomy and the pressures for collective conformity. Individual acts of heroism were suspect. Group work and group think were the ideals. Success was measured by how much individuals submerged themselves into some larger mass (society, bureaucracy) over which they had little individual control. The rewards of status, popularity, and acceptance came with conformity to the group. In the films of the period, people who did not sacrifice individual desires for general social needs were fated to die, commit suicide, be outcast, or simply go mad.

Popular books like Riesman's *The Lonely Crowd*, William Whyte's *The Organization Man*, and Vance Packard's *The Status Seekers* showed how the traditional model of the hard working, rugged individualist was being rejected for a world of the group—big universities, big suburbs, big business, and big media. Such harmony as existed resulted from the artificial ordering to an agreed upon surface norm. After the scarcity of the Depression came the affluence of the 1950s—complete with its never-ending routine

of conspicious consumption. Out of the victory for democracy and freedom came a society more standardized, less free, more conformist, and less personal. Out of splitting the atom came the threat of instant annihilation.

The mid-1950s films portrayed people trying desperately to ward off failure in the face of overwhelming destructive forces of nature (horror films), technology (science fiction films), and human imperfection *(film noir)*. There were films about people being taken over or reincarnated: *The Search for Bridie Murphy* (1956), *I've Lived Before* (1956), *Back from the Dead* (1957), *The Undead* (1957), *Vertigo* (1956), *Donovan's Brain* (1953); about individuals in conflict with their societies: *High Noon* (1952), *The Phenix City Story* (1955), *No Place to Hide* (1956), *Not on this Earth* (1957); about superior forces beyond man's control: *Them* (1954), *Tarantula* (1956), *The Beast from 20,000 Fathoms* (1953), *This Island Earth* (1955), *Earth versus the Flying Saucers* (1956); about the apocalypse: *20,000 Leagues Under the Sea* (1954), *On the Beach* (1959), *The Thing* (1951). In these films, the world seemed menacing, fluid, chaotic, impersonal, composed of forces which one seldom understood, and certainly never controlled. Fear is centered on the unknown, unseen terrors that lurk beneath the surface normality.

Invasion's podism is depicted as a malignant evil, as a state of mind where there is no feeling, no free will, no moral choice, no anger, no tears, no passion, no emotion. Human sensibility is dead. The only instinct left is the instinct to survive. Podism meant being "reborn into an untroubled world, where everyone's the same." "There is no need for love or emotion. Love, ambition, desire, faith—without them, life is so simple." A metaphor for communism? Perhaps! But, more directly, podism spoke to a society becoming more massified, more technological, more standardized.

The motto of the pods was "no more love, no more beauty, no more pain." Emotionless, impersonal, regimented, they became technological monsters. But they were not the irrational creatures of blood lust and power—they were just nonhuman. They became tranquil and obedient. They spoke to the fear of the 1950s—not the fear of violence, but the fear of losing one's humanity. As Susan Sontag argued, "the dark secret behind human nature used to be the upsurge of the animal—as in *King Kong* (1933). The threat to man, his availability to dehumanization, lay in his own animality. Now the danger is understood to reside in man's ability to be turned into a machine." The body is preserved, but the person is entirely reconstituted as the automated replica of an "alien" power.

The attraction of becoming a pod in the 1950s was all too real. But although dangling the carrot of conformity, *Invasion* opts ultimately for the stick of painful individuality. The possibility of moral uncertainty was the price we must pay for continued freedom. As Miles says: "Only when we have to fight to stay human do we realize how precious our humanity is." Podism, an existence without pain or fear or emotion, is seen as no existence at all. The fear of man becoming a machinelike organism, losing his humanity, was centered around the ambiguous dual legacy of an increasingly technological civilization. The atomic bomb was both a testament to man's increased control over his universe and a clear symbol of man's fallibility. *Invasion* mirrors this duality. It praises the possibility of a society without pain, yet it raises the spectre of a society without feeling. Security at what price?—the price of freedom and individualism. The rise of technology at what costs?—the cost of humanness itself. Although *Invasion* is ambiguous on this issue, demonstrating the positive effects of "podism" at the same time as condemning its consequences, this confusion, this ambiguity, is very much at the heart of the American cultural issues of the period—the internal conflict between the urge for conformity and the painful need for individuality, between an antiheroic loner and an institutionalized, bureaucratized system of mindless automated pods.

In his struggle to remain his own master, Miles fights against control by first falling back on the traditional notions inherited from the past. He appeals to friends—only to be betrayed. He appeals to the law—only to be pursued by it. He appeals to the system—only to be trapped by it. He appeals to love—only to be disappointed by losing it. All betray him. All become his enemy. Not because they are corrupt, or evil, but because they have become pods, because they have given up their individuality, their ability to choose.

If there is a 1950 vision of historical reality in *Invasion*, there is also a system of film technique designed to reinforce this vision. The language and technique of *Invasion* come out of the social reality of the period and speak directly to that context.

One of the major themes of life in the 1950s was the feeling of constraint—people feeling enclosed within boundaries. People were cut off from options, limited in their choices. There was a closing down of dissent, a shrinking of personal freedom. Silence became the acceptable response to oppression.

Invasion is a film about constraints. It is the story of a man whose ability to make sense of the world decreases and diminishes to the point of madness and frenzy. The film's action takes place within enclosed physical spaces and the physical spaces in the film induce a sense of isolation and constraint. The sleepy California town of Santa Mira is surrounded by hills. When Miles tries to escape he must run up a series of ladderlike stairs to flee the pod-people and reach the open highway that separates the town from the outside world. Miles and Becky are constantly running—in and out of small rooms, darkened cellars illuminated only by matches, large but empty nightclubs, miniature greenhouses, closets, low-ceilinged dens, abandoned caves. The giant seed pods are found in basements, closets, car trunks, greenhouses. The main actors are claustrophobically framed by doorways and windows photographed from low angles, and spend much of their time running down and up endless stairs, into locked doors, and beneath towering trees. The narrative structure of *Invasion* resembles a series of self-contained Chinese boxes and is designed to tighten the tension of

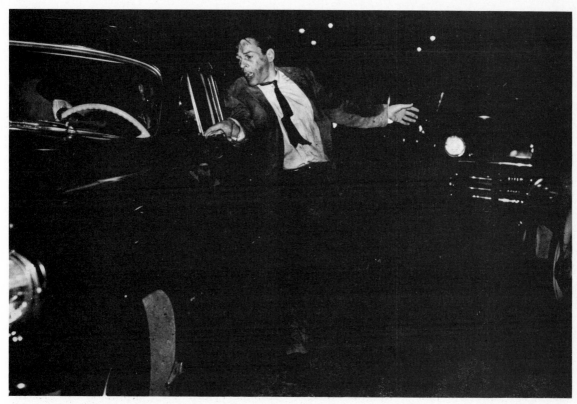

■ ■ *Still photo from the film* Invasion of the Body Snatchers. *This movie was made in 1956, a time when Hollywood began taking a look at the push for conformity and the collective paranoia about conspiracies that characterized the era.*

the story at every step. Though Miles returns from his convention on a sunny morning and the film ends in a confused mixture of daylight and darkness, the main section of the film takes place in darkness—at night.

The whole film is enclosed within a framing device of prologue and epilogue. Siegel's original version had not included this frame, but the addition of a prologue and epilogue, making the film narrative appear as an extended flashback, has the unintended effect of constricting the narrative—itself contained in a rigidly enclosed time frame—even further. Within this framing device, Siegel also uses the technique of repeating a situation at the end of the film that mirrors a sequence presented at the beginning. In the final flashback episode, Siegel has Miles running in panic down the road and being pursued by a

whole town of pod-people. This scene mirrors the opening scene when we see little Jimmy Grimaldi running down the road being pursued by his "podized" mother.

The effect of these devices is to keep the narrative tight in order to heighten tension and suspense. The use of flashback, prologue and epilogue, repeated scenes, interplay of lightness and darkness, all keep the narrative constrained within a carefully defined filmic space. The unbelievable tension is released only in the epilogue, when Miles finally finds someone who believes his story. The ending is not about the FBI's ability to counteract the threat of the pods but about the fact that Miles has finally made contact with another human—and that he is not alone. The film is more about being an alien, an outsider, an individualist, than about the "invasion" by aliens. When Dr. Bassett and his staff finally believe Miles's story, the enclosing ring of constraint is broken, and Miles collapses, relaxing for the first time in the film, knowing that at least he has been saved from a horror worse than death—the loss of identity. The final line—"Call the F.B.I."—is the signal that he is not alone and acts as an affirmative answer to the shout heard at the opening of the film—"I'm not insane." Up to the point when the doctor finally believes Miles's story, the film is actually about a man going insane.

Time is also a constant constraint on humanity, and Siegel emphasizes the fact that time is running out for Miles. The whole film is not only a race against madness, but also against time—of time slipping away. Time in *Invasion* is circumscribed by the fact that sleep is a danger. Miles needs to escape Santa Mira before he falls asleep. He takes pills, splashes his and Becky's face in a constant battle to stay awake. Sleep is not comfort and safety but the instrument of death.

Siegel uses a whole arsenal of filmic techniques to reinforce the feelings of enclosure, isolation, and time running out. His shot set-ups focus on isolated action. People are photographed in isolation standing beneath street lamps, in doorways, alone at crowded railway stations. A background of black velvet darkness and a direct artificial light are used to highlight objects which in isolation take on an "evil clarity." In the film, objects are always illuminated, people's faces are not. Shadows dominate people's space and obscure personality. Diagonal and horizontal lines pierce bodies.

Darkness is combined with a landscape of enclosure to increase the feeling of fear. There is a stressed relationship between darkness and danger, light and safety. Those who wish to remain free of the pods must not only keep awake, but must constantly keep themselves close to direct light. For example, when Miles discovers Becky's pod-like double in the basement of her home, he hurries upstairs into her darkened bedroom and carries her out of the dark house into his car which is parked directly beneath a bright street lamp.

Tension in the film is not only created by lighting techniques and camera setups, but most significantly by the contrast in how the actors play their roles. Miles is frenzied, harried, hard-driving, always running. The robot-like, affectless pod people stare out at the camera with vacant eyes, openly unemotional, unbelievably calm, rational, logical. They appear to be normal, and Miles appears to be insane; however, the reverse is true. The pod's blank expression, emotionless eyes mask their essential deadness.

The whole film texture is based on the internal contrast between normal and alien. The hot dog stands, used-car lots, small office buildings, friendly cops, sleepy town square, and neighborhood gas stations only create the illusion of normalcy played against the mounting terror.

The mise-en-scène, lighting, acting styles, physical presence, props, and Carmen Dragon's unrelenting, spine-chilling musical score keep the audience in a constant state of tension. The same is true of the constant introjection of siren sounds, cuckoo clocks, screams in the middle of the night, and the use of distorting lenses, claustrophobic close-ups, juxtaposed long shots, and low-angled shots that establish a mood of vague disquiet. All help to create a basic tension between the normal and the fearful, the familiar and the sinister, and to result in a film designed to give the audience a sense of isolation, suspense, and feeling of constraint.

Historians will debate the actual nature of the 1950s for a long time. But through the films of a period we can see how a particular society treated the period, viewed it, experienced it, and symbolized it. Few products reveal so sharply as the science fiction/horror films of the 1950s the wishes, the hopes, the fears, the inner stresses and tensions of the period. Directly or indirectly, *Invasion* deals with the fear of annihilation brought on by the existence of the A-bomb, the pervasive feeling of paranoia engendered by an increasing sense that something was wrong, an increasing fear of dehumanization focused around an increased massification of American life, a deep-seated expression of social, sexual, and political frustration resulting from an ever-widening gap between personal expectation and social reality, and a widespread push for conformity as an acceptable strategy to deal with the confusion and growing insecurity of the period. It is a film that can be used by historians, sociologists, and psychologists to delineate these problems and demonstrate the way American society experienced and symbolized this crucial decade.

■ ■ ■

STUDY QUESTIONS

1. How can films be viewed as ideological statements? Does a film have to be overtly political to be ideological?

2. Out of what sort of political, social, and intellectual atmosphere did *Invasion of the Body Snatchers* emerge? Why were science fiction and horror films popular in the 1950s?

3. How does *Invasion* suggest the theme of conformity in the 1950s? What made Americans retreat from individualism during the decade? What is meant by the shift from "inner-directed" to "outer-directed" individual?

4. How does *Invasion* suggest the themes of conspiracy and paranoia in the 1950s?

5. How does *Invasion* suggest the theme of alienation in the 1950s? Why was podism a very real fear during the decade?

6. How did director Don Siegel shoot the film in order to emphasize the feeling of constraint? What technical duties did he use to reinforce this general theme?

BIBLIOGRAPHY

A number of books deal intelligently with movies and the film industry during the Cold War. The most thoughtful and provocative is Victor Navasky, *Naming Names* (1980). Nancy Lynn Schwartz, *The Hollywood Writers' War* (1982), discusses the role of the Screen Writers Guild in the political battles in Hollywood. The blacklisting of film artists is treated in David Cants, *The Great Fear: The Anti-Communist Purge Under Truman and Eisenhower* (1978); Larry Ceplair and Steven Englund, *The Inquistition in Hollywood* (1980); Bruce Cook, *Dalton Trumbo* (1977); Sterling Hayden, *Wanderer* (1963); Lillian Hellman, *Scoundrel Time* (1976); Stefan Kanfer, *A Journal of the Plague Years* (1973); and Robert Vaughn, *Only Victims: A Study of Show Business Blacklisting* (1972). Two recent books that discuss the films themselves in a lively manner are Peter Biskind, *Seeing is Believing: How Hollywood Taught Us to Stop Worrying and Love the Fifties* (1983), and Nora Sayre, *Running Time: Films of the Cold War* (1982). Finally, Stuart A. Kaminsky, *Don Siegel: Director* (1974), and Alan Lovell, *Don Siegel: American Cinema* (1975), discuss the director of *Invasion of the Body Snatchers*.

Part Seven

COMING APART:
1960–1990

The era began innocently enough. In an extremely close election, John F. Kennedy defeated Richard M. Nixon for the presidency and quickly became one of the most admired men in the country. Blessed with brains, charisma, money, and a lovely, young family, Kennedy epitomized America, particularly the rise and triumph of the immigrant. In public rhetoric, he cultivated a tough idealism, one which offered a courageous challenge to the Russians and hope for democracy and prosperity in the rest of the world. When Kennedy assumed the presidency in 1961, Americans believed their moral hegemony would last forever. They believed that their values deserved to govern the world by virtue of their success—an equality of opportunity and a standard of living unparalleled in human history. In closing his inaugural address, Kennedy even invoked the divine by claiming that ''God's work must truly be our own.''

What few people realized was that Kennedy was sitting on a powder keg, both at home and abroad. His liberal idealism, so self-righteous and yet so naive, barely survived his own life. From the mid-1960s through the mid-1970s, the country passed through a period of intense turmoil and doubt. Smug convictions about the virtues of equality and opportunity in the United States succumbed to the shrill criticisms of racial, ethnic, and sexual groups. Beliefs in the virtues, safeguards, and stability of the American government were shattered by the lies exposed in the controversies over Watergate and the Pentagon Papers. By the late 1960s and early 1970s the explosion in oil prices, the appearance of stagflation, and the worries about the future of the environment all undermined the prevailing confidence

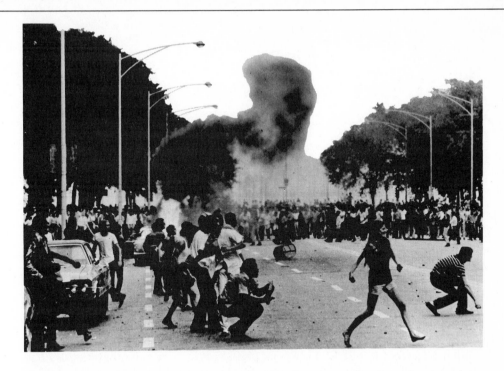

about the American economy. Finally, the moral complacency so endemic to Kennedy liberalism died in the jungles of Southeast Asia. Like few other events in American history, the Vietnam War tore the country apart. At home, America was characterized by bitterness, demonstrations, and widespread disaffection from the country's leaders. A counterculture of young people scornful of conventional values appeared, and the symbols of their rebellion were drugs and rock and roll. As far as world opinion was concerned, the country seemed to be a superpower out of control, employing the latest military technology in a futile effort to impose democracy on a nation barely out of the stone age.

Between 1964 and 1977, four American presidents struggled with these overwhelming problems. Lyndon Johnson's Great Society was eventually destroyed by what he called "that bitch of a war." Richard Nixon left the White House in disgrace after the Watergate tapes proved his complicity in perjury and obstructing justice. Gerald Ford failed in his "WIN" campaign—"whip inflation now"—and then watched helplessly as the last Americans, fleeing the invading North Vietnamese and Viet Cong troops, took off in helicopters from the roof of the United States embassy in Saigon. Jimmy Carter left the White House in 1977 after trying unsuccessfully to get Americans to accept the idea of austerity, shortages, and reduced expectations. The hostage crisis in Iran seemed the final symbol of American impotency. Not until the late 1970s, with Vietnam receding into history, oil prices dropping, inflation subsiding, and Ronald Reagan in the White House, did the United States recapture its legendary optimism about the future.

JOHN F. KENNEDY AND THE BLACK REVOLUTION

David Burner

On the morning after his election in 1960, no one had any idea of how completely John F. Kennedy would capture the American imagination. When he stated in his inaugural address that "the torch had been passed to a new generation of Americans," he became the symbol of a youth culture that would soon come to dominate American society and politics. By the early 1960s the first of the post–World War II baby boomers graduated from high school. Soon they filled colleges and universities, spearheading the crusades against racism, environmental pollution, and the Vietnam war. Raised during a time of unprecedented prosperity, and extraordinarily idealistic in outlook, they needed a political figure they could idolize.

John Fitzgerald Kennedy, for a brief period of time, became that idol. He had been tested in battle against the Japanese during World War II, and his exploits as commander of PT–109 had made him a hero. Kennedy had all the ingredients for stardom. Young and athletic, he exuded sexuality, at least for a major politician. His wife Jacqueline also enjoyed star qualities. Sexually appealing herself, she was at the same time refined and elegant. Small children romped in the White House for the first time since the administration of Theodore Roosevelt, and the public loved it. JFK's tragic death in 1963 only further endeared him to the American public.

However, by the early 1970s, Kennedy's image was changing. He was accused of having been lukewarm on civil rights, a belligerent "cold warrior," and a friend of the business community. Rumors of his sexual escapades with several women became national gossip. Instead of the young hero trying to shape a new world, Kennedy began to look like a calculating politician obsessed with the possibility of his own greatness. In "John F. Kennedy and the Black Revolution," David Burner looks at the record of the Kennedy administration in the area of civil rights, analyzing the political environment in which the young president operated and the extent to which his own views shaped—and limited—the federal response to the civil rights movement.

"No statesman," Abraham Lincoln wrote in the mid-1850s as the Civil War approached, "can safely disregard" the moral aversion people increasingly felt toward slavery. That, argues Richard Hofstadter in a famous essay on the Great Emancipator, was the "key to Lincoln's growing radicalism. As a practical politician he was naturally very much concerned with those public sentiments no statesman can safely disregard." A similar compounding of political and moral sensibilities moved John Kennedy to speak for the first time with unmistakable moral anger about racial injustice in 1963: "No city or state or legislative body can prudently choose to ignore . . . the fires of frustration and discord . . . burning in every city."

The civil rights movement had been stirring for years. Foreshadowed in government appeals for national unity during World War II and then in President Harry Truman's desegregation of the armed services and his establishment of a comprehensive study of social discrimination, the civil rights movement gained a major impetus in the Supreme Court decision of 1954, *Brown v. Board of Education of Topeka, Kansas*. The case repealed the longstanding criterion of "separate but equal" under which public schools had been allowed to practice segregation. In 1955 when Rosa Parks refused to move from her seat on a bus in Montgomery, Alabama, and the black community there waged a successful boycott of the city's buses, an invisible line had been crossed. In 1957 President Dwight Eisenhower sent federal troops to force the court-ordered desegregation of Central High School in Little Rock, Arkansas. By so doing he probably lost the South for the Republican Party in 1960. During the winter just preceding Kennedy's election, black and white students in defiance of segregation ordinances sat down and

drank coffee together at Southern lunch counters, first in Greensboro, North Carolina, and then within a few weeks throughout much of the South. In the summer of the next year, white racists assaulted freedom riders on their journey by bus to desegregate Southern transportation routes, a journey revolutionary not only in its rejection of racial customs but in its nonviolent resistance new to the staid conventions of twentieth-century American politics. In the fall of 1962 Mississippi's governor Ross Barnett fulminated against the enrollment of the first black student, James Meredith, at Ole Miss, where mobs took over the principal state campus and killed two men. In Birmingham the following spring Alabama's chief policeman, Bull Conner, turned police dogs and fire hoses on blacks; and then that September Klansmen dynamited four black children to death in the basement of a Baptist Church while they were singing a hymn in Sunday school class.

The civil rights movement bespoke a nearly miraculous liberation of minds and institutions from racial conventions seemingly set in iron. This movement for sudden freedom, which desegregated a bus or a train in an instant, had little in common with a president who appeared completely opportunistic and utilitarian on the race issue, a politician who twice voted to weaken civil rights bills in the 1950s and who spent more than two years in the White House before proposing any civil rights legislation. In his vice-presidential and presidential bids Kennedy relied for support on the South's most outspokenly segregationist governors, and he omitted civil rights from a list of the "real issues of 1960." Partly the conjunction of Kennedy and civil rights was a matter of coming to the presidency at the right moment. The civil rights movement had been stirring since the Montgomery bus boycott late in 1955 and the forced integration of Little Rock's Central High School in 1957. By the time of the Kennedy administration the movement was on the brink of a moral reformation. When Kennedy spoke his strong words about racial injustice in 1963, his

"Fires of Frustration," pp. 114–135, *John F. Kennedy and a New Generation* by David Burner, 1988. Reproduced by permission of Scott, Foresman.

presidency, now an active if nervous partner in the movement, gained thereby a moral high ground it had not anticipated. That transformation was not entirely accidental.

Kennedy's trust went to technology and experts, forces that would seem far distant in spirit from those of the civil rights rebellion. But new technological forces had great power in the 1960s. Television, for example, which greatly affected the course of the civil rights movement, enabled Kennedy to present himself less as a politician and more as an independent force for moral reformation. Television allowed the Kennedy family to enter the homes of all the nation's other families, a bit toney, perhaps, but gracious guests nonetheless. Television in good part rendered the major events of the early sixties into public phenomena significant not only in their purpose and their results but in the fact of being phenomena. The police dogs and fire hoses at Birmingham were such collective events, and seeing them in turn set the president angrily against the racists. The picture of a police dog attacking a black woman made him "sick," he told reporters. The Kennedy inaugural address, with its calls to growth and combat, had itself been a public event. James Meredith said that speech had spurred him to apply to the University of Mississippi the very next day, and some freedom riders remembered that stirring speech with its elevated rhetoric as spurring their dangerous treks. Yet the address said nothing beyond a general call for "human rights at home and around the world"; and during the presidential campaign the religious controversy had overshadowed the race issue. But in the early sixties the media portrayed the civil rights movement as the major news event that it deserved to be.

The inaugural was but the first occasion in a collective stream of experience that the nation associates with the Kennedy presidency. "His actual, tangible impact on history," Louise FitzSimons observes in the course of her severe commentary on Kennedy's foreign policy, "was not significant enough to explain his enormous psychological impact, the indefinable way in which John F. Kennedy touched people throughout the world." Why was it that in villages of India photographs of Gandhi, Nehru, and Kennedy hung side by side? Kennedy's death also won him a place in the memory of his own nation, as the central public figure in a confident time. This memorable quality that Kennedy conveyed was felt particularly by black Americans. One black woman would later remember, "Like a good book the life of John F. Kennedy steals inside and has somehow made me different. . . . Everyone I know loved him with a sort of possessiveness." The adulation of most blacks for Kennedy angers many serious American leftists. For what had this president done to deserve such love, so cautious in his recognition of a movement that, in retrospect, appears to constitute the visible and inescapable moral imperative of his presidential years?

On his own initiative, he did nothing striking. But his administration came at a time when political issues offered more of the hope and less of the distress that was to characterize issues thereafter, when the country seemed poised, in its science and technology as well as its social arrangements, at the edge of some futuristic transformation. The witness of the civil rights demonstrations, rooted in Southern evangelical churches, and the cold efficient promise of the space program demarcated polar opposites in American culture, but together they gave energy to the moment of Kennedy's administration. His presidency had a style consonant with that moment, and perhaps it had also the shrewdness along with the conscience to connect with it by some appropriate political gestures. The Kennedy style made government service and public commitment particularly appealing to young people, who became increasingly active in the civil rights movement, the Peace Corps, and public debates of many kinds. Many more young people wrote letters to this president than to any other president. "The biggest single influence that helped the formation of SDS [Students for a Democratic Society]," recalls

Robert Greenblatt, an early member, "was John F. Kennedy."

For blacks the new freedom had the press of a nation's history behind it. The Civil War did not eliminate slavery or degradation, and blacks were subjected to decades of massive oppression; after the "Jim Crow" segregation laws of the 1890s it almost seemed as though the South was the winner of that war. However, the civil rights movement reversed the nation's course and gave a new vitality to morally aware Americans. For a growing number of people this new freedom brought a sense that life could be immediately more promising, that America had not forgotten its idealistic heritage.

When Kennedy took office, he found the economy ready for stimulus, public schools in need of reform, and the Supreme Court ready to implement a major change in Southern custom—in the face of billboards that sprang up across the South after 1954 calling for Chief Justice Earl Warren's impeachment. In the next decade many victories came to progressive Americans who brought some optimism to national problems: the civil rights acts and poverty programs; massive federal funds spent on education, housing, and hospital care; tax cuts that generated larger revenues; and American astronauts who reached the moon. The legislative work of a generation was accomplished in about three years under a Kennedy–Johnson coalition founded on the symbolic memory of John Kennedy.

But the last Congress of the Eisenhower years, though Democratic by 280 to 155 in the House and by 66 to 34 in the Senate, had defeated a Medicare bill sponsored by Kennedy and also rejected a public housing law, minimum wage legislation, and aid to schools. The Democratic platform of 1960, drafted by the liberal Chester Bowles, promised action on civil rights, including power for the attorney general to seek court injunctions to enforce existing laws. Then in a short congressional session after the conventions, liberal Democrats joined conservative Southerners to table a civil rights bill

that Republicans had introduced to embarrass Kennedy. In response he and other senators promised to offer a bill in the first postelection session to "implement the pledge of the Democratic platform." The candidate even added a separate statement: "In order to implement this pledge and assure prompt action, I have asked Senator [Joseph] Clark and Representative [Emanuel] Celler to constitute a committee to prepare a comprehensive civil rights bill, embodying our platform commitments, for introduction at the beginning of the next session." The president in fact never proposed new laws until 1963. When Celler introduced a bill in the House in 1961, the White House press secretary pointedly backed away from giving it official support. Perhaps Kennedy would have lost Southern votes on other social legislation had he pushed a civil rights bill before it was certain to pass. Indeed social funding bills lost votes in the South after Kennedy supported a new civil rights law in 1963; congressmen even voted against funding that would benefit their own districts. His defenders explain that the narrowness of his election victory and of his party's margin in Congress gave him second thoughts. About 40 percent of the 261 Democrats in the new House were conservative Southerners. "The reason," Ted Sorensen wrote apologetically for not pushing liberal bills such as civil rights, "was arithmetic." In the presidential campaign itself, moreover, Kennedy had increasingly made promises to take direct executive action on civil rights. The trouble is that he delayed for eighteen months on the most symbolically and practically important of his campaign promises: to outlaw segregation in federally supported housing.

Kennedy himself, drawn to adventure stories, to James Bond novels, and elite military exploits, was—at least when he had the patience for it—also drawn to the slow arts of political compromise. Even if he entered the presidency as a liberal, he was apparently comfortable with a national legislature that could not be hurried into progressive laws. Nor did his background promise an assault on racial discrimination. *Profiles in Courage* purveys the stereotype of Reconstruction as a military occupation imposed on the war-ravaged South. No president before John Kennedy, Abraham Lincoln included, could meet more than the smallest test for racial justice, or for open discussion of the issue, on the terms later largely accepted. But no president had been put to the test by any movement as highly visible and moral as the civil rights forces of the sixties. They demanded absolute and uncompromised equality, an end to private and public discrimination, to stereotypes, to the range of nightmares and cruelties that have attended racism in this country. Indisputably, the Kennedy administration was alien at its roots from the work of protesters in the South and especially the courageous civil rights workers in the Southern back country. Neither rejection of his Irish ancestors by Boston Brahmins nor the recurring story that he had been rejected at Groton Preparatory School for being Irish seems to have much bothered John Kennedy.

Certainly an optimistic liberalism was foreign to his character. "There is always some inequality in life," he mused at a press conference in Greenfield, Massachusetts, on March 21, 1962. "Some men are killed in war, and some are wounded, and some men never leave the country, and some men are stationed in the Antarctic and some men are stationed in San Francisco. It is very hard in military or personal life to assure complete equality." A detached skepticism could inform, indeed toughen, a commitment to civil rights, which means a commitment to resist the downward drag of human nature and the appetites of the mob. But it is not in the typical style of twentieth-century liberalism.

Kennedy's first presidential actions did not suggest militancy on the issue. After the election and before he took office, he appointed a task force to study just about every problem except that of discrimination. He was more conscious of how America's treatment of blacks looked in the third world than he was of the moral questions at home. But he was conscious enough of the problem to appoint forty-one blacks to important posts within two months. Kennedy must have thought the chances of new legislation hopeless for the moment, inasmuch as he could not even get the appointment of the black economist, Robert C. Weaver, to be Secretary of Urban Affairs with cabinet rank. The civil rights movement perceived the administration as cautious and unfriendly; yet by 1963 its activity through the Justice Department made it the most hated federal administration in the deep South for a century.

The president did not choose for assistant attorney general for civil rights the dedicated Harris Wofford, who had proposed his telephoning Coretta King during the campaign when her husband, Martin Luther King, was imprisoned because of his civil rights work in the South. Instead he acted on the advice of his old professional football player friend Byron White, who was a conservative Rhodes scholar from Yale and Washington, a corporate lawyer, later a Kennedy appointee to the Supreme Court, and one of this century's most conservative members of the Court. At White's recommendation Kennedy selected Burke Marshall, also of Yale Law School.

Marshall captured the Kennedy administration's approach to civil rights. A patient negotiator, he had been a member of the American Civil Liberties Union and had early argued for the use of federal registrars to enroll Southern black voters. Few were registered under the Voter Education Project that the administration backed. Yet the effort brought money into the hands of the movement, awakening some black activism and giving it organizational structure. But voter registration was hardly safe work for young civil rights workers: rural Georgia, let alone Mississippi and Alabama, could hold a grim fate for them. Like Kennedy himself, who treated Southern congressmen with a degree of deference, Marshall disliked the use of federal power to coerce civil rights, much preferring the mode of compromise and agreement. He opposed the Civil Rights Commission's plan to hold hearings in Mississippi to publicize conditions there, and he objected as well to the Commission's wish to withhold federal funds from offending states. He labeled as "essentially negative and punitive" the withholding of funds from segregated school districts. He recoiled from any efforts to integrate housing nationwide ("a pretty drastic step legally and constitutionally"), and in 1964 at Columbia University he argued that the central government's police power could not deal effectively with the complex race problem without destroying the federal system. For decades legal conservatives, or legal realists as they are sometimes called, had similarly refrained from using the government to challenge unjust social institutions, and so the injustices continued. As late as the mid-1980s at a forum on Long Island, Marshall was to argue that the introduction of civil rights legislation in 1961 and 1962 had been useless "political posturing" and a waste of congressional time since a filibuster could have killed it.

One black woman has remembered of the early sixties that "when you had JFK, you had two Presidents—JFK and RFK." Attorney General Robert Kennedy was by turns passionate and prudent. Like his father he delighted in using whatever power he could lay his hands on, against radicals in the McCarthy era or against labor racketeers, about whom he published a book, *The Enemy Within*. But later, against an enemy within that was more deeply defiant of American justice, he made only selective use of the weapons of the federal government; the reason civil rights took so much of his time was mainly that it was so explosive an issue. Robert brought a few black attorneys into the Justice Department, along with Ramsey Clark, John Seigenthaler, John Doar, and Archibald Cox. He made a strong early speech at the University of Georgia in May 1961 praising two newly integrated black students as freedom fighters. No other attorney general had spoken on civil rights in the South in the twentieth century. One of the students, Charlayne Hunter, much later became a nationally prominent tele-

vision newscaster. The speech announced RFK's determination to work for racial justice. Yet he did not endorse the Democratic party's strong campaign platform on civil rights, and he feared the example of Eisenhower's employment of federal troops at Little Rock.

Beginning that spring, James Farmer's Congress of Racial Equality sent its courageous members on freedom rides through the South in buses, defying state and local statutes requiring segregation of bus terminals. Farmer even sent an itinerary of the rides to Kennedy, the FBI, and the Greyhound and Trailways Bus Lines but got no response. "Emotionally, I am totally in sympathy with them," Robert Kennedy said, but he feared that the testing would force federal intervention. Still, he did act to protect the riders, if not to give countenance to their journey. When a freedom bus was firebombed in Anniston, Alabama, and its occupants roughed up by Klansmen, he ordered J. Edgar Hoover's FBI to investigate, resulting in four arrests within a week. When the riders arrived in Birmingham, Robert Kennedy's administrative assistant, Seigenthaler, flew south to watch over them and successive groups, providing whatever defense against mob violence the Justice Department could furnish.

New riders, coming along the same route, had been promised protection by Alabama Governor John Patterson. Though a distinguished opponent of political corruption and a racial moderate by Southern standards at the time, Patterson decided against giving adequate protection to the riders and by his remarks incited that state's rednecks. Freedom riders proceeded from Birmingham to Montgomery, where the local police, stationed just two blocks away, did not appear at the terminal to protect them as promised by the state. Seigenthaler, who had accompanied the freedom riders, was hit on the head with an iron pipe while trying to rescue a black woman demonstrator, and lay unconscious on the ground for almost half an hour. To Robert Kennedy's later disgust the FBI men on the scene only took notes.

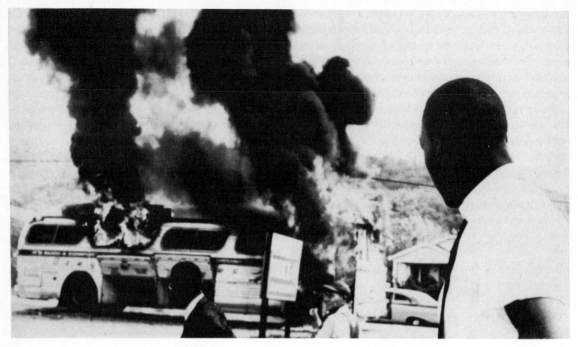

■ ■ *A Greyhound bus carrying "freedom riders" was set afire outside Anniston, Alabama, in May of 1961 by an angry mob of white men. Passengers, who were testing bus station segregation in the South, escaped without serious injury. The bus was destroyed.*

At this point the federal government acted briefly with real initiative. The president deputized immigration agents and prison guards as federal marshals under Byron White. That night the marshals protected the Reverend Martin Luther King, Jr., at a local church, which was surrounded by a mob. Finally Governor Patterson called up the National Guard to restore order. White, who believed that blacks needed money more than they needed civil rights, announced that marshals would not intervene if police arrested the freedom riders: the Justice Department, in its obvious discomfort over the whole business of the rides, apparently looked on police detention as a form of custodial care. On White's invitation, the state police arrested the riders when they tried to desegregate the bus terminal in Jackson, the capital. Since all this activity was very procedural, White was satisfied that justice and the safety of the riders were being served. A true conservative, he observed

that they would get adequate counsel. Segregationist federal judges refused to dismiss the arrests, which the Supreme Court later reversed in 1965. Both Kennedys desperately wanted to defuse the situation, and even Martin Luther King agreed to a moment's pause—a "lull" as he termed it.

The demonstrations, and more arrests, resumed later in the summer. In September 1961, the Interstate Commerce Commission began enforcing the Supreme Court mandate of desegregation in interstate transportation terminals, which Robert Kennedy had asked for as early as May. Some areas, however, refused to obey. In Albany, Georgia, 700 blacks were arrested that December, among them Reverend King. Burke Marshall obtained the release of the prisoners and an agreement to desegregate public transportation facilities. But the city reneged and the problem continued to fester. The community wide black movement in Albany would be copied elsewhere, notably in Birmingham in 1963.

The administration never pushed the South hard; the Kennedys thought calls for immediate freedom were irresponsible, and no more likely of realization than the cries for segregation forever. Finding not a single black district court judge in the United States, Kennedy did appoint a few, but segregationist judges continued to reach the bench in the South in accord with the tradition of approval from the states' senators for such appointments. Had Kennedy challenged the custom, the Senate Judiciary Committee, then headed by James Eastland of Mississippi, would probably never have cleared the appointment of Thurgood Marshall—who argued the Brown case in 1954 and who would later be appointed to the Supreme Court—and four other blacks to the federal courts. In addition, the administration got eight integrationists onto the famous Fifth Circuit that included the deep South. And in extenuation of the appointment of William A. Cox, who spoke of "niggers" and "chimpanzees" in open court, it should be observed both that the American Bar Association had given him its best ("Extremely Well Qualified") rating and that before his appointment he had promised the attorney general that he would enforce the law of the land.

The contradiction between a segregationist judiciary and a voter registration program dependent on the courts for its enforcement only slowly dawned on Marshall and Robert Kennedy. No government contracts were canceled because of job discrimination; the administration ran away from that idea as if it were a rattlesnake, said a member of the Civil Rights Commission. John Kennedy had criticized Eisenhower for tolerating segregation in federally funded housing, but it took him almost two years before he eliminated it by executive order. He was about to sign the order eight months after taking office but held back for fear of jeopardizing Robert Weaver's appointment to the cabinet; when he did sign, the scope was narrowed, because the administration knew

how explosive an issue housing was throughout the country. Quite a few Northern liberal Democrats from suburban districts even urged Kennedy to delay the order until after the midterm elections, which he did.

The Kennedy record on civil rights has bright moments, and its tone was superior to that of the Eisenhower years—though President Eisenhower's military enforcement of school desegregation in Little Rock, in contravention of the will of the governor of Arkansas, was of incalculable importance as a break with a longstanding federal practice of allowing the South to defy the Constitution.

As early as his inauguration day the president telephoned a cabinet secretary to ask why there had been no blacks in the Coast Guard marching band and was astonished to find that no blacks were enrolled in the entire Coast Guard Academy; vigorous recruiting efforts began forthwith. At Kennedy's insistence a policy of minority recruiting spread to all government agencies. In May 1961, before the freedom rides, Robert Kennedy wrote to forty-five law school deans asking for names of black lawyers and black law students the Justice Department might recruit. In a notable innovation, Marshall sent lawyers into the South to investigate violations of voting rights and permitted them to initiate remedial actions. No doubt this approach was eminently conservative, since it was only defending a constitutional right. But even so cautious a step as this inflamed Alabama and Mississippi. The administration persuaded Maryland to pass a public accommodations law and persuaded its governor to apologize to black diplomats turned away from a restaurant in that state while traveling from New York to the capital. In Washington, D.C., the president appointed the first black district commissioner.

Robert Kennedy asked Congress to forbid literacy tests for voting and instead use a sixth-grade education as the criterion. That a bill to this effect failed to pass no doubt indicated the fate a general civil rights bill would have met. But at the president's request and through a carefully crafted plan, Congress sent to the states for later passage the Twenty-fourth Amendment outlawing the poll tax. The government told universities that federal funds might be withheld if there was evidence of discrimination. Through the appointment in March 1961 of another President's Committee on Equal Employment Opportunity chaired by Vice President Johnson, the administration won some agreements from businesses to improve their minority hiring practices. But at least until 1963 the group relied too heavily on voluntary compliance and accomplished little. Johnson recommended that the civil rights bill of 1963 await passage of the tax reform bill, but he also advised the president to cast his message for rights in such a way that "it almost make[s] a bigot out of nearly anybody that's against him." Johnson himself made a strong speech at Gettysburg that May arguing for civil rights—and speaking in a Southern accent. Activists were appointed to the Civil Rights Commission, most notably the deans of Harvard and Howard law schools. The White House press pool and its photographers' association were at last desegregated. The president withdrew his application to the District's Cosmos Club when membership was denied a prominent black. And, unlike Eisenhower, Kennedy regularly entertained blacks in the White House, as did Robert Kennedy in his Virginia home. The president insisted that the Civil Service Commission establish minority recruitment visits to colleges and that all government departments increase their hiring of blacks at professional levels.

The "moral leadership" on civil rights that Kennedy had promised during the campaign was an attempt to lead by example, not by new legislation or even speeches. This was perhaps impressive for 1961 or even in 1962, but by 1963 Kennedy himself learned that there was no time left.

The administration also tried to get J. Edgar Hoover's Federal Bureau of Investigation involved, and the agency accomplished more on civil rights than is commonly supposed. Hoover

even transferred Southern-born agents out of Southern offices, for example. But he had a problem apart from his own conservatism and his strong belief in federalism: local police forces in the South were infiltrated by members of the Ku Klux Klan along with unaffiliated racists. Hoover's FBI had been careful to establish a cooperative relationship with local police that he did not wish to jeopardize. He had only a few blacks in his agency, among them his personal drivers and bodyguards; the Justice Department itself had only ten black lawyers out of some 1,000. Hoover was not the irresponsible psychopath television docudramas have made him out to be, and for many years the FBI maintained at least the appearance of a procedurally careful investigative force, a buttress rather than a threat to constitutional restrictions on federal power (privately Hoover had a habit of collecting potentially damaging information about politicians). It was a way of winning popular favor for the bureau; there are very few countries where the central police have enjoyed the public affection that the FBI received. But along with this carefully guarded demeanor went a temperamental stodginess that had little tolerance for public demonstrations, civil disobedience, and staged violations of social customs.

While Robert Kennedy pushed Hoover toward greater involvement in protecting civil rights workers and integrating the FBI, Hoover was able to convince the Justice Department civil rights lawyers, and through them the Kennedys, that Martin Luther King was consorting with known Communists. On learning this the president feared that an alliance with King would taint him with radicalism. He spoke to King in the White House Rose Garden in mid-1963 and warned him against his leftist friends as well as possible surveillance. The question revolved principally about a close friend of King, Stanley Levison, who had been very active in the Communist Party less than a decade earlier. Although there was no hard proof, the Justice Department thought Levison might have infiltrated the civil rights movement to promote communism. Subsequently, Hoover discovered that King was continuing his association with ex-Communists despite his promise to the president. Because of King's refusal to desert Levison, the FBI, with permission from the attorney general, began monitoring King's private conversations in late 1963.

Hoover also monitored an affair between the president and a woman who was also the mistress of a prominent Mafia leader. After a warning from the FBI leader, the relationship between Kennedy and Judith Exner was abruptly terminated. James MacGregor Burns has written that public character "turns on criteria of persistence, commitment, courage. . . . In the old days, leadership related to a president's pursuing of lofty ends, as in the case of [Jefferson and Wilson]. More recently moral leadership has been defined more often as relating to the president setting some kind of personal standard of morality. . . . I believe that the former concept is the more relevant one." (Before he died in November 1963 Kennedy's very amorous life was confined to a Vassar graduate, Mary Pinchot of the Pinchot family, renowned in American history. To her he revealed how much the word *liberal* made him gag. He apparently longed to be a college professor after his presidency, but the idea of associating with pretentious, pompous liberals deeply troubled him, he told her.) Kennedy, however, was a paragon neither in public nor in private. He secretly tape recorded much of what was said in the Oval Office, unbeknownst even to most of his closest advisors. He also ordered wiretaps on at least one congressman, and the administration prevailed on the Internal Revenue Service to audit groups it wanted to harass.

In 1963 the Kennedys were still signaling the South that they desired to maintain good relations at the same moment that the government was responding to blacks for almost the first time in nearly a century. The policy might have taken its natural course, with each small government gesture a step toward a formal reality the South could not avoid. But Southern

bigots forced the administration to act directly against them.

After a federal court ordered state officials to admit James Meredith to the University of Mississippi in the fall of 1962, some 550 federal marshals were under siege in a pitched battle with hinterland rednecks. The Kennedys would have cooperated with any reasonable plan to admit Meredith, but Governor Barnett, at great risk to the peace and safety of the campus, tried to maintain his popularity with the state's voters. He told a crowd of 46,000 at the Old Miss football game, "I love Mississippi. I love our people. I love our customs." The football team participated in the subsequent rioting almost en masse. A confused retired army general, Edwin Walker, encouraged the rioters, having discovered a connection among communism, integration, and the fall of Western civilization. After the mob killed two people and wounded twenty-eight marshals with gunfire, the president responded by sending some 23,000 federal troops. There would probably have been more bloodshed had the president allowed the marshals to use their firearms, but Kennedy was finally doing what Eisenhower had done five years before at Little Rock. Soldiers would remain on the campus for months. At last it was definite and clear that the federal government would enforce the law. The Mississippi State Senate passed a toothless motion expressing its "complete, entire and utter contempt for the Kennedy administration and its puppet courts."

In the spring of 1963 federal soldiers also protected two students enrolling at the University of Alabama. Here the president acted more swiftly, this time against a segregationist governor, George Wallace, who knew that compromise need not destroy his reputation. Against the advice of his staff, the president spoke to the nation, again calling the matter of race a "moral issue," and as soon as Wallace had performed his ritual act of "standing in the schoolhouse door," Kennedy summoned the National Guard to ensure compliance. Some 375 business executives in Alabama were phoned for help in avoiding trouble. Robert Kennedy, in Alabama for a press conference, was asked if he was a member of the Communist party and was jabbed with a nightstick by a state trooper.

Worse violence also came to Birmingham that same spring of 1963 when massive demonstrations by blacks for better jobs brought massive retaliation: electric cattle prods, police dogs, fire hoses. Burke Marshall, ever the negotiator, joined with other officials to win at least a part of the business community to the side of peace, but rioting meant that the civil rights movement had ended its nonviolent phase. Robert Kennedy objected to the protesters' use of children in their demonstrations, to which King countered that greater injury would come from continued discrimination. Soon violence would spread to the North, and the civil rights movement would lose much of its original nonviolent character.

On television an angry President Kennedy spoke eloquently and almost extemporaneously on morality and justice. Finally in full public support of the movement, he was a hero to most American blacks, although many black leaders and white allies thought his support came too late. In a 1963 poll blacks generally favored Kennedy against a Nelson Rockefeller Republican candidacy in 1964 by 89 to 3 percent and against the conservative Barry Goldwater by 91 to 2 percent. The supposed drift by blacks to the Republicans under President Eisenhower had been stemmed.

The White House sent Congress its first civil rights bill in February 1963, before Birmingham. It was a very weak measure, but at last the nation's president was plainly calling race discrimination wrong. Most of his advisors, including Vice President Johnson, thought the new bill could not pass. But in 1963 Kennedy worked hard to enact civil rights legislation, strengthening it enormously after riots in Birmingham by adding a ban on discrimination in public accommodations. Even voting rights provisions were included, but they did not become law until 1965. Mississippi's Senator James Eastland termed the bill a ''complete blueprint for a

totalitarian state.'' The president enlisted not only Johnson's help but also that of Representative Charles Halleck and Senator Everett Dirksen, the two Republican leaders in Congress. When Dirksen agreed in November not to support a filibuster, passage of a bill seemed certain, though a sizable minority of House Republicans opposed it. Before Kennedy's assassination the House Judiciary Committee had cleared the bill for a vote. Almost all members of Congress received pleas from the White House to favor the bill, and the president spoke with groups of national business, religious, legal, and labor leaders who might aid in its passage. If moderate blacks did not achieve what they legitimately wanted, the Kennedys warned, extremist groups would win civil rights leadership. Robert Kennedy repeatedly urged a new law to get black protesters ''off the streets and into the courts.'' Southerners like Johnson and Dean Rusk of Georgia pleaded with wavering senators.

The laws that passed in 1964 and 1965 went further than the president's bill, but the Kennedys labored hard for civil rights in 1963, and they began to lose some public support on it. Twice as many Americans thought that the administration was moving too fast as thought its progress too slow, and Kennedy's popularity plummeted throughout the white South where in June he received only a 33 percent approval rating. His likely opponent Goldwater did well in the South in 1964, and a chilly reception for the president in Philadelphia the year before had given premonitions of a white backlash in the North. The administration feared that King's March on Washington scheduled for August 1963 might turn violent, giving the South the chance to argue that it was being threatened by unruly mobs.

Failing the previous June to get the march canceled, the White House embraced it, ''I'll look forward to being there,'' the president said at his July 17 presidential news conference, and the administration persuaded the theologically conservative Roman Catholic archbishop of Washington, Patrick O'Boyle, to attend. As the day of the march approached one of its leaders said of Kennedy: "He almost smothered us [with support]. We had to keep raising our demands to keep him from getting ahead of us." The march was a heartening gathering of a quarter million blacks and whites—the largest crowd ever to assemble in American history. Joan Baez sang "We Shall Overcome" and then joined Peter, Paul, and Mary in a moving rendition of Bob Dylan's "Blowin' in the Wind." Dylan, Odetta, and Mahalia Jackson also performed. The president met afterward for coffee in the White House with ten major black leaders, recalling his serving coffee to a group of pacifist picketers in front of the White House during 1961.

On August 28 King delivered his famous and moving "I Have a Dream" speech, which was a counterpoise to the ugliness and violence of Birmingham. "I have a dream," he orated, "that one day . . . when we let freedom ring, when we let it ring from every village and every hamlet, from every state and every city, we will be able to speed up that day when all God's children, black men and white men, Jews and Gentiles, Protestants and Catholics, will be able to join in the words of that old Negro spiritual 'Free at last, Free at last, Thank God almighty, we are free at last.'" John and Robert Kennedy had not really joined him in visualizing that dream, but the white South and most of the nation's blacks saw them in league. Their approaches differed. The Kennedy brothers believed in a gradual, incremental resolution of issues in preference to dangerous confrontation. Robert particularly favored federal pressure, a strategy-tempered idealism. The right to vote, the president and his attorney general thought, would be the most effective goal. Liberals in Congress, a memoir by Robert Kennedy observes, preferred failure to a reasonable bill: "An awful lot of them, as I said then, were in love with death." They thought only of their own goals, he wrote, rather than of the needs of others or of practical problems. This moralistic denunciation of moralistic liberals came from a man in whom virtuous anger

seemed always close to the surface. Quite possibly a desire to go beyond practical limits might have had the effect of widening them. But Robert Kennedy made a good case against the virtuousness that thirsts after purity, even at the cost of defeat. The Kennedys believed in a federal power that could be used calculatingly against racism. It was the task of the Kennedy administration, more than of any other in the history of civil rights, to act for that part of the democratic process that restrained an unjust popular will.

Hesitancy not only kept the Kennedys from full participation in the largest movement of their time for social justice, but also marked their temperamental distance from its peculiar character, a character that is as important morally as its technical goals. The civil disobedience and the peaceful walks through angry crowds were more than protests against segregation. They were in themselves acts of spiritual integration, a stepping through the violence of the mob and of the racist tradition. They repressed the human urge to violence within the protesters themselves and instead emphasized peace and civility.

The rights demonstrators also raised questions of confrontation between law and conscience. That confrontation was not sharp and absolute, since the rights forces claimed (correctly) to be working to enforce the Constitution. But in style and sometimes in substance they were making a choice for conviction and against the immediate agents of legal authority. The peaceful act of conscience in the face of law or custom had an ancestry in abolitionism. But in more recent times the notion had nearly atrophied. The civil rights movement reawakened it, the antiwar protests nourished it, and it remained a dilemma for a small but significant number of Americans who had to learn that conscience may simultaneously require the upholding of a system of laws and yet the defiance of an unjust law.

The Kennedys were outside all this, although Robert would later acquire some affinity with the antiwar movement. But an administration is the sworn defender of institutions; it is supposed to respect informal political procedures, effect compromises, and preserve tranquility. The Kennedy presidency was behaving within that understanding of its role. In so doing, it succeeded in translating into some solid policies and laws the objectives of a movement that looked beyond law and policy to the uncompromisable demands of justice.

■ ■ ■

STUDY QUESTIONS

1. While he was serving as a United States senator from Massachusetts in the 1950s, what kind of a civil rights record did John F. Kennedy accumulate?

2. During his presidency, John F. Kennedy was extraordinarily popular among black Americans. Why? Did his own record on civil rights justify that popularity?

3. How did the split between the Northern and Southern wings of the Democratic party affect Kennedy's approach to civil rights and social welfare legislation? Could he have achieved more if he had been bolder and less concerned with Southern opinion?

4. What role did Robert Kennedy play in the administration's approach to civil rights?

5. Who were the Freedom Riders? How much impact did they have on the Kennedy administration?

6. Historians and critics have labeled John F. Kennedy as a conservative, a radical, or a moderate. Based on his civil rights record, what would you say about Kennedy's political philosophy?

BIBLIOGRAPHY

For favorable portraits of Kennedy and his administration, see Arthur M. Schlesinger, Jr., *A Thousand Days* (1965); Theodore M. Sorensen, *Kennedy* 1973); Herbert Parment, *Jack: The Struggles of John F. Kennedy* (1980) and *JFK: The Presidency of John F. Kennedy* (1983). Also see Henry Farlie, *The Kennedy Promise* (1973). For harsh criticisms of the Kennedy administration, see Bruce Miroff, *Pragmatic Illusions: The Presidential Politics of John F. Kennedy* (1976) and Garry Wills, *The Kennedy Imprisonment* (1982). For views of the Kennedy family, see Doris Kearns Goodwin, *The Fitzgeralds and the Kennedys: An American Saga* (1987) and Nancy Gager Clinch, *The Kennedy Neurosis: A Psychological Portrait of an American Dynasty* (1973). David Burner's *John F. Kennedy and a New Generation* (1987) is a short but excellent biography.

For studies of the civil rights movement of the 1960s, see Carl Bauer, *John F. Kennedy and the Second Reconstruction* (1977) and Harris Wofford's *Of Kennedys and Kings* (1980). Also see Robert E. Gilbert, "John F. Kennedy and Civil Rights for Black Americans," *Presidential Studies Quarterly* 12 (Summer 1982), pp. 386–399.

DR. STRANGELOVE (1964): NIGHTMARE COMEDY AND THE IDEOLOGY OF LIBERAL CONSENSUS

Charles Maland

Occasionally history repeats itself, although not nearly as frequently as many people assume. A good case, however, for the "cycles of history" is the preoccupation with nuclear war in the 1980s. Such films as *The Day After, Testament,* and *Operation Looking Glass* in 1983 and 1984 are reminders of similar concerns in the early 1960s. Films about nuclear war became classics then too, particularly such movies as *On the Beach, Fail Safe,* and *The Bedford Incident.* But the best of the genre, a film just as biting and relevant today as it was during its release in 1964, is Stanley Kubrick's *Dr. Strangelove or: How I Learned to Stop Worrying and Love the Bomb.* Produced during the Kennedy administration, well before the war in Vietnam injected cynicism into American political culture, the movie rejected the liberal consensus, particularly its naive faith in science and technology.

During the early 1960s, the legacy of American history was still working its magic on public policy. The legendary American sense of mission, first proclaimed by the Puritans in the seventeenth century, was as powerful as ever, but now it was reinforced by the technology of nuclear weapons. John Kennedy's "New Frontier" and Lyndon Johnson's "Great Society" proposed to eliminate poverty and discrimination at home while protecting the world from Soviet aggression. They approached world affairs with confidence and assertiveness, convinced that people everywhere were anxiously waiting for the expansion of American institutions to reach them. Nuclear weapons were the trump card guaranteeing the triumph of American values, even though their use would destroy American life as nothing else could. Stanley Kubrick agonized over that irony and produced *Dr. Strangelove* as his antidote for the insanity he saw in Washington, D.C. In the following essay, Charles Maland looks at the film and its critique of American ideology in the early 1960s.

D r. Strangelove or: How I Learned to Stop Worrying and Love the Bomb (Stanley Kubrick,
1964) is one of the most fascinating and important American films of the 1960s. As a sensitive
artistic response to its age, the film presents a
moral protest of revulsion against the dominant
cultural paradigm in America—what Geoffrey
Hodgson has termed the Ideology of Liberal
Consensus. Appearing at roughly the same time
as other works critical of the dominant paradigm—Catch 22 is a good literary example of the
stance—Dr. Strangelove presented an adversary
view of society which was to become much more
widely shared among some Americans in the
late 1960s. This essay will examine the Ideology
of Liberal Consensus, demonstrate how Dr.
Strangelove serves as a response to it (especially to
its approach to nuclear strategy and weapons),
and look at how American culture responded to
its radical reassessment of the American nuclear
policy in the early 1960s.

The American consensus to which Dr.
Strangelove responds was rooted in the late 1930s
and in the war years. When Americans in the
late 1930s began to feel more threatened by the
rise of foreign totalitarianism than by the economic insecurities fostered by the stock market
crash, a previously fragmented American culture
began to unify. A common system of belief
began to form, a paradigm solidified during
World War II, when American effort was directed toward defeating the Axis powers. Fueled by
the success of the war effort and the economic
prosperity fostered by the war, this paradigm
continued to dominate American social and
political life through the early 1960s.

The 1950s are commonly remembered as an
age of conformity typified by the man in the gray
flannel suit, the move to suburbia, and the

blandness of the Eisenhower administration.
There were, of course, currents running counter
to the American consensus in the 1950s—C.
Wright Mills challenging the power elite and the
era's "crackpot realism"; James Dean smoulder-
ing with sensitive, quiet rebellion; the Beats
rejecting the propriety and complacency of the
era—yet most people remained happy with
America and its possibilities. Much more than a
passing mood or a vague reaction to events, this
paradigm—the Ideology of Liberal Consensus—
took on an intellectual coherence of its own.
According to Geoffrey Hodgson, the ideology
contained two cornerstone assumptions: that
the structure of American society was basically
sound, and that Communism was a clear danger
to the survival of the United States and its allies.
From these two beliefs evolved a widely accepted view of America. That view argued its position in roughly this fashion: the American economic system has developed, softening the inequities and brutalities of an earlier capitalism,
becoming more democratic, and offering abundance to a wider portion of the population than
ever before. The key to both democracy and
abundance is production and technological
advance; economic growth provides the opportunity to meet social needs, to defuse class conflict, and to bring blue-collar workers into the
middle class. Social problems are thus less explosive and can be solved rationally. It is necessary
only to locate each problem, design a program to
attack it, and provide the experts and technological know-how necessary to solve the problem.

The only threat to this domestic harmony, the
argument continued, is the specter of Communism. The "Free World," led by the United
States, must brace itself for a long struggle
against Communism and willingly support a
strong defense system, for power is the only language that the Communists can understand. If
America accepts this responsibility to fight Communism, while also proclaiming the virtues of
American economic, social, and political democracy to the rest of the world, the country will
remain strong and sound. Hodgson sums up the

paradigm well when he writes: "Confident to the verge of complacency about the perfectability of American society, anxious to the point of paranoia about the threat of Communism—those were the two faces of the consensus mood."

These two assumptions guided our national leadership as it attempted to forge social policy in an era of nuclear weapons. After the Soviet Union announced in the fall of 1949 that it had successfully exploded an atomic bomb, President Truman on January 31, 1950 ordered the Atomic Energy Commission to go ahead with the development of a hydrogen bomb. By late 1952 the United States had detonated its first hydrogen bomb, 700 times more powerful than the atomic bomb dropped on Hiroshima. Less than a year later, on August 8, 1953, the Soviets announced that they, too, had a hydrogen bomb. The arms race was on.

About the time that Sputnik was successfully launched in 1957—leading to national fears about the quality of American science and education—some American intellectuals began to refine a new area of inquiry: nuclear strategy. Recognizing that nuclear weapons were a reality, the nuclear strategists felt it important to think systematically about their role in our defense policy. Henry Kissinger's *Nuclear War and Foreign Policy* (1957), one of the first such books, argued that the use of tactical nuclear weapons must be considered by decision makers. More widely known was the work of Herman Kahn, whose *On Thermonuclear War* (1960) and *Thinking About the Unthinkable* (1962) presented his speculations on nuclear war and strategy, most of which stemmed from his work for the RAND Corporation during the 1950s. Kahn was willing to indulge in any speculation about nuclear war, including such topics as the estimated genetic consequences of worldwide doses of radioactive fallout, the desirable characteristics of a deterrent (it should be frightening, inexorable, persuasive, cheap, non-accident prone, and controllable), and the large likelihood of vomiting in postwar fallout shelters.

Though the professed intent of the nuclear strategists was to encourage a rational approach to foreign policy in a nuclear age, the mass media seemed intent on making the public believe that thermonuclear war might be acceptable, even tolerable. A few examples illustrate that some mass magazines believed that nuclear war would not really be that bad. *U.S. News and World Report* carried a cover article, "If Bombs Do Fall," which told readers that plans were underway to allow people to write checks on their bank accounts even if the bank were destroyed by nuclear attack. The same issue contained a side story about how well survivors of the Japanese bombings were doing. *Life* magazine placed a man in a reddish fallout costume on its cover along with the headline, "How You Can Survive Fallout. 97 out of 100 Can Be Saved." Besides advising that the best cure for radiation sickness "is to take hot tea or a solution of baking soda," *Life* ran an advertisement for a fully-stocked, prefabricated fallout shelter for only $700. The accompanying picture showed a happy family of five living comfortably in their shelter. I. F. Stone suggested in response to this kind of writing that the media seemed determined to convince the American public that thermonuclear warfare was "almost as safe as ivory soap is pure." While all this was going on, a RAND corporation study released in August 1961 estimated that a 3000 megaton attack on American cities would kill 80 percent of the population.

This paradoxical, bizarre treatment of the nuclear threat can be explained in part as an attempt by journalists to relieve anxiety during a time when the Cold War was intensifying. A number of events from 1960 to 1963 encouraged this freeze in the Cold War. Gary Powers, piloting a U-2 surveillance plane, was shot down over the Soviet Union in May 1960. In 1961, the Bay of Pigs fiasco occurred in May, President Kennedy announced a national fallout shelter campaign on television in July, and in August, the Berlin Wall was erected and the Soviet Union announced that they were resuming atmospheric testing of nuclear weapons. Worst of all, the Cuban Missile Crisis of October 1962 carried the world to the brink of nuclear war, thrusting the dangers of nuclear confrontation to the forefront of the public imagination. Though the crisis seemed to be resolved in favor of the United States, for several days nuclear war seemed imminent.

One result of this intensification was to erode the confidence of some Americans in the wisdom of American nuclear policy. Though there had been a small tradition of dissent regarding American nuclear policy in the 1950s—led by people like J. Robert Oppenheimer, Linus Pauling, Bertrand Russell, and C. Wright Mills, and groups like SANE (the National Committee for a Sane Nuclear Policy)—these people were clearly a minority, prophets crying in the wilderness. But Edmund Wilson's warning in 1963 that our spending on nuclear weapons may be one of mankind's final acts, and H. Stuart Hughes' impassioned challenge to deterrence strategy and his support of disarmament in the same year, were both symptomatic of a growing dissatisfaction of some Americans with the federal government's nuclear policy. Judged from another perspective, outside the assumptions of the Ideology of Liberal Consensus, the threat posed by the Soviet Union did not at all warrant the use of nuclear weapons. In the same vein, the realities of America itself—as the defenders of the Civil Rights movement were pointing out—did not live up to the rhetoric about the harmonious American democracy so prevalent in the 1950s. By 1962 and 1963, when *Dr. Strangelove* was being planned and produced, the Ideology of Liberal Consensus seemed increasingly vulnerable. In fact, it is not unfair to say that an adversary culture opposed to the hypocrisies and inconsistencies of the dominant paradigm was beginning to form.

Stanley Kubrick, director of *Dr. Stangelove,* played a part in extending that adversary culture. Born in 1928 to a middle-class Bronx family, Kubrick was from an early age interested in chess and photography. It is not hard to move

from his fascination with chess, with the analytical abilities it requires and sharpens, to the fascination with technology and the difficulties men have in controlling it which Kubrick displays in *Dr. Strangelove* and *2001: A Space Odyssey.* Photography became a pasttime when Kubrick recieved a camera at age thirteen, and a profession when *Look* magazine hired him at age eighteen as a still photographer. From there Kubrick became interested in filmmaking and made a short documentary on middleweight boxer Walter Cartier called *Day of the Fight* (1950). He followed this with a second documentary for RKO, *Flying Padre* (1951), after which he made his first feature film, *Fear and Desire* (1953). From then on Kubrick was immersed in making feature films.

In his mature work Kubrick has returned constantly to one of the gravest dilemmas of modern industrial society: the gap between man's scientific and technological skill and his social, political, and moral ineptitude. In Kubrick's world view, modern man has made scientific and technological advances inconceivable to previous generations but lacks the wisdom either to perceive how the new gadgetry might be used in constructive ways or, more fundamentally, to ask whether the "advance" might not cause more harm than good. Kubrick first faced this problem squarely in *Dr. Strangelove.*

Kubrick's films before 1963 do hint at interests which he was to develop more fully in *Dr. Strangelove. The Killing* shows a group of men working toward a common purpose under intense pressure and severe time limitations. *Paths of Glory*—one of a handful of classic anti-war films in the American cinema—vents its anger at the stupidity of military leaders, their callous disregard for other human lives, and their own lust for power. Released in 1957 in the midst of the Cold War, *Paths* was a courageous film made slightly more palatable for audiences because of its setting and situation: World War One and the evils of French military leaders.

It is not totally surprising, then, that Kubrick should make a film about military and civilian leaders trying to cope with accidental nuclear war. Actually, Kubrick had developed an interest in the Cold War and nuclear strategy as a concerned citizen in the late 1950s, even before he thought of doing a film on the subject. In an essay on *Dr. Strangelove* published in mid-1963, a half year before the release of the film, Kubrick wrote: "I was very interested in what was going to happen, and started reading a lot of books about four years ago. I have a library of about 70 or 80 books written by various technical people on the subject and I began to subscribe to the military magazines, the Air Force magazine, and to follow the U.S. naval proceedings." One of the magazines he subscribed to was the *Bulletin of the Atomic Scientist*, which regularly published articles by atomic scientists (Oppenheimer, Edward Teller, and Leo Szilard) and nuclear strategists (Kahn, Bernard Brodie, and Thomas Schelling). The more he read on the subject, the more he became engrossed in the complexities of nuclear strategy and the enormity of the nuclear threat:

I was struck by the paradoxes of every variation of the problem from one extreme to the other—from the paradoxes of unilateral disarmament to the first strike. And it seemed to me that, aside from the fact that I was terribly interested myself, it was very important to deal with this problem dramatically because it's the only social problem where there's absolutely no chance for people to learn anything from experience. So it seemed to me that this was eminently a problem, a topic to be dealt with dramatically.

As his readings continued, Kubrick began to feel "a great desire to do something about the nuclear nightmare." From this desire came a decision to make a film on the subject. In preparation, he talked with both Thomas Schelling and Herman Kahn, gradually coming to believe that a psychotic general could engage in what Kahn termed "unauthorized behavior" and send bombers to Russia.

Kubrick found the literary work upon which his film was based almost by accident. When he requested some relevant readings from the Institute of Strategic Studies, the head of the Institute, Alastair Buchan, suggested Peter George's *Red Alert*, a serious suspense thriller about an accidental nuclear attack. The book contained such an interesting premise concerning accidental nuclear war that even a nuclear strategist like Schelling could write of it that "the sheer ingenuity of the scheme . . . exceeds in thoughtfulness any fiction available on how war might start." Kubrick, likewise impressed with the involving story and convincing premise, purchased rights to the novel.

However, when author and screenwriter started to construct the screenplay, they began to run into problems, which Kubrick describes in an interview with Joseph Glemis:

I started work on the screenplay with every intention of making the film a serious treatment of the problem of accidental nuclear war. As I kept trying to imagine the way in which things would really happen, ideas kept coming to me which I would discard because they were so ludicrous. I kept saying to myself: "I can't do this. People will laugh." But after a month or so I began to realize that all the things I was throwing out were the things which were most truthful.

By trying to make the film a serious drama, Kubrick was accepting the framework of the dominant paradigm, accepting Cold War premises and creating the gripping story within these premises. This was the approach of *Red Alert* as well as of *Fail Safe*, a popular film of late 1964 adapted from the Burdick and Wheeler novel. But after studying closely the assumptions of the Cold War and the nuclear impasse, Kubrick was moving outside the dominant paradigm. Kubrick's fumbling attempts to construct a screenplay provide an example of what Gene Wise, expanding on Thomas Kuhn, has called a "paradigm revolution" in the making: a dramatic moment when accepted understandings of the world no longer make sense and new ones are needed.

Kubrick describes in an interview how he

resolved his difficulties with the screenplay: "It occurred to me I was approaching the project in the wrong way. The only way to tell the story was as a black comedy, or better, a nightmare comedy, where the things you laugh at most are really the heart of the paradoxical postures that make a nuclear war possible. After deciding to use nightmare comedy in approaching his subject, Kubrick hired Terry Southern to help with the screenplay. This decision connects Kubrick to the black humor novelists of the early 1960s. Writers like Southern, Joseph Heller (*Catch 22*), Kurt Vonnegut (*Mother Night*), and Thomas Pyncheon (*V* and *The Crying of Lot 49*) shared with Kubrick the assumption of a culture gone mad, and responded to it with a similar mixture of horror and humor. Morris Dickstein's comment that "black humor is pitched at the breaking point where moral anguish explodes into a mixture of comedy and terror, where things are so bad you might as well laugh," describes quite accurately the way Kubrick came to feel about the arms race and nuclear strategy.

The premise and plot of the film are, paradoxically, quite realistic and suspenseful, which in part accounts for why the nightmare comedy succeeds. At the opening of the film a narrator tells us that the Russians have built a Doomsday device which will automatically detonate if a nuclear weapon is dropped on the Soviet Union, destroying all human life on the planet—a case of deterrence strategy carried to the absurd. A paranoid anti-Communist Air Force general, unaware of the Russian's ultimate weapon, orders a fleet of airborne SAC B-52s to their Russian targets. The President of the United States finds out, but soon learns that the jets cannot be recalled because only the general knows the recall code. Moving quickly into action, the President discusses the problem with his advisors, calls the Russian Premier, and assists the Russians in their attempts to shoot down the B-52s. Finally, all the planes are recalled but one, which drops its bombs on a secondary target, setting off the Russian retaliatory Doomsday device. *Dr. Strangelove* concludes in apocalypse.

After the narrator's initial mention of a Doomsday device, Kubrick subtly begins his nightmare comedy by suggesting that man's warlike tendencies and his sexual urges stem from similar aggressive instincts. He does this by showing an airborne B-52 coupling with a refueling plane in mid-air, while the sound track plays a popular love song, "Try a Little Tenderness." The connection between sexual and military aggression continues throughout the film, as when an otherwise nude beauty in a *Playboy* centerfold has her buttocks covered with a copy of *Foreign Affairs,* but it is most evident in the names given the characters by the screenwriters. Jack D. Ripper, the deranged SAC general, recalls the sex murderer who terrorized London during the 1880s. The name of Army strategist Buck Turgidson is also suggestive: his first name is slang for a virile male and his last name suggests both bombast and an adjective meaning "swollen." Major King Kong, pilot of the B-52, reminds viewers of the simple-minded beast who fell in love with a beautiful blonde. Group Captain Lionel Mandrake's last name is also the word for a plant reputedly known for inducing conception in women, while both names of President Merkin Muffley allude to female genitals. Appropriately, Ripper and Turgidson are hawks, while Muffley is a dove. Other names—Dr. Strangelove, the Soviet Ambassador De Sadesky, and Premier Dmitri Kissov—carry similar associations. These sexual allusions permeate the film, providing one level of the film's nightmare comedy.

More important than these sexual allusions, however, is *Dr. Strangelove's* frontal assault on the Ideology of Liberal Consensus. Above all else, *Dr. Strangelove* uses nightmare comedy to satirize four dimensions of the Cold War consensus: anti-Communist paranoia; the culture's inability to realize the enormity of nuclear war; various nuclear strategies; and the blind faith modern man places in technological progress.

The critique of American anti-Communist paranoia is presented primarily through General Ripper, played by Sterling Hayden. Kubrick portrays Ripper as an obsessed member of the radical right. Convinced that the Communist conspiracy has not only infiltrated our country but also, through fluoridation, contaminated our water, Ripper decides to take action by sending the B-52s to bomb Russia. Cutting off all communication to the outside world, he then orders his men to fight anyone attempting to capture the base.

The most grimly ominous character in the film, Ripper dominates its action in the first half, and Kubrick underlines this action stylistically, often shooting Ripper from a low camera angle. But Ripper's words also characterize his paranoia. Kubrick once agreed that whereas *2001* develops its focus visually, *Dr. Strangelove* does so much more through its dialogue. Early in the film, Ripper reveals his fears to Mandrake (Peter Sellers, in one of his three roles):

Mandrake, have you ever seen a Communist drink a glass of water? Vodka, that's what they drink, isn't it? Never water—on no account will a Commie ever drink water, and not without good reason . . . Mandrake, water is the source of life: seven-tenths of this earth's surface is water. Why, do you realize that 70 percent of you is water? And as human beings, you and I need fresh, pure water to replenish our precious bodily fluids. . . . Have you never wondered why I drink only distilled water or rain water and only pure grain alcohol? . . . Have you ever heard of a thing called fluoridation? Do you realize that fluoridation is the most monstrously conceived and dangerous Communist plot we've ever had to face?

Later Ripper mentions that fluoridation began in 1946, the same year as the postwar international Communist conspiracy. By portraying this paranoid officer willing to obliterate the world because of fluoridation, Kubrick lays bare the irrational American fear of Communism as one source of the cultural malaise of the early 1960s.

The second object of attack through satire—the failure to realize how nuclear weapons have changed the nature of war—is carried out primarily on one of General Ripper's B-52s. The pilot of the plane, Major King Kong (Slim Pickens), gives evidence of outmoded notions about war in his pep talk to the crew after they have received the "go" code:

Now look boys—I ain't much of a hand at makin' speeches. . . . I got a fair idea of the personal emotions that some of you fellas may be thinkin'. Heck, I reckon you wouldn't even be human bein's if you didn't have some pretty strong feelin's about nuclear combat. But I want you to remember one thing. The folks back home is a-countin' on you and, by golly, we ain't about to let 'em down. I'll tell you something else: if this thing turns out to be half as important as I figger it just might be, I'd say you're all in line for some important promotions and personal citations when this thing's over with. And that goes for every last one of you, regardless of yer race, color, or yer creed.

Such a pep talk might be appropriate for a World War II film—in fact, most films about that war contained some such scene—but Kong's blindness to what he is being asked to do is almost complete. The fact that Kong wears a cowboy hat while making the speech, connecting him to the frontier heritage, and that "When Johnny Comes Marching Home"—a patriotic American war tune—plays on the soundtrack in the background, reinforces the conception of Kong as a dangerous anachronism.

To drive this point home, Kubrick has Kong go through the contents of a survival kit. It includes, among other items, a pistol, nine packs of chewing gum, several pairs of nylon stockings, a miniature combination Bible and Russian phrase book, and, of course, an issue of prophylactics. Besides parodying what every soldier shot down over enemy territory might need, the scene reasserts that Kong is fighting another war at another time, never having realized that if his bomber goes down after dropping its atomic load, the crew will not have to worry much about survival, to say nothing of survival kits. Kubrick, perhaps responding to the media articles which made light of the nuclear war may not actually be that bad.

National strategies also come under attack.

Here the satire is particulary pointed; the various strategic positions taken by characters in the War Room correspond quite closely to positions taken by military and civilian strategists.

General Turgidson (George C. Scott) is a "hardliner." His position is even more severe than that of John Foster Dulles, who announced the policy of "massive retaliation" in 1954. Turgidson secretly favors a first-strike policy—he would like to see the U.S. obliterate the Russians offensively. After learning that the planes have been accidentally sent to their Russian targets, Turgidson urges the President to intensify the attack with even more planes:

T: *It is necessary now to make a choice, to choose between two admittedly regrettable but nevertheless distinguishable postwar environments. One, where you got twenty million people killed and the other where you got 150 million people killed.*

M: *(Shocked) You're talking about mass murder, general, not war.*

T: *I'm not saying we wouldn't get our hair mussed. But I do say no more than ten to twenty million killed, tops—depending on the breaks.*

M: *(Angrily) I will not go down in history as the greatest mass murderer since Adolph Hitler.*

T: *Perhaps it might be better, Mr. President, if you were more concerned with the American people than with your image in the history books.*

Scott delivers these lines with zestful enthusiasm, and his animated features suggest that he can hardly wait for the annihilation to begin. In rhetoric distressingly similar to the arguments occurring occasionally in the journals, Turgidson advises "total commitment," sacrificing a "few lives" for what he believes would be a more secure and satisfactory "post-war environment."

President Muffley's position is the most reasonable of any in the War Room. He is neither a fanatic nor a warmonger. Unfortunately, he's also nearly totally ineffectual as he tries to implement his goal: attempting to avoid catastrophe at all costs through communication with the Soviets. Peter Sellers plays this role with a bald wig,

in part to differentiate himself visually from his two other roles, in part to remind audiences of Adlai Stevenson, the quintessential liberal of the 1950s, twice-unsuccessful candidate for the Presidency. When Muffley negotiates with Premier Kissov over the hot line to Moscow, he appears ridiculous. After Kissov says Muffley should call the People's Central Air Defense Headquarters at Omsk, Muffley asks, "Listen, do you happen to have the phone number on you, Dmitri? . . . What? . . . I see, just ask for Omsk information." Muffley argues with Kissov about who is sorrier about the mistake, insisting that he can be just as sorry as Dmitri. Such small talk amidst the enormity of the crisis is ludicrous. By appearing both ridiculous and ineffectual, Muffley furthers Kubrick's nightmare comedy. For if the person who has the most rational strategy (and who also happens to be the commander in chief) is unable to control nuclear weapons and his military advisors, citizens really have something to worry about.

Although Dr. Strangelove does not speak until the last third of the film, the creators seem to have taken a great deal of care in creating Strangelove as a composite of a number of pundits in the new "science" of nuclear strategy. As a physicist involved in weapons research and development, he invites comparisons to Edward Teller. Not only was Teller involved in the creation of the atomic bomb, but he was also a strong anti-Communist who pushed hard for development of the much powerful hydrogen bomb in 1949 and 1950. In his background, accent, and some of his dialogue, Strangelove suggests Henry Kissinger. Like Kissinger, Strangelove came from Germany in the 1930s and still speaks with a German accent. With his wavy dark hair and sunglasses, he also bears a physical resemblance to Kissinger. Even his definition of deterrence—"the art of producing in the mind of the enemy the fear to attack you"—sounds remarkably like the definition Kissinger offered in his *Nuclear Weapons and Foreign Policy* (1957). Finally, Herman Kahn plays a part in the Strangelove composite, primarily as related to the Doomsday device. Strangelove tells the Pres-

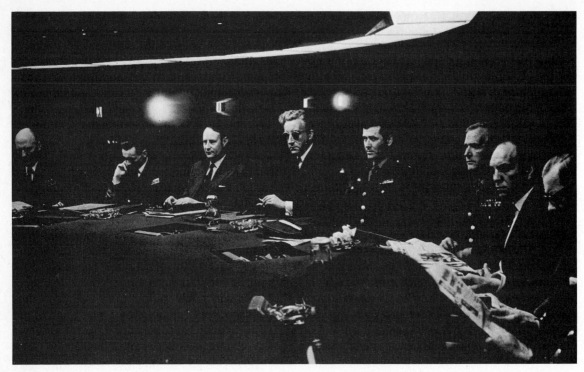

■ ■ *Stanley Kubrick's 1964 dark comedy Dr. Strangelove featured a mad nuclear strategist (played by Peter Sellers, shown in dark glasses) with unmistakable physical and speech resemblances to German scientists and geopoliticians, Nazi war criminals, and Washington D.C. think tank theorists.*

ident that he recently commissioned a study by the Bland corporation (Kahn worked for RAND) to examine the possibility of a Doomsday device. The study found the device technologically feasible; it would be hooked to a computer and programmed to detonate under certain prescribed circumstances. However, Strangelove found the machine impractical as a deterrent because it would go off even if an attack was accidental. All these details are similarly discussed in Kahn's *On Thermonuclear War*, with Kahn similarly concluding that though the device would contain most of the characterisitics of a deterrent, it would not meet the final characteristics of being controllable. As a mixture of Teller, Kissinger, and Kahn, and probably a number of others (Werner Von Braun is another possibility), Strangelove becomes a significant symbol. Es-

sentially, he is the coldly speculating mind, not unlike one of Nathaniel Hawthorne's calculating and obsessed scientists. Like them, Strangelove is devoid of fellow feeling. He proves this near the end of the film: even after the American B-52 gets through to bomb its target, Strangelove has ideas. He offers a plan to take all military and political leaders (along with attractive women at a ratio of ten women to one man) into a mine shaft in an effort to survive the virulent radioactivity produced by the Doomsday device. Clearly, none of the strategic postures presented by Kubrick—Turgidson's militarism, Muffley's tender-minded rationality, of Strangelove's constant speculations—are able to control the inexorable march of nuclear holocaust.

Although *2001* is more famous for its exploration of technology, Kubrick shows a fascination with machines in *Dr. Strangelove*. Most prominent is the stimulation of the B-52 cockpit, which Kubrick—after the Air Force denied him any assistance in making the film—had built from an unauthorized photograph he discovered in an aviation magazine. Throughout the B-52 scenes, Kubrick keeps viewer interest by alternating close-ups of various panel controls with shots of crew members expertly carrying out their orders. Besides those in the B-52, many other machines—telephones, radios, the electronic wall chart in the War Room—play important parts in the film.

Kubrick develops his attitude toward technology in *Dr. Strangelove* by making use of both machines of destruction and machines of communication; the problem in the film is that while people handle the machines of destruction with great alacrity, the more neutral machines of communication are either ineffectual or turned toward destructive purposes. Through a misuse of radio codes, Ripper sends the B-52s on their destructive mission; DeSadesky uses a camera to take pictures of the War Room, presumably for purposes of intelligence. When people try to use the neutral machines to prevent destruction, however, they prove to be ineffective. During President Muffley's call to Kissov, for example, social amenities and small talk hinder attempts to stop the B-52s, as does the slowness of the process. Likewise, when Mandrake tries to call the President after he has discovered the recall code, he cannot because he does not have a dime for the pay phone.

Though people can't use neutral machines effectively, they handle the machines of destruction with deadly efficiency. This includes not only the conventional weaponry at the Air Force base, where Army infantry and artillery attempt to take over the base, but also, more distressingly, the nuclear weapons. The whole crew of the B-52 expertly manipulate their machines, even after the explosion of an anti-aircraft missile damages the plane. Kong, to the dismay of the audience, shows great ingenuity in repairing damaged circuits in time to open the bomb doors

over the target. Kubrick is not really suggesting that machines are dominating men. Rather, he seems to perceive a human death instinct. Arising from a nearsighted rationality, this death instinct leads man first to create machines, then to use them for destroying human life. In questioning the "progress" inherent in technology, Kubrick was challenging a fundamental assumption of the dominant paradigm. This challenge to technology—both to the stress on technique in society and to the increasing importance of machines in modern life—was to become a dominant theme in the late 1960s, important in several works of social criticism during that era, including Theodore Roszak's *The Making of A Counter Culture* (1969), Lewis Mumford's *The Myth of the Machine: The Pentagon of Power* (1969), and Phillip Slater's *The Pursuit of Loneliness* (1970).

The film's final scene underlines Kubrick's attack on the Ideology of Liberal Consensus. Mushroom clouds billow on the screen, filling the sky, exuding both an awesome power and a perverse beauty. Simultaneously, a light, sentimental love song from the late 1940s—Vera Lynn's "We'll Meet Again"—provides a contrasting aural message in an excellent use of film irony. Its opening lines are: "We'll meet again, don't know where, don't know when, but I know we'll meet again some sunny day." If we go on with the world view of the postwar era, Kubrick ironically suggests, we will never meet again, because there will be no one left on earth. Retaining the conflict between image and sound throughout the final credit sequence, Kubrick hopes to prod his viewers to reflect on all that they have seen.

Taken as a whole, *Dr. Strangelove* fundamentally challenges the Ideology of Liberal Consensus by attacking anti-Communist paranoia, American adherence to outmoded notions of heroism, various nuclear strategies, and faith in social salvation through technological expertise. The Cold War foreign policy so strongly supported by Americans in the late 1940s and 1950s rested on the belief that America was a fundamentally just society threatened only by the germs of "Godless" Communism. *Dr. Strange-love*, though it certainly does nothing to imply that the Soviet leaders are any wiser than their American counterparts, suggests that no nation-state has a monopoly on foolishness and that the backstage strategies of military and political leaders are simply exercises in paranoia. The nightmare comedy presented a disturbing and deeply wrought challenge to America in 1963 and 1964.

The film would not be so important were it not so *un*characteristic in the way it treated the Cold War. The House Un-American Activities Committee investigated Hollywood in two waves, once in 1947 (resulting in the infamous Hollywood Ten trials) and later in the early 1950s. Hollywood responded not by fighting government interference—as it had in the mid-Thirties censorship controversies—but by coop-erating, blacklisting people who were suspected of leftist affiliations in the Thirties and making a spate of films which overtly or covertly support-ed the dominant paradigm.

The paradigm was overtly supported by a good number of anti-Communist melodramas from the late 1940s and early 1950s, of which *My Son John* (1952) may be the most famous example. These films were most popular between 1948 and 1953; in 1952 alone, twelve of them were released. Films about World War II, portraying the Nazis or the Japanese as vil-lians, tended also to divide the world into good (the Allies) and evil (the Axis powers) and thus to support the dominant paradigm. Here Kub-rick's anti-war *Paths of Glory* (1957) was clearly an anomaly. Even science fiction films, like *The Thing* (1951) or *War of the Worlds* (1952), by using threats from outer space as a metaphor of the Communist threat, covertly supported this conventional way of looking at and understand-ing the world. More directly related to *Dr. Strangelove* are a series of films through the 1950s and into the 1960s dealing with the bomb and especially with the Strategic Air Command.

Dr. Strangelove seems all the more amazing when one contrasts its iconoclasm and sharp sat-ire with *Above and Beyond* (1952), *Strategic Air Command* (1957), *Bombers B-52* (1957), *A Gath-ering of Eagles* (1963), and *Fail Safe* (1964). The first of these films concerns the story of Paul Tib-betts, commander of the group which actually dropped the first atomic bombs on Hiroshima and Nagasaki. Much of the story concerns Mrs. Tibbetts' gradual acceptance of her husband's secret yet important work. *Strategic Air Command* follows much the same vein. In it a major league baseball star and former World War II pilot, played by Jimmy Stewart, gives up the last years of his prime to return to active duty. Stewart's wife, at first upset at her husband's decision, realizes that it is necessary for the peace and well-being of the nation. Produced in the same year, *Bombers B-52* concerns a sergeant who resists the temptation to take a higher paying civilian job, and thus retains his wonderful exis-tence as an enlisted man.

Both *A Gathering of Eagles* and *Fail Safe* were released about the time of *Dr. Strangelove*, yet their approaches to their subjects are light years from that of *Strangelove*. General Curtis LeMay, commander of SAC, took a personal concern in *A Gathering of Eagles:* he stressed the need to explain how many safeguards had been created to prevent accidental war. The film concerns a young colonel who takes over a SAC wing that has failed a surprise alert and gradually trains his men so they are ever ready to go to war if the necessity arises. LeMay was pleased with the film, judging it "the closest any of [the Air Force films] ever came to showing the true picture of what the military was all about."

Fail Safe, released less than a year after *Dr. Strangelove*, at first seemed quite similar to *Dr. Strangelove* in that both films, nuclear weapons are detonated by accident. But *Fail Safe* does nothing to suggest, as *Strangelove* does, that national policy is ridiculous. Instead it portrays the President (Henry Fonda) as a responsible and competent man caught in a tragic, yet controllable circumstance. His decision—to obliterate New York City in exchange for the accidental destruction of Moscow—prevents the destruction of the world and is powerfully rendered without a touch of irony: in the final moments, we see freeze frames of people on New York streets just before the bomb explodes. Despite its powerful cinematic ending, the film is, as Julian Smith has suggested, "a morally and intellectually dangerous film because it simplifies and romanticizes the issues of national responsibility."

All these films present a common respect for national and military leaders. Though bad apples may show up occasionally, though accidents may cause some difficulties, each film ends with control being reestablished, the viewer reassured that the American way is the best course and that the military is doing the best job possible to shield us from the Communist menace. None hint, as does *Dr. Strangelove*, that we may need protection against ourselves.

A look at how reviewers and the public responded to *Dr. Strangelove* can give us some indication of how Kubrick's adversary views were accepted. Since a feature film most often must reinforce the cultural values and attitudes of its viewers if it expects to be popular, it is understandable that neither critics nor the public were swept away by the film. Though few critics of mass magazines or political journals panned the film, a number of them, thinking within the bounds of the dominant paradigm, came up with strange interpretations. The critic for the right-wing *National Review*, for example, suggested that *Dr. Strangelove's* theme was that all ideology should be abandoned. He went on to defend American ideology "with its roots thrust deep in Greek political thought," closing curiously with a hope that Kubrick might make a film criticizing Stalinism. *Saturday Review's* Hollis Alpert gave a generally favorable review, concluding with these comments: "No one thinks our ingeniously destructive world-destroying bombs are a laughing matter. Certainly director Kubrick doesn't. But on some fairly safe planet out of

view, maybe this is the way they would view our predicament." Alpert seems to miss Kubrick's point. No one accepting the dominant paradigm would see nuclear weapons as a laughing matter, but Kubrick, after studying the arms race, the Cold War, and the idea of deterrence carefully, realized the insanity of the situation and found that the only way he could possibly approach the material was through the satirical thrust of nightmare comedy. By having the audience laugh at the situation, he hoped not that they would realize its seriousness but rather that they would perceive its absurdity. Alpert, evidently, misunderstood the social rhetoric.

Two observers who thought highly of the film were Stanley Kauffmann and Lewis Mumford. Writing for *The New Republic*, Kauffmann—a critic notoriously harsh on most American films—thought *Dr. Strangelove* the best American film in fifteen years. The film showed "how mankind, its reflexes scored in its nervous system and its mind entangled in orthodoxies, insisted on destroying itself." This is a keen analysis: the entangling orthodoxies were those of the Liberal Consensus. Mumford's response to the film came in a letter to the *New York Times* defending the film, and he was as perceptive as anyone about the film's thrust when he wrote: "What the wacky characters in *Dr. Strangelove* are saying is precisely what needs to be said: this nightmare eventuality that we have concocted for our children is nothing but a crazy fantasy, by nature as horribly crippled and dehumanized as Dr. Strangelove himself. It is not this film that is sick: what is sick is our supposedly moral, democratic country which allowed this policy to be formulated and implemented without even the pretense of public debate." In a particularly acute comment, Mumford went on to argue that the film represented "the first break in the catatonic cold war trance that has so long held our country in its rigid grip." It is no surprise that Mumford, who had been a perceptive cultural critic of America at least since *The Golden Day* (1926), would later offer one of the most articulate criticisms of America's worship of technology in *The Pentagon of Power* (1969), still one of the most sensitive and persuasive studies of America to emerge during the late 1960s.

Like the critical observations, the box-office figures on *Dr. Strangelove* suggest a mixed response. Though figures for film rentals are notoriously rough, they seem to indicate that after doing a very stong business in New York and some other large cities, *Dr. Strangelove* slowed down and failed to live up to its early returns. It opened at the Victoria and the Baronet in New York, setting house records in the Baronet (an "art" theater) and providing the best business in years for the first week at the Victoria. Business remained strong at both theaters for at least nine weeks, yet when the final box-office tabulations were in for 1964, *Dr. Strangelove* ranked 14th, after such films as *The Carpet Baggers, It's a Mad . . . World, The Unsinkable Molly Brown, Charade, Good Neighbor Sam,* and *The Pink Panther*. Right above *Dr. Strangelove* in the 1964 box-office ratings was the Beatles/Richard Lester Production, *A Hard Day's Night,* which is at least symbolically significant. For what was beginning to happen in the film industry in the 1960s was that the audience for films was getting younger and more iconoclastic. Since *Dr. Strangelove* did very well in New York—the center for our cultural trendmakers—and not so well in smaller cities, the box-office figures seem to indicate that the adversary attitude toward dominant values expressed in films like *Dr. Strangelove* was still puzzling to many people in 1964. Nevertheless, this attitude was strangely attractive to those becoming disaffected with American society.

Dr. Strangelove is a watershed film. By rejecting the Ideology of Liberal Consensus through the iconoclastic perspective of nightmare comedy, it established a stance which was to become widespread in American movies in the late 1960s. Its alternating tone of comedy and horror was to reappear in *Bonnie and Clyde* and *Little Big Man*. Its critical attitude toward dominant social values was to be expanded in *The Graduate, Easy Rider,* and *Five Easy Pieces*. Its disdain for military leaders and war found its way to *M*A*S*H*. Its notion that technological change was not necessarily social progress appeared in such diverse films as *Butch Cassidy and the Sundance Kid, McCabe and Mrs. Miller,* and *A Clockwork Orange*. Its importance as a groundbreaking film in the history of American movies can hardly be overestimated.

Yet the film is also important in a broader cultural sense. Lionel Trilling once wrote that at its base, art is a criticism of life. *Dr. Strangelove,* in the way it attacks the "crackpot realism" of American culture in the 1950s and early 1960s, is as important a cultural document as the Port Huron Statement of 1962, Martin Luther King's "I Have a Dream" speech at the March on Washington in 1963, Herbert Marcuse's *One-Dimensional Man* (1964), or Malcolm X's *Autobiography* (1965). Anyone seeking to understand the breakdown of the American consensus in the early and mid-1960s, and the new iconoclasm which was challenging it, can learn a good deal from the nightmare comedy of *Dr. Strangelove*.

■ ■ ■

STUDY QUESTIONS

1. Describe the "Liberal Consensus" which the film rejects. What were its origins? How does the film attack this idea?

2. How significant was the fear of Communism in the United States during the 1950s and early 1960s?

3. One of Kubrick's criticisms of nuclear policy in the late 1950s and early 1960s was that it seemed to be based on premises from earlier wars. How did Kubrick express that idea in the film?

4. Stanley Kubrick was particularly concerned that too many Americans believed a nuclear war was "winnable." Why did that concept concern him? Do you agree with Kubrick? Why or why not? How does Kubrick express his conviction that nuclear war is not "winnable"?

5. The film is laced with sexual metaphors. Give some examples of those metaphors and explain why Kubrick used them.

6. Describe the character of Dr. Strangelove. The character is a composite figure of several people. Who are those people and why did Kubrick compose the character around them?

BIBLIOGRAPHY

For a good introduction to the history of the Cold War see Walter LaFeber, *America, Russia, and the Cold War* (1980). On the origins of the Cold War, see John L. Gaddis, *The United States and the Origins of the Cold War* (1972), and Daniel Yergin, *Shattered Peace* (1977). Robert Divine, *Eisenhower and the Cold War* (1981), describes the immediate foreign policy background to the production of *Dr. Strangelove*. An excellent discussion of the origins of American nuclear policy is Norman Moss, *Men Who Play God: The Story of the H-Bomb and How the World Came to Live With It* (1968). For books on the strategy of nuclear war, which Kubrick found particularly frightening, see Henry Kissinger, *Nuclear War and Foreign Policy* (1957), and Herman Kahn, *On Thermonuclear War* (1961). Stanley Kubrick's career is described in Norman Kagan, *The Cinema of Stanley Kubrick* (1972), and Gene Phillips, *Stanley Kubrick: A Film Odyssey* (1975).

THE WOUNDED GENERATION: THE TWENTY-SEVEN MILLION MEN OF VIETNAM

Lawrence M. Baskir and William A. Strauss

The American quagmire in Southeast began quietly in 1965 when United States infantry went to South Vietnam. Sporadic antiwar demonstrations began shortly thereafter. In those first months, people had no idea of the catastrophe looming ahead. The challenge seemed simple. Aggressive Communist forces, led by dictator Ho Chi Minh but orchestrated by an international Soviet conspiracy, were bent on crushing the democratic government of South Vietnam. And just as in Greece and Turkey in 1946 and Korea in 1950, the United States committed its resources to stem the tide of Communist aggression. South Vietnam was a little country filled with little people, and President Lyndon Johnson and most of his military advisers anticipated a brief "police action" and an overwhelming victory. After all, who in the world could stand up to American military power?

Three years later, after the famous Tet offensive of 1968, Lyndon Johnson announced his decision not to seek reelection. National outrage over the war was so intense that his chances for political redemption were nonexistent. The Viet Cong and North Vietnamese were proving to be tenacious adversaries, while the South Vietnamese were often unreliable and corrupt. Tens of thousands of American soldiers were dead, hundreds of thousands wounded, and millions more psychologically affected by the war. At home, millions of other Americans lost faith in their own leaders and became disillusioned about the American destiny. In the steaming jungles of South Vietnam, Americans confronted the underside of their history. Self-righteously committed to the export of American values, United States policymakers had confused communism with nationalism, applying a Cold War formula to an internal rebellion. In the process, the United States became the enemy, not only to the Viet Cong and North Vietnamese, but to most of the world, including tens of millions of its own citizens. In "The Wounded Generation," Lawrence M. Baskir and William A. Strauss assess the toll exacted by the war.

When John F. Kennedy was inaugurated President on January 20, 1961, the new President told the nation and the world that "the torch has been passed to a new generation of Americans," under whose leadership America would "pay any price, bear any burden . . . to assure the survival and the success of liberty." These were brave words, very well received.

This "new generation," described by Kennedy as "tempered by war, disciplined by a hard and bitter peace," consisted of World War II veterans then in their late thirties and forties. Their "best and brightest" would later steer the nation through a very different, much more controversial war in Vietnam. Yet this time it was not they who had to do the fighting. Fewer than five hundred members of this generation died in Southeast Asia, most from accident, disease, and other causes which had nothing to do with combat. The rest helped pay the taxes to finance this $165-billion venture. It was their children, the baby-boom generation—the product of an enormous jump in the birth rate between 1946 and 1953—who paid the real price in Vietnam.

Fifty-three million Americans came of age during the Vietnam War. Roughly half were women, immune from the draft. Only six thousand women saw military duty in Vietnam, none in combat. But as sisters, girl friends, and wives, millions of draft-age women paid a heavy share of the emotional cost of the war.

For their male counterparts, the war had devastating consequences. Twenty-six million eight hundred thousand men came of draft age between August 4, 1964, when the Tonkin Gulf Resolution marked the nation's formal entry into the war, and March 28, 1973, when the last American troops left. Fifty-one thousand died in Vietnam—17,000 from gunshot wounds, 7,500 from multiple fragmentation wounds, 6,750

"The Wounded Generation: The 27,000,000 Men of Vietnam" by Lawrence M. Baskir and William A. Strauss, *American Heritage 29* (April/May, 1978). Reprinted by permission.

from grenades and mines, 10,500 from other enemy action, 8,000 from "nonhostile" causes, and 350 by suicide. Another 270,000 were wounded, 21,000 of whom were disabled. Roughly 5,000 lost one or more limbs in the war. A half-million were branded as criminals. More than two million served in the war zone. Millions had their futures shaped by the threat of going to war.

These were the sons of parents reunited after a long but victorious war, parents who, in columnist George Will's description, "were anxious to turn from the collective task of history-making to the private task of family-making. Like Studebakers and toothpaste, the next batch of children would be 'new and improved.' " Having themselves faced depression and war, this generation of parents wanted their children to know nothing but peace and prosperity. As William Manchester noted in *The Glory and the Dream*, their offspring would be "adorable as babies, cute as grade school pupils, and striking as they entered their teens. After high school they would attend the best colleges and universities in the country, where their parents would be very, very proud of them." The children were the Dr. Spock generation, the Sputnik generation, and eventually the Woodstock generation. But above all else, they became the Vietnam generation.

As children and teen-agers, they had grown accustomed to the existence of the draft. Some looked forward to military service as an exciting and potentially valuable experience—a chance to demonstrate their manhood, serve their country, and get some adventure before settling down. Others saw the draft as an unpleasant, but nonetheless tolerable demand on two years of their lives. Many, especially those from well-to-do families, looked upon the draft as something to avoid, an unwelcome interference with their personal plans. But most never thought much about it. Consciously or unconsciously, they put the draft out of their minds; it was something that happened to someone else, never to them.

But when the generation and the Vietnam War collided, the draft became of pre-eminent

concern. In 1966 a survey of high school sopho-
mores found that only seven per cent mentioned
the draft or Vietnam as one of "the problems
young men your age worry about most." But
when the same question was asked of the same
individuals after their high school graduation in
1969, that number had grown to 75 per cent.
Few nineteen- to twenty-six-year-olds were
eager to risk their lives in Vietnam. Many saw
the draft as a means of coercing them to fight a
war they found politically or morally repugnant.
To others, the war simply had no meaning.

Although only six per cent of all young men
were needed to fight, the Vietnam draft cast the
entire generation into a contest for individual
survival. The draft was not, however, an arbi-
trary and omnipotent force, imposing itself like
blind fate upon men who were powerless to
resist. Instead, it worked as an instrument of
Darwinian social policy. The "fittest"—those
with background, wit, or money—generally
managed to escape. Through an elaborate structure of deferments, exemptions, legal technicali-
ties, and noncombat military alternatives, the
draft rewarded those who manipulated the system to their advantage.

For most of the members of this generation,
fighting for one's country was not a source of
pride; it was misfortune. Going to Vietnam was
the penalty for those who lacked the wherewith-
al to avoid it. A 1971 Harris survey found that
most Americans believed that those who went to
Vietnam were "suckers, having risked their lives
in the wrong war, in the wrong place, at the
wrong time."

Much of this sentiment reflected the public's
growing disenchantment with American involvement in Vietnam. The outspoken antiwar
views of many young people helped sway public
opinion and turn around the nation's policies.
Their activism often involved moral courage, but
little concreted sacrifice. Except for occasional
individuals who, on principle, abandoned deferments and exemptions to go to prison or take
exile, opposing the war was in every draft-age
man's self-interest. The sooner the war ended,

the less likely it was that he would bear personal
hardship.

This sense of self-interest was best illustrated
by the attitude of antiwar collegians toward their
student deferments. Harvard College graduate
James Glassman recalled that in 1966, before the
draft calls began to rise, "students complained
that the system was highly discriminatory, favor-
ing the well-off. They called the 2-S [the student
deferment] an unfair advantage for those who
could go to college." But as the war escalated,
"the altruism was forgotten. What was most
important now was saving your own skin." In
1967, when graduate school deferments were
abolished, the Harvard *Crimson* published an editorial entitled "The Axe Falls," accusing the government of "careless expediency" which was
"clearly unfair to students."

Many students defended their deferments—
and their draft avoidance—with a measure of
class arrogance. A Rhodes scholar, now a corporate lawyer, observed that "there are certain
people who can do more good in a lifetime in
politics or academics or medicine than by getting
killed in a trench." A University of Michigan student commented that "if I lost a couple of years,
it would mean $16,000 to me. I know I sound
selfish, but, by God, I paid $10,000 to get this
education."

These attitudes were shared by millions of
draft-age men with other deferments and
exemptions. "I got a good steady job," a Dela-
ware defense worker said. "I'm making good
money and having a ball every weekend. Why
the hell should I want to go?" Why indeed?
Vietnam veterans were held in little esteem, and
the fate of the nation hardly lay in the balance.

"The result," as former Yale University President Kingman Brewster noted, was "a cynical
avoidance of service, a corruption of the aims of
education, a tarnishing of the national spirit, . . .
and a cops and robbers view of national obligation." Avoiding Vietnam became a generation-
wide preoccupation. According to a Notre Dame
survey, approximately fifteen million (60 per

cent) of the draft-age men who did not see actual combat took positive steps to help fate along. More than half of all men who escaped the draft, and almost half of all servicemen who escaped combat, believe today that the actions they took were wholly or partly responsible for keeping them away from the fighting.

Avoiding Vietnam did not necessarily mean emerging unscathed. For one in four, it meant hurried marriages, unwanted children, misdirected careers, or self-inflicted physical impairments. But millions emerged untouched, triumphant in what New Orleans draft counselor Collins Vallee called a "victory over the government." They never went to war, and they never faced the costly alternatives of prison, exile, or court-martial.

Avoidance was available to everyone. Ghetto youths side-stepped the draft by failing to register. High school dropouts married and had children. Young workingmen sought "critical" occupations. But by far the greatest number of escape routes were open to youths from privileged backgrounds. Through educational, employment, or hardship deferments, physical exemptions, or safe enlistments, they had little difficulty staying far from Vietnam. Even doctors, who were subject to special draft calls, were seldom involved in the war. Fewer than one of every ten medical school graduates were drafted; many of the rest found refuge in the National Institute of Health, the Public Health Service, or the reserves.

The young men who fought and died in Vietnam were primarily society's "losers," the same men who get left behind in school, jobs, and the rest of life's competition. The discriminatory social, economic, and racial impact of Vietnam cannot be fairly measured against other wars in American history, but certainly the American people were never before so conscious of how unevenly the obligation to serve was distributed. Few of the nation's elite had sons or close friends who did any fighting. Professor and critic Leslie Fiedler, commenting about his university community, wrote that he "had never known a sin-

gle family that had lost a son in Vietnam, or indeed, one with a son wounded, missing in action, or held prisoner of war. And this despite the fact that American casualties in Vietnam are already almost equal to those of World War I. Nor am I alone in my strange plight: in talking to friends about a subject they seem eager not to discuss, I discover they can, they must, all say the same. . . ."

Racial inequities became a major scandal of the late 1960's. The late General S.L.A. Marshall commented that he had seen "too many of our battalions come out of line after hard struggle and heavy loss. In the average rifle company, the strength was 50 per cent composed of Negroes, Southwestern Mexicans, Puerto Ricans, Guamanians, Nisei, and so on. But a real cross-section of American youth? Almost never."

At the end of World War II, blacks composed 12 per cent of all combat troops; by the start of the Vietnam War, their share had grown to 31 per cent. In 1965 blacks accounted for 24 per cent of all Army combat deaths. The Defense Department undertook a concerted campaign to reduce the minorities' share of the fighting. That share was reduced to 16 per cent in 1966, 13 percent in 1968. In 1970 the figure for all services was under 9 per cent.

Throughout the course of the war, minorities unquestionably did more than their share of the fighting and dying. Yet the most serious inequities were social and economic. Poorly educated, low-income whites and poorly educated, low-income blacks together bore a vastly disproportionate share of the burdens of Vietnam. The Notre Dame survey found that men from disadvantaged backgrounds were about twice as likely as their better-off peers to serve in the military, go to Vietnam, and see combat. These were the men President Eisenhower once called "sitting ducks" for the draft.

During the war, the government never undertook any studies of the social and economic incidence of military service. The only contemporary evidence was scattered and anecdotal. A 1965–66 survey discovered that college graduates made up only 2 per cent of all draftees. Congressman Alvin O'Konski took a personal survey of one hundred inductees from his northern Wisconsin district. Not one of them came from a family with an annual income of over five thousand dollars. A Harvard *Crimson* editor from the class of 1970 tallied his twelve hundred classmates and counted only fifty-six who entered the military, just two of whom went to Vietnam. By contrast, thirty-five men from the Harvard class of 1941 died in World War II, and hundreds more saw combat duty. Not many Vietnam-era troops were college graduates, and even the relatively few who joined the service had a better-than-normal chance of avoiding Vietnam.

After the war was over, however, the evidence began to mount. Postwar Army records showed that an enlisted man who was a college graduate had a 42 per cent chance of going to Vietnam, versus a 64 per cent chance for a high school graduate and a 70 per cent chance for a high school dropout. Surveys in Long Island, Wisconsin, and Salt Lake City found a very heavy incidence of combat deaths among disadvantaged youths. In the most significant study thus far, sociologists Gilbert Badillo and David Curry analyzed casualties suffered by Chicago neighborhoods with different socioeconomic characteristics. They discovered that youths from low-income neighborhoods were three times as likely to die in Vietnam as youths from high-income neighborhoods. They also found youths from neighborhoods with low educational levels to be four times as likely to die in Vietnam as youths from better-educated neighborhoods.

During World War II, conscription and combat service were matters of personal honor. Men bent the rules to get into military service. Patriotism knew no class boundaries; Winthrop Rockefeller and the president of the New York Stock Exchange were among the first ten thousand to submit voluntarily to induction. Returning veterans were public heroes. But among the tragic ironies of Vietnam was the fact that the only real heroes of the war were POW's. Most were not members of the younger generation;

they were Air Force and Navy pilots, officers well beyond draft age. Returning combat troops were easily forgotten.

America was not winning the war, and many people were ashamed of what was happening. With the war calling into question so much of America's self-esteem, and with so many young men resisting the war, the nation needed assurance that patriotism still had meaning. Draft resisters and deserters thus became the folk villians of the times. John Geiger of the American Legion spoke for a great many Americans when he called these young men "a mixture of victims of error, deliberate conspirators, and professional criminals." Their detractors insisted that their numbers were small—Richard Nixon referred to them as "those few hundreds"—and that the judicial system dealt with them swiftly and severely. None of this was true, but it helped reaffirm traditional values.

The national conscience was also salved by comparing the cowardice of draft resisters and deserters with the courage of combat soldiers. This helped blind the nation to the fact that twenty-five million draft-age men did not serve in Vietnam, and that relatively few Americans were touched directly by the sacrifices of those two million who did.

After the fighting was over, draft resisters and deserters served one last, tragic purpose. They became scapegoats—much like Eddie Slovik, the only soldier executed for desertion in World War II. Slovik was a weak man, a misfit totally incapable of being a combat soldier. He performed so poorly in basic training that his commanding officer tried, without success, to get him discharged or transferred to a noncombat unit. Slovik never actually ran away, but he confessed to desertion as a way of staying out of the fighting. On the day of his execution, a few months before the end of the war, Slovik told a reporter: "They are not shooting me for deserting the U.S. Army. Thousands of guys have done that. They just need to make an example out of somebody, and I'm it."

In the same way, those who feel a deep, unarticulated resentment about what happened in Vietnam have made whipping boys of the draft resisters and deserters. They are the ones to blame for the tragedy of a lost war and lost illusions, symbols of the nation's lack of resolve to win. For those who condemn the anti-authoritarian values of the generation, the resisters and deserters represent the worst of a bad lot. For those who suffered personal tragedies in the war, these are the men who should have gone in place of loved ones.

As important a symbol as the draft resisters and deserters have been, Americans know little about them. They are, like the Vietnam combat veterans, society's losers—disproportionately black, poorly educated youths from low-income families. Had they been better advised or more clever, most could have found one of the escape routes used by so many others. The disadvantaged not only did more than their share of the fighting; they also have paid much of the penalty for not fighting.

Vietnam-era draft and military offenders number more than a million. An estimated 570,000 men committed draft violations that could have sent them to prison for five years. Yet fewer than half were reported to federal prosecutors, 25,000 were indicted, and fewer than 9,000 convicted. Only 3,250 went to prison, most of whom were paroled within a year. In the military, a quarter of a million men were punished with Undesirable, Bad Conduct, or Dishonorable Discharges, branding them as deserters or military criminals of other sorts. Yet only 13 per cent of them were convicted by court-martial, and even they seldom spent more than a few months in prison. Another 300,000 sevicemen were sent home with General Discharges which label their service as less than fully honorable and handicap their ability to find jobs.

A great many escaped the brunt of the law because of legal or administrative problems. Over 100,000 draft cases were dismissed because of draft boards' failure to obey court-imposed rules. The overburdened military justice system gave 130,000 servicemen Undesirable Dis-

charges as plea bargains, sparing the armed forces the expense of trying and imprisoning them. But in part, this leniency reflected the views of many prosecutors, judges, and military officers that these individuals did not deserve the stiff punishments the public thought they were getting.

It would be inaccurate to say that the "evaders," as a group, did anything fundamentally worse than their twenty-four million peers who also escaped Vietnam, but by legal means. The term "evader" says little about each individual's attitude toward his responsibility to serve in the military. A great many men who legally avoided combat service would have been evaders had the necessity arisen; the Notre Dame survey found that 15 per cent of all draft avoiders would have seriously considered breaking the law if that had been their only recourse. As one resister commented, "Almost every kid in this country [was] either a draft evader, a potential draft evader, or a failed draft evader." According to Michael Brophy, a Milwaukee draft counselor, the epithet had been misapplied: "To evade is to avoid something by deceitful means. The draft evaders are in the Reserves and the National Guard, seminaries, and other educational institutions. . . . A man who [breaks the law] may do so to avoid the draft, but he is not deceiving anyone."

The opprobrium of "evader" is inappropriate for large categories of Vietnam-era offenders. About one-third of all draft resisters could have avoided the draft through deferments, exemptions, and legal loopholes, but they insisted on accepting exile or punishment as the consequence of their beliefs. One-fifth of all deserters never evaded Vietnam service. They finished full combat tours before running afoul of military discipline back home, often because of postcombat readjustment problems.

The law has worked its will on the offenders. By the mid-1970's all but a few thousand had paid the legal price of their actions. They were prosecuted, punished, and officially forgiven. Still, the question remains whether the American people will continue to condemn them.

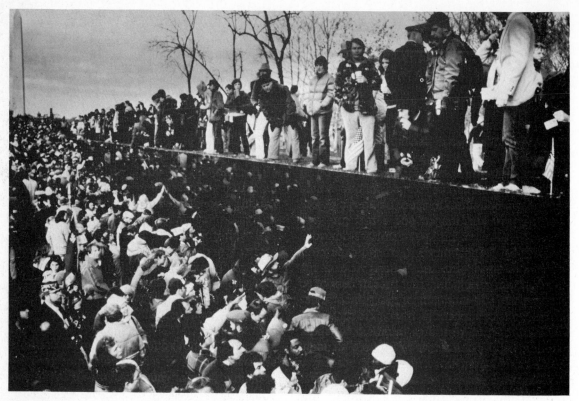

■ ■ *When the last helicopter left Saigon in 1975, Americans suffered a kind of collective amnesia about the Vietnam War. It took ten years to erect a national monument, shown here, to honor those who served in the war.*

Until Americans evaluate the conduct of these men in the context of the entire generation's response to the war, there can never be any real understanding of the tragedy of Vietnam. The memory of the war may be too bitter for anyone to be cast as a hero. But perhaps the American people can begin to understand the extent to which so many young men, veterans and law-breakers alike, were victims. And, with the passage of time, critics of the generation may stop setting victim against victim, fixing blame that only exacerbates the tragedy of the war.

Vietnam wrought havoc on millions of lives in a manner which most Americans may never understand. The war was, at root, the personal calamity of the generation called upon to fight it. They are the ones who faced the terrible choices, and they are the ones who suffered. "You were

damned if you did go and damned if you didn't," said Ursula Diliberto, whose son was killed in Vietnam two weeks before the end of his tour. "My son was a victim, my family was a victim, all boys of draft age were victims in one way or another."

The members of the Vietnam generation are now in their late twenties and thirties. Vietnam was and always will be their war, just as World War II belonged to their parents, and World War I to their grandparents. The war stories of older generations—stories about mustard gas, Guadalcanal, or the liberation of little French towns—have little meaning for those who came of age during Vietnam. . . . These twenty-seven million men have their own stories, but they are seldom told with pride. Their battles were with the police, their narrow escapes involved draft boards and courts, and the enemy was their own government. Some feel guilty, others lucky. Many have a faint sense of disquiet from having been involved but not really involved, from having left the fighting and dying to others.

The war affected them in complex ways, but it engendered a strong sense of kinship. Vietnam was a crisis they all faced—whether in the barracks, on the campus, or in the streets. Unlike other Americans, most members of the Vietnam generation seem reluctant to judge a man by his personal response to the war. They feel that the labels—sucker, opportunist, evader, deserter—are part of the tragedy of Vietnam.

■ ■ ■

STUDY QUESTIONS

1. Describe the ''baby-boom'' generation which ended up with fighting and dying in Vietnam.

2. How did this generation view the draft? How were their opinions about military service different from those of their parents? Why were their views different?

3. Explain the major reasons why so many young men tried to avoid military service. What groups of Americans actually served in Vietnam?

4. Describe the racial dimensions of service in Vietnam.

5. Did the burden of service fall equitably on all Americans? Why or why not?

6. Of the 570,000 men who violated draft laws during the Vietnam War, how many actually served prison terms? Why was the number so few? Should more of them have been prosecuted and imprisoned? Why or why not?

BIBLIOGRAPHY

A number of books have recently appeared detailing the history of the American involvement in Southeast Asia. An indispensable primary source is *The Pentagon Papers,* which now exists in a number of editions. David Halberstam's *The Best and the Brightest* (1972), is an excellent journalistic account of American public life in the 1960s. For views of the Vietnam War which attempt to justify the American commitment there, see Guenter Lewy, *America in Vietnam* (1972), and Norman Podhoretz, *Why We Were in Vietnam* (1982). For a discussion of the draft during the Vietnam War, see Lawrence H. Baskir and William Strauss, *Chance and Circumstance* (1978). Domestic opposition to the war is described in Thomas Powers, *The War at Home* (1973), and Irwin Unger, *The Movement* (1974). For the best general studies of the Vietnam War, see Francis Fitzgerald, *Fire in the Lake* (1972); George Herring, *The Longest War* (1979); and Stanley Karnow, *Vietnam* (1982).

THE ELVIS PRESLEY PHENOMENON

Greil Marcus

Elvis. His last name is used only to give balance to his first. There is no need to use it as a point of identification. The history of rock'n'roll is the story of a series of overnight wonders, performers who rose fast, achieved momentary fame, and then drifted into obscurity, only to be revived years later on golden oldies concerts. But not Elvis Presley. His fame lasted. Even his death has not diminished it. He was one of a kind.

Why? He didn't discover or invent rock'n'roll. He wasn't the first white singer to blur the lines between race and hillbilly music. Elvis's career took off in 1956. Five years earlier, disc jockey Alan Freed began his "Moon-dog's Rock-and-Roll Party" on station WJW in Cleveland. Several years before anyone heard of Elvis, Bill Haley and the Comets reached the Top Ten with "Rock Around the Clock." But Elvis was different, and he was better.

Elvis defies easy description. He was modest and soft-spoken, shy around women and deferential to his elders. He was raised in the shadow of the Pentecostal First Assembly of God Church, and gospels were the first songs he sang. "He grew up," noted one music critic, "schooled in all the classic virtues of small-town America: diffident, polite, sirring and ma'aming his elders. . . ." But there was another side to Elvis, a wild impulsive side. On stage, his movements shocked middle-class white America, and his voice was hungry and sensual. In the following selection, Greil Marcus beautifully describes the culture and times that produced Elvis.

They called Elvis the Hillbilly Cat in the beginning; he came out of a stepchild culture (in the South, white trash; to the rest of America, a caricature of Bilbo and moonshine) that for all it shared with the rest of America had its own shape and integrity. As a poor white Southern boy, Elvis created a personal culture out of the hillbilly world that was his as a given. Ultimately, he made that personal culture public in such an explosive way that he transformed not only his own culture, but America's. I want to look at that hillbilly landscape for a bit—to get a sense of how Elvis drew on his context.

It was, as Southern chambers of commerce have never tired of saying, A Land of Contrasts. The fundamental contrast, of course, could not have been more obvious: black and white. Always at the root of Southern fantasy, Southern music, and Southern politics, the black man was poised in the early fifties for an overdue invasion of American life, in fantasy, music, and politics. As the North scurried to deal with him, the South would be pushed farther and farther into the weirdness and madness its best artists had been trying to exorcise from the time of Poe on down. Its politics would dissolve into night-riding and hysteria; its fantasies would be dull for all their gaudy paranoia. Only the music got away clean.

The North, powered by the Protestant ethic, had set men free by making them strangers; the poor man's South that Elvis knew took strength from community.

The community was based on a marginal economy that demanded cooperation, loyalty, and obedience for the achievement of anything resembling a good life; it was organized by religion, morals, and music. Music helped hold the community together, and carried the traditions and shared values that dramatized a sense of place. Music gave pleasure, wisdom, and shelter.

"It's the only place in the country I've ever been where you can actually drive down the highway at night, and if you listen, you hear music," Robbie Robertson once said. "I don't know if it's coming from the people or if it's coming from the air. It lives, and it's rooted there." Elegant enough, but I prefer another comment Robbie made. "The South," he said, "is the only place we play where evertbody can clap on the off-beat."

Music was also an escape from the community, and music revealed its underside. There were always people who could not join, no matter how they might want to: tramps, whores, rounders, idiots, criminals. The most vital were singers: not the neighbors who brought out their fiddles and guitars for country picnics, as Elvis used to do, or those who sang in church, as he did also, but the professionals. They were men who bridged the gap between the community's sentimentalized idea of itself, and the outside world and the forbidden; artists who could take the community beyond itself because they had the talent and the nerve to transcend it. Often doomed, traveling throughout the South enjoying sins and freedoms the community had surrendered out of necessity or never known at all, they were ambitious, ornery, or simply different to fit in.

The Carter Family, in the twenties, were the first to record the old songs everyone knew, to make the shared musical culture concrete, and their music drew a circle around the community. They celebrated the landscape (especially the Clinch Mountains that ringed their home), found strength in a feel for death because it was the only certainty, laughed a bit, and promised to leave the hillbilly home they helped build only on a gospel ship. Jimmie Rodgers, their contemporary, simply hopped a train. He was every boy who ever ran away from home, hanging out in the railroad yards, bumming around with black minstrels, pushing out the limits of his life. *He* celebrated long tall mamas that rubbed his back and licked his neck just to cure the cough that killed him; he bragged about gunplay on Beale Street; he sang real blues, played jazz with Louis Armstrong, and though there was melancholy in his soul, his smile was a good one. He sounded like a man who could make a home for himself anywhere. There's so much *room* in this country, he seemed to be saying, so many things to do— how could an honest man be satisfied to live within the frontiers he was born to?

Outside of the community because of the way they lived, the singers were tied to it as symbols of its secret hopes, of its fantasies of escape and union with the black man, of its fears of transgressing the moral and social limits that promised peace of mind. Singers could present the extremes of emotion, risk, pleasure, sex, and violence that the community was meant to control; they were often alcoholic or worse, lacking a real family, drifters in a world where roots were life. Sometimes the singer tantalized the community with his outlaw liberty; dying young, he finally justified the community by his inability to survive outside of it. More often than not, the singer's resistance dissolved into sentiment. Reconversion is the central country music comeback strategy, and many have returned to the fold after a brief fling with the devil, singing songs of virtue, fidelity, and God, as if to prove that sin only hid a deeper piety—or that there was no way out.

By the late forties and early fifties, Hank Williams had inherited Jimmie Rodgers' role as the central figure in the music, but he added an enormous reservation: that margin of loneliness in Rodgers' America had grown into a world of utter tragedy. Williams sang for a community to which he could not belong; he sang to God in whom he could not quite believe; even his many songs of good times and good lovin' seemed to lose their reality. There were planty of jokes in his repertoire, novelties like "Kawliga" (the tale of unrequited love between two cigar store Indians); he traveled Rodgers' road, but for Wil-

liams, that road was a lost highway. Beneath the surface of his forced smiles and his light, easy sound, Hank Williams was kin to Robert Johnson in a way that the new black singers of his day were not. Their music, coming out of New Orleans, out of Sam Phillips' Memphis studio and washing down from Chicago, was loud, fiercely electric, rausous, bleeding with lust and menace and loss. The rhythmic force that was the practical legacy of Robert Johnson had evolved into a music that overwhelmed *his* reservations; the rough spirit of the new blues, city R&B, rolled right over his nihilism. Its message was clear: "What life doesn't give me, I'll take."

Hank Williams was a poet of limits, fear, and failure; he went as deeply into one dimension of the country world as anyone could, gave it beauty, gave it dignity. What was missing was that part of the hillbilly soul Rodgers had celebrated, something Williams' music obscured, but which his realism could not express and the community's moralism could not contain: excitement, rage, fantasy, delight—the feeling, summed up in a sentence by W. J. Cash from *The Mind of the South*, that "even the Southern physical world was a kind of cosmic conspiracy against reality in favor of romance"; that even if Elvis's South was filled with Puritans, it was also filled with natural-born hedonists, and the same people were both.

To lie on his back for days and weeks [Cash writes of the hillbilly], storing power as the air he breathed stores power under the hot sun of August, and then to explode, as that air explodes in a thunderstorm, in a violent outburst of emotion—in such a fashion would he make life not only tolerable, but infinitely sweet.

In the fifties we can hardly find that moment in white music, before Elvis. Hank Williams was not all there was to fifties country, but his style was so pervasive, so effective, carrying so much weight, that it closed off the possibilities of breaking loose just as the new black music helped open them up. Not his gayest tunes, not

"Move It on Over," "Honky Tonkin'," or "Hey Good Lookin'," can match this blazing passage from Cash, even if those songs share its subject:

To go into the town on Saturday afternoon and night, to stroll with the throng, to gape at the well-dressed and the big automobiles, to bathe in the holiday cacaphony . . . maybe to have a drink, maybe to get drunk, to laugh with the passing girls, to pick them up if you had a car, or to go swaggering or hesitating into the hotels with the corridors saturated with the smell of bicloride of mercury, or the secret, steamy bawdy houses; maybe to have a fight, maybe against the cops, maybe to end, whooping and goddamning, in the jailhouse. . . .

The momentum is missing; that will to throw yourself all the way after something better with no real worry about how you are going to make it home. And it was this spirit, full-blown and bragging, that was to find its voice in Elvis's new blues and the rockabilly fever he kicked off all over the young white South. Once Elvis broke down the door, dozens more would be fighting their way through. Out of nowhere there would be Carl Perkins, looking modest enough and sounding for all the world as if he was having fun for the first time in his life, chopping his guitar with a new kind of urgency and yelling: "Now Dan got happy, and he started ravin'"—He jerked out his razor but he wasn't shavin.' "

Country music (like the blues, which was more damned and more honestly hedonistic than country had ever been) was the music for a whole community, cutting across lines of age, if not class. This could have meant an openly expressed sense of diversity for each child, man, and woman, as it did with the blues. But country spoke to a community fearful of anything of the sort, withdrawing into itself, using music as a bond that linked all together for better or for worse, with a sense that what was shared was less important the crucial fact of sharing. How could parents hope to keep their children if their

kids' whole sense of what it meant to live—which is what we get from music when we are closest to it—held promises the parents could never keep?

The songs of country music, and most deeply, its even narrow sound, had to subject the children to the heartbreak of their parents: the father who couldn't feed his family, the wife who lost her husband to a honky-tonk angel or a bottle, the family that lost everything to a suicide or a farm spinning off into one more bad year, the horror of loneliness in a world that was meant to banish that if nothing else. Behind that uneasy grin, this is Hank Williams' America; the romance is only a night call.

Such a musical community is beautiful, but it is not hard to see how it could be intolerable. All that hedonism was dragged down in country music; a deep sense of fear and resignation confined it, as perhaps it almost had to, in a land overshadowed by fundamentalist religion, where original sin was just another name for the facts of life.

Now, that Saturday night caught by Cash and Perkins would get you through a lot of weekdays. Cash might close it off—"Emptied of their irritations and repressions, left to return to their daily tasks, stolid, unlonely, and tame again"—and he's right, up to a point. This wasn't any revolution, no matter how many cops got hurt keeping the peace on Saturday night. Regardless of what a passport to that Southern energy (detached from the economics and religion that churned it up) might do for generations of restless Northern and British kids, there is no way that energy can be organized. But the fact that Elvis and the rest could trap its spirit and send it out over a thousand radio transmitters is a central fact of more lives than mine; the beginning of most of the stories in this book, if nothing near the end of them.

For we are treading on the key dividing line that made Elvis *King of Western Bop* (they went through a lot of trouble finding a name for this

music) instead of just another country crooner or
a footnote in someone's history of the blues: the
idea (and it was just barely an ''idea'') that Saturday night could be the whole show. You had
to be young and a bit insulated to pull it off, but
why not? Why not trade pain and boredom for
kicks and style? Why not make an escape from a
way of life—the question trails off the last page
of *Huckleberry Finn*—into a way of life?

You might not get revered for all time by
everyone from baby to grandma, like the Carter
Family, but you'd have more fun. Reality would
catch up sooner or later—a pregnant girlfriend
and a fast marriage, the farm you had to take
over when your daddy died, a dull and pointless
job that drained your desires until you could
barely remember them—but why deal with reality before you had to? And what if there was a
chance, just a chance, that you *didn't* have to
deal with it? ''When I was a boy,'' said Elvis not
so long ago, ''I was the hero in comic books and
movies. I grew up believing in a dream. Now I've
lived it out. That's all a man can ask for.''

Elvis is telling us something quite specific:
how special he was; how completely he captured and understood what for most of us is only
a tired phrase glossing the surfaces of our own
failed hopes. It is one thing, after all, to dream of
a new job, and quite another to dream of a new
world. The risks are greater. Elvis took chances
dreaming his dreams; he gambled against the
likelihood that their failure would betray him,
and make him wish he had never dreamed at all.
There are a hundred songs to tell that story, but
perhaps Mott the Hoople, chasing the rock 'n'
roll fantasy Elvis made of the American dream,
said it best: ''I wish I'd never wanted then/What
I want now twice as much.''

Always, Elvis felt he was different, if not better, than those around him. He grew his side-
burns long, acting out that sense of differentness,
and was treated differently: in this case, he got
himself kicked off the football team. Hear him
recall those days in the midst of a near-hysterical
autobiography, delivered at the height of his
comeback from the stage at the International

Hotel in Las Vegas: ''. . . Had pretty long hair for
that time and I tell you it got pretty weird. They
used to see me comin down the street and they'd
say, 'Hot dang, let's get him, he's a squirrel, he's
a squirrel, get him, he just come down outta the
trees.' ''

High school classmates remember his determination to break through as a country singer;
with a little luck, they figured, he might even
make it.

Out on the road for the first time with small-
change country package tours, though, Elvis
would plot for something much bigger—for
everything Hollywood had ever shown him in its
movies.

On North Main in Memphis, as Harmonica
Frank recalls Elvis, this was nothing to put into
words. Talking trash and flicking ash, marking
time and trying to hold it off, what did Elvis have
to look forward to? A year or so of Saturday
nights, a little local notoriety, then a family he
didn't quite decide to have and couldn't support? It would be all over.

Elvis fancied himself a trucker (if there
weren't any Memphis boys in the movies, there
were plenty on the road), pushing tons of
machinery through the endless American night;
just his version of the train whistle that called out
to Johnny B. Goode and kept Richard Nixon
awake as a boy. If it is more than a little odd that
what to Elvis served as a symbol of escape and
mastery now works—as part of his legend—as a
symbol of everything grimy and poor he left
behind when he did escape, maybe that only
tells us how much his success shuffled the facts
of his life, or how much he raised the stakes.

You don't make it in America—Emerson's
mousetrap to the contrary—waiting for someone to come along and sign you up. You might
be sitting on the corner like a Philly rock 'n'
roller and get snatched up for your good looks,
but you'll be back a year later and you'll never
know what happened. Worst of all, you may not
even care. What links the greatest rock 'n' roll
careers is a volcanic ambition, a lust for more
than anyone has a right to expect; in some cases,

a refusal to know when to quit or even rest. It is that bit of Ahab burning beneath the Huck Finn rags of "Freewheelin'" Bob Dylan, the arrogance of a country boy like Elvis sailing into Hollywood, ready for whatever kind of success America had to offer.

So if we treat Elvis's words with as much respect as we can muster—which is how he meant them to be taken—we can see the first point at which his story begins to be his own. He took his dreams far more seriously than most ever dare, and he had the nerve to chase them down.

Cash's wonderful line—"a cosmic conspiracy against reality in favor of romance"—now might have more resonance. Still, if the kind of spirit that romance could produce seems ephemeral within the context of daily life, you would not expect the music it produced to last very long either. Not even Elvis, as a successful young rocker, could have expected his new music to last; he told interviewers rock 'n' roll was here to stay, but he was taking out plenty of insurance, making movies and singing schmaltz. You couldn't blame him; anyway, he liked schmaltz.

Within the realm of country music, the new spirit dried up just like Saturday fades into Monday, but since rock 'n' roll found its own audience and created its own world, that hardly mattered. Rock 'n' roll caught that romantic conspiracy on records and gave it a form. Instead of a possibility with a music, it became the essence; it became, of all things, a tradition. And when that form itself had to deal with reality—which is to say, when its young audience began to grow up—when the compromise between fantasy and reality that fills most of this book was necessary to preserve the possibility of fantasy, the fantasy had become part of the reality that had to be dealt with; the rules of the game had changed a bit, and it was a better game. "Blue Suede Shoes" had grown directly into something as serious and complex, and yet still offhand, still take-it-or-leave-it-and-pass-the-wine, as the

Rolling Stones' "You Can't Always Get What You Want," which asks the musical question, "Why *are you* stepping on my blue suede shoes?"

Echoing through all of rock 'n' roll is the simple demand for peace of mind and a good time. While the demand is easy to make, nothing is more complex than to try to make it real and live it out. It all sounds simple, obvious; but that one young man like Elvis could break through a world as hard as Hank Williams', and invent a new one to replace it, seems obvious only because we have inherited Elvis's world, and live in it.

Satisfaction is not all there is to it, but it is where it all begins. Finally, the music must provoke as well as delight, disturb as well as comfort, create as well as sustain. If it doesn't, it lies, and there is only so much comfort you can take in a lie before it all falls apart.

The central facts of life in Elvis's South pulled as strongly against the impulses of hedonism and romance as the facts of our own lives do against the fast pleasures of rock 'n' roll. When the poor white was thrown back on himself, as he was in the daytime, when he worked his plot or looked for a job in the city, or at night, when he brooded and Hank Williams' whippoorwill told the truth all too plainly, those facts stood out clearly: powerlessness and vulnerability on all fronts. The humiliation of a class system that gave him his identity and then trivialized it; a community that for all its tradition and warmth was in some indefinable way not enough; economic chaos; the violence of the weather; bad food and maybe not enough of that; diseases that attached themselves to the body like new organs—they all mastered him. And that vulnerability produced—along with that urge to cut loose, along with that lively Southern romance—uncertainty, fatalism, resentment, acceptance, and nostalgia: limits that cut deep as the oldest cotton patch in Dixie.

Vernon Presley was a failed Mississippi sharecropper who moved his family out of the country with the idea of making a go in the city; it's not so far from Tupelo to Memphis, but in some ways, the journey must have been a long one—scores of country songs about boys and girls who lost their souls to the big town attest to that. Listen to Dolly Parton's downtown hooker yearning for her Blue Ridge mountain boy; listen to the loss of an America you may never have known.

They don't make country music better than that anymore, but it's unsatisfying, finally; too classical. This country myth is just one more echo of Jefferson pronouncing that, in America, virtue must be found in the land. I like myths, but this one is too facile, either for the people who still live on the land or for those of us who are merely looking for a way out of our own world, for an Annie Green Springs utopia. The myth is unsatisfying because the truth is richer than the myth.

"King Harvest (Has Surely Come)," the Band's song of blasted country hopes, gives us the South in all of its earthly delight and then snuffs it out. All at once, the song catches the grace and the limbo of the life that must be left behind.

The tune evokes a man's intimacy with the land and the refusal of the land to respond in kind. The music makes real, for the coolest city listener, a sense of place that is not quite a sense of being at home; the land is too full of violence for that. One hears the farmer's fear of separating from the land (and from his own history, which adhering to the land, is not wholly his own); one hears the cold economic necessities that have forced him out. The melody—too beautiful and out of reach for any words I have—spins the chorus into the pastoral with a feel for nature that is *really* hedonistic, and a desperate, ominous rhythm slams the verses back to the slum streets that harbor the refugees of the pastoral disaster: "Just don't judge me by my shoes!" Garth Hudson's organ traces the circle of the song, over and over again.

The earliest picture of Elvis shows a farmer, his wife, and their baby; the faces of the parents

are vacant, they are set, as if they cannot afford an unearned smile. Somehow, their faces say, they will be made to pay even for that.

You don't hear this in Elvis's music; but what he left out of his story is as vital to an understanding of his art as what he kept, and made over. If we have no idea of what he left behind, how much he escaped, we will have no idea what his success was worth, or how intensely he must have wanted it.

Elvis was thirteen when the family left Tupelo for Memphis in 1948, a pampered only child; ordinary in all respects, they say, except that he liked to sing. True to Chuck Berry's legend of the Southern rocker, Elvis's mother bought him his first guitar, and for the same reason Johnny B. Goode's mama had in mind: keep the boy out of trouble. Elvis sang tearful country ballads, spirituals, community music. On the radio, he listened with his family to the old music of the Carter Family and Jimmie Rodgers, to current stars like Roy Acuff, Ernest Tubb, Bob Wills, Hank Williams, and to white gospel groups like the Blackwood Brothers. Elvis touched the soft center of American music when he heard and imitated Dean Martin and the operatics of Mario Lanza; he picked up Mississippi blues singers like Big Bill Broonzy, Big Boy Crudup, Lonnie Johnson, and the new Memphis music of Rufus Thomas and Johnny Ace, mostly when no one else was around, because that music was naturally frowned upon. His parents called it "sinful music," and they had a point—it was dirty, and there were plenty of blacks who would have agreed with Mr. and Mrs. Presley—but Elvis was really too young to worry. In this he was no different from hundreds of other white country kids who wanted more excitement in their lives than they could get from twangs and laments—wanted a beat, sex, celebration, the stunning nuances of the blues and the roar of horns and electric guitars. Still, Elvis's interest was far more casual than that of Jerry Lee Lewis, a bad boy who was sneaking off to black dives in his spare time, or Carl Perkins, a musician who was consciously working out a synthesis of blues and country.

The Presleys stumbled onto welfare, into public housing. Vernon Presley found a job. It almost led to the family's eviction, because if they still didn't have enough to live on, they were judged to have too much to burden the county with their troubles. Elvis was a loner, but he had an eye for flash. He sold his blood for money, ushered at the movies, drove his famous truck, and divided the proceeds between his mother and his outrageous wardrobe. Looking for space, for a way to set himself apart.

Like many parents with no earthly future, the Presleys, especially Gladys Presley, lived for their son. Her ambition must have been that Elvis would take all that was good in the family and free himself from the life she and her husband endured: she was, Memphian Stanley Booth wrote a few years ago, "the one, perhaps the only one, who had told him throughout his life that even though he came from poor country people, he was just as good as anybody."

On Sundays (Wednesdays too, sometimes) the Presleys went to their Assembly of God to hear the Pentecostal ministers had down a similar message: the last shall be first. This was democratic religion with a vengeance, lower class and gritty. For all those who have traced Elvis's music and his hipshake to his religion (accurately enough—Elvis was the first to say so), it has escaped his chroniclers that hillbilly Calvinism was also at the root of his self-respect and his pride: the anchor of his ambition.

His church (and the dozens of other Pentecostal sects scattered throughout the South and small-town America) was one part of what was left of the old American religion after the Great Awakening. Calvinism had been a religion of authority in the beginning; in the middle-class North, filtered through the popular culture of Ben Franklin, it became a system of tight money, tight-mindedness, and gentility; in the hillbilly South, powered by traveling preachers and their endless revivals, the old holiness cult produced a

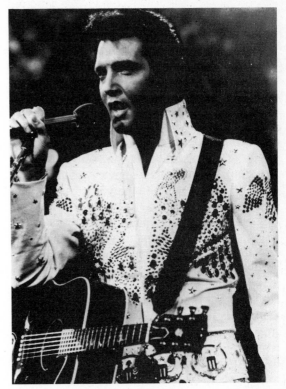

■ ■ *One of the sources of Elvis Presley's ''rockabilly'' rhythms with their energy, tension, and power, was the intensity of the music of the Assembly of God, a Pentacostal church of Elvis's childhood.*

faith of grace, apocalypse, and emotion, where people heaved their deepest feelings into a circle and danced around them. Momentum scattered that old authority; all were sinners, all were saints. Self-consciously outcast, the true faith in a land of Philistines and Pharisees, it was shoved into storefronts and tents and even open fields, and no less sure of itself for that.

Church music caught moments of unearthly peace and desire, and the strength of the religion was in its intensity. The preacher rolled fire down the pulpit and chased it into the aisle, signifying; men and women rocked in their seats, sometimes onto the floor, bloodying their fingernails scratching and clawing in a lust for absolute sanctification. No battle against oppression, this was a leap right through it, with tongues babbling toward real visions, negating stale red earth, warped privvies, men and women staring from their sway-backed porches into nothingness. It was a faith meant to transcend the grimy world that called it up. Like Saturday night, the impulse to dream, the need to escape, the romance and the contradictions of the land, this was a source of energy, tension, and power.

Elvis inherited these tensions, but more than that, gave them his own shape. It is often said that if Elvis had not come along to set off the changes in American music and American life that followed his triumph, someone very much like him would have done the job as well. But there is no reason to think this is true, either in strictly musical terms, or in any broader cultural sense. It is vital to remember that Elvis was the first young Southern white to sing rock 'n' roll, something he copied from no one but made up

on the spot; and to know that even though other singers would have come up with a white version of the new black music acceptable to teenage America, of all that did emerge in Elvis's wake, none sang as powerfully, or with more than a touch of his magic.

Even more important is the fact that no singer emerged with anything like Elvis's combination of great talent and conscious ambition, and there is no way a new American hero could have gotten out of the South and to the top—creating a whole new sense of how big the top was, as Elvis did—without that combination. The others—Perkins, Lewis, Charlie Rich—were bewildered by even a taste of fame and unable to handle a success much more limited than Presley's.

If Elvis had the imagination to come up with the dreams that kept him going, he had the music to bring them back to life and make them real to huge numbers of other people. It was the genius of his singing, an ease and an intensity that has no parallel in American music, that along with his dreams separated him from his context.

■ ■ ■

STUDY QUESTIONS

1. What role did country music traditionally play in Southern culture and society?

2. How did the Southern singers help to define the boundaries and limits of community life?

3. In what way was Hank Williams a "poet of limits, fears, and failure?" How was he similar to or different from Elvis Presley?

4. What factors explain the success of rock'n'roll?

5. How did Elvis Presley change the course of American, and particularly Southern, music?

6. How was Elvis Presley different from the other Southern rock'n'roll singers of his day?

BIBLIOGRAPHY

The above selection is from Greil Marcus' insightful *Mystery Train* (1975). Throughout the volume, Marcus demonstrates and traces the relationships of rock'n'roll, blues music, and American culture. There are several readable histories of rock'n'roll. Among the best are such popular studies as Carl Belz, *The Story of Rock* (1972); Nik Cohn, *Rock from the Beginning* (1969); John Gabree, *The World of Rock* (1968); Ralph Gleason, *The Jefferson Airplane and the San Francisco Sound* (1969); Jerry Hopkins, *The Rock Story* (1970); and Arnold Shaw, *The Rock Revolution* (1970). Charlie Gillett, *The Sound of the City* (1970), is more scholarly and contains a wealth of information about early rock music and the industry of music. Pete Guralnick, *Feel Like Going Home* (1971), is outstanding on the Southern origins of rock'n'roll. The best biography of Elvis Presley is Jerry Hopkins, *Elvis* (1971). Bill Malone, *Country Music U.S.A.* (1968), surveys the world that produced Elvis.

PERFECT BODIES, ETERNAL YOUTH: THE OBSESSION OF MODERN AMERICA

Randy Roberts and James S. Olson

The message comes at Americans from every direction, every hour of the day. Cher appears on television touting the miraculous benefits of the President's First Lady exercise salons. Lynn Redgrave comes on a few minutes later delivering superlatives about Weight Watchers' frozen entree foods. Jane Fonda's exercise videotapes confront shoppers in supermarkets and video stores. Victoria Principal and Raquel Welch write diet and fitness books, both of which become best sellers. Plastic surgeons advertise in newspapers and on television, urging Americans to get rid of what they hate or acquire what they want for their bodies. Every issue of *Family Circle, Woman's Day*, and *The Enquirer* contains some new article about the latest weight-loss panacea.

Sports programming dominates television, as if Americans have an insatiable need to watch football, baseball, basketball, bowling, bodybuilding, and a host of other competitions. Future linguists and anthropologists will study what have become the highlights of contemporary American popular culture—diet sodas, lite beers, Lean Cuisine, sugarless gum, half-the-calories bread, Nautilus, jogging, Iron Man, marathons, "fun runs," tennis, bicycling, 10K races, Superbowls, play-offs, World Series, Grand Slams of golf and tennis, Little League, Pop Warner football, and championship after championship.

Modern America is not the first society to indulge in the emptiness of narcissism, but no other society has ever had such resources to spend on a fruitless crusade to prevent aging and deny death. In "Perfect Bodies, Eternal Youth: The Obsession of Modern America," Randy Roberts and James S. Olson examine the preoccupation with health, fitness, and youth in the United States, explaining how and why the members of an entire culture have become infatuated with their own bodies.

Fewer and fewer people these days argue that running shortens lives, while a lot of people say that it may strengthen them. If that's all we've got for the time being, it seems a good enough argument for running. Not airtight, but good enough.

—JIM FIXX

It was a perfect July day in Vermont—clear and cool. Jim Fixx, on the eve of a long-awaited vacation, put on his running togs and headed down a rural road for his daily run, expecting to do the usual twelve to fifteen miles. At fifty-two years of age, Fixx was a millionaire, the best-selling author of *The Complete Book of Running*, and the reigning guru of the American exercise cult. In 1968 he had weighed 214 pounds, smoked two packs of cigarettes a day, and worried about his family health history. Fixx's father had died of a heart attack at the age of forty-three. So Fixx started running and stopped smoking. He lost 60 pounds and introduced America to the virtues of strenuous exercise: longevity, freedom from depression, energy, and the "runner's high." He regularly ran 80 miles a week. When he hit the road on July 21, 1984, Fixx weighed 154 pounds and seemed the perfect image of fitness. Twenty minutes into the run he had a massive heart attack and died on the side of the road. A motorcyclist found his body later that afternoon.

Fixx's death shocked middle- and upper-class America. Of all people, how could Jim Fixx have died of a heart attack? Millions of joggers, runners, swimmers, cyclists, tri-athletes, walkers, weightlifters, and aerobic dancers had convinced themselves that exercise preserved youth and postponed death. It was the yuppie panacea; "working out" made them immune to the ravages of time.

The autopsy on Fixx was even more disturbing. In spite of all the running, his circulatory system was a shambles. Fixx's cholesterol levels had been dangerously high. One coronary artery was 98 percent blocked, a second one 85 percent blocked, and a third one 50 percent blocked. In the previous two to eight weeks, the wall of his left ventricle had badly deteriorated. On that clear Vermont day, Jim Fixx shouldn't have been running; he should have been undergoing triple-bypass surgery.

Even more puzzling, Fixx had been complaining for months of chest pains while running—clear signs of a deadly angina, the heart muscle protesting lack of oxygen. Friends had expressed concern and urged him to get a check-up. He resisted, attempting to will good health. In January 1984 he had agreed to a treadmill test, but he skipped the appointment that afternoon, running 16 miles instead. Why had someone so committed to health ignored such obvious warnings? How had sports, exercise, and fitness become such obsessions in the United States?

Modern society was the culprit. In an increasingly secular society, church membership no longer provided the discipline to bind people together into cohesive social groups. Well-integrated neighborhoods with long histories and strong identities had given way after World War II to faceless suburbs. Corporate and professional elites tended to be highly mobile, relocating whenever a pay raise was offered. The new American community had become fifty suburban homes and a 7-11 convenience store. New organizations, especially business and government bureaucracies, had assumed power in the United States, but those were hardly places where most Americans could feel comfortable and in control. Blessed with money but deprived of community in the 1970s and 1980s, Americans began to use sports to rebuild their sense of community and fitness and to define individual happiness and individual pleasure, creating a culture of competitive narcissism supported by a host of therapeutic panaceas, such as EST, psychotherapy, Scientology, and strenuous exercise.

Roberts, Randy and James S. Olson, *Winning Is the Only Thing*. The Johns Hopkins University Press, Baltimore/London, 1989, pp. 213–234.

For individuals, families, groups, and communities, sports had become a new cultural currency, a common ground upon which a diverse people could express their values and needs. Unlike European society, where such traditional institutions as the church, the aristocracy, and the monarchy had maintained order through established authority, America had been settled by lower-class working people and small farmers. The traditional institutions anchoring European society were absent. Without those same moorings, America had always confronted the centrifugal forces of individualism, capitalism, Protestantism, and ethnicity, using the culture of opportunity to stave off social disintegration. Social mobility, the westward movement, the abundance of land, and ruralism helped stablilize a highly complex society.

But in the twentieth century, when industrialization, urbanization, and the disappearance of the frontier changed the definitions of opportunity and progress, the values of individualism, community, and competition had to find new modes of expression, and sports became a prominent one. At the local, regional, and national levels, sports evolved into one of the most powerful expressions of identity. Outside observers marveled, for example, at the "religion" of high school football in the more than eleven hundred independent school districts of Texas. When viewed simply as sport, of course, the obsession with football seems absurd, but when viewed in terms of community identity, it becomes more understandable. In hundreds of rural areas, where scattered farms surround tiny county seats, the local high school, with its arbitrarily drawn district lines, was the central focus of community life. Rural Texans passionately opposed school district consolidations, even when it made good economic sense, because it threatened the high school, high school football, and community identity. For hundreds of small Texas towns—and rural areas throughout much of the rest of the country—high school athletics was literally the cement of community life.

It wasn't just high school sports which provided new identities in the United States. After World War II, social and economic pressures worked against the nuclear family. More and more women were working outside the home; more and more men were working at job sites long commutes from the suburbs; and divorce rates were way up. Childhood play became less spontaneous and more organized as schools, government, and communities assumed roles once played by the family. The most obvious consequence was the appearance of organized youth sports. Little League grew by leaps and bounds beginning in the 1950s; child's play, once the domain of the home and immediate neighborhood, became a spectator sport complete with uniforms, umpires, scoreboards, leagues, play-offs, drafts, and championships. By the 1980s, Little League was competing for time with Pop Warner football, Little Dribblers basketball, soccer, and swimming, with organized competition beginning in some sports at the age of three. In 1987 sports sociologists estimated that thirty million children under sixteen years of age were competing in organized sports.

Sports functioned as identity on the regional level as well. In an age when television, movies, and mass culture threatened regional distinctiveness, sports emerged as the single most powerful symbol of localism and community loyalty. That was obviously true of high school and college sports, but even in professional sports, when ownership shifted away from local businesses and entrepreneurs to conglomerates and national corporations, the regional identity of teams remained critically important to gate receipts and television revenues. The rivalries between the Chicago Bears and the Green Bay Packers, or the Boston Red Sox and the New York Yankees, or the Boston Celtics and the Los Angeles Lakers, filled stadiums, arenas, and living rooms with fans desperate for the home team to win. Five hundred years ago, European cities dedicated all their surplus capital over the course of 100 to 200 years to build elaborate cathedrals to God. In the United States during the 1970s and 1980s, the modern equivalent of the medieval cathedral was the domed stadium. For sports, not for God, American communities would sell bonds and mortgage themselves for the next generation.

Even on the national level, sports competition reflected and promoted American nationalism. Sports was a mirror of federalism, at once local in its community loyalties but national in its collective forms. The 1984 Olympic Games in Los Angeles did not just expose a rising tide of patriotism and national pride; they became a major force in stimulating a new American nationalism. Unlike the recent Olympic Games in Montreal, Moscow, and Seoul, the Los Angeles Games did not accumulate billion-dollar deficits and require the resources of national governments to prop them up. In 1984, "free enterprise capitalism" organized and conducted the Games, used existing facilities, and turned a profit. The Los Angeles Coliseum was filled with flag-waving Americans cheering every native athlete winning a medal. On television back home, Europeans watched the proceedings with astonishment and not a little fear, worrying about the burst of American patriotism, nationalism, and even chauvinism. Nearly a decade after the debacle in Vietnam, American pride and optimism were on the rebound, and the 1984 Olympic Games was center stage for the resurrection of the American sense of mission.

Modern sports in the United States also provided a sense of identity cutting across class, racial, and ethnic lines. In penitentiaries throughout the country, intense struggles were waged every evening over television and radio programming, black convicts wanting to watch soul stations and black sit-coms and whites demanding MTV or white sit-coms. But there was no trouble or debate on Sunday afternoon or Monday nights during the fall. It was football, only football, and blacks and whites watched the programs with equal enthusiasm. On Monday evenings in the fall, whether in the poorest ghetto tenement of the South Side of Chicago or the most tastefully appointed living room in the

Lake Forest suburbs, televisions were tuned in to football, and discussions at work the next morning revolved around the game, who won and who lost, and why.

For ethnic minorities and immigrants, sports similarly became a way of identifying with the new society, a powerful form of acculturation. During the 1980s, for example, Los Angeles became the second largest Mexican city in the world, behind only Mexico City in Spanish-speaking population and larger now than Guadalajara in terms of Mexican residents. At Dodger Stadium in Los Angeles, Mexicans and Mexican Americans became an increasingly large part of the evening box office, helping to sustain Dodger attendance at its three million-plus levels each year. In September 1986, when Dodger pitcher Fernando Valenzuela won his twentieth game of the season, the Spanish cable network SIN broke into its regular programming nationwide for live interviews. The fact that sports was making its way to the headlines and front pages of major newspapers was no accident in the United States. It had become, indeed, a new cultural currency in modern America, a way to interpret change and express traditional values.

Women, too, used sports as a vehicle in their drive for equality and identity. The development of women's and men's sports in America has varied considerably. From the first, men's sports have emphasized fierce competition and the ruthless pursuit of expertise. Early male and female physical educators, however, believed women were uncompetitive and decided that women's sports should promote a woman's physical and mental qualities and thus make her more attractive to men. They also believed that sports and exercise should sublimate female sexual drives. As renowned nineteenth-century physical educator Dudley A. Sargent noted, "No one seems to realize that there is a time in the life of a girl when it is better for her and for the community to be something of a boy rather than too much of a girl."

But tomboyish behavior had to stop short of abrasive competition. Lucille Eaton Hill, director of physical training at Wellesley College, urged women to "avoid the evils which are so apparent . . . in the conduct of athletics for men." She and her fellow female physical educators encouraged widespread participation rather than narrow specialization. In short, women left spectator and professional sports to men. Indeed, not until 1924 were women allowed to compete in Olympic track and field events, and even then on a limited basis.

During the 1920s the tennis careers of Suzanne Langlen and Helen Wills were used to demonstrate the proper and improper pursuit of victory by athletic women. Tennis, for the great French champion Langlen, was not only a way of life: it was life. Her only object on a tennis court was to win, and between 1919 and 1926, when she turned professional, Langlen lost only two sets of singles and won 269 of 270 matches. But at what cost? Bulimic in her eating habits and subject to dramatic swings in emotions, she suffered several nervous breakdowns and lived in fear of losing. In addition, male critics noted that, far from keeping her looking young, tennis cruelly aged Langlen. Journalist Al Laney remarked that by the mid-1920s Langlen looked thirty years older than she actually was and that her complexion had turned dull and colorless. Her friend Ted Tinling agreed that before she turned twenty-five, "her face and expression had already the traces of deep emotional experiences far beyond the normal for her age."

In contrast, Helen Wills was a champion of great physical beauty. Before Wills, Americans tended to agree with journalist Paul Gallico that "pretty girls" did not excel in sports and that outstanding female athletes were simply compensating for their lack of beauty. Summarizing this school of thought, Larry Engelmann observed: "Athletics was their way of getting attention. If Suzanne Langlen were really beautiful, for instance, she wouldn't be running around like crazy on the tennis courts of Europe. She would have been quietly at home, happily married. Athletics proved a refuge and a last chance for the desperate female ugly duckling."

Yet Wills was beautiful, and she was great, winning every set of singles competition she played between 1927 and 1933. Journalists explained Wills' success and beauty by stressing the fact that tennis was only a game for her, not a way of life and certainly not life itself. Losses did not worry her. She always appeared composed. "My father, a doctor," she explained, "always told me not to wince or screw up my face while I was playing. He said it would put lines on my face." And no victory was worth a line.

Women were not fully emancipated from the older ideal until the 1970s, when they asserted their right to be as ruthless and competitive in athletics as men. Tennis champion Billy Jean King symbolized on the court as well as off this new attitude. Like Langlen, she single-mindedly pursued victory. And she was no more concerned with sweating and grimacing than Pete Rose. Unlike Wills, King was not interested in art or starting a family. When asked why she was not at home, she replied, "Why don't you ask Rod Laver why he isn't at home?" It was as eloquent a statement of athletic liberation as could be asked for.

To develop fully as an athlete, King had to earn money. Along with Gladys Heldman and Philip Morris Tobacco Company, King helped to organize the Virginia Slims women's tennis circuit in 1971. That year she became the first female athlete to earn $100,000 in a single year. More importantly, she labored to get women players a bigger share of the prize money at the major championships. In the early 1970s women's purses at Wimbledon and the U.S. Open were about 10 percent of the men's. By the mid-1980s the prize money split was equal. As if to punctuate the point that women's tennis had arrived, King defeated the former Wimbledon triple-crown champion (1939) Bobby Riggs 6–4, 6–3, 6–3, in a highly publicized match in the Houston Astrodome in 1973.

Even more important than King for the future of women's athletics was Title IX of the 1972 Educational Amendments Act. It outlawed sexual discrimination by school districts or colleges and universities which received federal aid. Certainly, athletic budgets in high schools and universities are not equally divided between male and female athletics. But women have made significant gains. Before Title IX less than 1 percent of athletic budgets went to women's sports. By the 1980s that figure had increased to over 10 percent. No longer is there a serious argument over the road women's sports should travel. Instead, the battle is over what portion of that pie they should receive.

But it wasn't just countries, cities, colleges, small towns, high schools, and ethnic groups which turned to sports in the 1980s as the most powerful way of defining their values. The most extraordinary development in contemporary popular culture was the extent to which individuals turned to athletics, exercise, and body image as a way of finding meaning in an increasingly dislocated society. In the mid-1980s, a Louis Harris poll indicated that 96 percent of all Americans found something about their bodies that they didn't like and would change if they could. Harris said that the "rampant obsessions of both men and women about their looks have produced an obvious boon for the cosmetics industry, plastic surgery, diet doctors, fitness and shape advisers, fat farms, and exercise clubs." The cult of fitness and the cult of individual happiness went hand in hand. Politicans used international sports at the Olympic level to confirm the superiority of various political systems or prove the equality of their Third World cultures; they mustered professional sports to project the quality of life in major American cities; collegiate sports touted the virtues of different universities; and in the 1970s and 1980s, millions of Americans embraced the cult of fitness to discover the meaning of life, retreating into the fantasy that they are how they look.

The cult of fitness and preoccupation with physical appearance first emerged in the United States during the John Kennedy administration. In the election of 1960, Kennedy used television as it had never been used before when he challenged Richard Nixon to a series of debates. Kennedy faced formidable odds. Young, handsome, and wealthy, he was considered perhaps too young, too handsome, and too wealthy to make an effective president. His Roman Catholicism seemed another albatross. Behind the polls, Kennedy needed a boost. The televised debates were perfect.

Nixon arrived in Chicago for the first debate looking tired and ill. He had injured his knee six weeks before, and a hospital stay had weakened him. On the eve of the debate a chest cold left him hoarse. He looked like a nervous corpse— pale, twenty pounds underweight, and haggard. Make-up experts suggested covering his heavy beard with a thick powder, but Nixon accepted only a thin coat of Max Factor's "Lazy Shave," a pancake cosmetic.

Kennedy looked better, much better. He arrived at Chicago from California with a suntan. He didn't need make-up to look healthy, nor did he need special lighting to hide a weak profile. He did, however, change suits. He believed that a dark blue rather than a gray suit would look better under the bright lights. Kennedy was right, of course, as anyone who watches a nightly news program must realize. Once the debate started, Kennedy intentionally slowed down his delivery and watered down his ideas. His face was controlled and cool. He smiled with his eyes and perhaps the corners of his mouth, and his laugh was a mere suggestion of a laugh. Although Nixon marshalled a mountain of facts and closely reasoned arguments, he looked bad. Instead of hearing a knowledgeable candidate, viewers saw a nervous, uncertain man, one whose clothes didn't fit and whose face looked pasty and white. In contrast, Kennedy *looked* good, scored a victory in the polls, and went on to win the election by a razor-thin margin.

The first president born in the twentieth century, Kennedy had claimed in his inaugural address that "the torch had been passed to a new generation of Americans . . . tempered by war, disciplined by a hard and bitter peace, proud of our ancient heritage." Life around the

White House soon reflected the instincts of a new generation. It wasn't just little Caroline and later John-John frolicking on the White House lawn. The Kennedys were fiercely competitive and obsessed with sports. At the family compound at Hyannisport or Robert Kennedy's "Hickory Hill" home in Virginia, the days were filled with tennis, golf, sailing, isometric exercise, swimming, horseback riding, badminton, and a brutal form of touch football, which overweight and overaged visitors dreaded, since the Kennedys expected everyone to give it a try. An atmosphere of youthful virility surrounded the Kennedy administration. To impress the Kennedys, one associate remembered, you had to "show raw guts, fall on your face now and then. Smash into the house once in a while going after a pass. Laugh off twisted ankles or a big hole torn in your best suit."

The whole country became infatuated with the sense of vitality, and the fifty-mile hike became the symbol of fitness. Marine Corps commandant General David M. Shoup, whom Kennedy especially admired, accepted Kennedy's challenge to see if his marines could duplicate a feat of Theodore Roosevelt's 1908 marines—march fifty miles in less than twenty hours. Shoup met the challenge, as did Attorney General Robert Kennedy, who walked his fifty miles along the path of the C & O canal. Kennedy's secretaries took up the challenge, and once the newspapers had picked up the story, tens of thousands of Americans tried it too. The spring of 1963 became the season of the fifty-mile hike.

These were also years of giddy infatuation with the Mercury astronauts, whose crew-cut fitness first came to public attention at their introductory press conference in 1959. All of them were military pilots, and John Glenn of Ohio emerged as their leader. Square-jawed with ramrod perfect posture, Glenn had a personality and value system to match. He was the ultimate "goody-goody," and America loved him. The country was also astounded at his daily fitness regimen—vigorous calisthenics followed by a two-mile jog along the beach. Two miles—every day! Even when it rained.

If John Glenn was the leading jogger of the 1960s, the scientific father of running was Kenneth Cooper, an Air Force physician. A high school track star in Oklahoma City, Cooper finished medical school and joined the Air Force as a physician at the School of Aerospace Medicine in San Antonio. He tested fitness levels in thousands of potential Air Force pilots and in the process developed new standards of conditioning. To really benefit from exercise, Americans had to get their heart rate above 130 beats a minute for a sustained period. Jogging, running, racquetball, squash, cycling, walking, and swimming were the best exercises.

To please an increasingly technical, postindustrial clientele whose faith in science was unrivaled, Cooper even charted fitness, providing a quantified methodology to guarantee fitness. An aerobically fit person had to "earn 30 points a week." He or she could do this by walking three miles in no more than forty-one minutes five times a week; by swimming 700 yards in fifteen minutes five times a week; or by running a mile in eight minutes only twice a week. To measure fitness, Cooper recommended the "twelve minutes test." If a person can run or walk less than a mile in twelve minutes, he or she is in "very poor shape"; 1 to 1.25 miles is "poor"; 1.25 to 1.5 miles is "fair"; 1.5 to 1.75 miles is "good"; and more than 1.75 miles is "excellent." Cooper also warned people to watch out if their pulse rate exceeded 80 beats a minute. Fewer than 60 beats was "excellent." Vigorous exercise would reduce the heart rate. In Cooper's own words, "You might just save your heart some of those 20,000 to 30,000 extra beats you've forced on it every day."

The country was more than ready for Cooper's message. Early in the 1960s the first of the baby-boom generation hit college. The "don't trust anyone over thirty" culture had appeared, protesting war and inequality and proclaiming the virtues of brotherly love and sexual liberation. In 1961 half the American population was

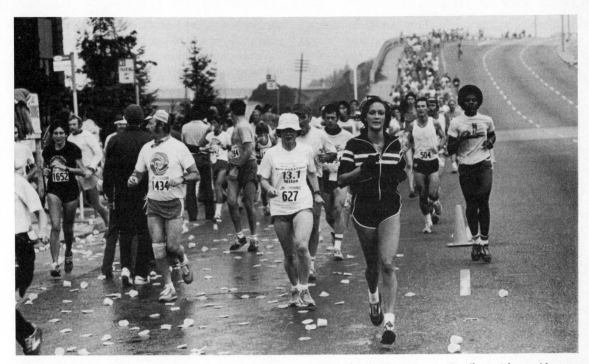

■ ■ *According to tradition, the marathon commemorates the messenger who, in 490 B.C., ran 20 miles to Athens with news of the Greek victory at Marathon. Running marathons has gained popularity in recent years: In 1986 some 20,000 runners entered New York City's marathon and 19,412 finished it.*

under thirty. By 1964 the median age had dropped to twenty-seven and in 1966 to twenty-five. America fell in love with youth, health, sex, and pleasure. Hippies, protests, "love-ins," "teach-ins," Woodstock, drugs, rebellion, and loud, self-righteous rejections of materialism emanated from college campuses.

But in 1967 the first baby-boom class graduated from college. The transformation of hippies into "yuppies" was underway. By 1971 those 1946 babies were twenty-five years old. The cruel tricks of gravity and heredity commenced. Bellies started to thicken, hairlines to recede. Women with babies looked despairingly at abdominal stretch marks and the faint beginnings of "crow's feet." The youth culture still survived, but individual youth was proving to be a temporary state. Middle age loomed as large as death.

Dr. Kenneth Cooper had the answer. Late in 1968, he coined a new word and wrote a book

by the same name—*Aerobics*. By 1972 the book had sold nearly three million copies to anxious yuppies bent on postponing the inevitable. By the early 1970s, Cooper had an estimated eight million Americans, including astronaut John Glenn, adding up their weekly points, counting their pulse, testing their speed, taking their blood pressure, and weighing their bodies.

Throughout the 1970s and 1980s the cult of fitness reached extraordinary dimensions in the United States. More than twenty million Americans regularly exercised, and along with the running boom came a boom in racquetball, tennis, swimming, cycling, weightlifting, and "aerobic" dancing. In 1970 only 125 people entered the first New York City marathon, which took runners over a 26-mile course through all four boroughs; but in the 1986 marathon, 20,000 officially entered the race, and 19,412 finished it. The race was so popular that organizers had to reject thousands of applicants. Marathons became common events on every weekend all across the country.

The triathlon endurance was an even better gauge of the fitness cult. Known as the ultimate of the "ultrasports," the triathlon combined a 2-mile swim with a 112-mile cycle ride and a 26-mile run. In 1986 more than one million Americans competed in triathlon events around the country. And in what can only be considered the absurd limit of the fitness craze, Stu Mittleman won the "Sri Chinmey 1,000 Mile Marathon" in New York City in 1986. His time of just under fifteen days "was my best ever."

The cult of fitness was rivaled only by the obsession with youth and body image which swept through American culture in the 1970s and 1980s. To be sure, this was nothing new. Americans had long been preoccupied with their bodies, and attempts to stay young had centered on staying thin, as if slenderness were in itself a foundation of youth. In the 1860s Harriet Beecher Stowe had written: "We in America have got so far out of the way of a womanhood that has any vigor of outline or opulence of physical proportion, that, when we see a woman made as a woman ought to be, she strikes us as a monster. Our willowy girls are afraid of nothing so much as growing stout."

To stay thin, nineteenth-century American women dieted and corseted their bodies. "It ain't stylish for young courting gals to let on like they have any appetite," admitted one female. And through tightlacing their corsets, women could maintain the proper girlish waistline of eighteen inches, with only such acceptable side effects as headaches, fainting spells, and uterine and spinal disorders.

If tightlacing and dieting led to serious health problems, illness was in itself admired. Consumptive women were romanticized and imbued with spiritual qualities. Little Eva in *Uncle Tom's Cabin*, Beth in *Little Women*, Mimi in *La Bohème*—all were thin, romantic consumptives who radiated spirituality and sensuality. Perhaps the ideal was the romantic ballerina—

thin, ethereal, pale, pure, as certain to die young as poor broken-hearted Giselle.

Throughout the twentieth century, thinness has largely remained the feminine ideal, although sickliness generally declined as an attractive characteristic. The Gibson Girl of the turn of the century touted athletics, and during the 1920s the flapper exuded energy, vitality, and youth. And if the breast-bound flapper did not survive the 1929 stock market crash, an emphasis on thinness did. Indeed, only during the 1950s, when Marilyn Monroe was at her height was there a serious challenge to the slender ideal.

Post–World War II culture has enshrined both thinness and youth for men as well as women. Advertisers have aided the process. Since photographers maintain that clothes look best on lean bodies, leading fashion models have always been thin and generally young. But since the 1960s, advertisers have used youth and thinness to sell other products as well. The evolution of Pepsi-Cola slogans illustrates this point:

1935: "Twice as Much"
1948: "Be Sociable—Have a Pepsi."
1960: "Now it's Pepsi for those who think young."
1965: "The Pepsi Generation."
1984: "Pepsi: The Choice of a New Generation."

Appeals to abundance ("twice as much") and social interaction ("be sociable") were replaced by the promise of eternal youth. As if to reinforce this appeal, Pepsi paid magnificent amounts to two thin, youthful Michaels as spokesmen: Michael Jackson and Michael J. Fox. Far from being sociable, Jackson is a virtual recluse, obsessed with personality change through plastic surgery. And Fox, as sure as Peter Pan, is the perpetual adolescent.

To fit the culture's procrustean mold, advertisers encourage Americans to binge and purge, consume and diet. Consume because "you are someone special" and "you can have it all." Diet because "you can never be too thin or too rich."

In his perceptive book *Never Satisified*, Hillel Schwartz argues that "dieting is an essentially nostalgic act, an attempt to return to a time when one *could* be satisfied, when one *was* thinner, when the range of choices in the world neither bewildered nor intimidated. To restrict one's range of choices, as all dieters must do, is not so much deficient as it is regressive. . . . Imagining a miraculous future, the dieter is always looking back."

In a secular, materialistic age, dieting has become an ascetic religion, Seventeenth-century poet and preacher John Donne wrote, "The flesh that God hath given us is affliction enough, but the flesh that the devil gives us, is affliction upon affliction and to that, there belongs a woe." To be fat in America has become a religious as well as a secular sin. Christian diet books emphasize John 3:30 "He must increase, but I must decrease."

In 1957 Charlie Shedd in his *Pray Your Weight Away* confessed, "We fatties are the only people on earth who can weigh our sin." His book inspired some Christians to lose weight and others to write diet books. Such works as Deborah Price's *I Prayed Myself Thin*, John Cavanaugh's *More of Jesus and Less of Me*, Reverend H. Victor Kane's *Devotion for Dieters*, and Francis Hunter's *God's Answer to Fat—Lose It!* emphasized that godliness is in league with thinness. Capturing the temper of her times, columnist Ellen Goodman wrote in 1975 that "eating has become the last bona fide sin left in America." And on this point, religion and secular humanism are in complete accord.

The fitness boom and body-image obsession financed a huge growth industry. To support their new interest in fitness, Americans needed equipment and clothes—shoes, shorts, shirts, racquets, bicycles, balls, paddles, bats, cleats, gloves, goggles, weights, scales, blood-pressure cuffs, timing watches, clubs, socks, headbands, wristbands, and leotards. Between 1975 and 1987 sporting goods sales in the United States increased from $8.9 billion to $27.5 billion. Americans spent $4 billion on athletic shoes

alone in 1987. Health clubs, once the domain of the wealthy and a small clique of bodybuilders, multiplied in number from 350 in 1968 to more than 7,000 in 1986. Gross revenues in 1987 exceeded $650 million.

Exercise and fitness revenues were matched by those of the weight loss industry. Jean Nidetch founded Weight Watchers in 1962 and eventually franchised it, making sure that group leaders had been through the diet program and reached "maintenance" levels. Attendance doubled between 1983 and 1987, and gross revenues went past $200 million that year. Sybil Ferguson's Diet Center, Inc., founded in 1969, had two thousand franchises in 1987 and nearly $50 million in gross revenues. Americans spent $6 billion for diet soda in 1986, $5 billion for vitamins and health foods, and $350 million for diet capsules and liquid protein. The President's Council on Physical Fitness estimated that 65 million Americans were dieting in 1987. Diet Coke, Diet Pepsi, Diet Dr. Pepper, Lean Cuisine, Bud Light, Miller Lite, lite bread, sugarless gum, NutraSweet, Cambridge, and a host of other diet products entered American popular culture.

What dieting and exercise couldn't fix, plastic surgery could. Americans went on a plastic surgery binge in the 1980s—not to repair real damage to their bodies or birth defects, but to improve their appearance cosmetically and recapture the illusion of youth. In 1987 more than 500,000 Americans underwent cosmetic plastic surgery. The most popular procedures were abdominoplasty (tummy tucks), breast augmentation, liposuction (fat removal), blepharoplasty (eyes), and rhinoplasty (nose). Plastic surgeons were also beginning to perform "total body contour" procedures. To postpone middle age, yuppies made plastic surgery a $3 billion industry.

Americans also changed a number of their habits in the 1970s and 1980s. Cigarette consumption began to decline in 1982. In 1965, 52 percent of men and 34 percent of women smoked. By 1985 only 33 percent of men and 28 percent of women smoked, and at the end

of 1987 the American Cancer Society estimated that only 27 percent of Americans were
still smoking. Per capita whiskey consumption dropped nearly 20 percent between
1976 and 1986 as Americans turned to lower-
alcohol-content beer and wine coolers. Beef
and pork consumption dropped in favor of
chicken and fish when cholesterol-conscious
Americans turned away from "red meat." Caffeine was also suspect. Americans under twenty-
five drank only a third of the coffee their parents
did; sales of decaffeinated coffee and drinks
like Pepsi Free and Pepper Free symbolized the
new health consciousness.

The results were impressive, even though
some of the gains had to be attributed to better
drug therapy, the rise of heart bypass surgery,
and improvement of cardiac care units in American hospitals. But the bottom line was that
between 1950 and 1985, the death rate per
100,000 people from cardiovascular and cere-
brovascular disease declined from 511 to 418, a
dramatic improvement. The cult of fitness
seemed to be paying dividends.

But there was an underside to the cult of
fitness, an obsessive perfectionism which was
the antithesis of good health. Jim Fixx and his
daily runs in spite of chest pains were one
example. Kathy Love Ormsby was another. The
North Carolina State University junior, who
held the U.S. collegiate women's record for
10,000 meters, had difficulty dealing with failure. In the 1986 NCAA championships, after
6,400 meters, she was struggling along in fourth
place, running a bad race. Then, as she approached a turn, she decided to keep going
straight. She ducked under a railing and ran
stright past Wisconsin team coach Peter Tegen.
"It was eerie," he said. "Her eyes were focused
straight ahead." She kept going—out of Indiana
University's track stadium in Indianapolis,
across a softball diamond, over a seven-foot
fence, down New York Street, toward the bridge
that spans the White River. Seventy-five feet
onto the bridge she stopped, climbed over the
railing, and jumped. After falling thirty-five feet,

she landed on the soggy ground close to the
river. She broke a rib, collapsed a lung, and
fractured a vertebrae. The doctor who attended
her said that she would be permanently para-
lyzed from the waist down: "Given the distance
that she fell, she's very lucky she's not a
quadriplegic," Dr. Peter Hall noted. "She could
have easily died."

Why? Ormsby was a high school valedicto-
rian, a straight-A student, the record holder for
the 800, 1,600, and 3,200 meters. At North
Carolina State she was a track star and promising premed student. She was raised in a strong
Christian family and was deeply religious herself. After her record-breaking 10,000-meter
run, she told a reporter: "I just have to learn to
do my best for myself and for God and to turn
everything over to Him." Her leap had turned
everything over to Him.

Some observers blamed Ormsby's consuming
pursuit of perfection. Others blamed the pressure of world-class sport competition. Her father
commented, "I believe . . . that it had something
to do with the pressure that is put on young
people to succeed." Certainly society's emphasis
on the importance of sports places tremendous
strains on young athletes. Often isolated from
the world outside gyms and tracks and stadiums,
they begin to think that their world has real,
lasting meaning. Failure, then, becomes equated
with death itself.

Such obsessive perfectionism also affected
millions of other people, only a tiny fraction of
whom were competitive athletics. For many
people, exercise and weight loss became forms
of psychological discipline, proof that the individual was in charge of his or her life. A 1986
Gallup Poll estimated that three million Americans, most of them women, suffered from eating
disorders—anorexia nervosa and bulimia. In
anorexia nervosa, victims virtually starve themselves to death, using laxatives, exercise, and
absurdly low calorie intake to lose body weight.
Most psychologists attribute the eating disorder
to a sense of powerlessness in the victim. They
strive for a sense of weightlessness, and in that

weightlessness they find a sense of control missing from other areas of their lives. In 1984 the soft-rock vocalist Karen Carpenter brought the disease to national attention when she died of a heart attack induced by extreme weight loss. Even when their weight drops below 85 pounds and they resemble concentration-camp victims, anorectics still look in the mirror and see themselves as fat, with round faces and flabby skin. Breasts disappear, menstruation stops, and their bodies return momentarily, just before death, to preadolescence.

Bulimia is a related disorder. The Gallup Poll concluded that nearly 10 percent of all American women between the ages of sixteen and twenty-five practice bulimia, an eating disorder characterized by huge calorie intake followed by self-induced vomiting. The Food and Drug Administration said that bulimia may last up to eight hours, with an intake of 20,000 calories (an equivalent of 210 brownies, or 6 layer cakes, or 35 "Big Macs"), involve 25 to 30 vomiting episodes, and cost up to $75 a day for food purchases. If untreated, the disease causes irregular heartbeats, cramps, fatigue, and seizures by destroying the body's electrolyte balance. The gastric acid from vomiting will also erode teeth away.

In a country which historically has been keenly competitive and has periodically affirmed a belief in perfectionism, the idea of a better life through sports has been carried to obsessive lengths. Often the object of physical fitness has not been to produce health and well-being but to test or even to escape the limits of one's body. Ultra-distance runner Stu Mittleman, one of the leaders in his field during the 1980s, was the epitome of this tendency. For him a 26-mile marathon was unsatisfactory, a flat, almost meaningless endeavor. The 100-mile event was better, and in the early 1980s he established the American record with a 12:56:34 run. Better still was the six-day event, in which his 488 miles was also an American record.

In ultra-distance running Mittleman saw man rediscovering his lost past. "Our culture forces us to eliminate sensory input so that we can cope," he observed. "Sports re-sensitizes. I want to live life intensely. . . . Long slow running has a heritage in hunting and gathering. Sprinting is based on retreat, on flight." Life, then, is best experienced at the limits of endurance, well past what is good for one's health. Yet, sometimes even that does not seem enough. As Mittleman told an interviewer, "I plan to do a 12-hour run tomorrow. You know, it seems like so little now."

Among world-class athletes, performance is more important than health. During the nineteenth century athletes occasionally took drugs to enhance their performances. Cyclists, in particular, used drugs to extend their pain and endurance barriers. As early as 1869 some cyclists used "speed balls" of heroin and cocaine to increase endurance. Others used caffeine, alcohol, nitroglycerine, ethyl ether, strychnine, and opium to achieve the same effect.

Of course, not all athletes survived such experimentation. And in the twentieth century, as drug use became more frequent, the casualty rate climbed. In 1960 Danish cyclist Knut Jensen collapsed and died during the Rome Olympics. He had taken amphetamines and nicotinyl tartrate to improve his chances of victory. In 1967 Thomas Simpson died during the ascent of Mount Ventoux in the Tour de France. Amphetamines were discovered in his jersey pockets and luggage.

Since World War II, however, stimulants have done less damage than muscle-building drugs. During the 1920s American scientists isolated the male hormone testosterone. By the 1940s testosterone was being hailed as a potential fountain of youth. Science writer Paul de Kruif in *The Male Hormone* (1945) noted that the newly developed synthetic testosterone" did more than give [the subjects] more energy and a gain in weight. . . . It changed them, and fundamentally. . . . after many months on testosterone, their chest and shoulder muscles grew much heavier and stronger. . . . in some mysterious manner, testosterone caused the human body to synthesize protein, it caused the human body to be able to build the very stuff of its own life." There is evidence that during World War II testosterone was administered to German storm troopers to increase their strength and aggressiveness.

In 1945 de Kruif speculated, "It would be interesting to watch the productive power of [a] . . . professional group [of athletes] that would try a systematic supercharge with testosterone.", By the 1952 Helsinki Olympics the Soviet Union had embarked on just such a campaign. That year Soviet weightlifters won seven Olympic medals, and U.S. Olympic weightlifting coach Bob Hoffman told reporters, "I know they're taking the hormone stuff to increase their strength."

At the 1954 World Weightlifting Championships in Vienna, a Soviet team physician confirmed Hoffman's belief. Upon returning home, Dr. John Ziegler, the U.S. team physician, acquired some testosterone and tested it on himself, Hoffman, and several American lifters. Concerned about the hormone's side effects— heightened aggression, increased libido, prostatic problems, and hirsutism—Ziegler approached the CIBA pharmaceutical company about producing a drug that would have testosterone's anabolic (muscle-building) effects without its androgenic (masculine characteristics) problems. The unsatisfactory result was the anabolic steroid Dianabol, a drug intended to aid burn victims and certain postoperative and geriatric patients.

Dianabol soon became the candy of the athletic world. By the 1960s nearly every world-class weightlifter was taking some form of anabolic steroid. In fact, steroids became the *sine qua non* of lifting. American superheavyweight weightlifting champion Ken Patera announced in 1971 that he was anxious to meet his Russian counterpart Vasily Alexiev in the 1972 Olympics: "Last year, the only difference between me and him was that I couldn't afford his pharmacy bill. Now I can. When we hit Munich next year, I'll weigh in at about 340, maybe

350. Then we'll see which are better—his steroids or mine."

Track and field athletes, football players, and bodybuilders similarly improved their performances with the aid of drugs. Jay Sylvester, a member of the 1972 U.S. Olympic track and field team, polled his teammates and found that 68 percent had used steroids to prepare for the Games. They believed that without them they would be at a competitive disadvantage. The same was true in football. One San Diego Charger player told team psychiatrist Arnold J. Mandell, "Doc, I'm not about to go out one-on-one against a guy who's grunting and drooling and coming at me with big dilated pupils unless I'm in the same condition."

Testosterone and anabolic steroids have led to athletes' experimenting with other performance-enhancing drugs. One of the more popular recent additions to this drug array is human growth hormone (hGH), a hormone manufactured from the pituitary. As the authors of *The Underground Steroid Handbook* claimed, hGH could "overcome bad genetics. . . . We LOVE the stuff." Of course, it may also cause elongation of the chin, feet, and hands; thickening of the rib cage and wrists; and heart problems.

Risk is part of taking drugs. Anabolic steroids can cause a rare, fatal type of kidney tumor, high blood pressure, sterility, intestinal bleeding, hypoglycemia, heart problems, acne, a deepened voice, and a change in the distribution of body hair. Steroids and testosterone also make users more aggressive and irritable. One NFL player confessed that testosterone "definitely makes a person mean and aggressive. . . . On the field I've tried to hurt people in ways I never did before. . . . A lot of guys can't handle it. I'm not sure I can. I remember a while back five of the guys on our team went on the juice at the same time. A year later four of them were divorced and one was separated. I've lost a lot of hair from using it, but I have to admit it's great for football. . . . I lost my family, but I think I'm a better player now. Isn't that a hell of a trade-off?"

By the 1970s steroids had become part of America's drug culture, and athletes asserted the right to decide what could or could not go into their own bodies. Frederick C. Hatfield in *Anabolic Steroids: What Kind and How Many* (1982) wrote: "As pioneers, these athletes carefully weigh the risk-to-benefit ratio and proceed with caution and with open minds. Can there be much wrong with getting bigger and/or stronger?" Users, then, have been transformed into pioneers, "adventurers who think for themselves and who want to accomplish something noble before they are buried and become worm food."

Ironically, however, most of the users are not world-class athletes. In the 1980s use of steroids expanded out of the realm of world-class athletes to college and high school playing fields. An estimated one million young American men and women were consuming large amounts of anabolic steroids in 1987. The praise they received for "bulking up" was irresistible. When they reduced steroid use and lost muscle tissue, friends immediately commented on how "much smaller you are," and they would return to the pills. Like bulimia and anorexia nervosa, anabolic steroids were addictions linked inseparably with body image.

Steroid use was most pronounced in the subculture of bodybuilding. Most of these men and women are not competitive athletes trying to break a world record or win an Olympic gold metal—"to accomplish something noble"—but people who want to look "pumped." Like dieting and cosmetic surgery, steroid use has become a means to a better-looking body, and looks—not health—is the real objective.

The quest for the "ideal" body has been taken to its furthest pharmaceutical extremes by bodybuilders. Not only do they take steroids to build up muscle mass, but they also diet and take diuretics to achieve maximum muscular striation, or the "cut up" look. For weeks or even months before an important competition, bodybuilders eat as little as 1,000 calories a day and still work out eight or more hours a day. The

result may be "the picture of health," but there is no reality behind the image. As one professional commented, "When we walk on stage we are closer to death than we are to life." And after a contest, in a bulimic binge, bodybuilders "pig out," often putting on fifteen pounds in one evening of eating.

Furthermore, to support their quest, many bodybuilders resort to homosexual "hustling." In theory, male bodybuilders have enshrined heterosexuality. Charles Atlas advertisements emphasized that the prize for the biggest biceps was the woman in the bathing suit. *Muscle and Fitness*, the leading bodybuilder magazine, reinforces this mythology by always picturing beautiful women hanging onto the biceps and thighs of "pumped," oiled men. "Ya know," said *Muscle and Fitness* editor Joe Weider, "in every age the women, they always go for the guy with the muscles, the bodybuilder. [The women] never go for the studious guy."

In fact, gay men have been a continual source of financial support for bodybuilders. Since serious bodybuilding is a full-time pursuit, the men involved need some source of income. Anthropologist Alan M. Kline estimated that 50 to 75 percent of southern California bodybuilders "hustle" the gay community for living expenses. Hustling ranges from posing for "beefcake" photographers and dancing nude at all-male events to pornography and sexual acts. Most bodybuilders, however, insist that they are not homosexual, that they have to hustle only to finance their bodybuilding habit. And besides, they insist, almost everyone does it. "People don't realize," noted one bodybuilder, "that in any given line-up of twenty competitors ten are hustling."

Many serious bodybuilders sacrifice heterosexual relationships as well as good health for their obsession. As one admitted, "On any given day I can go out with a woman, but it is not very satisfying. . . . Women demand time. I don't have that right now." Time, commitment, women, and even other men—all are obstacles to be mastered or avoided in the pursuit of a narcissistic ideal. To echo Michael Jackson's popular 1988 song, life for these bodybuilders starts and ends with the man in the mirror.

By the end of the 1980s, sports had become the secular religion of America. The stadiums, tanning salons, health spas, and gymnasiums had become the new cathedrals; jogging, running, aerobic dancing, cycling, weightlifting, and dieting the new rituals; and televised events, newspapers, radio talk shows, and sports and health magazines the new liturgies. The most obsessive athletes have a disciplined devotion that even the most ascetic medieval saints would have envied. Alberto Salazar, the world-class marathoner, bragged about his willingness to run 105 miles a week on stress-fractured legs. In the heat of one marathon, he kept running even when his body temperature had reached 108 degrees, collapsed in heat prostration, and while being packed in ice, received the last rites of the Roman Catholic Church.

Sports in the 1980s holds out secular salvation for nations, communities, and individuals. In competition and fitness, they locate the holy grail, the meaning of life in a world where God, church, and state no longer reign supreme. In *The Complete Book of Running*, Jim Fixx wrote: "It is here with my heart banging against my ribs that I discover how far beyond reason I can push myself. Furthermore, once a race has ended, I know what I am truly made of. Who can say how many of us have learned life's profoundest lessons while aching and gasping for breath?" On that Vermont road in 1986, with his body aching, his lungs gasping for breath, and his heart pounding against his ribs, Jim Fixx may have discovered the meaning of life.

■ ■ ■

Study Questions

1. Why did sports assume such an important dimension in American culture after World War II?

2. To what extent does sports in America reflect the aggressive, competitive spirit of the larger culture?

3. What are the advantages and disadvantages to the new American obsession with sports?

4. In rural areas, why does high school sports become so important to the community?

5. Why has plastic surgery become so popular in modern America?

6. How can anorexia nervosa and bulimia be seen as cultural, not merely physical, extremes?

7. What does the concept "cultural currency" mean? How does sports assist American society in transcending ethnic and religious divisions?

8. What is the connection between the cult of fitness and the post–World War II baby boom generation of "yuppies"?

BIBLIOGRAPHY

For an extraordinary look at American values in the contemporary period, see Christopher Lasch, *The Culture of Narcissism: American Life in the Age of Diminishing Expectations* (1975). Also see Peter Clecak, *America's Quest for the Ideal Self* (1983). Randy Roberts and James S. Olson analyze the American obsession with sports in *Winning Is the Only Thing* (1989). Studs Terkel's *American Dreams: Lost and Found* (1980) is an oral history of how Americans coped with the social and economic changes of the 1970s and 1980s. Hillel Schwartz's *Never Satisfied. A Cultural History of Diets, Fantasies and Fat* (1986) is an outstanding examination of the American preoccupation with youth and body image. Also see Kim Chernin, *The Obsession: Reflections on the Tyranny of Slenderness* (1981). For the dangerous, pathologic dimension of weight consciousness in history, see Rudolph M. Bell, *Holy Anorexia* (1985).